Chinese Herbal Medicine

Chinese Herbal Medicine

Editor: Patrick Lampard

Callisto Reference
www.callistoreference.com

Callisto Reference,
118-35 Queens Blvd., Suite 400,
Forest Hills, NY 11375, USA

Visit us on the World Wide Web at:
www.callistoreference.com

ISBN: 978-1-63239-964-9 (Hardback)

The publisher's policy is to use permanent paper from mills that operate a sustainable forestry policy. Furthermore, the publisher ensures that the text paper and cover boards used have met acceptable environmental accreditation standards.

Printed in China.

Cataloging-in-Publication Data

Chinese herbal medicine / edited by Patrick Lampard.
p. cm.
Includes bibliographical references and index.
ISBN 978-1-63239-964-9
1. Medicine, Chinese. 2. Herbs--Therapeutic use. I. Lampard, Patrick.
R602 .C45 2018
610.951--dc23

Table of Contents

Preface

The main aim of this book is to educate learners and enhance their research focus by presenting diverse topics covering this vast field. This is an advanced book which compiles significant studies by distinguished experts in the area of analysis. This book addresses successive solutions to the challenges arising in the area of application, along with it; the book provides scope for future developments.

Chinese medicine is an ancient practice that originated in China that is used to cure diseases like chronic pain, infertility, liver diseases, hormonal imbalance, etc. It includes methods like acupuncture, exercise, massage and herbal medicine. This book outlines the processes and applications of Chinese medicine in detail. It provides thorough information about the various methods used in this practice. This text explores all the important aspects of Chinese medicine in the present day scenario. Those in search of information to further their knowledge will be greatly assisted by it.

It was a great honour to edit this book, though there were challenges, as it involved a lot of communication and networking between me and the editorial team. However, the end result was this all-inclusive book covering diverse themes in the field.

Finally, it is important to acknowledge the efforts of the contributors for their excellent chapters, through which a wide variety of issues have been addressed. I would also like to thank my colleagues for their valuable feedback during the making of this book.

Editor

1

Radix *Puerariae lobatae* (*Gegen*) suppresses the anticoagulation effect of warfarin: a pharmacokinetic and pharmacodynamics study

Beikang Ge[†], Zhen Zhang[†] and Zhong Zuo[*]

Abstract

Background: Radix *Salvia miltiorrhiza* (*Danshen*) and Radix *Puerariae lobatae* (*Gegen*) are used in Traditional Chinese Medicine to treat cardiovascular diseases. However, adverse herb-drug interactions were observed between warfarin and herbal remedies containing *Danshen* and *Gegen*. This study aims to investigate the pharmacokinetic and pharmacodynamic interactions between warfarin and the different components found in *Danshen* and *Gegen*.

Methods: Sixty Sprague–Dawley rats were used to investigate the effects of warfarin (0.2 mg/kg), *Danshen* (240 or 480 mg/kg) and *Gegen* (240 or 480 mg/kg) both in isolation and combination. The rats in the warfarin and *Danshen/Gegen* combination groups were given an oral dose of *Danshen* or *Gegen* 2 h after being given an oral dose of warfarin. After five consecutive days of treatment, the pharmacokinetic interactions between *Danshen/Gegen* and warfarin were investigated by simultaneously monitoring and comparing the cytochrome P450 (CYP) activities, mRNA and protein expression levels in the livers of the rats from the different treatment groups. The pharmacodynamic interactions were evaluated by monitoring and comparing the vitamin K epoxide reductase (VKOR) activities, mRNA and protein expression levels in the livers of rats from the different groups, as well as the thrombomodulin (TM) activities, mRNA and protein in the lungs of these animals. The rat plasma soluble thrombomodulin concentrations of the different treatment groups were also evaluated. Microsomes incubation, Real Time-Polymerase Chain Reaction and Western blot was applied respectively to study the activity, mRNA expression and protein expression of CYP, VKOR and TM.

Results: The activities and expression levels of the CYP and VKOR enzymes in the warfarin-*Gegen* combination groups increased by nearly 30 % ($P = 0.02$) compared with the warfarin-alone group, whereas those of TM decreased by almost 25 % ($P = 0.02$). The administration of *Danshen* did not lead to any changes in the activities or the expression levels of the CYP, VKOR or TM enzymes compared with those of the control group. *Gegen* induced several warfarin-metabolizing CYP enzymes and neutralized the effects of warfarin towards VKOR and TM.

Conclusion: *Gegen*, rather than *Danshen* at the same tested dosage, offsets the anticoagulant effects of warfarin by accelerating the phase I liver metabolism of warfarin, as well as increasing the activity, mRNA and protein expression of VKOR while decreasing those of TM.

Background

The use of the anticoagulant warfarin in combination with herbal remedies has caused several safety concerns because of the narrow therapeutic window of warfarin [1]. According to reports from pharmacists in the United Kingdom, about 58 % of patients prescribed warfarin also regularly consumed herbal medicines to manage their conditions [2, 3]. A racemic mixture of warfarin consists of a 1:1 mixture of its *R*- and *S*-enantiomers, which differ considerably in terms of their potency and the rate at

*Correspondence: joanzuo@cuhk.edu.hk

[†]Beikang Ge and Zhen Zhang contributed equally to this work

School of Pharmacy, Faculty of Medicine, The Chinese University of Hong Kong, Shatin, New Territories, Hong Kong, China which they are metabolized [4]. Both of the enantiomers of warfarin are metabolized by cytochrome P450 (CYP) enzymes in a region- and stereo-selective manner, to afford the corresponding 6-, 7-, 8-, 10- and 4′-hydroxywarfarin compounds as the major metabolites [5]. The ingestion of certain plant materials such as grapefruit [6] and garlic [7, 8] can have a pronounced effect on the activity and/or expression of the CYP enzymes, which could have serious consequences for the metabolism of warfarin. The co-administration of herbs and drugs can also affect the activity and expression of vitamin K epoxide reductase (VKOR), which is the target protein of warfarin in terms of its anticoagulant effects. Although there were two separate studies pertaining to the inhibitory activities of the drug-warfarin interactions of paracetamol and sodium dehydroacetate (DHA-S) towards VKOR [9, 10], there were studies concerning the impact of herbs on the activity or expression of VKOR. In addition to VKOR, plasma-soluble thrombomodulin TM (sTM), which is the cleavage product of cellular TM [11], could be used as a potential biomarker for identifying patients at high risk of bleeding during warfarin treatment [12–14]. Notably, Salvianolic acid B led to an increase in the activity and expression of TM in vitro [15]. *Danshen-Gegen* formula (DGF), which is a herbal medicine containing Radix *Salvia miltiorrhiza* (*Danshen*) and Radix *Puerariae lobatae* (*Gegen*), led to a 5.36-fold increase in the mRNA expression of TM [16].

DGF, which is the aqueous extract derived of a 7:3 (w/w) mixture of *Danshen* and *Gegen*, was recently developed in Hong Kong [17]. DGF contains a variety of active components, including danshensu, salvianolic acid B (SAB), protocatechuic aldehyde (PCA), puerarin, daidzin and daidzein [18], and was reported to be an effective agent for the treatment of cardiovascular diseases [19–21]. The results of our previous in vivo study in rats demonstrated that the co-administration of DGF with warfarin led to pronounced herb-drug interactions [22], including a significant decrease in the C_{max}, area under curve (AUC) and the prothrombin (PT) time of warfarin. Although these changes in the pharmacokinetic properties of warfarin were attributed to the DFG-mediated induction of the CYP enzymes, the precise nature of the herbal components responsible for these induction effects were identified.

Danshen was reported to improve microcirculation, cause coronary vasodilation, suppress the formation of the thromboxane and inhibit the adhesion and aggregation of platelets. Based on its many interesting biological properties, *Danshen* has been widely used to treat coronary artery disease and numerous other cardiovascular diseases in China, Korea and Japan, as well as several other Asian countries [23–25]. Although the results of several previous studies suggested that *Danshen* interacts with warfarin by changing its pharmacokinetic and pharmacodynamic parameters [26–29], these studies generally fail to provide dosage information for *Danshen.* Furthermore, there are several inconsistencies in the findings of these studies. Preclinical studies in this area not reached an agreement on the effects of *Danshen* on the PT time of warfarin after the co-administration of these agents [30, 31]. The discrepancies observed in these pre-clinical and clinical research data could be explained in terms of the differences in the administration routes, dosages and *Danshen* preparations used in the different studies. In this study, we used an ex vivo approach to mimic the clinical behaviors of warfarin and *Danshen* and investigate the underlying mechanism of interaction between these two agents. Compared with *Danshen,* there were very few reports pertaining to the herb-drug interactions of *Gegen,* which is another major component of DGF. In a similar manner to *Danshen, Gegen* was reported to improve micro-circulation, increasing blood flow and preventing coronary artery disease [32]. Puerarin and *Gegen* extract were reported to regulate the activity of certain CYP enzymes in rats [33]. Furthermore, the results of a recent clinical study showed that puerarin induced the activity of CYP1A2 and inhibited the activity of CYP2D6 [34], which indicated that there could be potential interactions between warfarin and *Gegen.*

Existing mechanistic studies mainly focused on the impact of changes in the pharmacokinetics of warfarin rather than its pharmacodynamics, despite the fact that changes in the latter account for 79.9 % of all the identifiable herb-drug interaction mechanisms [35]. This study aims to investigate the pharmacokinetic and pharmacodynamic interactions between warfarin and *Danshen/Gegen.* To achieve these goals, we applied an ex vivo approach to investigate the effects of *Danshen/Gegen* on the different CYP enzymes involved in the metabolism of warfarin (for pharmacokinetic analysis). We also monitored the effects of *Danshen/Gegen* on the activities and mRNA and protein expression levels of VKOR and TM (for pharmacodynamic analysis).

Methods

Herbs

The concentrated Chinese medicine granules of *Danshen* (Batch No. 1007) and *Gegen* (Batch No. 1027) with the extraction ratio of 1:5 were purchased from Nong's Company Limited (Hong Kong). The raw herbs were morphologically authenticated by an in-house herbalist and chemically by the thin layer chromatography in accordance with the Chinese Pharmacopoeia 2005 [36]. The plant names in current study were used according to the latest revision in "The Plant List" (http://www.theplantlist.org).

Reagents

Racemic warfarin, diclofenac sodium and naringin (internal standards) were purchased from Sigma-Aldrich (St. Louis, MO, USA). The standards of sodium danshensu, protocatechuic aldehyde, SAB, puerarin, daidzin and daidzein were purchased from Zhongxin Innova Laboratories (Tianjin, China). Phenobarbital (PB), beta-naphthoflavone (BNF), cyclophosphamide monohydrate (CPA), bovine serum albumin, S-2238 and human thrombin were purchased from Sigma-Aldrich (St. Louis, MO, USA). Vitamin K_1 purchased from Sigma was used to prepare vitamin K_1 2, 3-epoxide (VKO) by the method of Tishler [37]. Hirudin was purchased from Calbiochem (La Jolla, California, USA). Acetic acid and ethyl acetate were obtained from BDH Laboratory (Poole, England). Acetonitrile and methanol (HPLC grade) were obtained from Tedia Company Inc. (Fairfield, USA) and Fisher Scientific UK Limited (Leicestershire, UK), respectively. All other reagents were analytical or HPLC grade. Distilled and deionized water was used for the preparation of all solutions. *S*-warfarin, *R*-warfarin, and racemic standards of 4′-, 6-, 7-, 8- and 10-OH-warfarin were purchased from Ultrafine Chemicals (Manchester, UK). Both the primary and secondary antibodies of CYP1A1, CYP2B1/2B2, CYP2C6, CYP2C11, VKOR, TM and GAPDH were purchased from Abcam (Abcam Inc., Cambridge, MA). ELISA kits for detecting sTM plasma concentration were purchased from Life Science Inc.

Animals

Healthy male SD rats (220–250 g) were supplied by the Animal Service Center at the Chinese University of Hong Kong and fasted overnight before use. The experiments were carried out under the approval by the Animal Ethics Committee of the Chinese University of Hong Kong with an approval number of (12-538) in DH/HA&P/8/2/1 Pt.26 (Additional file 1).

Instruments for sample analyses

The LC/MS/MS system, used for sample analyses of warfarin and its monohydroxylated metabolites, were performed with an ABI 2000 tandem triple quadruple LC/MS spectrometer equipped with an electrospray ionization source (ESI), two Perkin-Elmer PE-200 series micro-pumps and auto-sampler (Perkin-Elmer, Norwalk, CT, USA). The liquid chromatographic sample analyses instrument for detecting VK and VKO was a Waters HPLC system (Waters, Milford, MA,USA) equipped with 996 photodiode-array detector and 2695 separation module (pump and auto sampler). The chromatographic separation was performed at ambient temperature by X-Bridge™ C_{18} column (150 × 4.6 mm i.d., 3.5 μm particle size). The auto-sampler was set at 4 °C. Acetonitrile/isopropanol/water in a ratio of 100/8/2 (*v*/*v*/*v*) was used as mobile phase, with the flow rate of 1.2 mL/min. Absorbance of the eluting materials was measured at 250 nm. The Bio-Rad microplate reader from BioRad (Benchmark, Japan) was used to analyze the optical destiny of samples from ELISA and TM activity tests.

Standardization of Danshen and Gegen granules

Identification and quantification of the major components in *Danshen* and *Gegen* granules were performed by Waters HPLC according to our previous study with modifications [22]. The chromatographic separation of the analytes was achieved by an Agilent Eclipse XDB-C18 column (250 × 4.6 mm i.d., 5 μm particle size). The mobile phase consisting of 0.5 % acetic acid in acetonitrile (solvent A) and 0.5 % acetic acid in water (solvent B) was run with gradient elution at a flow rate of 1 mL/min. The linear gradient elution was carried out as follows with a total running time of 90 min: solvent A was kept at 5 % for the first 5 min, and then increased to 10, 17, 35 and 90 % in the next 13, 12, 10 and 30 min, respectively, then returned to 5 % in 5 min and equilibrated for 15 min before the next injection. HPLC analyses indicated that the marker compounds (μg/100 mg granules, mean ± SD, n = 3) for *Danshen* granules were danshensu (1140.3 ± 24.6), SAB (821.3 ± 33.1), PCA (82.2 ± 4.6), and that for *Gegen* granules were puerarin (1314.9 ± 44.1), daidzein (74.4 ± 9.4) and daidzin (89.2 ± 7.2), respectively.

Animal treatments

The dosage of *Danshen* and *Gegen* for rats were both 240 mg/kg/day (twice a day), which were calculated from its respective clinical therapeutic dose recommended by Chinese Pharmacopeia [36]. Since the clinical therapeutic dosage of warfarin in common use was 1–2 mg/day for a person, the equivalent rats dosage was calculated to be 0.2 mg/kg (human equivalent dosage in rat = human dosage/60 kg × 6.2), once daily [38]. Healthy male SD rats were divided into nine groups (n = 6) and each group was treated for five consecutive days with different substance, including *Danshen* single dose (*Danshen*×1: 240 mg/kg/day), *Danshen* double dose (*Danshen*×2: 480 mg/kg/day), warfarin plus *Danshen* single dose (War + *Danshen*×1: 0.2 + 240 mg/kg/day), warfarin plus *Danshen* double dose (War + *Danshen*×2: 0.2 + 480 mg/kg/day), *Gegen* single dose (*Gegen*×1: 240 mg/kg/day), *Gegen* double dose (*Gegen*×2: 480 mg/kg/day), warfarin plus *Gegen* single dose (War + *Gegen*×1: 0.2 + 240 mg/kg/day), warfarin plus *Gegen* double dose (War + *Gegen*×2: 0.2 + 480 mg/kg/day) and warfarin alone (War: 0.2 mg/kg/day). *Danshen/Gegen* was given to rats twice daily. In the combination groups, Danshen/Gegen was given to rats 2 h after the oral dosing of warfarin. In addition to the drug-treated groups, H_2O, phenobarbital (PB 60 mg/kg/day), beta-naphthoflavone (BNF 40 mg/kg/day) and cyclophosphamide (CPA 40 mg/kg/day) were also given orally for five consecutive days to rats that formed into one vehicle control and three positive controls (for determining the activity and expressions of CYPs) respectively. Specifically, BNF for CYP1A1, PB for CYP2B1 and CYP2C6 and CPA for CYP2C11, were used to validate the assay. For the determining the activity and expressions of VKOR and TM, warfarin was regarded as the positive control for the assay validation. Two hours after the last dosing, rats were sacrificed by decapitation. Livers, lungs and plasma were obtained from each rat for further treatment and assay.

Tissue sample preparations

Rat liver microsome (RLM) preparation

The rat livers were perfused by saline before being excided surgically on ice and cut into pieces for storage at −80 °C. The liver microsomes were prepared by series centrifugation as described previously [39]. Briefly, liver samples were thawed and weighed before homogenization medium were added. The tissue was chopped using scissors and homogenized with an automatic homogenizer at 500 rpm (IKA Labortechnik, Staufen, Germany). The resultant homogenates were transferred to clean centrifuge tubes, and centrifuged (Beckman Colter, Inc, Fullerton, CA, USA) at 20,000×*g* for 20 min at 4 °C. The supernatant was collected and further centrifuged at 100,000×*g* for 1 h under 4 °C by the L8-70 Beckman ultracentrifuge. The obtained microsomal pellet was re-suspended with homogenization medium and stored at −80 °C. Protein concentrations of the prepared liver microsomes were determined by the Bio-Rad protein assay kit (Bio-Rad Pacific Ltd, Hong Kong) and analyzed by the micro-plate reader (Benchmark, Japan) [40].

Extraction of TM from rat lungs

Rat lungs were perfused by saline before being excided surgically on ice and cut into pieces for storage at −80 °C. Pieces of lung were then homogenized in a glass tissue grinder of 50 mL at 4 °C. Centrifuge was performed at 30,000×*g* for 40 min at 4 °C to get the pellet, which was re-suspended in 250 mL buffer (0.25 M sucrose, 0.02 M Tris–HCl and 1 mM benzamidine-HCl, pH 7.5), homogenized, and centrifuged again as described above. The TM was finally extracted from the pellet by homogenization in 0.25 M sucrose, 0.02 M Tris–HCl, 1 mM benzamidine-HCl, and 0.5 % (*v*/*v*) Triton X-100, pH 7.5. This process was repeated three times and TM activity was assessed in the resulting extract [41]. The protein concentration of the extract was measured with Bio-Rad protein assay kit and adjusted to 100 ng/mL.

Methods for pharmacokinetic studies

CYP activities, mRNA and protein expressions in rat liver

Rat liver microsomal activities for mono-hydroxylation of warfarin

The activities of rat liver microsomes for metabolizing warfarin were detected according to methods from our previous study [22]. A typical incubation (100 µL) contained 50 mM Tris–HCl buffer (pH 7.4), 10 mM $MgCl_2$, 1.0 mg/mL microsomal protein, and racemic-, *R*- or *S*-warfarin as substrate respectively (5 µM for *R*- and *S*-warfarin, 10 µM for racemic warfarin). The mixture was pre-warmed in a 37 °C water bath with gentle shaking for 10 min before addition of NADPH (final concentration of 1.0 mM) into the mixture to initiate the reaction. About 0.1 mL ice-chilled acetonitrile containing internal standard (2.0 µg/mL of diclofenac sodium) was added and incubated for another 30 min. After the mixture centrifugation, the supernatant was subjected to LC/MS/MS to compare the mono-hydroxywarfarin metabolites (4′-, 6-, 7-, 8- and 10-hydroxywarfarin) among different treatment groups. The activities of CYPs could be expressed as the amount of mono-hydroxywarfarin metabolites formed.

CYP mRNA expression

Approximately 30 mg of rat livers were homogenized, and RNA was isolated with the Qiagen RNA extraction kit (Valencia, CA, USA). The quality of RNA was evaluated by measuring the 260/280 ratio (˃1.9) with an ultraviolet light spectrophotometer (Shimadzu, Japan). The sequence of the sense and antisense primers for rat CYP1A1 (FP: CCAAACGAGTTCCGGCCT; RP: TGCC CAAACCAAAGAGAATGA) [42], CYP2B1 (FP:AACCC TTGATGACCGCAGTAAA; RP: TGTGGTACTCCAAT AGGGACAAGATC) [42], CYP2C6 (FP: ATAAGACGCT TTACCCTCAC; RP: GATTTTCCTGCTTCCACTTA) [43], CYP2C11 (FP: TGCCCCCTTTTTACGAGGCT; RP: GGAACAGATGACTCTGAATTCT) [44] and GAPDH (FP: CAAGGTCATCCATGACAACTTTG; RP: GGGCC ATCCACAGTCTTCTG) [42] gene were designed as described previously. The reaction mixture system (final volume 20 µL) was prepared as follow: 4 units multiscribe reverse transcriptase, 1×RT buffer, 1 mM random hexamer primers, 0.5 mM each of dATP, dGTP, dCTP and dTTP, and 10 mL total mRNA extract. The PCR involved an initiating heating for 10 min at 95 °C, 40 cycles consisting of 10 s at 95 °C, 20 s at 60 °C, and a final extension step of 30 s at 72 °C. The fold change of target gene expression level in different drug treatment groups (after correction with the level of GAPDH) was determined by the following equation: Fold change $= 2^{-\Delta(\Delta Ct)}$, where $\Delta Ct = Ct(target) - Ct(GAPDH)$ and $\Delta(\Delta Ct) = \Delta Ct(treated) - \Delta Ct(vehicle\ control)$ [22]. The Ct (cycle threshold) in the equation was defined as the number of cycles required for the fluorescent signal to cross the threshold.

CYP protein expression

The levels of CYP1A1, 2B1/2, 2C6, 2C11 and GAPDH proteins in rat liver microsomes obtained from different treatment groups were determined by Western blotting. Sodium dodecyl sulfate (SDS)–PAGE was performed by a Mini-Protean II system (Bio-Rad) as described previously [45]. After denaturing with sample buffer, rat liver microsomal proteins were separated in a 10 % (*w*/*v*) SDS–polyacrylamide gel and blotted onto a PVDF membrane (Immobilon transfer membrane, Millipore, Billerica, MA, USA). The membrane was blocked in 5 % defatted milk which was then incubated with the primary and secondary antibodies (horseradish peroxidase labeled anti-mouse or anti-rabbit IgG). The membrane was then immersed in the enhanced chemiluminescence solution (Millipore, Billerica, MA, USA) for 60 s. Digital chemiluminescence images were captured and analyzed by FluorChem Q Imaging System (Alpha Innotech Corporation, Santa Clara, CA, USA).

Methods for pharmacodynamic studies

VKOR activity, mRNA and protein expression in rat livers

VKOR activity

Rat liver microsomes of different treatment groups were rinsed and re-suspended in the 0.02 M Tris–HCl buffer (pH 7.4) to obtain a microsomal protein concentration of 5 mg/mL 0.02 mL of this microsomal suspension was mixed with 0.071 mL of the 0.02 M Tris–HCl buffered solution (pH 7.4). The mixture was pre-incubated for 3 min at 30 °C. Tris–HCl buffered solution (pH 7.4, 2 μL 0.02 M) containing 0.1 M DTT (Sigma-Aldrich, St. Louis, MO, USA) were added, mixed and incubated for 5 min at 30 °C. Synthesized VKO (10 nM) in 2 μL of isopropanol was also added and subsequently incubated for 60 min at 30 °C. The reaction was stopped by the addition of 0.1 mL of ice-chilled isopropanol. Tocopheryl acetate (2.5 μg; Sigma-Aldrich, St. Louis, MO, USA) in 0.2 mL of hexane was added as the internal standard. After vortex for 1 min, the mixture was centrifuged at 15,000×*g* for 5 min. The hexane phase was evaporated to dryness with nitrogen [39]. The residue was dissolved in 150 μL mixed buffer containing acetonitrile/isopropanol/water (100/8/2: *v*/*v*/*v*), and 10 μL was analyzed by HPLC. The amount of vitamin K_1 formed was determined from the peak height ratio between vitamin K_1/internal standard and a calibration graph. VKOR activity was expressed as the amount of vitamin K_1 formed.

VKOR mRNA and protein expression

The sequence of the sense and antisense primers for rat VKOR gene (VKORC1) used in RT-PCR was designed as described previously [46]. RT-PCR procedures for detecting mRNA expression of VKORC1 were same as that described for CYP mRNA expression. VKOR protein expression detection was conducted with the same operations for CYP protein expression.

TM activity, mRNA and protein expression in rat lung

TM activity

The ability of TM to accelerate protein C activation by thrombin was tested by a chromogenic assay as follow: 0.5 M of purified protein C (Stago) in 100 μL of buffer was activated by 10 nM (1 NIH unit) of human thrombin (Sigma-Aldrich, St. Louis, MO, USA) in 10 μL of buffer in the presence of 5 mM calcium, 3 mg/mL of bovine serum albumin and of 50 μL of lung extracts from different substance treated groups. The final volume was 200 μL. Incubation of the mixture lasted 30 min at 37 °C. The activation phase was stopped by adding 2 units of hirudin. The hydrolytic activity of the activated protein C (APC) thus generated was assessed by spectrophotometric measurement at 405 nm of the rate of hydrolysis of D-Phe-Pip-Arg-pNA·2HCl, that is, S-2238. For this purpose, 800 μL of Tris–HCl buffer, pH 7.5, containing 0.1 mM of S-2238 was added to the mixture (final volume: 1 mL). The changes in optical density per minute were converted into units of APC formed by referring to a standard curve constructed with concentrations of 20, 40, 80, 160 and 320 n of standard APC (Stago). The activity of TM could be expressed as the amount of APC formed during incubation [47].

TM mRNA and protein expression

TM mRNA and protein (extracted from rat lung) expression were detected as that described for CYP. The sequence of the sense and antisense primers for rat TM used in RT-PCR was designed as described previously [48].

sTM plasma concentration analysis

After the animal treatment described previously, blood was collected using 3.8 % sodium citrate (sodium citrate: blood = 1:9) as an anticoagulant. Plasma was obtained by centrifuging the blood at 15,000×*g* for 3 min. The plasma samples were frozen and stored at −80 °C until the assay. An enzyme-linked immunosorbent assay (ELISA) was used to measure the plasma concentration of sTM. Standard sTM was series diluted to make a calibration curve. The concentration of sTM was determined from the optical density of each sample at 450 nm against a calibration graph.

Statistical analysis
Data were expressed as the mean ± SD. Differences between two groups were analyzed by an unpaired student's *t* test. Differences between groups for continuous variables were evaluated by one way ANOVA with post hoc Tukey (when variances were equal according to Levene's test) or Games-Howell test (when variances were not equal according to Levene's test) [49]. *P* value less than 0.05 was considered as statistically significant.

Results

Pharmacokinetic mechanisms of warfarin-*Gegen* interaction

Gegen induced the activities and mRNA expressions of different CYPs in rat liver

Induction on CYP activities for warfarin metabolism When *R*-warfarin was used as the substrate (5 μM), the formation of all five mono-hydroxylated warfarin metabolites in the *Gegen*×1 and *Gegen*×2 groups increased significantly by 19–31 % ($P = 0.03$) and 24–30 % ($P = 0.03$), respectively, relative to the vehicle control group. Compared with the combined amount of all five mono-hydroxylated warfarin metabolites formed in the warfarin-alone group, there were significant increases in both of the combination groups (i.e., War + *Gegen*×1 and War + *Gegen*×2) of 19–49 % ($P = 0.02$) and 22–49 % ($P = 0.03$), respectively. No significant differences were observed in the amounts of the mono-hydroxylated metabolites formed between the vehicle control and *Danshen* groups. In the positive control groups, the formation of 7- and 8-hydroxylated warfarin increased by 281 % ($P < 0.001$) and 242 % ($P < 0.001$) when the animals were treated with PB and BNF (positive controls for the activities of rat CYP2C6 and CYP1A1, respectively, contributing to the formation of 7- and 8-hydroxylated warfarin) [22], respectively, compared with the results of the vehicle control group (Fig. 1).

When *S*-warfarin was used as a substrate (5 μM), the formation of the three detectable mono-hydroxylated warfarin metabolites (i.e., 4′-, 6- and 7-hydroxylated warfarin) increased significantly by 14–16 % ($P = 0.04$) and 16–19 % ($P = 0.03$) in the *Gegen*×1 and *Gegen*×2 groups, respectively, compared with the vehicle control group. Compared with the combined amount of the 4′-, 6- and 7-monohydroxylated warfarin metabolites formed in the warfarin-alone group, we observed significant increases of 17–19 % ($P = 0.04$) and 17–22 % ($P = 0.03$) in the formation of these metabolites in the *Gegen*×1 and *Gegen*×2 groups, respectively. No inductive effects were observed in the *Danshen*-treated groups based on a comparison of the warfarin metabolites formed in this group with those in the vehicle control group. In the positive control groups, the formation of 7-hydroxywarfarin increased by 237 % ($P < 0.001$) when the rats were treated with PB (positive controls for rat CYP2C6, contributing to the formation of 7-hydroxywarfarin) compared with the vehicle control group (Fig. 2).

When racemic warfarin was used as the substrate (10 μM containing 5 μM of the *R*- and *S*-enantiomers) there were significant increases of 21–28 % ($P = 0.03$) and 24–39 % ($P = 0.02$) in the formation of the 4′-, 6-, 7-, 8- and 10-hydroxywarfarin metabolites in the *Gegen*×1 and *Gegen*×2 groups, respectively, compared with the vehicle control group. Compared with the warfarin-alone group, the co-administration of *Gegen*×1 and *Gegen*×2 with warfarin led to significant increases in the formation of all five mono-hydroxylated warfarin metabolites by 21–27 % ($P = 0.03$) and 20–29 % ($P = 0.03$), respectively. No inductive effect was observed when for the warfarin metabolites formed in the *Danshen*-treated groups based on a comparison of these results with those of the vehicle control group. In the positive control groups, the formation of the 7- and 8-hydroxywarfarin metabolites increased by 251 % ($P < 0.001$) and 209 % ($P < 0.001$) when the rats were treated with PB and BNF, respectively, compared with the vehicle control group (Fig. 3).

Induction of the mRNA expression of CYP1A1, CYP2B1, CYP2C6 and CYP2C11 Compared with the vehicle control group, there were significant increases of 260 % ($P < 0.001$) and 220 % ($P < 0.001$) in the mRNA expression levels of CYP1A1 and CYP2B1 in the *Gegen*×1 group, respectively. Similar increases of 250 % ($P < 0.001$) and 290 % ($P < 0.001$) were also observed in the *Gegen*×2 group, respectively (Fig. 4). However, these increases were small in size compared with those of the positive control groups. For example, BNF afforded a 8761-fold increase, whereas PB gave a 2812-fold increase. Compared with the mRNA expression ratio of CYP1A1 to CYP2B1 in the warfarin-alone group, there were significant increases ($P < 0.001$) in the counterpart ratios of both combination groups (i.e., War + *Gegen*×1 and War + *Gegen*×2). For example, the former of these two groups (i.e., War + *Gegen*×1) showed 2.8- and 2.1-fold increases for CYP1A1 and CYP2B1, respectively, whereas the latter group (i.e., War + *Gegen*×2) showed 4.0- and 1.9-fold increases for CYP1A1 and CYP2B1, respectively. No inductive effects were observed in the mRNA expression levels of CYP1A1 and CYP2B1 when the *Danshen*-treated group was compared with the vehicle control group.

PB was used as a positive control to detect the mRNA expression of CYP2C6. Compared with the vehicle control group, there was a significant increase of 420 % ($P < 0.001$)

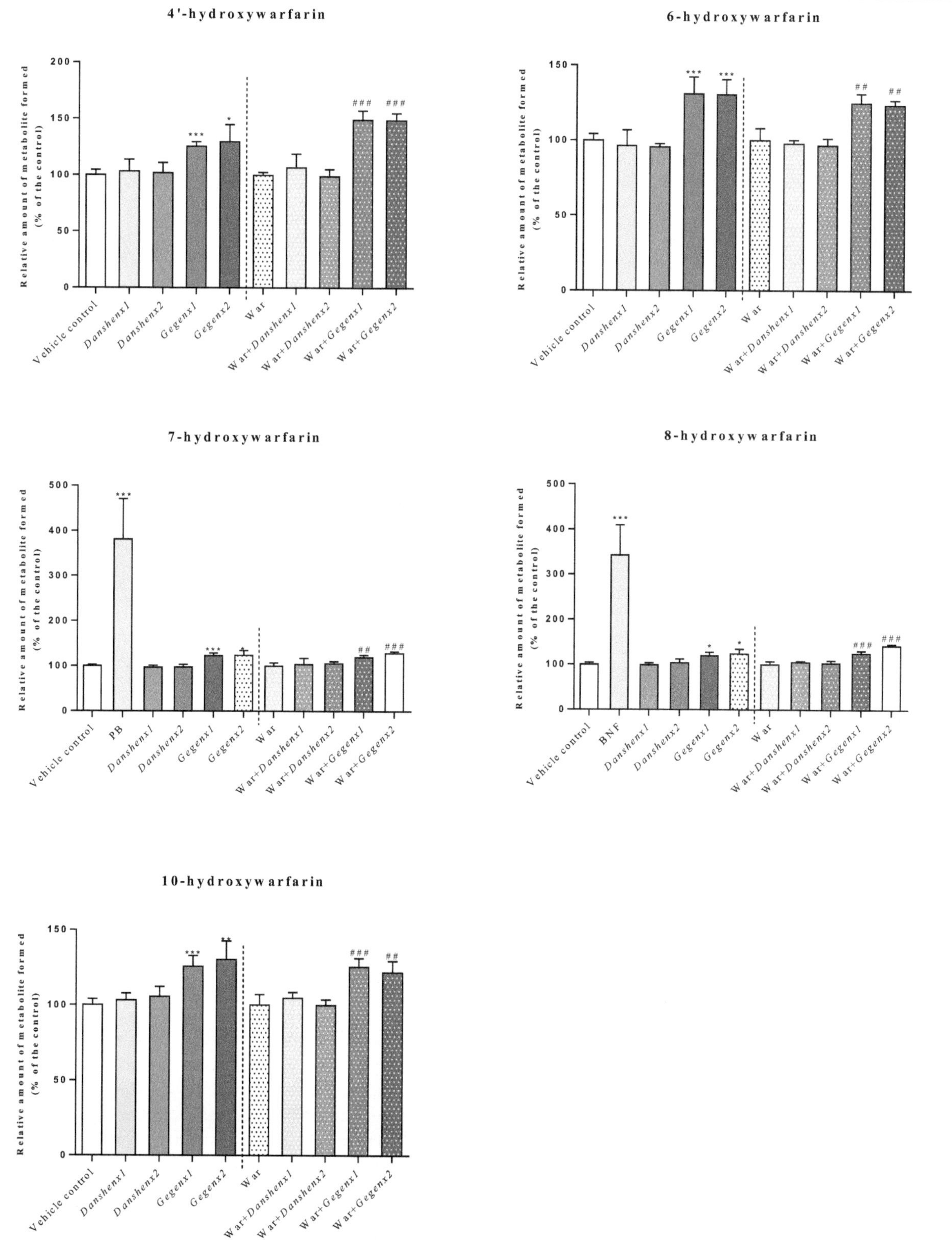

Fig. 1 Relative amount of formed monohydroxywarfarin (% of control) from different treatment groups. Using *R*-warfarin as substrate. **P* < 0.05; ***P* < 0.01; ****P* < 0.001, compared with the vehicle control group. #*P* < 0.05; ##*P* < 0.01; ###*P* < 0.001, compared with the warfarin alone group. &*P* < 0.05; &&*P* < 0.01; &&&*P* < 0.001, compared within same groups of different doses. Each point represents the mean ± SD (n = 6)

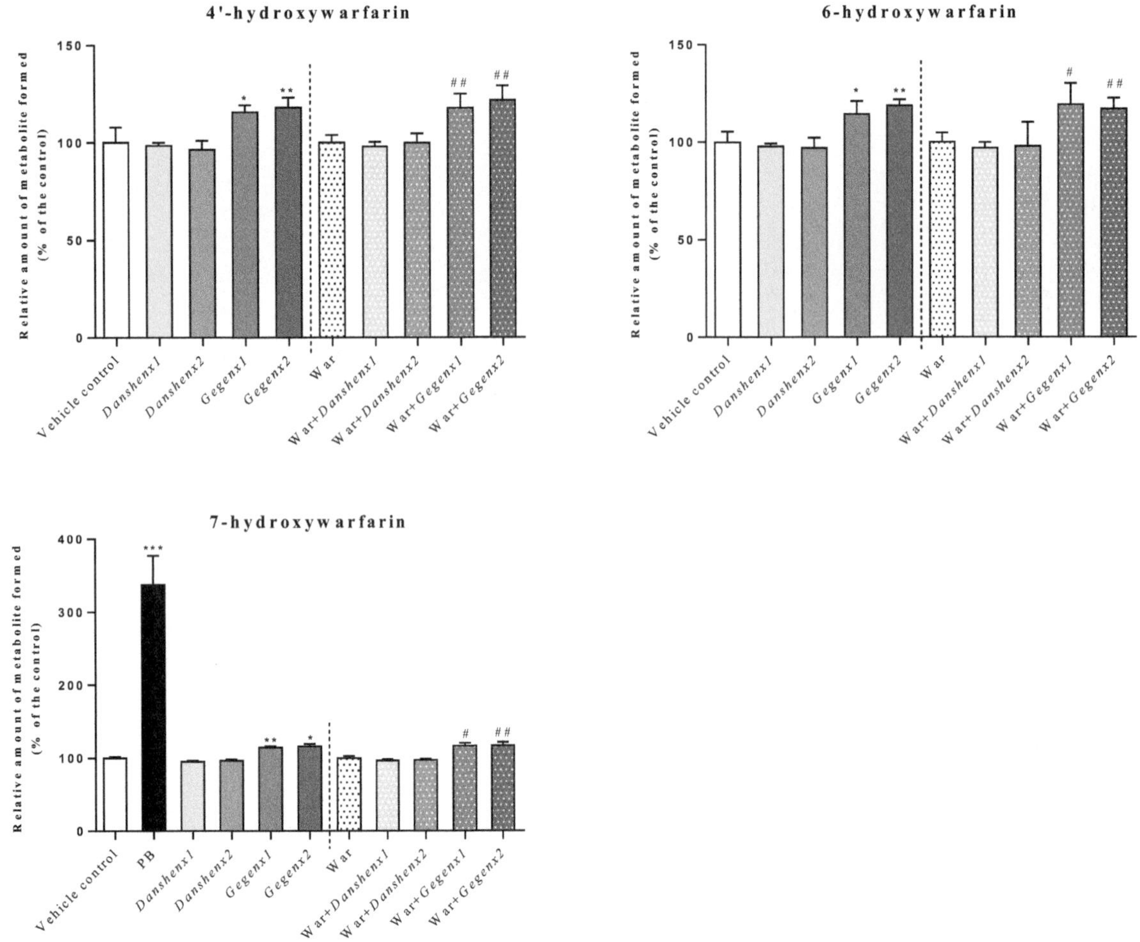

Fig. 2 Relative amount of formed monohydroxywarfarin (% of control) from different treatment groups. Using S-warfarin as substrate. $^{*}P < 0.05$; $^{**}P < 0.01$; $^{***}P < 0.001$, compared with the vehicle control group. $^{\#}P < 0.05$; $^{\#\#}P < 0.01$; $^{\#\#\#}P < 0.001$, compared with the warfarin alone group. $^{\&}P < 0.05$; $^{\&\&}P < 0.01$; $^{\&\&\&}P < 0.001$, compared within same groups of different doses. Each point represents the mean ± SD (n = 6)

in the mRNA expression ratio of CYP2C6 in the positive control group. Furthermore, the mRNA expression levels of CYP2C6 increased significantly by 1.4- and 1.5-fold in the *Gegen*×1 ($P = 0.03$) and *Gegen*×2 ($P = 0.02$) groups, respectively, compared with the vehicle control group. A significant 1.4-fold ($P = 0.03$) increase in the mRNA expression level of CYP2C6 was also observed in both of the *Gegen* combination groups (i.e., War + *Gegen*×1 and War + *Gegen*×2), compared with the warfarin-alone group. No significant differences were observed in the CYP2C6 mRNA expression ratios between the *Gegen*×1 and *Gegen*×2 groups. Furthermore, no inductive effects were observed in the mRNA expression level of CYP2C6 for both doses of *Danshen* compared with the vehicle control group.

In terms of the mRNA expression of CYP2C11, we observed a slight increase of 1.07-fold in the *Danshen*×1 group ($P = 0.04$) compared with the vehicle control group. A small increase of 117 % ($P = 0.02$) was also observed in the mRNA expression of CYP2C11 in the War + *Gegen*×1 group compared to the warfarin-alone group.

No significant effects on the rat liver CYP protein expressions Changes in the protein expression levels of the target CYP isozymes were determined to be minor compared with those observed for the metabolic activity and mRNA expression levels (Fig. 5). In the *Gegen*×1 and *Gegen*×2 groups, the expression level of CYP2C6 protein appeared to increase compared with the vehicle control group, but this increase was not statistically significant. No inductive effects were observed in the expression levels of any of the target CYP proteins in the *Danshen*-treated groups compared with the vehicle control group. In the positive control groups, the expression levels of the CYP1A1, CYP2B1/2B2 and CYP2C6 proteins increased significantly by 6.1- ($P < 0.001$), 5.6- ($P < 0.001$) and 1.7-fold ($P = 0.003$), respectively, compared with the vehicle control group.

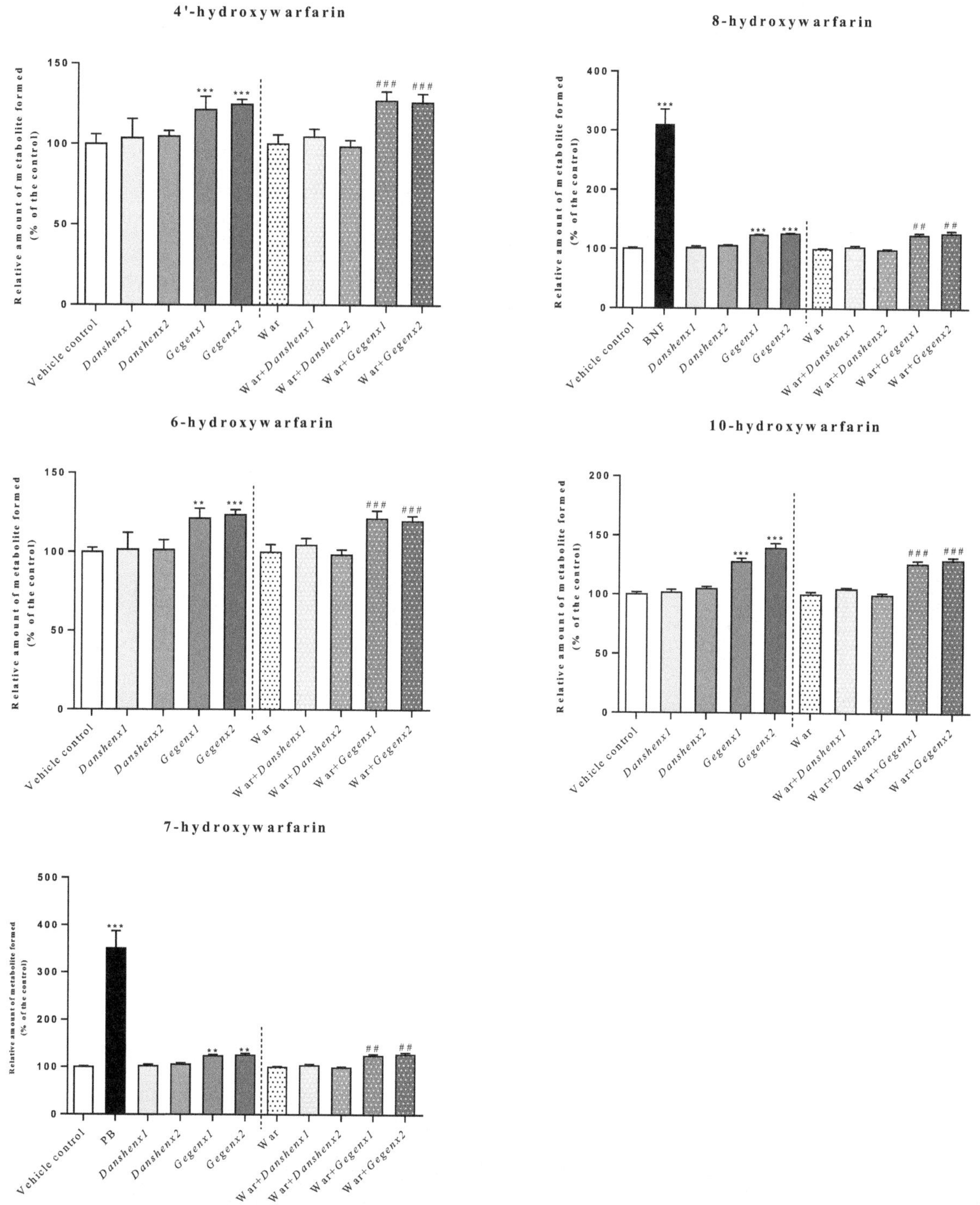

Fig. 3 Relative amount of formed monohydroxywarfarin (% of control) from different treatment groups. Using racemic warfarin as substrate. *$P < 0.05$; **$P < 0.01$; ***$P < 0.001$, compared with the vehicle control group. #$P < 0.05$; ##$P < 0.01$; ###$P < 0.001$, compared with the warfarin alone group. &$P < 0.05$; &&$P < 0.01$; &&&$P < 0.001$, compared within same groups of different doses. Each point represents the mean ± SD (n = 6)

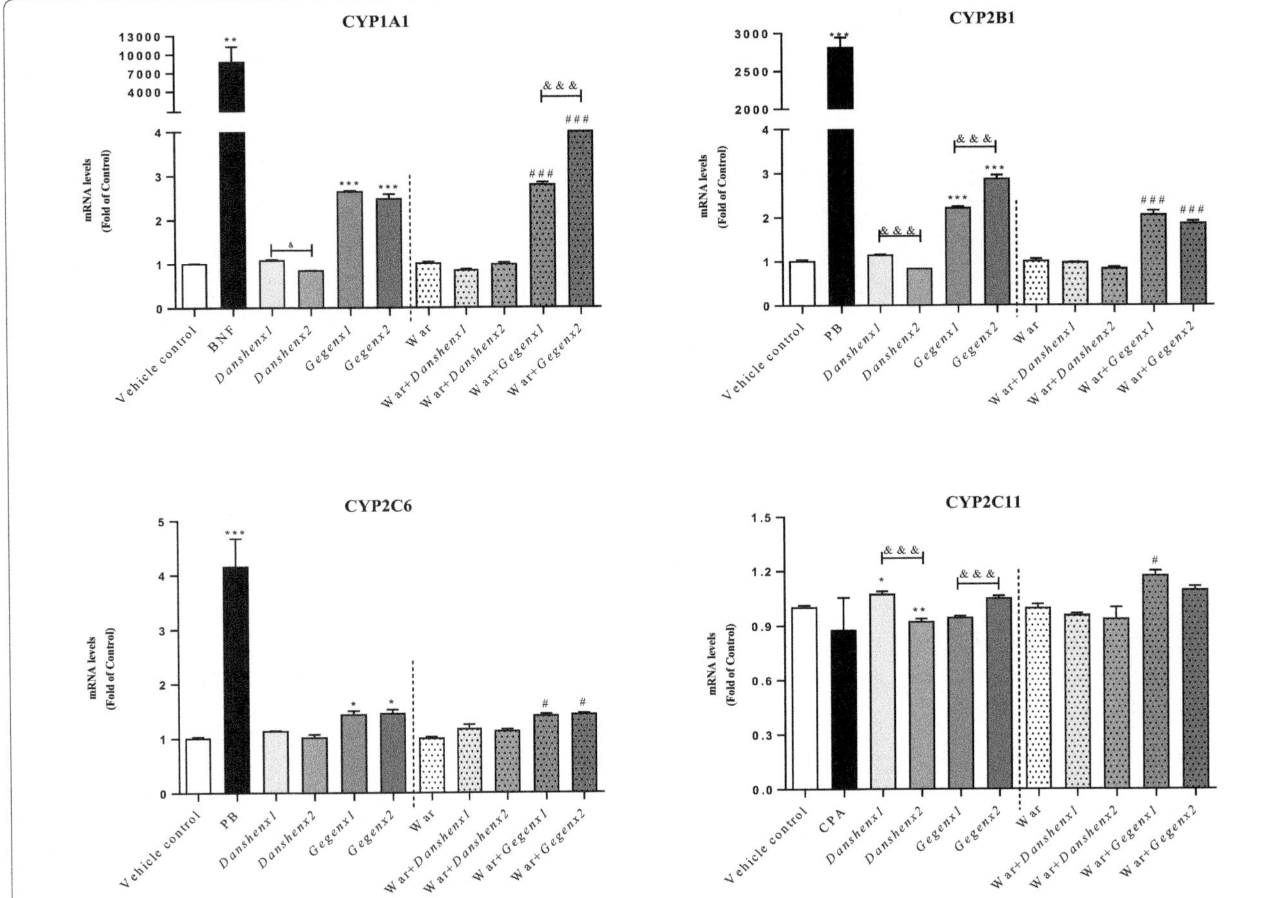

Fig. 4 Rat liver mRNA expression (Fold of Control) for target CYP isoforms from different treatment groups. *$P < 0.05$; **$P < 0.01$; ***$P < 0.001$, compared with the vehicle control group. #$P < 0.05$; ##$P < 0.01$; ###$P < 0.001$, compared with the warfarin alone group. &$P < 0.05$; &&$P < 0.01$; &&&$P < 0.001$, compared within same groups of different doses. Each point represents the mean ± SD (n = 6)

Pharmacodynamic mechanisms of the warfarin-*Gegen* interaction

Gegen led to an increase in the activity, as well as the mRNA and protein expression levels of VKOR in rat liver

Induction on VKOR activity

Compared with the vehicle control group, the *Danshen*×1 and *Danshen*×2 groups showed no significant changes in their VKOR activity. In contrast, there were significant increases of 124.4 ± 6.3 % ($P < 0.001$) and 131.1 ± 12.9 % ($P < 0.001$) in the VKOR activities of the *Gegen*×1 and *Gegen*×2 groups, respectively. Warfarin reduced the activity of VKOR by 52.4 ± 5.1 % ($P < 0.001$) compared with the vehicle control group, which was consistent with its therapeutic effect. A comparison of the warfarin-alone group with the four different combination groups (i.e., War + *Danshen*×1; War + *Danshen*×2; War + *Gegen*×1; War + *Gegen*×2) revealed that *Danshen* had no impact on the VKOR activity during warfarin treatment. In contrast, the co-administration of *Gegen* with warfarin led to significant increases of 35.9 ± 4.9 % ($P < 0.001$) and 36.2 ± 6.9 % ($P < 0.001$) in the VKOR activities of the War + *Gegen*×1 and War + *Gegen*×2 groups, respectively. However, it was not possible to completely offset the inhibitory activity of warfarin towards VKOR using *Gegen* (Fig. 6).

Up-regulation in the mRNA and protein expression levels of VKOR

Compared with the vehicle control group, there were no significant changes in the mRNA and protein expression levels of VKOR in the *Danshen*×1 and *Danshen*×2 groups. In contrast, there were significant increases of 116.1 ± 6.6 % ($P < 0.001$) and 123.0 ± 10.8 % ($P < 0.001$) in the mRNA expression of VKOR in the *Gegen*×1 and *Gegen*×2 groups, respectively, compared with the vehicle control group. Significant increases of 123.9 ± 2.9 % ($P = 0.002$) and 127.8 ± 5.7 % ($P = 0.002$) were also observed in the expression levels of the VKOR protein in the *Gegen*×1 and *Gegen*×2 groups, respectively, compared with the vehicle control group. Warfarin led to significant reductions of 43.7 ± 13.9 % ($P < 0.001$) and

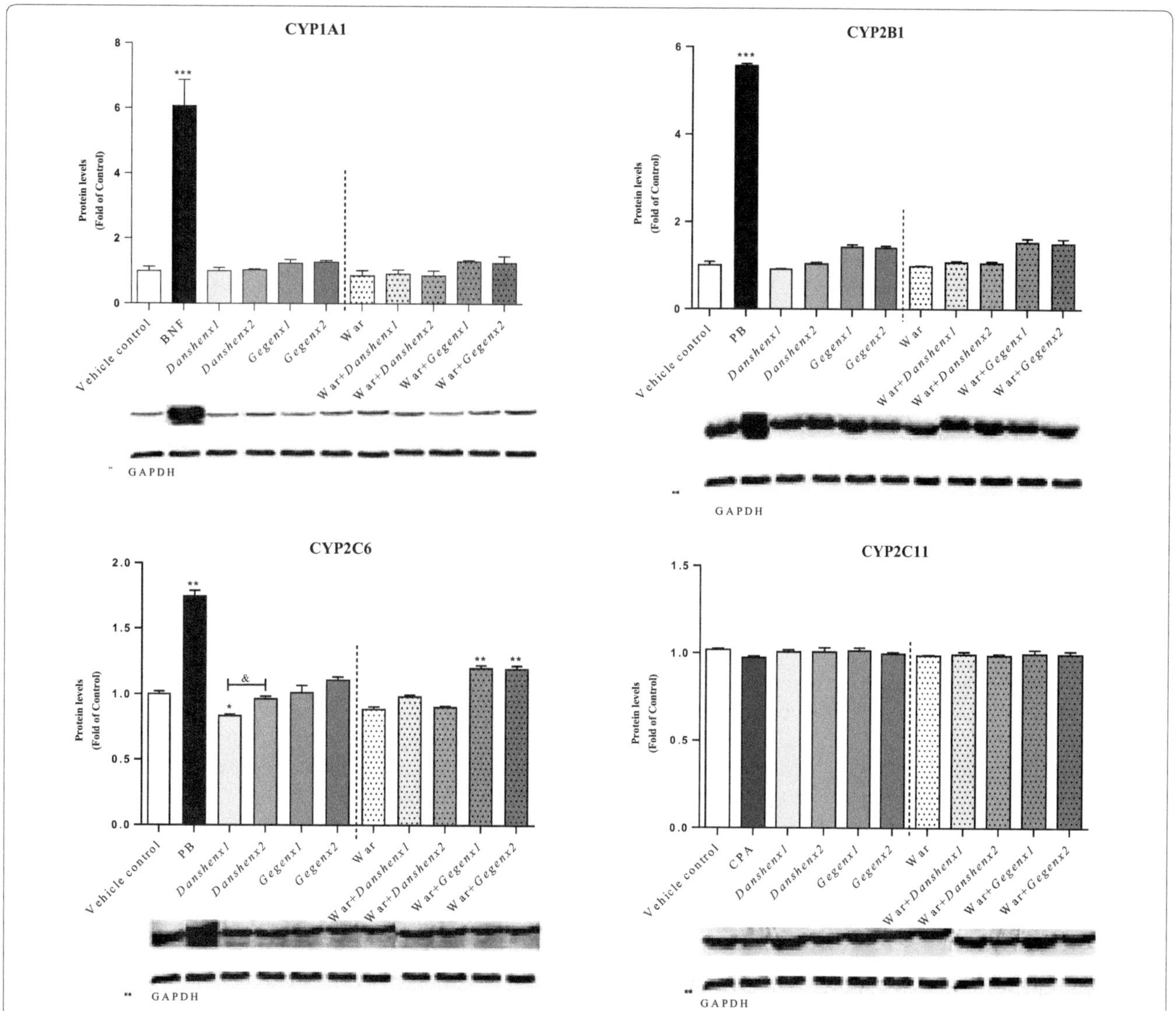

Fig. 5 Protein level (Fold of Control) for target rat liver CYP isoforms from different treatment groups. *P < 0.05; **P < 0.01; ***P < 0.001, compared with the vehicle control group. #P < 0.05; ##P < 0.01; ###P < 0.001, compared with the warfarin alone group. &P < 0.05; &&P < 0.01; &&&P < 0.001, compared within same groups of different doses. Each point represents the mean ± SD (n = 6)

71.6 ± 11.4 % (P = 0.004) in the mRNA and protein expression levels of VKOR, respectively compared with the vehicle control group. Compared with the mRNA and protein expression levels of VKOR in the warfarin-alone group, there were significant increases ($P < 0.001$) of 27 % (mRNA expression) and 25 % (protein expression) in the corresponding *Gegen* combination groups, respectively. However, the co-administration of *Danshen* with warfarin had no discernible impact of the mRNA or protein expression of VKOR (Fig. 7).

Gegen *reduced the activity, as well as the mRNA and protein expression levels of TM in rat lung*

Inhibition of the TM activity

Compared with the vehicle control group, there were no significant changes in the TM activities of the groups treated with *Danshen* or *Gegen*, although there did appear to be a decrease in the TM activities of the *Gegen*×1 and *Gegen*×2 groups. Warfarin led to a significant increase of 125.7 ± 4.2 % ($P < 0.001$) in the TM activity compared with the vehicle control group. A

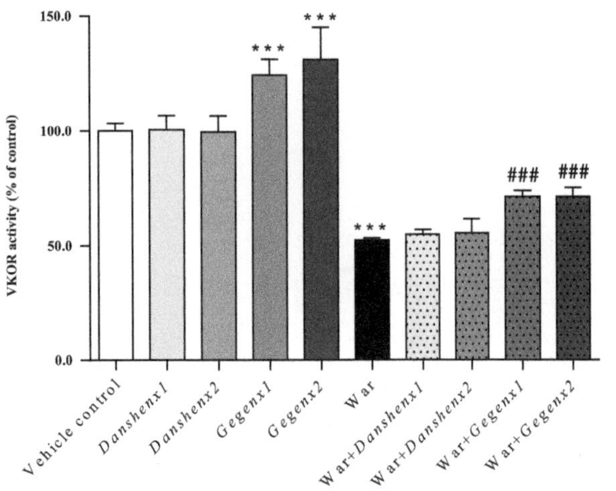

Fig. 6 Fold of change in VKOR activity from different treatment groups. $^{*}P < 0.05$; $^{**}P < 0.01$; $^{***}P < 0.001$, compared with the vehicle control group. $^{\#}P < 0.05$; $^{\#\#}P < 0.01$; $^{\#\#\#}P < 0.001$, compared with the warfarin alone group. $^{\&}P < 0.05$; $^{\&\&}P < 0.01$; $^{\&\&\&}P < 0.001$, compared within same groups of different doses. Each point represents the mean ± SD (n = 6)

comparison of the warfarin-alone group with the combination groups (i.e., War + *Danshen*×1; War + *Danshen*×2; War + *Gegen*×1; War + *Gegen*×2) showed that *Danshen* did not affect the activity of TM during warfarin treatment. In contrast, the co-administrating of *Gegen* with warfarin led to significant decreases of 83.1 ± 3.2 % ($P = 0.003$) and 80.6 ± 2.9 % ($P = 0.003$) in the TM activities of the War + *Gegen*×1 and War + *Gegen*×2 groups, respectively. *Gegen* could therefore be used to offset the induction effect of warfarin towards TM activity (Fig. 8).

Down-regulation of the mRNA and protein expression levels of TM

Compared with the vehicle control group, no significant change was observed in the expression of the TM protein in the *Danshen* group, but we did observe an increase of almost 125 % ($P = 0.02$) in the mRNA expression of TM. In contrast, significant decreases of 66.3 ± 1.5 % ($P = 0.03$) and 63.3 ± 7.5 % ($P = 0.03$) were observed in the mRNA expression levels of TM in the *Gegen*×1 and *Gegen*×2 groups, respectively, compared with the vehicle control group. We also observed significant decreases of 67.6 ± 12.5 % ($P = 0.03$) and 63.3 ± 7.5 % ($P = 0.03$) in the expression levels of the TM protein in the *Gegen*×1 and *Gegen*×2 groups, respectively, compared with the vehicle control group. Significant increases of 141.9 ± 17.8 % ($P = 0.003$) and 158.6 ± 8.2 % ($P = 0.002$) were observed in the mRNA and protein expression levels of TM in the warfarin-alone group compared with the vehicle control group. Compared with the mRNA and protein expression levels of TM in the warfarin-alone group, we observed decreases of nearly 25 % ($P = 0.03$, mRNA expression) and 12 % ($P = 0.04$, protein expression), respectively, in the *Gegen* combination groups. Notably, the co-administration of *Danshen* with warfarin had no discernible impact on the mRNA or protein expression levels of TM compared with the warfarin-alone group (Fig. 9).

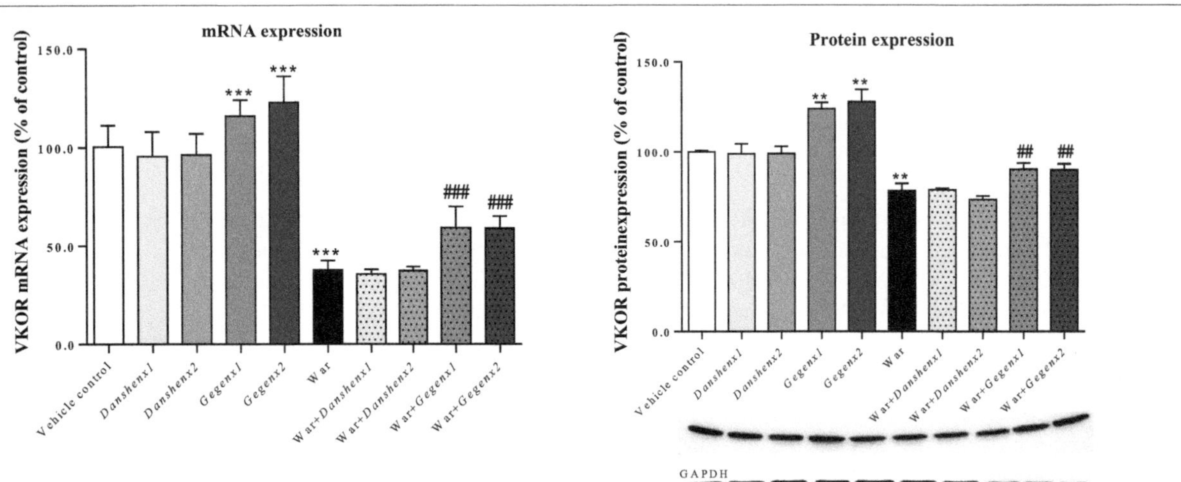

Fig. 7 Fold of change in VKOR mRNA (*left*) and protein (*right*) expression from different treatment groups. $^{*}P < 0.05$; $^{**}P < 0.01$; $^{***}P < 0.001$, compared with the vehicle control group. $^{\#}P < 0.05$; $^{\#\#}P < 0.01$; $^{\#\#\#}P < 0.001$, compared with the warfarin alone group. $^{\&}P < 0.05$; $^{\&\&}P < 0.01$; $^{\&\&\&}P < 0.001$, compared within same groups of different doses. Each point represents the mean ± SD (n = 6)

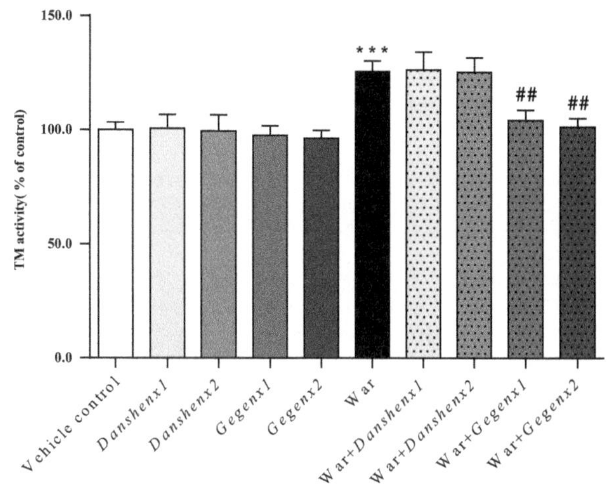

Fig. 8 Fold of change in TM activity from different treatment groups. *$P < 0.05$; **$P < 0.01$; ***$P < 0.001$, compared with the vehicle control group. #$P < 0.05$; ##$P < 0.01$; ###$P < 0.001$, compared with the warfarin alone group. &$P < 0.05$; &&$P < 0.01$; &&&$P < 0.001$, compared within same groups of different doses. Each point represents the mean ± SD (n = 6)

Gegen led to a decrease in the plasma concentration of sTM

Compared with the vehicle control group, there were no discernible changes in the plasma concentration of sTM in the *Danshen*×1 and *Danshen*×2 groups. In contrast, significant decreases of 86.3 ± 1.5 % ($P = 0.01$) and 86.5 ± 1.8 % ($P = 0.01$) were observed in the plasma concentrations of sTM in the *Gegen*×1 and *Gegen*×2 groups, respectively. Warfarin led to an increase in the plasma concentration of sTM to 112.0 ± 3.2 % ($P = 0.03$) compared with the vehicle control group. A comparison of the warfarin-alone group with the different combination groups (i.e., War + *Danshen*×1; War + *Danshen*×2; War + *Gegen*×1; War + *Gegen*×2) showed that *Danshen* had no discernible impact on the plasma concentration of sTM during warfarin treatment. In contrast, significant decreases of 11.4 ± 1.7 % ($P = 0.03$) and 10.2 ± 1.5 % ($P = 0.03$) were observed in the plasma concentrations of sTM for the War + *Gegen*×1 and War + *Gegen*×2 groups, respectively (Fig. 10).

Discussion

Danshen and *Gegen* elicit their effects by improving microcirculation and inhibiting platelet aggregation [24, 32], whereas warfarin exerts its anticoagulant effect by inhibiting the activity of VKOR and inducing TM.

In the healthy Sprague–Dawley rats used in the current study, *Gegen* rather than *Danshen* interacted with warfarin to offset its anticoagulant effects. In the *Gegen*-warfarin interaction, *Gegen* could induce the phase I metabolism of warfarin in the liver by increasing the activities and mRNA expression levels of the different CYP isozymes, as well as inducing the activity and expression levels of VKOR and inhibiting those of TM. The results of our previous study showed that the administration of a DFG-warfarin combination led to a reduction in the warfarin plasma concentration and PT time

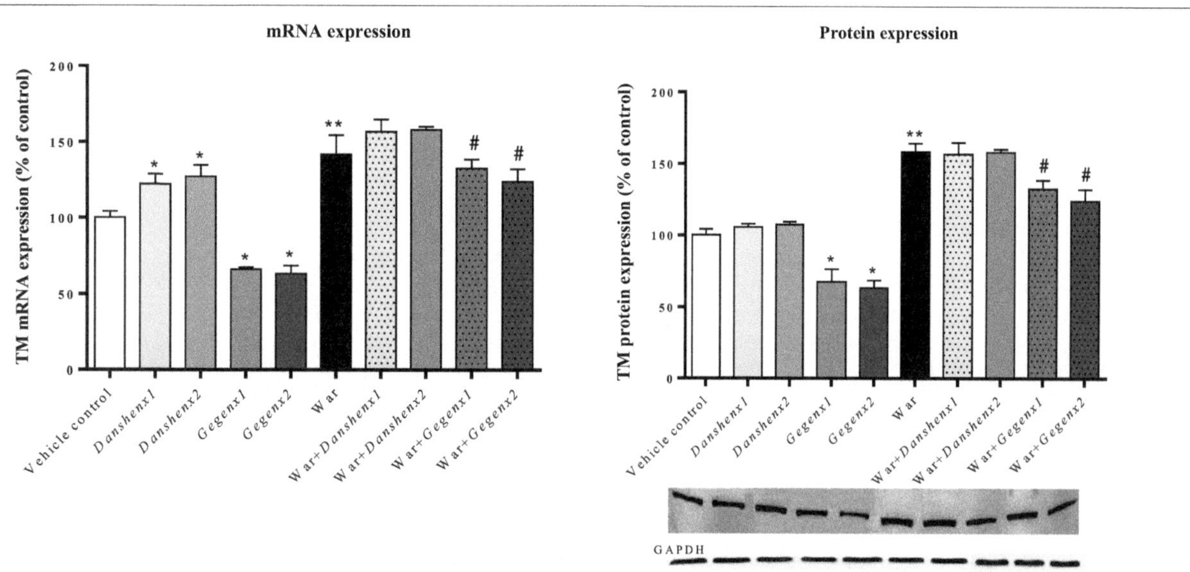

Fig. 9 Fold of change in TM mRNA (*left*) and protein (*right*) expression from different treatment groups. *$P < 0.05$; **$P < 0.01$; ***$P < 0.001$, compared with the vehicle control group. #$P < 0.05$; ##$P < 0.01$; ###$P < 0.001$, compared with the warfarin alone group. &$P < 0.05$; &&$P < 0.01$; &&&$P < 0.001$, compared within same groups of different doses. Each point represents the mean ± SD (n = 6)

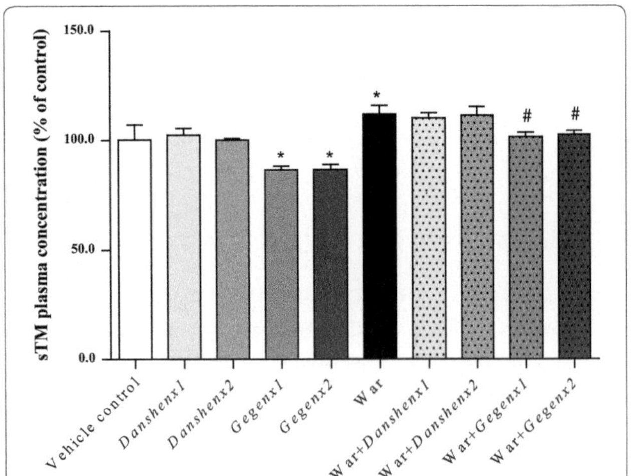

Fig. 10 Fold of change in sTM plasma concentration from different treatment groups. $^{*}P < 0.05$; $^{**}P < 0.01$; $^{***}P < 0.001$, compared with the vehicle control group. $^{\#}P < 0.05$; $^{\#\#}P < 0.01$; $^{\#\#\#}P < 0.001$, compared with the warfarin alone group. $^{\&}P < 0.05$; $^{\&\&}P < 0.01$; $^{\&\&\&}P < 0.001$, compared within same groups of different doses. Each point represents the mean ± SD (n = 6)

of rats [23, 32]. Taken together with the results of the current study, it seems clear that these effects could be attributed to the *Gegen* present in DFG.

Although there were no clinical reports in the literature pertaining to the interactions between *Gegen* and warfarin, the results of several case reports indicated that *Danshen* can interact with warfarin in humans [20–22]. However, these reports are inconsistent with our current findings. This discrepancy could be caused by several different factors, including (1) the use of different sources and preparations of *Danshen* (e.g., differences in the quality of the herbal medicines/contamination profiles); (2) a lack of adequate information in the documented case report (e.g., only one case report failed to infer a causal relationship); and (3) differences in the nature of the animals used in the different studies (e.g., rats versus humans). CYP enzymes represent some of the most highly conserved entities among different species, with relatively small differences in the primary amino acid sequences of the CYP enzymes across different species [50, 51]. Human CYP2C9, CYP2C19, CYP1A1 and CYP1A2 play important roles in warfarin metabolism, especially CYP2C9 [5], whereas the corresponding enzymes in rats are CYP2C11, CYP2C6, CYP1A1 and CYP2B1 (Fig. 11) [52]. Rat CYP1A1 shows a high level of conservation among species with greater than 80 % sequence identity compared with the corresponding enzyme in humans [50, 51]. The 6-, 7- and 8-mono-hydroxylated warfarin metabolites are formed by the CYP1A1 enzymes in rats and humans [50, 51]. Furthermore, gene sequence similarities of 74–80 % were reported for the CYP2C11 and CYP2C6 enzymes in rats compared with the human enzymes belonging to the

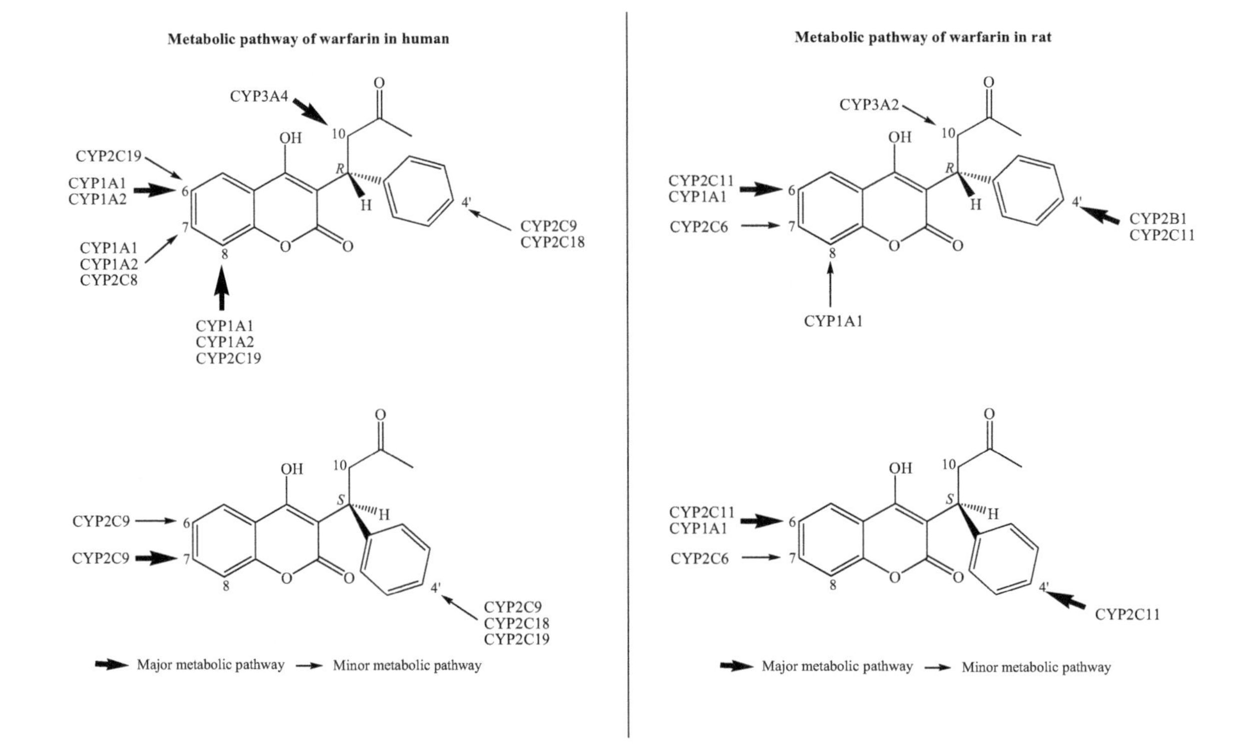

Fig. 11 CYPs involved in warfarin metabolism in human and rat

CYP2C subfamily (mainly CYP2C9 and 2C19) [50, 51]. The 4′-, 6- and 7-mono-hydroxylated warfarin metabolites are mainly formed by CYP2C11 and CYP2C6 in rats. In humans, however, these metabolites are formed by CYP2C9, CYP2C19 and CYP2C18. Notably, a genetic similarity of 78 % was reported between the rat and human CYP2B1 enzymes, which are responsible for the formation of 4′-mono-hydroxylated warfarin [50, 51]. Based on the details provided above, CYP2C11, CYP2C6, CYP1A1 and CYP2B1 were selected in the current study to investigate warfarin-related interactions in a rat model. Although these isoforms are expressed in several different species, a high degree of similarity in their gene sequences between rats and human may not automatically result in similar levels of catalytic specificity and activity.

As well as assessing the impact of warfarin on the activities of CYPs, we also investigated the variability in the effects of warfarin in humans caused by polymorphisms in the CYP2C9 and VKORC1 genes [53]. Algorithms that integrate the relevant genetic and physical factors into comprehensive, individualized predictive models were used to predict warfarin dose [54]. Furthermore, physiological-based pharmacokinetic (PBPK) modeling and simulation software, including Simcyp, PK-Sim, GastroPlus and MATLAB Sim-Biology, were recently made available to quantitatively predict the drug/herb-drug interactions of warfarin in humans based on rat data [54].

The results of an in vitro study using HepG2 cells indicated that tanshinones could be used to induce the expression of CYP1A1 and CYP1A2 [55]. The treatment of rats with *Danshen*, which mainly consists of danshensu, SAB and tanshinones, led to an increase in the activity and protein expression of CYP1A2. However, the activity of CYP1A2 did no change when rat hepatocytes were treated with danshensu or SAB in isolation [56]. Furthermore, CYP1A-, CYP2C- and CYP3A-inducing agents were found in the ethyl acetate extract, but not in the aqueous extract of *Danshen* [57]. Taken together, the results of these previous studies indicate that the lipophilic tanshinones in *Danshen*, rather than the hydrophilic components, were responsible for inducing the activity and enhancing expression of the different CYP isozymes. We found that the major components in *Danshen* granules were hydrophilic compounds, including danshensu (1140.3 ± 24.6 μg/100 mg granules), SAB (821.3 ± 33.1 μg/100 mg granules) and PCA (82.2 ± 4.6 μg/100 mg granules), which might explain why *Danshen* showed no effect on the CYP activities or expression levels. This finding is also supported by Yueng's study, where the major tanshinone components rather than the aqueous extract of *Danshen* showed effects on warfarin hydroxylation in vitro and in vivo [58].

Although paracetamol and sodium dehydroacetate (DHA-S) were reported to interact with warfarin by inhibiting VKOR activity, leading to hemorrhage in Sprague–Dawley rats, similar studies pertaining to the VKOR activity have never been conducted in context of herb-warfarin interactions [9, 10]. Regarding the results of previous studies on TM, the treatment of H9c2 cells with DFG led to a 5.36-fold up-regulation in the mRNA expression of TM compared with a control system [16]. Furthermore, SAB led to an 1.25- and 1.8-fold increases in the activity and mRNA expression of TM, respectively, over the control levels in human umbilical vein endothelial cells [15]. In our study, the mRNA expression of TM in the *Danshen*-treated group was slightly higher than that of the vehicle control group. However, there were no significant differences in the activity and protein expression levels of TM between these two groups. The inconsistencies observed between our own findings and those reported by other researchers could be attributed to differences in the nature of the experiments. For example, SAB was directly loaded onto the cells used in Shi's study at a high concentration (0.0125–0.5 mg/mL) [15]. However, SAB was reported to be poorly absorbed in animal studies and has an extremely low systemic bioavailability [59]. In our study, although SAB was used as a major component of the *Danshen* granules, the in vivo effects were very different to those observed in cells because of the poor absorption and bioavailability of SAB. Moreover, the other components in the herbs could also act on the CYP, VKOR and TM enzymes. All of these factors could therefore be considered as potential explanations for the discrepancies observed between the in vitro and in vivo results.

Conclusion

Gegen, rather than *Danshen* at the same tested dosage, offsets the anticoagulant effects of warfarin by accelerating the phase I liver metabolism of warfarin, as well as increasing the activity, mRNA and protein expression of VKOR while decreasing those of TM.

Abbreviations

CYP: liver cytochrome P450; VKOR: vitamin K epoxide reductase; VKO: vitamin K_1 2, 3-epoxide; VK: vitamin K; TM: thrombomodulin; DGF: Danshen–Gegen Formula; SAB: salvianolic acid B; PB: phenobarbital; BNF: beta-naphthoflavone; CPA: cyclophosphamide; ELISA: enzyme-linked immunosorbent assay.

Authors' contributions

BKG, ZZh and ZZu conceived and designed the study. BKG and ZZh performed the experiments. BKG, ZZh and ZZu analyzed the data. BKG, ZZh and. ZZu wrote the manuscript. All authors read and approved the final manuscript.

Acknowledgements
This work was supported by the Health and Medical Research Fund 6903483 from the Food and Health Bureau, Hong Kong SAR, China.

Competing interests
The authors declare that they have no competing interests.

References

1. Ge BK, Zhang Z, Zuo Z. Updates on the clinical evidenced herb-warfarin interactions. Evid Based Complement Alternat Med. 2014;2014:957362. doi:10.1155/2014/957362.
2. Ramsay NA, Kenny MW, Davies G, Patel JP. Complimentary and alternative medicine use among patients starting warfarin. Brit J Haematol. 2005;130:778–80.
3. Ernst E, Pittler MH, Stevinson C, White A. The desktop guide to complementary and alternative medicine. Br J Clin Pharmacol. 2002;54:454.
4. Hirsh J, Dalen JE, Anderson DR, Poller L, Bussey H, Ansell J, Deykin D. Oral anticoagulants: mechanism of action, clinical effectiveness, and optimal therapeutic range. Chest. 2001;119:8s–21s.
5. Kaminsky LS, Zhang ZY. Human P450 metabolism of warfarin. Pharmacol Ther. 1997;73:67–74.
6. Guo L, Yamazoe Y. Inhibition of cytochrome P450 by furanocoumarins in grapefruit juice and herbal medicines. Acta Pharmacol Sin. 2004;25:129–36.
7. Foster BC, Foster MS, Vandenhoek S, Krantis A, Budzinski JW, Arnason JT, et al. An in vitro evaluation of human cytochrome P450 3A4 and P-glycoprotein inhibition by garlic. J Pharm Pharm Sci. 2001;4:176–84.
8. Macan H, Uykimpang R, Alconcel M, Takasu J, Razon R, Amagase H, Niihara Y. Aged garlic extract may be safe for patients on warfarin therapy. J Nutr. 2006;136:793–5.
9. Sakaguchi Y, Suga S, Oshida K, Miyamoto-kuramitsu K, Ueda K, Miyamoto Y. Anticoagulant effect of sodium dehydroacetate (DHA-S) in rats. J Appl Toxicol. 2008;28:524–9.
10. Thijssen HH, Soute BA, Vervoort LM, Claessens JG. Paracetamol (Acetaminophen) warfarin interaction: NAPQI, the toxic metabolite of paracetamol, is an inhibitor of enzymes in the vitamin K cycle. Thromb Haemost. 2004;92:797–802.
11. Weiler H, Isermann BH. Thrombomodulin. J Thromb Haemost. 2003;1:1515–24.
12. Ikemoto T, Hojo Y, Kondo H, Takahashi N, Hirose M, Nishimura Y, Katsuki T, Shimada K, Kario K. Plasma endoglin as a marker to predict cardiovascular events in patients with chronic coronary artery diseases. Hear Vessel. 2012;27:344–51.
13. Takano S, Kimura S, Ohdama S, Aoki N. Plasma thrombomodulin in health and diseases. Blood. 1990;76:2024–9.
14. Dharmasaroja P, Dharmasaroja PA, Sobhon P. Increased plasma soluble thrombomodulin levels in cardioembolic stroke. Clin Appl Thromb Hem. 2012;18:289–93.
15. Shi CS, Huang HC, Wu HL, Kuo CH, Chang BI, Shiao MS, Shi GY. Salvianolic acid B modulates hemostasis properties of human umbilical vein endothelial cells. Thromb Res. 2007;119:769–75.
16. Fong CC, Wei F, Chen Y, Yu WK, Koon CM, Leung PC, Fung KP, Lau BS, Yang MS. Danshen-Gegen decoction exerts proliferative effect on rat cardiac myoblasts H9c2 via MAPK and insulin pathways. J Ethnopharmacol. 2011;138:60–6.
17. Chiu PY, Wong SM, Leung HY, Leong PK, Chen N, Zhou LM, Zuo Z, Lam PY, Ko KM. Long-term treatment with Danshen-Gegen decoction protects the myocardium against ischemia/reperfusion injury via the redox-sensitive protein kinase C-ε/mK(ATP) pathway in rats. Rejuv Res. 2011;14:173–84.
18. Chang Q, Sun L, Zhao RH, Chow MSS, Zuo Z. Simultaneous determination of ten active components in traditional Chinese medicinal products containing both Gegen (*Pueraria lobata*) and Danshen (*Salvia miltiorrhiza*) by high-performance liquid chromatography. Phytochem Anal. 2008;19:368–75.
19. Chook P, Tam WY, Chan LT, Qiao M, Cheng KF, Poon YK, Qiao M, Chan LT, Cheung SP, Cheng KF, Fung KP, Tang SL, Lau KM, Koon CM, Leung PC, Celermjer DS, Woo KS. Efficacy and safety of Danshen and Gegen as adjunctive secondary prevention therapy in coronary artery disease. South China J Cardio Vasc Dis. 2011;17:48–52.
20. Chook P, Tam LW, Poon PY, Qiao M, Chan LL, Cheung AS, Cheng KF, Fung KP, Tang SL, Koon CM, Leung PC, Celermjer DS, Woo KS. Danshen and Gegen as cardiovascular tonic in coronary patients: a novel strategy for secondary atherosclerosis prevention. South China J Cardio Vasc Dis. 2005;12:32.
21. Tam WY, Chook P, Qiao M, Chan LT, Chan TYK, Poon YK, Fung KP, Leung PC, Woo KS. The efficacy and tolerability of adjunctive alternative herbal medicine (*Salvia miltiorrhiza* and *Pueraria lobata*) on vascular function and structure in coronary patients. J Altern Complem Med. 2009;15:415–21.
22. Zhang Z, Ge BK, Zhou LM, Lam TN, Zuo Z. Induction of liver cytochrome P450 s by Danshen-Gegen formula is the leading cause for its pharmacokinetic interactions with warfarin. J Ethnopharmacol. 2014;154:672–86.
23. Zhou LM, Wang S, Zhang Z, Lau BS, Fung KP, Leung PC, Zuo Z. Pharmacokinetic and pharmacodynamic interaction of Danshen-Gegen extract with warfarin and aspirin. J Ethnopharmacol. 2012;143:648–55.
24. Cheng TO. Cardiovascular effects of Danshen. Int J Cardiol. 2007;121:9–22.
25. Wang BQ. Salvia miltiorrhiza: chemical and pharmacological review of a medicinal plant. J Med Plants Res. 2010;4:2813–20.
26. Chan TYK. Interaction between warfarin and Danshen (*Salvia miltiorrhiza*). Ann Pharmacother. 2001;35:501–4.
27. Izzat MB, Yim APC, El-Zufari MH. A taste of Chinese medicine! Ann Thorac Surg. 1998;66:941–2.
28. Tam LS, Chan TYK, Leung WK, Critchley JAJH. Warfarin interactions with Chinese traditional medicines: danshen and methyl salicylate medicated oil. Aust NZ J Med. 1995;25:258.
29. Yu C, Chan J, Sanderson J. Chinese herbs and warfarin potentiation by 'danshen'. J Inter Med. 1997;241:337–9.
30. La ACT, Chan K, Yeung JHK, Woo KS. The effects of Danshen (*Salvia miltiorrhiza*) on pharmacokinetics and pharmacodynamics of warfarin in rats. Eur J Drug Metab Pharmacokinet. 1992;17:257–62.
31. Chu Y, Zhang L, Wang X, Guo J, Guo Z, Ma X. The effect of compound Danshen dripping pills, a Chinese herb medicine, on the pharmacokinetics and pharmacodynamics of warfarin in rats. J Ethnopharmacol. 2011;137:1457–61.
32. Zhang Z, Lam TN, Zuo Z. Radix Puerariae: an overview of its chemistry, pharmacology, pharmacokinetics, and clinical use. J Clin Pharmacol. 2013;53:787–811.
33. Guerra MC, Speroni E, Broccoli M, Cangini M, Pasini P, Minghett A, Crespi-Perellino N, Mirasoli M, Cantelli-Forti G, Paolini M. Comparison between Chinese medical herb *Pueraria Lobata* crude extract and its main isoflavone puerarin antioxidant properties and effects on rat liver CYP-catalysed drug metabolism. Life Sci. 2000;67:2997–3006.
34. Zheng J, Chen B, Jiang B, Zeng L, Tang ZR, Fan L, Zhou HH. The effects of puerarin on CYP2D6 and CYP1A2 activities in vivo. Arch Pharm Res. 2010;33:243–6.
35. Tsai HH, Lin HW, Lu YH, Chen YL, Mahady GB. A review of potential harmful interactions between anticoagulant/antiplatelet agents and Chinese herbal medicines. PLoS ONE. 2013;8:e64255.
36. Chinese-Pharmacopoeia, 2010. Pharmacopoeia of the People's Republic of China Version 2010, vol. 1. Beijing: Chemical Industry Press; 2010.
37. Tishler M, Louis FF, Norman LW. Hydro, oxido and other derivatives of vitamin K_1 and related compound. J Am Chem Soc. 1940;62:2866–71.
38. Reagan-Shaw S, Nihal M, Ahmad N. Dose translation from animal to human studies revisited. FASEB J. 2008;22:659–61.
39. Wallin R, Martin LF. Warfarin poisoning and vitamin K antagonism in rat and human liver. Design of a system in vitro that mimics the situation in vivo. Biochem J. 1987;241:389–96.
40. Fong YK, Li CR, Wo SK, Wang S, Zhou L, Zhang L, Lin G, Zuo Z. In vitro and in situ evaluation of herb-drug interactions during intestinal metabolism and absorption of baicalein. J Ethnopharmacol. 2012;141:742–53.
41. Esmon NL, Owen WG, Esmon CT. Isolation of a membrane-bound cofactor for thrombin-catalyzed activation of protein C. J Biol Chem. 1982;257:859–64.
42. Baldwin SJ, Bramhall JL, Ashby CA, Yue L, Murdock PR, Hood SR, Ayrton AD, Clarke SE. Cytochrome P450 gene induction in rats ex vivo assessed

by quantitative real-time reverse transcriptase-polymerase chain reaction (Taqman). Drug Metab Dispos. 2006;34:1063–9.
43. Hoen PA, Bijsterbosch MK, van Berkel TJ, Vermeulen NP, Commandeur JN. Midazolam is a phenobarbital-like cytochrome p450 inducer in rats. J Pharmacol Exp Ther. 2001;299:921–7.
44. Rahmaniyan M, Patrick K, Bell NH. Characterization of recombinant CYP2C11: a vitamin D 25-hydroxylase and 24-hydroxylase. Am J Physiol Endocrinol Metab. 2005;288:e753–60.
45. Laemmli UK. Cleavage of structural proteins during the assembly of the head of bacteriophage T4. Nature. 1970;227:680–5.
46. Lasseur R, Longin-Sauvageon C, Videmann B, Billeret M, Berny P, Benoit E. Warfarin resistance in a French strain of rats. J Biochem Mol Toxicol. 2005;19:379–85.
47. He CJ, Kanfer A. Quantification and modulation of thrombomodulin activity in isolated rat and human glomeruli. Kidney Int. 1992;41:1170–4.
48. Yamashita T, Sekiguchi A, Iwasaki Y, Sagara K, Hatano S, Iinuma H, Aizawa T, Fu LT. Thrombomodulin and tissue factor pathway inhibitor in endocardium of rapidly paced rat atria. Circulation. 2003;108:2450–2.
49. Wong YC, Zuo Z. Brain disposition and catalepsy after intranasal delivery of Loxapine: role of metabolism in PK/PD of intranasal CNS drugs. Pharm Res. 2013;30:2368–84.
50. Martignoni M, Groothuis GMM, De Kanter R. Species differences between mouse, rat, dog, monkey and human CYP-mediated drug metabolism, inhibition and induction. Expert Opin Drug Metab Toxicol. 2006;2:875–94.
51. Fasco MJ, Silkworth JB, Dunbar DA, Kaminsky LS. Rat small intestinal cytochromes probed by warfarin metabolism. Mol Pharmacol. 1992;43:226–33.
52. Soucek P, Gut I. Cytochromes P-450 in rats: structures, functions, properties and relevant human forms. Xenobiotica. 1992;22:83–103.
53. Martin JH, Pharmacologist C, Physician G, Medicine D. Pharmacogenetics of warfarin—is testing clinically indicated ? Exp Clin Pharmacol. 2009;32:76–80.
54. Brantley SJ, Gufford BT, Dua R, Fediuk DJ, Graf TN, Scarlett YV, Fisher MB, Paine MF. Physiologically based pharmacokinetic modeling framework for quantitative prediction of an herb-drug interaction. CPT Pharmacometrics Syst Pharmacol. 2014;3:e107.
55. Zhang R, Sun J, Ma L, Wu X, Pan G, Hao H, Zhou F, Jiye A, Liu C, Shang LL, Ai H, Gao HY, Peng Y, Wu H, Wang GJ. Induction of cytochromes P450 1A1 and 1A2 by tanshinones in human HepG2 hepatoma cell line. Toxicol Appl Pharmacol. 2011;252:18–27.
56. Lee WYW, Zhou X, Or PMY, Kwan YW, Yeung JHK. Tanshinone I increases CYP1A2 protein expression and enzyme activity in primary rat hepatocytes. Phytomedicine. 2012;19:169–76.
57. Kuo YH, Lin YL, Don MJ, Chen RM, Ueng YF. Induction of cytochrome P450-dependent monooxygenase by extracts of the medicinal herb *Salvia miltiorrhiza*. J Pharm Pharmacol. 2006;58:521–7.
58. Wu WWP, Yeung JHK. Inhibition of warfarin hydroxylation by major tanshinones of Danshen (*Salvia miltiorrhiza*) in the rat in vitro and in vivo. Phytomedicine. 2010;17:219–26.
59. Zhou LM, Chow MSS, Zuo Z. Effect of sodium caprate on the oral absorptions of danshensu and salvianolic acid B. Int J Pharm. 2009;379:109–18.

2

Authentication of Acori Tatarinowii Rhizoma (*Shi Chang Pu*) and its adulterants by morphological distinction, chemical composition and ITS sequencing

Kelly Yin-Ching Lam[1], Chuen-Fai Ku[2], Huai-You Wang[1,3], Gallant Kar-Lun Chan[1], Ping Yao[1], Huang-Quan Lin[1,3], Tina Ting-Xia Dong[1,3], Hong-Jie Zhang[2] and Karl Wah-Keung Tsim[1,3*]

Abstract

Background: Acori Tatarinowii Rhizoma (ATR; rhizome of *Acorus tatarinowii* Schott) (*Shi Chang Pu*) is widely used in Chinese medicine (CM) to resuscitate, calm the mind, resolve *shi* (*dampness*) and harmonize the *wei* (*stomach*). Seven different species have been identified as belonging to the genus *Acorus*, all of which can be found in China. However, it can be difficult to distinguish the different species of *Acorus* because of their morphological similarities. The aim of this study was to authenticate *Acorus* species using macroscopic and microscopic techniques, chemical analysis and DNA authentication and to compare the resolution power and reliability of these different methods.

Methods: Four batches of ATR, Acori Graminei Rhizoma (AGR), Acori Calami Rhizoma (ACR) and Anemones Altaicae Rhizoma (AAR) (totaling 16 samples) were collected from Hong Kong and mainland China. The major characteristic features of these *Acorus* species were identified by macroscopic and microscopic examination. The identified samples were also analyzed by UHPLC analysis. Principal component analysis (PCA) and hierarchal clustering analysis (HCA) on UHPLC results were used to differentiate between the samples. An internal transcribed spacer (ITS) was selected as a molecular probe and a modified DNA extraction method was developed to obtain trace amounts of DNA from the different *Acorus* species. All extracted DNA sequences were edited by Bioedit and aligned with the ClustalW. And the sequence distances were calculated using the Maximum Parsimony method.

Results: Macroscopic and microscopic analyses allowed for AAR to be readily distinguished from ATR, AGR and ACR. However, it was difficult to distinguish between ATR, AGR and ACR because of their similar morphological features. Chemical profiling revealed that α- and β-asarone were only found in the ATR, AGR and ACR samples, but not in the AAR samples. Furthermore, PCA and HCA allowed for the differentiation of these three species based on their asarone contents. Morphological authentication and chemical profiling allowed for the partial differentiation of ATR, AGR ACR and AAR. DNA analysis was the only method capable of accurately differentiating between all four species.

Conclusion: DNA authentication exhibited higher resolution power and reliability than conventional morphological identification and UHPLC in differentiating between different *Acorus* species.

*Correspondence: botsim@ust.hk

[1] Division of Life Science, and Center for Chinese Medicine, The Hong Kong University of Science and Technology, Clear Water Bay Road, Hong Kong, China

Full list of author information is available at the end of the article

Background

The dried rhizome from *Acorus tatarinowii* Schott (*Shi Chang Pu*) is used as a Chinese medicine (CM), which is known as Acori Tatarinowii Rhizoma (ATR). *A. tatarinowii* is recorded in the Chinese pharmacopoeia (2015) as the official botanical source of ATR. ATR is produced in the Sichuan, Zhejiang, Jiangsu and Hunan provinces of China [1]. However, there are seven different species of plant belonging to the *Acorus* genus, which are distributed from the northern temperate areas of the globe to the sub-tropical regions. Notably, all seven of these species can be readily found in China. Three species of *Acorus*, including ATR, Acori Graminei Rhizoma (AGR; rhizome derived from the *A. gramineus* Soland; *Jin Qian Chang Pu*) and Acori Calami Rhizoma (ACR; rhizome derived from the *A. calamus* Linn; *Shui Chang Pu*) are widely used in CM.

The aerial parts and rhizomes of these three plants show similar morphological characteristics, and these plants have been described as herbal medicines in a variety of different national pharmacopoeia in Asia. For example, ATR is used for epilepsy, loss of consciousness, forgetfulness and insomnia in CM [2]. In Korea and Japan [3], AGR is used to treat convulsions and stomach aches, and this material is also used as a sedative in oriental medicine. In contrast, ACR is used to treat cognitive disorders, epilepsy, asthma, pain and diabetes in India [4, 5]. In addition, Anemones Altaicae Rhizoma (AAR; *Jiu Jie Chang Pu*), which is the rhizome from *Anemone altaica* Fisch. ex Mey, is a member of the ranunculaceae family, which has been used as a substitute for ATR to treat dreaminess, amnesia, rheumatoid arthritis and epilepsy [6]. These four CM herbs are all known by the same Chinese name "*Chang Pu*" and share several morphological similarities, making it difficult to differentiate between these plants based on their physical appearance.

The aim of this study was to develop a new method to authenticate *Acorus* species using a combination of macroscopic and microscopic examination, chemical analysis and DNA authentication, as well as comparing the resolution power and reliability of these different methods.

Methods

Chemicals, reagents and herbal materials

The chemical standards α- and β-asarone (purity ≥98 %) were purchased from TLCM (Hong Kong, China). Acetonitrile and ethanol (HPLC grade) for UHPLC analysis were purchased from Merck (Darmstadt, Germany). Ultra-pure water was obtained from a Milli-Q purification system (Millipore, Molsheim, France). Four batches of ATR, AGR, ACR and AAR (totaling 16 samples, which were numbered from 1 to 16) were collected from herbal markets in Hong Kong and mainland China (Table 1).

Table 1 ATR, AGR, ACR and AAR collected from different regions of China

Herbs	Sample	Voucher no.	Regions
ATR	1	ATR-1-2014	Liuzhou, Guangxi
	2	ATR-2-2014	Lingbao, Henan
	3	ATR-3-2014	Taiyuan, Shanxi
	4	ATR-4-2014	Tianshui, Gansu
AGR	5	AGR-1-2014	Bozhou, Anhui
	6	AGR-2-2014	Muyang, Jiangsu
	7	AGR-3-2014	Xian, Shanxi
	8	AGR-4-2014	Datian, Fujian
ACR	9	ACR-1-2014	Anxin, Hebei
	10	ACR-2-2014	Suqian, Jiangsu
	11	ACR-3-2014	Xiaoshan, Hangzhou
	12	ACR-4-2014	Muyang, Jiangsu
AAR	13	AAR-1-2014	Jiujiang, Jiangxi
	14	AAR-2-2014	Hanzhong, Shanxi
	15	AAR-3-2014	Zigong, Sichuan
	16	AAR-4-2014	Bozhou, Anhui

All of the samples were authenticated by Dr. Tina Dong [Hong Kong University of Science and Technology (HKUST)], according to their morphological characteristics and the descriptions of these materials found in the Chinese Pharmacopoeia (2015) and related documents [7, 8]. Voucher specimens were collected and deposited at The Centre for Chinese Medicine Research and Development, HKUST, under the accession numbers listed in Table 1.

Macroscopic and microscopic examination

The appearance, color, odor and taste characteristics of the samples were observed and recorded, together with digital color photographs of each sample [9]. Representative samples of the transverse section of each batch were fixed in formalin-acetic acid-alcohol for a minimum of 24 h. After fixing, the samples were dehydrated using a series of graded ethanol (50, 70, 80, 90 and 100 %) (Unichem Ltd, Chessington, UK) and xylene (50, 100 %) (VWR International, Lutterworth, UK) solutions, before being embedded in paraffin wax (Leica, Shanghai, China) using a previously reported technique [10]. The embedded materials were then cut into 15-μm-thick sections using a rotary microtome (Leica), and stained with safranin-T (Sigma-Aldrich, St Louis, MO, USA) and fast green FCF solution (Sigma-Aldrich). Finally, the stained sections were sealed with DPX-Mountant (Sigma-Aldrich). At least 20 different transverse sections from each sample were prepared. For the powder sections, samples of each of these crude drugs were powdered using a grinder and passed through a 300-μm sieve. The powdered materials were sealed with dilute glycerine and observed under a ZEISS Axio Scope A1 universal microscope (Zeiss Group, Jena, Germany). The powder of each sample was observed for at least 10 slides. The distinct characteristics of these materials were observed under light and polarized light microscopes using a ZEISS Axio Scope A1 universal microscope equipped with a reflector Axio-photo module (Zeiss Group, Jena, Germany) and a direct current (DC) camera.

Chemical analysis by UHPLC-DAD

Standard stock solutions were prepared at a concentration of 50 mg/L in ethanol, which was identified as the optimal solvent for the extraction of asarone. One gram of powdered sample material was accurately weighed and placed in a centrifuge tube with 10 mL of ethanol. After sonication in a Branson 5200 sonicator (Branson Ultrasonic Corp, Connecticut, USA) for 30 min, the mixture was centrifuged (Eppendorf centrifuge 5810R, Eppendorf, Hamburg, Germany) at 3000×*g* for 5 min. The supernatant was then transferred to a 25-mL volumetric flask and the extraction process was repeated once more. The combined supernatants were diluted to a total volume of 25 mL with ethanol and filtered through a 0.45-μm PTFE filter before being analyzed. UHPLC-DAD analysis was conducted on a Thermo Scientific™ UltiMate 3000 UHPLC System comprising a vacuum degasser, binary pump, auto-sampler, thermostatted column compartment and DAD (Thermo Fisher Scientific, Waltham, MA, USA), which was used for acquiring chromatograms and UV spectra. The samples were analyzed using a Kinetex C18 column (phenomenex, Torrance, CA, USA; 2.1 × 100 mm, 2.6 μm), which was eluted with a mobile phase consisting of water (A) and acetonitrile (B) according to the following gradient program: 30–45 % (B) 0–5 min; 45 % (B) 5–15 min; and 45–100 % (B) 15–25 min. The flow rate, detection wavelength and column temperature were set at 0.2 mL/min, 270 nm and 40 °C, respectively, with an injection volume of 1.0 μL.

DNA extraction and ITS sequence analysis

Samples of each plant were ground into a fine powder with a grinder and extracted using a DNeasy®Plant Mini Kit (Qiagen, Hilden, Germany) according to the manufacturer's protocol. DNA quantification was performed using a NanoDrop 2000 Spectrophotometer (Thermo Fisher Scientific). An absorbance (A260/A280) ratio of 1.8 indicated insignificant levels of contamination from unwanted proteins and polysaccharides. Five microliters of genomic DNA (~100 ng) was added to a master mix containing 10× PCR buffer (with Mg^{2+} at a concentration of 1.5 mM containing a bromophenol blue loading dye), 0.5 mM dNTP, 400 nM of the forward and reverse primers (ITS-S, AGG AGA AGT CGT AAC AAG; ITS-AS, GTT TCT TTT CCT CCG CT) [11] and 1.5 U of Taq Polymerase (KAPA Taq DNA Polymerase with dye, KAPA Biosystems, Woburn, MA, USA) for a 50 L PCR reaction. A GeneAmp 9700 thermal cycler (Applied Biosystems, Foster City, CA, USA) was used with the following program: 3 min at 95 °C, 30 s at 55 °C and 45 s at 72 °C, followed by 40 cycles of 30 s at 95 °C, 30 s at 55 °C and 30 s at 72 °C, with a final 10 min extension at 72 °C [12]. Ten microliters of the amplification product was collected and separated on a 1.2 % agarose gel, and detected under UV-light after staining with SYBR® Safe DNA gel stain (Thermo Fisher Scientific). The PCR product was purified with a PCR purification kit (Qiagen) according to the manufacturer's protocol. The cycle sequencing and sequence reactions were performed by an external company (Dragon Technology Limited, Hong Kong, China). All of the sequences were edited using a Biological Sequence Alignment Editor (Bioedit) and aligned with the ClustalW algorithm found in version 6.0 of the Molecular Evolutionary Genetics Analysis (MEGA 6) software (The Biodesign Institute, Arizona, MA, USA). All of the sequence distances were calculated using the Maximum Parsimony method (Kimura 2-parameter model, bootstrap = 1000 replicates) with MEGA 6.

Statistical analysis

Peaks above the S/N ratio of the chromatogram were labeled and manually integrated using version 7.2 of the Chromeleon Chromatography Data System software (Thermo Fisher Scientific) to distinguish between the different species of *Acorus*. Principal component analysis (PCA) and Hierarchical clustering analysis (HCA) of the relative peak areas were performed using the SPSS for Windows 16.0 software (SPSS Corporation, Armonk, NY, USA) to differentiate between the different peaks. Summary data were expressed as the mean ± standard deviation (SD) for $n = 4$.

Results

Macroscopic features

Sixteen samples of herbs corresponding to ATR, AGR, ACR and AAR were collected from different production sites and numbered from 1 to 16 (Table 1). The different samples were initially identified based on their morphological appearance. The unique features of these samples are described below.

ATR

Compressed-cylindrical, frequently tortuous, normally branched, 3–15 cm in length and 3–10 mm in diameter. Externally brown or greyish-brown, rough, with uneven annulations, internodes of 1–15 mm in length, with fine longitudinal wrinkles, occasionally with remnants of fibrous roots or rounded root scars; leaf scars triangular, arranged alternately, some with hairy and scaly remnants of the leaf bases (Fig. 1a). Odor, aromatic; taste, bitter and slightly pungent.

AGR
Almost the same as ATR, but smaller in size. Compressed-cylindrical, frequently tortuous, normally branched, 1–4 cm in length and 2–7 mm in diameter. Externally brown or pale green, rough, with uneven annulations, internodes of 1.5–4 mm long, with fine longitudinal wrinkles, occasionally with remnants of fibrous roots or rounded root scars; leaf scars triangular, arranged alternately, some with hairy and scaly remnants of the leaf bases (Fig. 1b). Odor, aromatic; taste, bitter and slightly pungent.

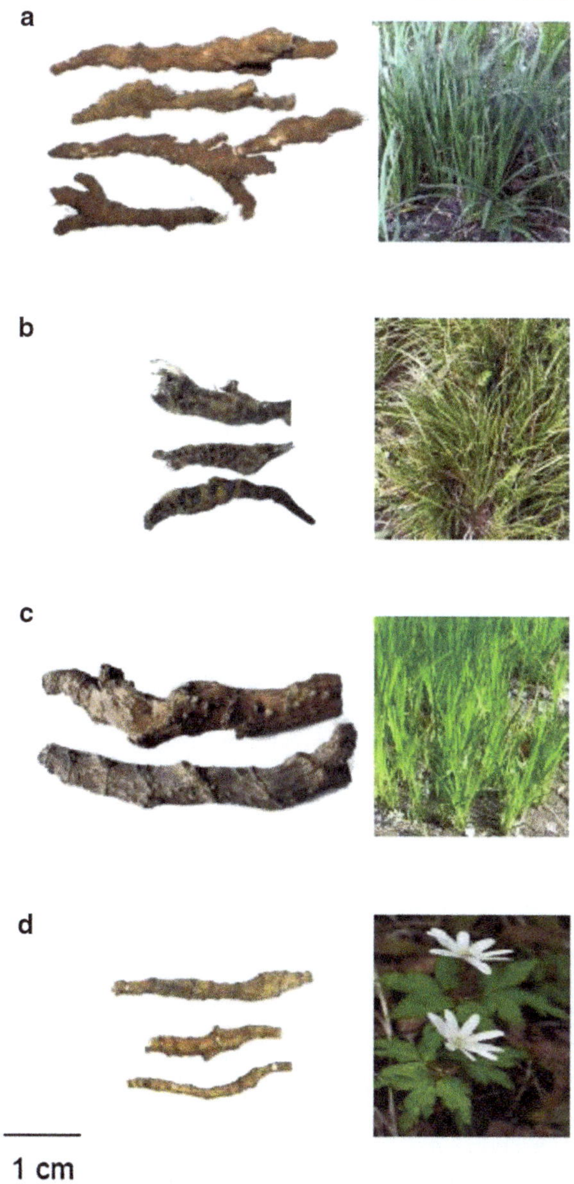

Fig. 1 Photographs of the rhizomes of *A. tatarinowii* and its adulterants. **a** *ATR* Acori Tatarinowii Rhizoma; **b** *AGR* Acori Graminei Rhizoma; **c** *ACR* Acori Calami Rhizoma; **d** *AAR* Anemones Altaicae Rhizoma

ACR
Similar to ATR, but larger in size. Cylindrical, flattened and branched at the nodes, 5–20 cm in length and 10–15 mm in diameter. Externally, the rhizomes appeared light brown to red, and the inner surface appeared pale brown. Fewer internodes than ATR, 4–15 mm in length with fine longitudinal wrinkles, occasionally with remnants of the fibrous roots or rounded root scars; large triangular leaf scars, arranged alternately, some with hairy and scaly remnants of the leaf bases (Fig. 1c). Strong aromatic odor, pungent taste.

AAR
Fusiform in shape, slightly curved, 1–4 cm in length and 3–5 mm in diameter. Externally, yellowish brown to brown in color. Nodes with numerous semi-circular protuberances and root scars (Fig. 1d). Odor slight, slightly sour taste with numbness.

Microscopic features of transverse sections

ATR
Epidermis consisting of one layer of brown cells with a thickened outer wall. Broad cortex with numerous scattered fiber bundles and leaf-trace vascular bundles. Endodermis distinct. Stele vascular bundles amphivasal or collateral, densely lined up in close proximity to the endodermis, gradually becoming larger and sparse going inward, vascular bundles with a distinct sheath. Parenchyma scattered with sub-rounded secretory cells, filled with secretions (Fig. 2a).

AGR
Almost the same as ATR, but smaller in size. Epidermis consisting of one layer of brown cells with a thickened outer wall. Broad cortex with numerous scattered fiber bundles and leaf-trace vascular bundles. Endodermis distinct. Stele vascular bundles amphivasal or collateral, densely lined up in close proximity to the endodermis, gradually becoming larger and sparse going inward, vascular bundles sheath distinct. Parenchyma scattered with sub-rounded secretory cells, filled with secretions (Fig. 2b).

ACR
Similar to ATR, but larger in size. Epidermis consisting of one layer of brown cells with a thickened outer wall.

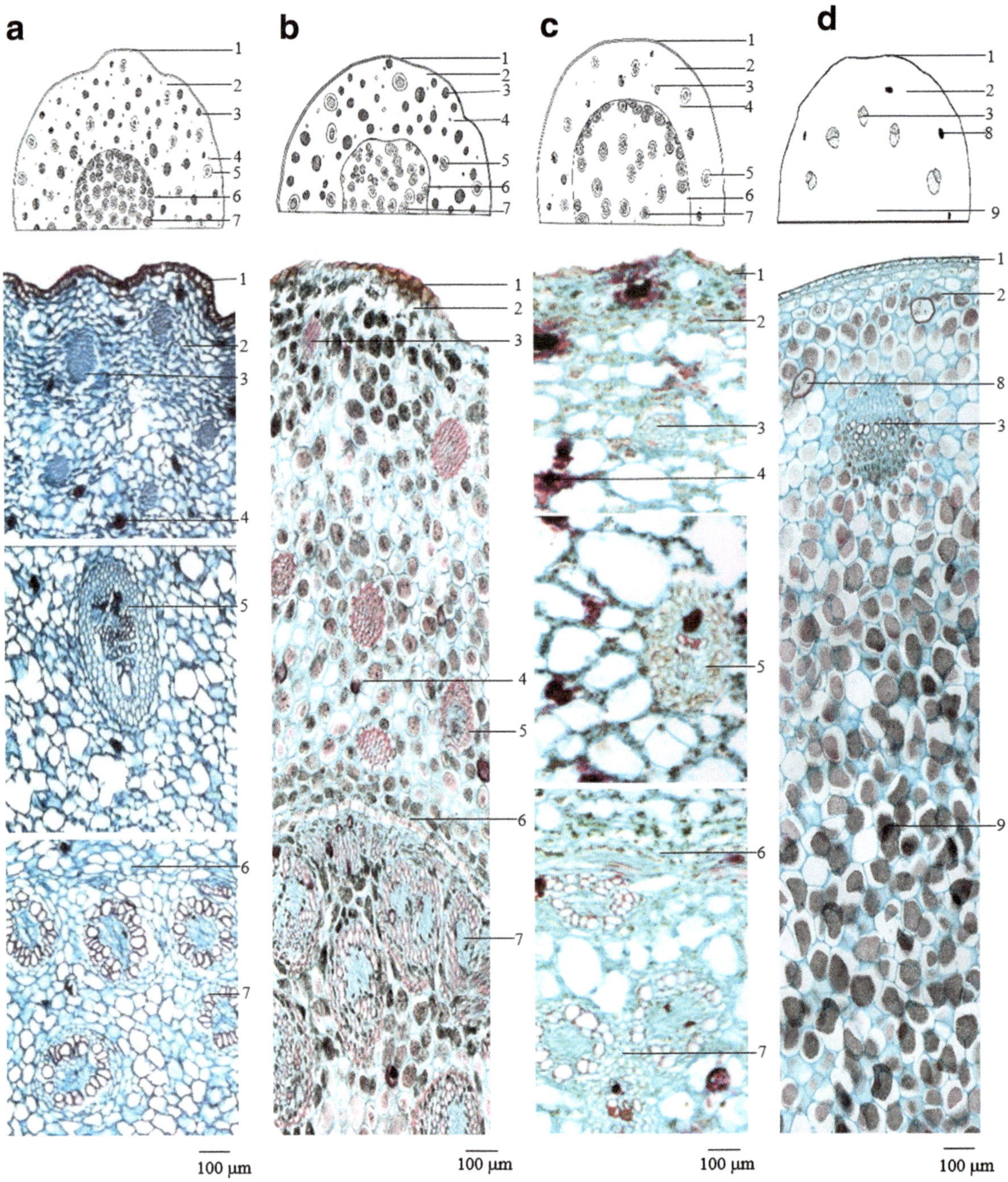

Fig. 2 Micrographs show transverse sections of ATR and its adulterants. **a** *ATR* Acori Tatarinowii Rhizoma; **b** *AGR* Acori Graminei Rhizoma; **c** *ACR* Acori Calami Rhizoma; **d** *AAR* Anemones Altaicae Rhizoma. Notations are: *1* epidermis; *2* cortex; *3* fiber bundles; *4* secretory cells; *5* leaf-trace vascular bundle; *6* endodermis; *7* stele vascular bundle; *8* stone cells; *9* pith

Broad cortex with numerous scattered fiber bundles and leaf-trace vascular bundles. Fewer fiber bundles compared with ATR. Distinct endodermis. Stele vascular bundles amphivasal or collateral, densely lined up in close proximity to the endodermis, gradually becoming larger and sparse going inward, vascular bundles sheath distinct. Parenchyma scattered with sub-rounded secretory cells, filled with secretions (Fig. 2c).

AAR

Epidermis consisting of one layer of flat cells with a thickened outer wall. Sub-spherical stone cells scattered across the outer part of the cortex. Collateral vascular bundles composed of 8–12 units arranged in a ring. Phloem cells flat and shrunken. Cambium indistinct. Xylem vessels polygonal or sub-rounded. Pith large. Parenchymatous cell filled with starch granules (Fig. 2d).

Microscopic features of powder sections

ATR, AGR and ACR

There were no significant differences in the microscopic features of the ATR, AGR and ACR powders. The fibers were mostly bundled, colorless or pale yellow in color, tapered towards the ends and lignified with distinct pit canals. Fibrous bundles surrounded by cells containing calcium oxalate prisms, which formed crystalline fibers. Polyhedral, sub-polygonal or polycone-like calcium oxalate prisms, which appeared yellowish-white or polychromatic under a polarized microscope. Simple starch granules, which were ellipsoid, spheroidal, long-ovoid, hilum pointed, V-shaped or short slit-shaped with indistinct striation marks; black and cruciate-shaped under a polarized microscope; compound starch granules composed of 2–20 units. Secretory cells abundant, sub-rounded or elongated-rounded, filled with orange-yellow secretions. The epidermal cells of the leaf sheath were greyish-green or pale yellowish-brown and rectangular in shape. The vessels were mainly reticulate (Fig. 3A–C).

AAR

Fibers mostly in bundles, yellowish-white or polychromatic under a polarized microscope. Numerous starch granules. Simple starch granules spherical to ovoid, with dotted, cleft or asteroidal hilum, compound granules composed of 2–4 units, black in color and cruciate-shaped under a polarized microscope. Stone cells, which were sub-rounded or oblong in shape. The vessels were mostly reticulate. Parenchymatous cells abundant (Fig. 3D).

Table 2 Characteristics of the ATR, AGR, ACR and AAR samples, as determined by microscopic analysis. These features could serve as parameters for the identification of these herbs.

Chemical analysis by UHPLC-DAD

α-Asarone and β-asarone, which are the most abundant chemicals in these plant species, were used as chemical markers for ATR. These chemicals have also been reported to exhibit biological functions [13–16]. The samples were analyzed using a DAD detector according to the popular criteria. The detection wavelength of the DAD detector was set to 270 nm to acquire the most abundant peaks. Typical chromatograms of ATR, AGR, ACR and AAR from samples 1–16 are shown in Fig. 4a. The results revealed that there were considerable differences in the chromatographic profiles of the ATR, AGR and ACR extracts compared with the AAR extract. The majority of the α-asarone and β-asarone components were eluted in less than 30 min from the ATR, AGR and ACR extracts. In contrast, the chromatogram of the AAR extract did not contain any α-asarone or β-asarone based on a comparison of its retention times and UV spectra with those of the standard compounds (Fig. 4a). The chromatographic fingerprints of all of the extracts were shown to be highly stable and reproducible using the "Similarity evaluation system for the chromatographic fingerprints of TCM" software, which was developed by the Chinese Pharmacopeia Commission. The application of PCA to the chromatographic fingerprints summarized most of the UHPLC-DAD data into the first two principle components, PC1 and PC2, with two-dimensional score plots showing clear differences between the different samples. It is noteworthy that PC1 and PC2 covered more than 90 % of the total variability. Data for α-asarone and β-asarone were found to be distinct from those of the main cluster profiles of the ATR, AGR, ACR and AAR extracts. The scatter points showed that the samples could be readily classified into four different groups, indicating that it was possible to differentiate between the different plants. The α-asarone and β-asarone contents of the different extracts could therefore be used to discriminate ATR from AGR, ACR and AAR (Fig. 4b). Hierarchical clustering analysis (HCA) was also applied to differentiate between the different extracts using Pearson's correlation as a measurement (Fig. 4c). In a similar manner to the PCA results, HCA allowed for most of the samples to be classified into two groups, including cluster 1 [samples 1–4 (ATR)] and cluster 2 [samples 5–16 (AGR, ACR and AAR)]. This clustering agreed well with the results of ATR and non-ATR samples. Taken together, these results suggest that ATR can be readily differentiated from the other three *Acorus* species based on differences in their asarone contents. PCA and HCA allowed for the different species to be partially distinguished by visual inspection for conventional quality control purposes.

DNA analysis by ITS sequence

Genomic DNA was isolated from the 16 different samples. The yields for the DNA extraction process were in the range of 50–300 ng of DNA from 50 mg of ATR,

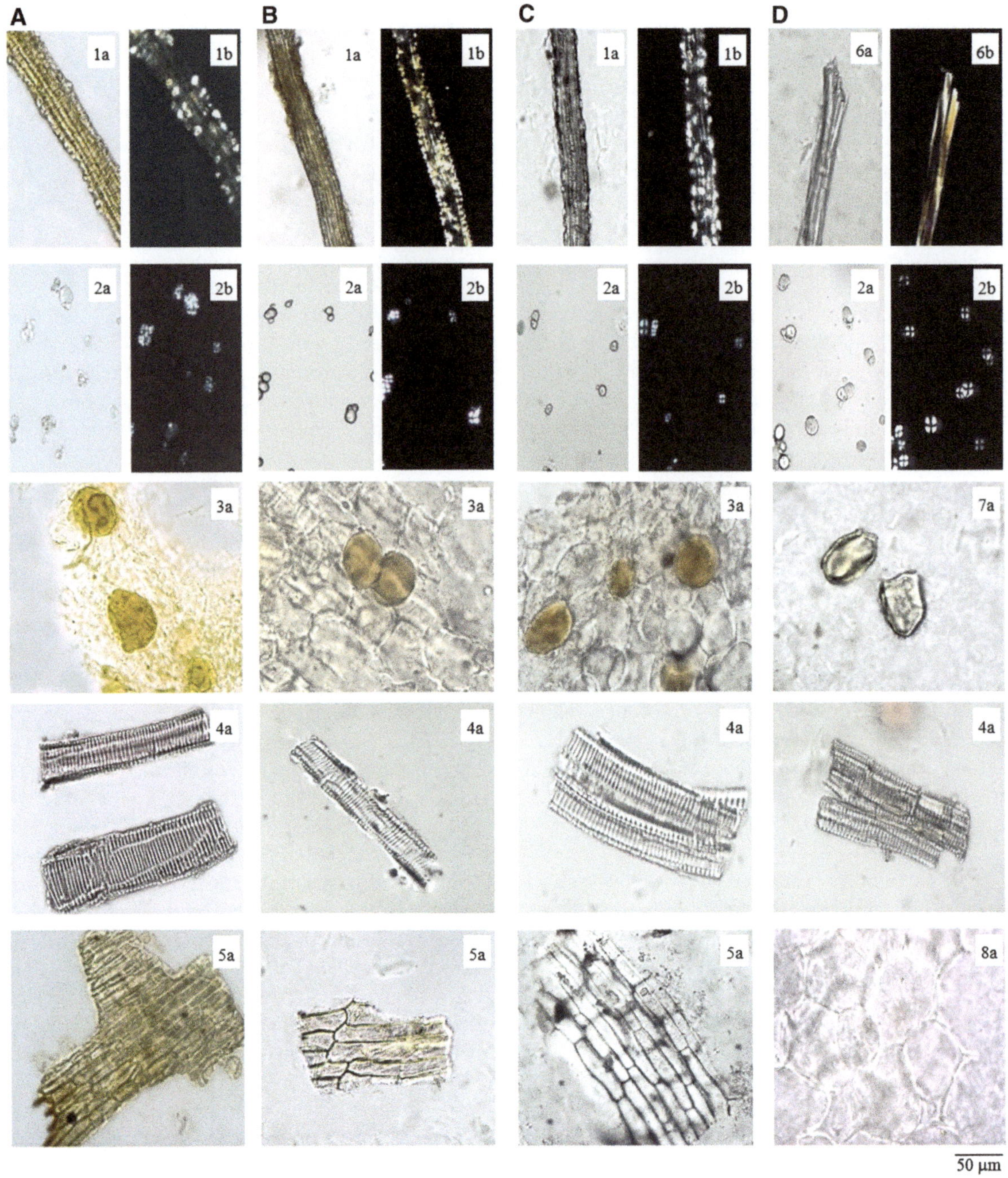

Fig. 3 Micrographs show powders of ATR and its adulterants. **A** *ATR* Acori Tatarinowii Rhizoma; **B** *AGR* Acori Graminei Rhizoma; **C** *ACR* Acori Calami Rhizoma; **D** *AAR* Anemones Altaicae Rhizoma. Notations are: *1* crystal fibers; *2* starch granules; *3* secretory cells; *4* vessels; *5* epidermal cells of leaf sheath; *6* fibers; *7* stone cell; *8* parenchymatous cell. *a* Indicated features under the light microscope; *b* Indicate features under the polarized microscope

AGR, ACR and AAR. Two flanking primers, ITS-S and ITS-AS, were used for the PCR experiments to allow for the identification of the ITS sequences. About 850 base pair were amplified and sequenced in each case (Fig. 5a). The results of the nucleotide sequence analysis experiments (Additional file 1), including the complete ITS1, ITS2 and 5.8S rRNA regions, revealed that the ITS sequences of these samples were highly homologous, regardless of their geographical origins. The ITS sequences of the 16 samples evaluated in the

Table 2 Summary of the macroscopic and microscopic features of ATR, AGR, ACR and AAR

	ATR	AGR	ACR	AAR
Morphology				
Shape	Flattish-cylindrical		Cylindrical	Fusiform
Length (cm)	3–15	1–4	5–20	1–4
Diameter (mm)	3–10	2–7	10–15	3–5
Fracture	Fibrous, numerous dotted vascular bundles and brown oil spots visible		Fibrous, numerous dotted vascular bundles visible	Granular protuberances, starchy
Odor	Aromatic; taste bitter and slightly pungent		Strong aromatic and taste pungent	Slight; taste slightly sour and numbness
Transverse section				
1. Epidermis	Sub-square brown cells			Flat square cells
2. Cortex	3. Fiber bundles, 4. Secretory cells and 5. Leaf-trace vascular bundle are scattered			3. Fiber bundles arrange in ring, 8. Stone cells, suborbicular, scattered
	Small intercellular spaces		Large intercellular spaces	
7. Stele vascular bundle	Amphivasal or collateral, densely lined up near the 6. Endodermis			N/A
9. Pith	N/A			Large
Powder				
1. Crystal fibers	Fiber bundles surrounded by cells containing prisms of calcium oxalate, forming crystal fibers			6. Fibers, not crystal fiber
2. Starch granules	Ellipsoid, spheroidal or long-ovoid, black and cruciate-shaped under the polarized microscope			
3. Secretory cells	Abundant, sub-rounded or elongated-rounded			N/A
4. Vessels	Mainly reticulate			
5. Epidermal cells of leaf sheath	Greyish-green or pale yellowish-brown, rectangular			N/A
7. Stone cells	N/A			Abundant
8. Parenchymatous cells	Less			Abundant

The number is referred to the notations in Fig. 2 (transverse section) and Fig. 3 (powder section)

current study were obtained and subjected to phylogenetic analysis using the maximum parsimony method (Fig. 5b). Two major clades were formed, with distance values ranging from 0.572 to 0.605. *A. calamus* formed a sub-clade by itself, whilst another taxon was formed that further divided into two sub-clades representing *A. tatarinowii* and *A. gramineus*. These results therefore demonstrate that the rRNA ITS region can be used to authenticate *Acorus* species.

Discussion

Substitutes and adulterants of CM could be introduced intentionally or accidentally, not only seriously attenuating therapeutic effects of these materials but also leading to poisoning. The development of an accurate method for the authentication of CM is therefore essential [17]. In this study, ATR and its adulterants were investigated using several promising methods, including macroscopic and microscopic examination, chemical analysis and DNA authentication. The results of the microscopic identification process revealed that AAR could be readily distinguished from the other species by the lack of crystal fibers (specific features of *Acorus* species) in AAR. Moreover, stone cells were only observed in AAR and not in the ATR, AGR or ACR. Morphological identification processes require botanical expertise for the unequivocal authentication of different plant samples because of similarities in the morphological features of related species [18]. Chemical analysis is a commonly used technique for rapid separation, identification and quantification of the chemical components of herbal materials. In this study, the peaks corresponding to α-asarone and β-asarone were used to differentiate between ATR, AGR and ACR, but not AAR. Furthermore, PCA and HCA provided partial visual differentiation according to their species based on these two chemicals.

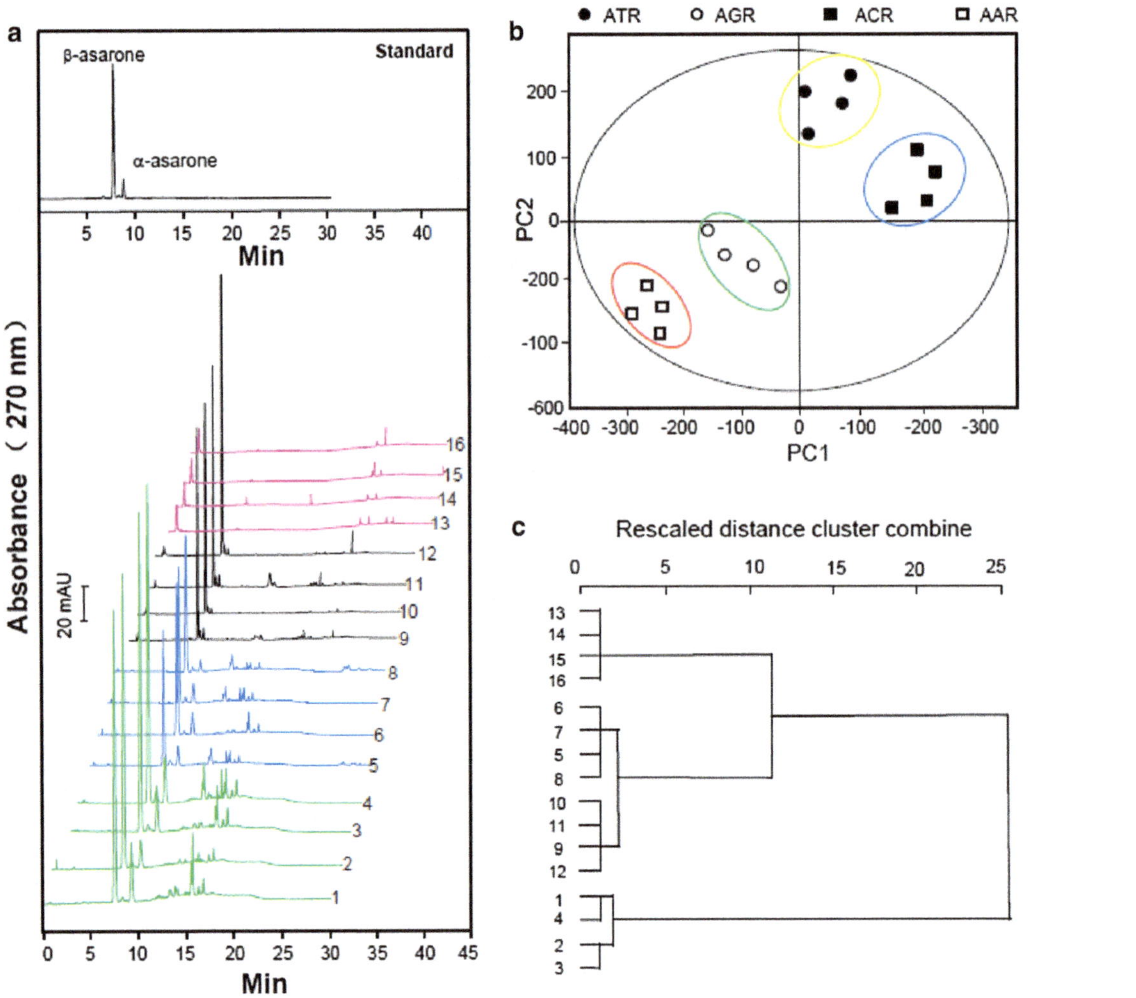

Fig. 4 UHPLC-DAD chromatograms of extracts from ATR and its adulterants. **a** UHPLC-DAD chromatograms of 16 samples (number 1–16 for different samples, shown in Table 1) at 270 nm were shown. *Upper panel* shows the *markers*, α-asarone and β-asarone. **b** Score plots for ATR and its adulterants, using peak areas of α-asarone and β-asarone as input data, were shown. **c** Hierarchical clustering analysis for the 16 samples. The loading plot was performed with the original peak areas of α-asarone and β-asarone as input data

Macroscopic and microscopic methods are labor intensive, whereas chemical fingerprinting techniques can be adversely affected by external factors. In contrast, genetic tools were more reliable and less demanding in sample amounts and external factors for the authentication of herbal materials at the DNA level. Various DNA-based molecular markers have been developed for the authentication of herbal medicines with an increasing number of applications in recent years [19–24]. ITS was used in the current study as a DNA marker to authenticate the *Acorus* species that were indistinguishable by neither morphological features nor phytochemical compositions. DNA authentication only requires a small amount of sample, exhibits high levels of stability and is largely unaffected by external factors.

This study showed that quality control for the *Acorus* species which was mainly dependent on qualitative characteristics (i.e., morphological authentication, chemical fingerprinting and genetic sequencing) could be used to generate quantitative hypotheses. The combination of quantitative and qualitative methods described in this study provided a new approach to enhancing the research in CM.

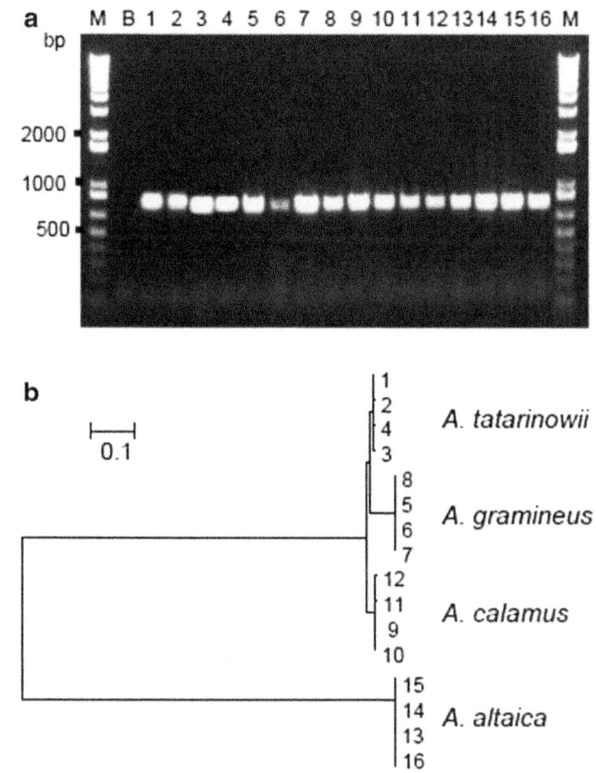

Fig. 5 ITS sequence of ATR and its adulterants. **a** Amplicons of ATR and its adulterants with ITS primers. **b** Blank (nuclease-free distilled water); *Lane* 1–4: ATR; *Lane* 5–8: AGR; *Lane* 9–12: ACR; *Lane* 12–16: AAR. All samples produced a band at ~850 bp, $n = 4$. **b** The ITS sequences were identified and matched fully from sequences of GenBank, i.e., *A. tatarinowii* (DQ008851), *A. gramineus* (DQ008849), *A. calamus* (DQ008853) and *A. altaica* (this study). DNA sequences of ITS fragment from 16 samples were submitted to phylogenetic study by Maximum Parsimony method. Two major clades were remarked. The distance corresponding to sequence divergence is indicated by the *bar*

Conclusion

DNA authentication exhibited higher resolution power and reliability than conventional morphological identification and UHPLC in differentiating between different *Acorus* species.

Abbreviations

ATR: Acori Tatarinowii Rhizoma; AGR: Acori Graminei Rhizoma; ACR: Acori Calami Rhizoma; AAR: Anemones Altaicae Rhizoma; CM: Chinese medicine; DAD: diode-array detector; HCA: hierarchical clustering analysis; ITS: internal transcribed spacer; PCA: principal component analysis; UHPLC: ultra high performance liquid chromatography.

Authors' contributions

TTXD and KWKT designed the study. HYW, PY and HQL collected the herbs. KYCL carried out the macroscopic and microscopic identification. CFK and HJZ performed the UPLC fingerprinting. KYCL and GKLC performed the ITS sequencing. KYCL and CFK wrote the manuscript. All authors read and approved the final manuscript.

Author details

[1] Division of Life Science, and Center for Chinese Medicine, The Hong Kong University of Science and Technology, Clear Water Bay Road, Hong Kong, China. [2] School of Chinese Medicine, Hong Kong Baptist University, Hong Kong, China. [3] HKUST Shenzhen Research Institute, Hi-Tech Park, Nanshan, Shenzhen, Guangdong Province, China.

Acknowledgements

Supported by Hong Kong Research Grants Council Theme-based Research Scheme (T13-607/12R), ITF (UIM/254), GRF (661110, 662911, 660411, 663012, 662713, M-HKUST604/13), TUYF12SC02, TUYF12SC03, TUYF15SC01, The Hong Kong Jockey Club Charities Trust (HKJCCT12SC01) and Foundation of The Awareness of Nature (TAON12SC01) to Karl Tsim, Shen Zhen Science and Technology Innovation (JCYJ20160229205726699, JCYJ20160229205812004, JCYJ20160229210027564). Kelly Yin-Ching LAM holds a Lee's Pharmaceutical-Kanya Kee Postgraduate Scholarship.

Competing interests

The authors declare that they have no competing interests.

References

1. Chinese Herbs Editor Board. Chinese herbs, vol. 8. Shanghai: Science and Technology Press; 1999.
2. Chinese Pharmacopoeia Commission. Pharmacopeia of the People's Republic of China. Beijing: China Medical Science and Technology Press; 2015.
3. Commission of Korea Food and Drug Administration. The Korean pharmacopoeia. Seoul: Yakup Daily; 2012.
4. Indian Pharmacopoeia Commission. Indian pharmacopoeia. Ghaziabad: National Institute of Science Communication and Information Resources; 2007.
5. Si MM, Lou JS, Zhou CX, Shen JN. Insulin releasing and alpha glucosidase inhibitory activity of ethyl acetate fraction of *Acorus calamus* in vitro and in vivo. J Ethnopharmacol. 2010;128:154–9.
6. Man J, Cai J, Cai C, Huai H, Wei C. Physicochemical properties of rhizome starch from a traditional Chinese medicinal plant of Anemone altaica. Carbohydr Polym. 2012;89(2):571–7.
7. Wu ZY, Peter HR, Co-Chairs of the Editorial Committee. Flora of China, vol. 23. Beijing, St. Louis: Science Press, Missouri Botanical Garden; 2000.
8. The State Administration of Traditional Chinese Medicine of Chinese Materia Medica Editorial Board. Chinese materia medica. Shanghai: Shanghai Science and Technology Publisher; 2004.
9. Zhao ZZ, Liang ZT, Guo P. Macroscopic identification of Chinese medicinal materials: traditional experiences and modern understanding. J Ethnopharmacol. 2011;134:556–64.
10. Ruzin SE. Plant microtechnique and microscopy. New York, Oxford: Oxford University Press; 1999.
11. Zhao KJ, Dong TT, Tu PF, Song ZH, Lo CK, Tsim KW. Molecular genetic and chemical assessment of radix Angelica (Danggui) in China. J Agric Food Chem. 2003;51:2576–83.
12. Lam KY, Chan GK, Xin GZ, Xu H, Ku CF, Chen JP, et al. Authentication of *Cordyceps sinensis* by DNA analyses: comparison of ITS sequence analysis and RAPD-derived molecular markers. Molecules. 2015;20:22454–62.
13. Wei G, Chen YB, Chen DF, Lai XP, Liu DH, Deng RD, et al. Beta-asarone inhibits neuronal apoptosis via the CaMKII/CREB/Bcl-2 signaling

pathway in an in vitro model and AβPP/PS1 mice. J Alzheimers Dis. 2012;33:863–80.
14. Yang YX, Chen YT, Zhou XJ, Hong CL, Li CY, Guo JY. Beta-asarone, a major component of *Acorus tatarinowii* Schott, attenuates focal cerebral ischemia induced by middle cerebral artery occlusion in rats. BMC Complement Altern Med. 2013;13:236.
15. Shi HX, Yang J, Yang T, Xue YL, Liu J, Li YJ, et al. Alpha-asarone protects endothelial cells from injury by angiotensin II. Evid Based Complement Alternat Med. 2014;2014:682041.
16. Kim BW, Koppula S, Kumar H, Park JY, Kim IW, More SV, et al. Alpha-asarone attenuates microglia-mediated neuroinflammation by inhibiting NF kappa B activation and mitigates MPTP-induced behavioral deficits in a mouse model of Parkinson's disease. Neuropharmacology. 2015;97:46–57.
17. Zhao Z, Hu Y, Liang Z, Yuen J, Jiang Z, Leung KSY. Authentication is fundamental for standardization of Chinese medicines. Planta Med. 2006;72:865–74.
18. Zhao ZZ, Yuen JPS, Wu J, Yu T, Huang W, Zhao ZZ, et al. Easily confused Chinese medicines in Hong Kong. Ann Acad Med. 2007;35(11):764–9.
19. Marieschi M, Torelli A, Bruni R. Quality control of saffron (*Crocus sativus* L.): development of SCAR markers for the detection of plant adulterants used as bulking agents. J Agric Food Chem. 2012;60:10998–1004.
20. Cui XM, Lo CK, Yip KL, Dong TT, Tsim KW. Authentication of *Panax notoginseng* by 5S-rRNA spacer domain and random amplified polymorphic DNA (RAPD) analysis. Planta Med. 2003;69:584–6.
21. Xin GZ, Lam YC, Maiwulanjiang M, Chan GK, Zhu KY, Tang WL, et al. Authentication of bulbus fritillariae cirrhosae by RAPD-derived DNA markers. Molecules. 2014;19:3450–9.
22. Chen S, Pang X, Song J, Shi L, Yao H, Han J, et al. A renaissance in herbal medicine identification: from morphology to DNA. Biotechnol Adv. 2014;32(7):1237–44.
23. Ma XC, Xie CX, Guan M, Xu XH, Miki E, Takeda O, et al. High levels of genetic diversity within one population of *Rheum tanguticum* on the Qinghai-Tibet Plateau have implications for germplasm conservation. Pharmaceut Crops. 2014;5:1–8.
24. Xin T, Li XJ, Yao H, Lin YL, Ma XC, Cheng RY, et al. Survey of commercial Rhodiola products revealed species diversity and potential safety issues. Sci Rep. 2015;5:8337.

3

Validation of the *qi blood yin yang deficiency* questionnaire on chronic fatigue

Jihye Kim, Boncho Ku and Keun Ho Kim*

Abstract

Background: Chronic fatigue (CF) reflects an imbalance of inter-organ functions or of the four essential physiological components *qi*, *blood* (*xue*), *yin*, and *yang*. CF can be subdivided into different patterns. However, there are no diagnostic methods for CF. This study aimed to clinically validate a pattern identification method by identifying correlations between CF and responses to the *qi blood yin yang deficiency* questionnaire (QBYY-Q).

Methods: Participants were recruited between May and June 2014 through the Kyung Hee University Korean Medicine hospital website and via posters and comprised 129 CF patients diagnosed with the United States Centers for Disease Control and Prevention (1994) criteria. Participants who had organic diseases that explained the CF were excluded. A total of 159 participants were asked to complete the QBYY-Q, the fatigue severity scale, and the Chalder fatigue scale. The latter two questionnaires were used to assess convergent validity with the QBYY-Q. Among the 129 CF participants, 70 and 59 had chronic fatigue syndrome and idiopathic chronic fatigue, respectively. Two Korean medical doctors independently assessed participants' *qi*, *blood*, *yin*, and *yang deficiency* patterns using QBYY deficiency pattern identification guidelines. Based on the results of a preliminary study of the QBYY-Q, we selected 32 reliable items for symptoms corresponding to each *deficiency* pattern. The items were used to estimate internal consistency and construct validity. Multinomial logistic regression analysis was performed for scores on each *deficiency* pattern.

Results: The data were means and standard deviations or numbers of participants and proportions for continuous and categorical variables, respectively. A statistical significance level of $P < 0.05$ was assumed. The QBYY-Q showed satisfactory internal consistency. Explanatory factor analysis extracted two factors for each *deficiency* pattern. The percentages of explained variance for *qi*, *blood*, *yin*, and *yang deficiency* were 45.1, 58.0, 52.2, and 63.4 %, respectively. Each QBYY-Q deficiency score was positively associated with each corresponding *deficiency* pattern. *Qi deficiency* was used as a reference category. Odds ratios of *blood*, *yin*, and *yang deficiency* were 10.97, 10.69, and 14.64, respectively.

Conclusion: The QBYY-Q was suitable for estimating the influences of *qi*, *blood*, *yin*, and *yang deficiencies* in CF.

Trial registration This trial was registered with the Korean Clinical Trial Register (KCT0001199)

Keywords: Pattern identification, Deficiency pattern, Questionnaire, *Qi blood yin yang deficiencies*, Chronic fatigue

Background

Fatigue is a state of subjective tiredness and can be subdivided into prolonged fatigue and chronic fatigue (CF). CF is a condition of subjective tiredness and is reported by nearly 10 % of the global population [1]; it can be categorized as either explained CF or unexplained CF. Unexplained CF is further subdivided into chronic fatigue syndrome (CFS) and idiopathic chronic fatigue (ICF) [2]. CFS is characterized by severe disabling fatigue and a combination of four additional symptoms that may include impairments in cognitive or neurological function, sleep dysfunction, musculoskeletal pain, and endocrine or immune dysfunction (Table 1). Additionally, alternative medical and psychiatric causes must have been excluded, and the condition must have persisted

*Correspondence: rkim70@kiom.re.kr
KM Fundamental Research Division, Korea Institute of Oriental Medicine, 1672 Yuseongdae-ro, Yuseong-gu, Daejeon 34054, Republic of Korea

Table 1 Diagnosis CDC-1994 criteria

Chronic fatigue syndrome symptoms
A. Major criteria (both criteria required)
1. Severe fatigue >6 months
a. Persistent or relapsing in course
b. Does not resolve with bed rest
c. Significant reduction in average daily activity (below 50 % of prior activity)
2. Other causes excluded
a. See fatigue causes
B. Minor criteria (4 or more present for 6 months)
1. Headache
a. New type, severity or pattern
b. Typically non-focal headache
2. Migratory polyarthralgias
a. Non-inflammatory (no swelling or erythema)
3. Myalgias
4. Postexertional malaise or fatigue
a. Duration >24 h
5. Short-term memory or concentration impaired
6. Pharyngitis
7. Tender cervical or axillary adenopathy
8. Non-restorative sleep

for at least 6 months. ICF meets all the criteria for CFS except for the four additional symptoms.

Studies of CFS and ICF indicate prevalence rates of approximately 10 and 1 % of the general population, respectively [3]. The estimated prevalence of CF in the Republic of Korea is between 0.6 and 2 % of the general adult population [4]. Several hypotheses have been proposed for the pathogenesis of CF, including oxidative stress, hypothalamic–pituitary–adrenal axis abnormalities, and immune dysfunction [5–7]. Western medicine offers no objective diagnostic methods or effective therapies for CF and the recommended drugs have many side effects [8–11]. CFS and ICF patients tend to be interested in complementary and alternative medicine treatments [9, 12, 13].

An individual's constitution and current health status can be conceptualized in terms of the balance between the *qi* and *blood* (*xue*) conditions of the internal organ functions and of the co-existing *yin* and *yang* (which constitute the physical form and functioning of the human body and its deficient and excessive energetic qualities) [9, 14, 15]. Treatments such as acupuncture, moxibustion, herbal medicine, and qigong restore the balance of the four essential components of the human body: *qi, blood, yin,* and *yang.*

Unexplained CF can be classified as either a *deficiency* syndrome or an *excess* syndrome; these syndromes refer to the *deficiency* or excess of *qi, blood, yin,* and *yang* [16, 17]. Unexplained CF is usually considered a *deficiency* pattern representing an imbalance of the four essential components; most cases are treated by invigorating *qi* and *yang* and nourishing *blood* and *yin* [9, 18, 19]. CF treatments are based on individual patterns of body constitution or pattern identification (PI); most patients are diagnosed according to four patterns of body constitution that involve the five major organs: the heart, liver, spleen, lungs, and kidney. These patterns are *qi deficiency* (QD, i.e., decreases in visceral functions and body resistance), *blood deficiency* (BD, i.e., failure to nourish the organs, tissues, and meridians), *yin deficiency* and *yang deficiency* (YnD and YgD, i.e., failure to maintain normal function of internal organs) [9, 11, 18].

This study aimed to clinically validate a PI diagnostic method by testing for correlations between CF and responses to the *qi blood yin yang deficiency* questionnaire (QBYY-Q).

Methods

Ethics

The study protocol was reviewed and approved by the Institutional Review Board of the Cheonan Oriental Hospital at Daejeon University (authorization number: 2014-A01-02) and was registered with the clinical research information service (registration number: KCT0001199) (Additional file 1).

Study design

This study was designed as a single-center, cross-sectional, case-controlled study, and it was performed at the Cheonan Oriental Hospital of Daejeon University in Cheonan, South Korea from May to June 2014. The procedures of this study were depicted in Fig. 1.

Participants

Participants were recruited by advertising on hospital websites and posters displayed in hospitals and local universities, Seoul, Republic of Korea from May to June 2014. They went through telephone pre-screening by the clinical study coordinator to ensure that CF patients met the inclusion criteria of "males and females aged 19–39" and "the presence of CF that is continuous and repetitive for more than 6 months". Then, participants visited the clinical study center and go through a more in-depth screening process to determine whether they satisfied the inclusion criteria.

Participants who worked at night or drank alcohol more than twice per week were excluded. We excluded the participants who had organic diseases for explained CF, such as acute or chronic liver disease (e.g., hepatitis, and liver cirrhosis); anemia; tuberculosis; chronic lung

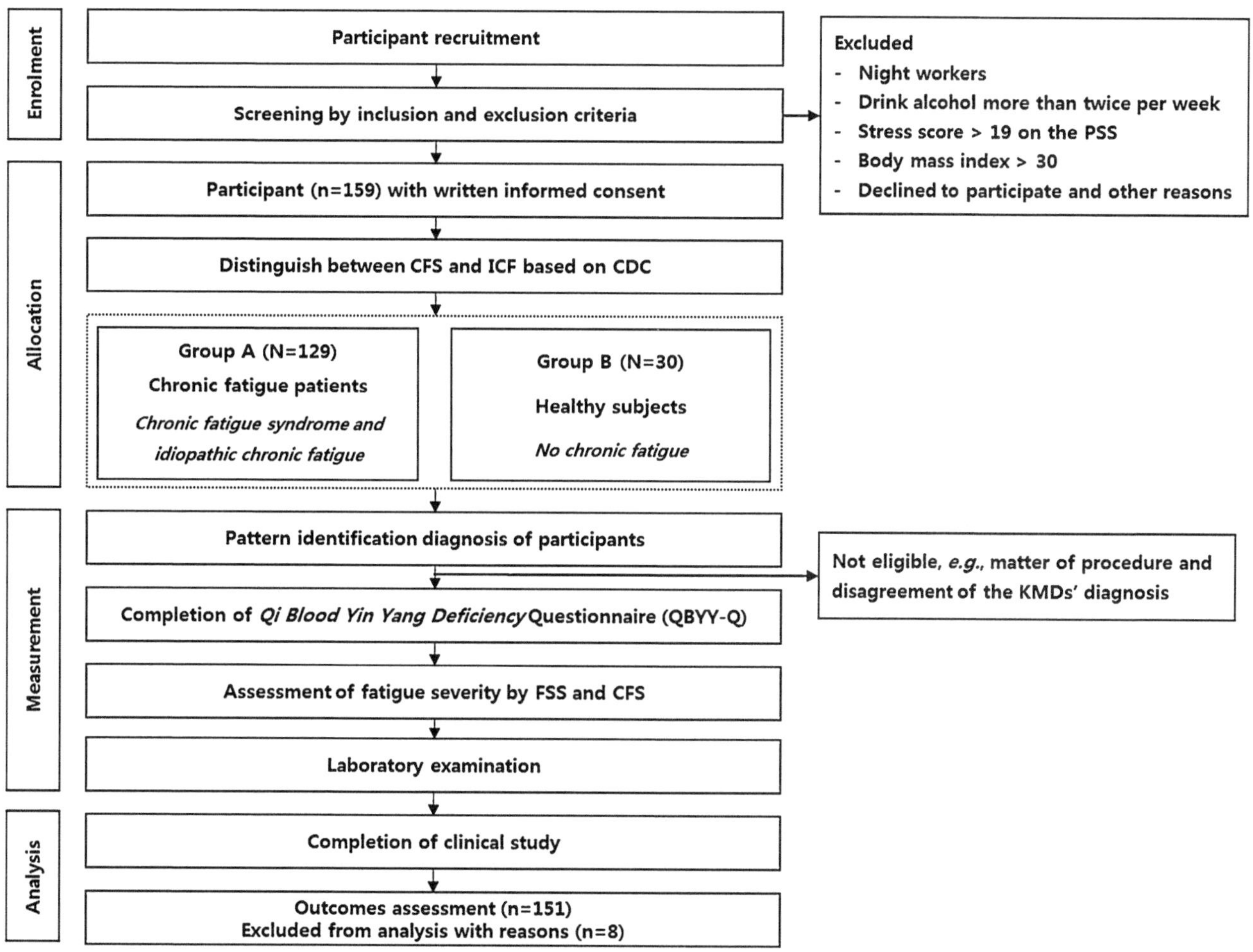

Fig. 1 Flow diagram of the procedures of the clinical study

disease; cardiovascular disease (e.g., heart failure, hypertension); endocrine/metabolic disease (e.g., diabetes, thyroid gland disease, and severe obesity); autoimmune disease (e.g., rheumatoid arthritis, systemic lupus erythematosus, and multiple sclerosis); malignant tumors; or infectious disease were excluded. In addition, CF patients with psycho-social diseases, such as depression, anxiety neurosis, recent severe stress, schizophrenia, alcoholism, or an eating disorder (e.g., anorexia nervosa, bulimia nervosa), were excluded [12, 13]. Cut-offs of BMI ($\geq$30 kg/m^2) have shown good specificity in diagnosing severe obesity, which is defined as BMI $\geq$30 kg/m^2 based on measured weight and height and is a type of metabolic disease [20, 21]. The participants were informed of the entire process of the clinical study and were asked to sign informed consent forms (Additional file 2).

The final participants included 129 patients with unexplained CF and 30 controls. The enrolled patients mainly suffered from fatigue lasting more than 6 months. The CDC-1994 criteria for CFS [22] were used to distinguish between CFS and ICF, using the cutoff of 4 among the 8 symptoms in the minor criteria, respectively (Table 1). CFS patients complained of major criteria symptoms and more than four of the minor criteria symptoms, and ICF patients complained of major criteria symptoms and less than four of the minor criteria symptoms. If a subject complained of fatigue lasting more than 6 months, headache and pharyngitis, the subject was diagnosed as ICF. Among the attending 129 CF patients, 70 and 59 were found to have CFS and ICF, respectively.

The control (30 healthy participants) came to the same clinic who worked at night and drank alcohol were excluded. The control group consisted of participants who satisfied the following criteria: (1) not meeting the CFS and ICF criteria from CDC-1994; (2) absence of organopathy; and (3) normal results of laboratory tests and radiological examinations.

Of the 159 participants, two participants were excluded due to noncompliance with the process described in the protocol; therefore, 157 participants were included in this study.

Pattern diagnosis

There is no "gold standard" for pattern diagnosis. Our previous study demonstrated discrepancies in the diagnoses of QD, BD, YnD, and YgD among Korean medical doctors (KMDs) [23]. To increase the internal consistency of KMD expert pattern diagnosis, we created PI guidelines for QD, BD, YnD, and YgD with PI experts, using data from previous studies [9, 24] and the standard Korean medical literature [22] 4 months before the study commenced. The developed PI guidelines were validated after consultation with experts. Based on the PI guidelines, two KMDs with 4 years of clinical experience independently diagnosed the participants' *deficiency* status; the KMDs were blinded to the results of the diagnoses. Participants for whom the KMD diagnoses disagreed were excluded from the analysis.

Measurements

QBYY-Q scales

In our previous studies, items related to QD, YnD, YgD, and BD were systematically reviewed [9, 25–27], and a QBYY-Q constructed by a panel of experts was selected for use in a pilot study. This QBYY-Q had been established by an expert panel of 27 KMDs in a previous study [28]. A pilot study was performed to determine the reliability and validity of the QBYY-Q for 100 participants with CF [23]. After these participants completed the QBYY-Q, the KMDs divided the patients into four groups: QD, BD, YnD, and YgD. After 3 weeks, the 100 participants were retested in the same way. The results from our pilot study showed that Cronbach's α coefficient was 0.916 for internal consistency of the QBYY-Q. Construct validity analyzed using exploratory factor analysis (EFA) produced four factors with eigenvalues greater than 1.0. Factors 1, 2, 3, and 4 were identified as QD, YnD, YgD, and BD, respectively. However, four items, "menstrual cycle slowdown," "decreased masculine energy," "damp and cold penis," and "decreased sexual desire," produced an item-total correlation of less than 0.5. Because the results indicated that the four items were not equivalent to the others, these items were excluded from the validity tests. Test–retest reliability was high (intraclass correlation coefficient = 0.699) [23]. Consequently, the final version of the QBYY-Q included 32 sign and symptom entries consisting of nine QD, eight BD, nine YnD, and six YgD pattern items. The order of the 32 QBYY-Q pattern items was reversed to reduce bias (Additional file 3). The QD pattern included two signs, enervation and shortage of *qi* or faint breathing, and the BD pattern included three signs, pale complexion, sweating during the day, and palpitations (a subjective sensation of rapid and forceful beating of the heart). The YnD pattern was divided into following two signs: (1) dry skin and mouth; and (2) heat vexation and fever accompanied by uneasiness or restlessness. The YgD pattern was divided into two signs, cold in the extremities up to the knees and elbows and diarrhea. The severity of each item was graded using the following 4-point scale: 1 = strongly disagree, 2 = disagree, 3 = agree, and 4 = strongly agree. The scores for each item were totaled, and QD-Q, BD-Q, YnD-Q, and YgD-Q scores calculated.

Fatigue severity scale (FSS)

The FSS is a self-rating questionnaire comprising nine items that are scored between 1 (completely disagree) and 7 (completely agree). The items assess the extent of fatigue symptoms and their impact on patient functioning (including motivation; exercise; physical functioning; ability to perform duties; and interference with work, family, or social life) [29]. Example items on the questionnaire are "exercise brings on my fatigue" and "my fatigue is very debilitating"; higher item scores indicate a greater degree of fatigue.

Chalder fatigue scale–Korean version (CFS-K)

The CFS is a self-reported questionnaire that measures fatigue intensity on a 4-point scale (0 = less than usual to 3 = much more than usual) [30]. Symptoms assessed by the scale are divided into two subcategories: seven items related to physical symptoms, and four items related to mental fatigue. Although the internal consistency of the CFS-K has not been fully reported, many studies using versions of the CFS in different languages have shown strong internal consistency for both the physical and mental symptoms of fatigue. Likert scoring with weights was used to score the magnitude of fatigue [30].

Statistical analysis

The data were represented as means ± standard deviations (SDs) or as numbers of participants and proportions for continuous and categorical variables, respectively. All statistical analyses were performed using R software (The R Foundation), version 3.1.1, on a Windows 7 platform. R software is a free software environment for statistical computing and graphics [31]. The level of significance was set at $P < 0.05$ for all analyses. Inter-rater agreement for the two KMDs' diagnoses of QD, BD, YnD, and YgD was evaluated using Cohen's κ coefficient. Differences between CF patients (CFS and ICF) and the non-CF group were tested using a one-way ANOVA for continuous variables and Pearson's Chi square test for categorical variables. The Keiser–Meyer–Olkin (KMO) test was used to test sample adequacy (considered acceptable if the KMO constant is >0.60) [32]. The KMO was used to check the matrix of correlations for the applicability of factorial analysis, and then a principal axis factoring extraction method was applied. Construct validity for each *deficiency* scale on the questionnaire was estimated by performing EFA with a combination of minimum residual extraction and promax rotation. For each *deficiency* scale, conceptual factors were identified by examining the factor loadings. The internal consistency of each *deficiency* scale was also tested using Cronbach's α coefficient. Convergent validity of *deficiency* scores derived from the four QBYY-Q scales and the total scores on the CFS-K and FSS was assessed using Spearman's correlation coefficient. The mean differences in *deficiency* scores between the CF and non-CF groups were examined using a one-way ANOVA test. In addition, binary logistic regression analysis was used to estimate the odds ratios (ORs) of CF (CFS + ICF versus no CF) in the KMD diagnoses of QD, BD, YnD, and YgD to confirm the associations between CF and PI. Both CF and PI could have been influenced by other confounding factors; therefore, age and sex were included to estimate the adjusted ORs for CF. Discriminative validity was determined using the ORs of the four *deficiency* scale scores derived from a multinomial logistic regression model.

Results

Demographic characteristics

Because of the absence of a gold standard for pattern diagnosis, six of the 157 participants showed discrepancies in pattern diagnoses and were excluded to increase the internal consistency. Therefore, 151 participants were included in the analysis. Table 2 shows the demographic characteristics of the 65 participants with CFS, the 56 participants with ICF, and the 30 control subjects in the non-CF group. For most of the characteristics, there were no significant differences among the CF groups (CFS and ICF) and the control group. However, the age and sex distributions showed significant differences among the three groups. The means and SDs for age were 29.7 ± 4.9 years for participants with CFS, 27.4 ± 5.2 years for participants with ICF, and 26.0 ± 3.7 years for the control group ($F = 7.09$, $P = 0.001$). The proportions of women in the CFS, ICF, and control groups were 64.6, 35.7, and 50.0 %, respectively ($\chi^2 = 10.07$, $P = 0.007$).

Table 2 Demographic characteristics of participants with CF (CFS and ICF) and controls

	Chronic fatigue		Controls (n = 30)	*P* value
	CFS (n = 6 5)	ICF (n = 56)		
Age (years)	29.7 ± 4.9	27.4 ± 5.2	26.0 ± 3.7	0.001
Sex (female)	42 (64.6)	20 (35.7)	15 (50.0)	0.007
BMI (kg/m^2)	22.8 ± 3.5	22.3 ± 3.0	21.8 ± 3.1	0.746
SBP (mm Hg)	116.3 ± 11.0	116.8 ± 10.2	119.2 ± 12.7	0.471
DBP (mm Hg)	69.5 ± 11.1	71.8 ± 9.0	71.2 ± 12.5	0.471
Pulse rate (beats/min)	71.4 ± 8.9	70.0 ± 6.3	72.0 ± 9.5	0.482
Body temperature (°C)	36.4 ± 0.2	36.4 ± 0.2	36.4 ± 0.2	0.601
Smoking	18 (27.7)	13 (23.2)	4 (13.3)	0.305
Regular exercise	20 (30.8)	27 (48.2)	12 (40)	0.145
Regular diet	36 (55.4)	33 (58.9)	19 (63.3)	0.76
Pattern identification				
QD	16 (24.6)	13 (23.2)	14 (46.7)	0.129
BD	13 (20)	18 (32.1)	6 (20)	
YnD	16 (24.6)	14 (25)	6 (20)	
YgD	20 (30.8)	11 (19.6)	4 (13.3)	

The data are represented as the means ± SDs or as numbers of participants and proportions; N (%) for continuous and categorical variables, respectively. One-way ANOVA was performed for continuous variables and Pearson's χ^2 test for categorical variables

CFS chronic fatigue syndrome, *ICF* idiopathic chronic fatigue, *SBP* systolic blood pressure, *DBP* diastolic blood pressure, *QD qi deficiency, BD blood deficiency, YnD yin deficiency, YgD yang deficiency*

Table 3 Agreement results in the KMD diagnoses (n = 157)

KMD diagnoses		KMD #1			
		QD	BD	YnD	YgD
KMD #2	QD	43	0	0	1
	BD	1	37	1	0
	YnD	1	2	36	0
	YgD	0	0	0	35

KMD Korean medical doctor, *QD qi deficiency, BD blood deficiency, YnD yin deficiency, YgD yang deficiency*

KMD inter-rater agreement

Cohen's κ coefficient was 0.95 ($Z = 20.69$, $P < 0.001$), which indicated that the agreement between the two KMDs was sufficiently strong. The two KMDs differed in their PI diagnoses for six (3.8 %) of the 157 participants (Table 3).

Internal consistency and construct validity of the QBYY-Q

The internal consistency and construct validity of each of the QBYY-Q scales were assessed by merging the current study and pilot study data (totaling 252 cases). The Cronbach's α coefficients of the nine QD items (QD-Q), the eight BD items (BD-Q), the nine YnD items (YnD-Q), and the six YgD items (YgD-Q) were 0.816, 0.826, 0.807, and 0.717, respectively.

KMO tests of sphericity confirmed that each QBYY-Q scale contained an eligible number of items and a sufficient sample size (QD-Q = 0.856, BD-Q = 0.833, YnD-Q = 0.807, YgD-Q = 0.702). Two factors were extracted for each QBYY-Q scale following EFA with minimum residual extraction and promax rotation. The EFA results for each QBYY-Q scale are shown in Table 4.

Convergent validity of the QBYY-Q

The convergent validity of each QBYY-Q scale was assessed with the FSS and CFS-K using pairwise Spearman's correlation coefficients (Table 5). Total *deficiency* scores for the QD-Q, BD-Q, YnD-Q, and YgD-Q were calculated by averaging all the items corresponding to each *deficiency* scale. Subscores for each *deficiency* scale were also obtained by averaging the items relevant to each factor, which were identified from the EFA. The QD-Q score correlated significantly with both the FSS ($r = 0.721$, $P < 0.001$) and the CFS-K ($r = 0.645$, $P < 0.001$). The BD-Q score also correlated significantly with the FSS

Table 4 Extracted factor loadings of items for each QBYY-Q and the variance explained by two factors

PI	Item	Sub-scale	QD-Q		BD-Q		YnD-Q		YgD-Q	
			FL1	FL2	FL1	FL2	FL1	FL2	FL1	FL2
QD	QD-Q 01	Fatigue	*0.821*	−0.054						
	QD-Q 02		*0.798*	−0.087						
	QD-Q 05		*0.824*	−0.033						
	QD-Q 06		*0.444*	0.043						
	QD-Q 07		*0.367*	−0.107						
	QD-Q 09		*0.287*	0.160						
	QD-Q 03	Weakened voice	−0.147	*1.098*						
	QD-Q 04		0.231	*0.330*						
	QD-Q 08		0.171	*0.433*						
	% of variance explained		27.90	17.20						
BD	BD-Q 01	Heart pounding			*0.831*	−0.081				
	BD-Q 02				*0.865*	−0.182				
	BD-Q 03				*0.537*	0.098				
	BD-Q 08				*0.537*	0.016				
	BD-Q 04	Pale and dry body			0.112	*0.499*				
	BD-Q 05				0.090	*0.617*				
	BD-Q 06				−0.222	*0.977*				
	BD-Q 07				0.308	*0.313*				
	% of variance explained				45.30	12.70				
YnD	YnD-Q 02	Rough and dry body					*0.508*	0.145		
	YnD-Q 05						*0.712*	−0.120		
	YnD-Q 06						*0.770*	−0.102		
	YnD-Q 07						*0.689*	−0.033		
	YnD-Q 01	Body steaming					0.243	*0.267*		
	YnD-Q 03						−0.042	*0.741*		
	YnD-Q 04						0.216	*0.448*		
	YnD-Q 08						−0.154	*0.848*		
	YnD-Q 09						0.054	*0.388*		
	% of variance explained						39.60	12.60		
YgD	YgD-Q 01	Preference for warm things							*0.821*	−0.120
	YgD-Q 02								*0.560*	0.012
	YgD-Q 03								*0.692*	−0.072
	YgD-Q 04								*0.417*	0.225
	YgD-Q 05	Diarrhea							−0.146	*0.939*
	YgD-Q 06								0.052	*0.646*
	% of variance explained								41.50	21.90

The italic letters represents the largest loading between two factors

PI pattern identification, *QD qi deficiency*, *QD-Q qi deficiency* questionnaire, *BD blood deficiency*, *BD-Q blood deficiency* questionnaire, *YnD yin deficiency*, *YnD-Q yin deficiency* questionnaire, *YgD yang deficiency*, *YgD-Q yang deficiency* questionnaire, *FL* factor loading

Table 5 Pairwise Spearman's correlation coefficients of QBYY-Q scores and sub-scales of the QD-Q, BD-Q, YnD-Q and YgD-Q with the CFS-K and FSS

	CFS-K	*P* value	FSS	*P* value
QD-Q score	0.645	<0.001	0.721	<0.001
QD-Q S1: Fatigue	0.653	<0.001	0.704	<0.001
QD-Q S2: Weakened voice	0.419	<0.001	0.484	<0.001
BD-score	0.467	<0.001	0.441	<0.001
BD-Q S1: Heart pounding	0.298	<0.001	0.366	<0.001
BD-Q S2: Pale and dry body	0.481	<0.001	0.411	<0.001
YnD-score	0.485	<0.001	0.408	<0.001
YnD-Q S1: Rough and dry body	0.387	<0.001	0.252	0.0018
YnD-Q S2: Body steaming	0.411	<0.001	0.433	<0.001
YgD-score	0.291	<0.001	0.403	<0.001
YgD-Q S1: Preference for warm things	0.295	<0.001	0.384	<0.001
YgD-Q S2: Diarrhea	0.083	0.314	0.152	0.063

CFS-K Korean version of the Chalder fatigue scale, *FSS* fatigue severity scale, *QD-score qi deficiency* score, *BD-score blood deficiency* score, *YnD-score yin deficiency* score, *YgD-score yang deficiency* score

($r = 0.44$, $P < 0.001$) and the CFS-K ($r = 0.47$, $P < 0.001$). The YnD-Q score correlated significantly with the FSS ($r = 0.41$, $P < 0.001$) and the CFS-K ($r = 0.48$, $P < 0.001$). The YgD-Q score also correlated significantly with the FSS ($r = 0.40$, $P < 0.001$) and the CFS-K ($r = 0.29$, $P < 0.001$). Most of the subscales for the *deficiency* scales were significantly correlated with both the CFS-K and the FSS, with correlations ranging from 0.295 to 0.704. However, YgD-S2 was not significantly correlated with either the CFS-K ($r = 0.083$, $P = 0.314$) or the FSS ($r = 0.152$, $P = 0.063$).

Least square means of QBYY-Q scores with CF status

The least square means of each QBYY-Q scale score with CF status were acquired after multivariate adjustment for sex and age. Each marginal mean corresponding to a QBYY-Q score was estimated from the linear mixed model. The least square means of each QBYY-Q scale for the CF and the control groups are shown in Fig. 2a. The total scores for the QD-Q, BD-Q, YnD-Q, and YgD-Q for the CFS patients were 1.962, 2.038, 1.928, and 1.767, respectively, and those for the control group were 1.615, 1.554, 1.530, and 1.411, respectively. Patients with a diagnosis of CFS showed significantly higher QD, BD, and YnD, and YgD scores than those diagnosed with ICF (QD-Q score: $P < 0.001$; BD-Q score: $P = 0.001$, YnD-Q score: $P = 0.002$; YgD-Q score: $P = 0.024$) or those in the control group (QD-Q score: $P = 0.042$; BD-Q score: $P = 0.001$; YnD-Q score: $P = 0.002$; YgD-Q score: $P = 0.008$). The profiles of the mean QBYY-Q scores among the control, ICF, and CFS groups are shown in Fig. 2b. The mean difference between the QD score and YgD score was significant for both the control ($P = 0.042$) and the CFS group ($P = 0.001$). There were no significant differences among QBYY-Q scores for the ICF group.

Association between PI and CF

To analyze the association between the KMD diagnosis and CF, the ICF and CFS groups were merged into one

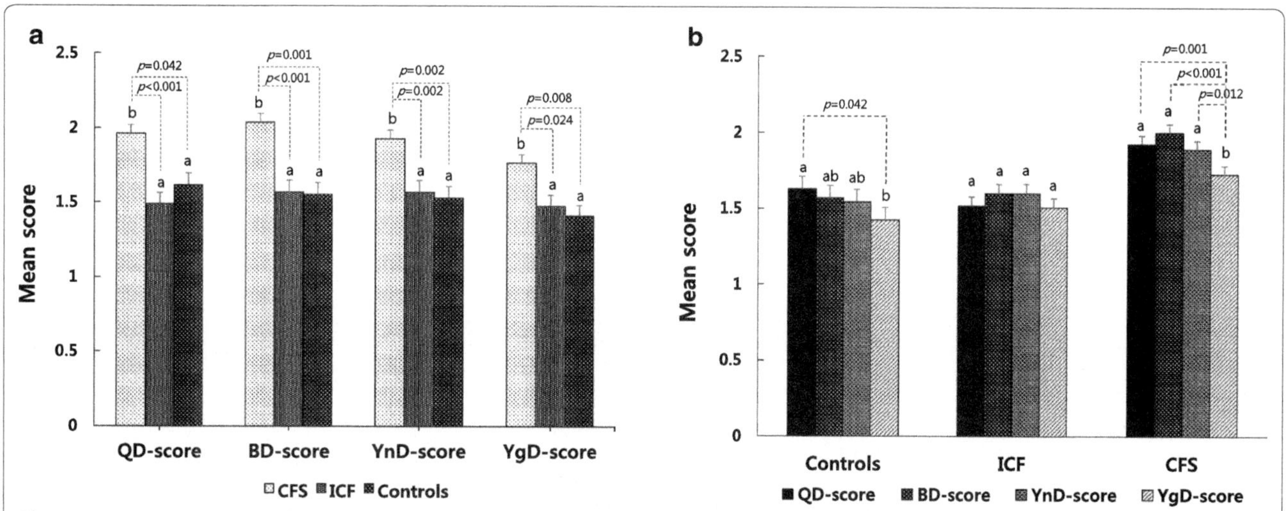

Fig. 2 Least mean square plot for QBYY-Q scores. **a** Least mean squares of each QBYY-Q score according to the control, ICF, and CFS groups; **b** Least mean squares of QBYY-Q scores among the control, ICF, and CFS groups after adjustment for sex and age. *Dotted lines* denote the significant pairwise comparisons in which the *P* value was less than 0.05. Alphabetic notations (i.e., a, ab and b) above the standard *error bars* indicate the homogeneous groups resulting from Tukey's HSD test for multiple comparisons

large CF group. Table 6 shows the crude and adjusted ORs for the association between the KMD PI diagnoses and CF, which were acquired through binomial logistic regression. The crude ORs for BD, YnD, and YgD were significantly higher than the OR for QD (2.49-, 2.41-, and 3.74-fold, respectively). The prevalence ORs of BD, YnD, and YgD in model 1 were 3.41-, 3.41-, and 4.68-fold higher, respectively, than the OR of QD. These results were statistically significant ($P < 0.05$).

Associations between PI and CFS and QBYY-Q scores

A multinomial logistic regression was used to examine associations between PI and QBYY-Q scores. The resulting values were ORs (95 % confidence intervals) with mean increments and are shown in Table 7. Using QD as a reference category for all PI scores, the BD, YnD, and YgD scale scores were positively associated with each corresponding *deficiency* pattern (adjusted ORs: BD-Q score = 5.877, YnD-Q score = 12.570, YgD-Q score = 13.558).

Table 6 Crude and adjusted odds ratios of CF by PI

PI	Crude	Model 1
QD	Reference	Reference
BD	2.49 (0.88, 7.85)	3.41 (1.10, 11.87)*
YnD	2.41 (0.85, 7.61)	3.41 (1.13, 11.48)*
YgD	3.74 (1.19, 14.40)*	4.68 (1.35, 19.65)*

Odds ratio OR (95 % confidence interval), *qi deficiency* was used as a reference category, *Model 1* adjusted for sex and age, *QD qi deficiency, BD blood deficiency, YnD yin deficiency, YgD yang deficiency, PI* pattern identification

* <0.05, ** <0.01, *** <0.001

Discussion

In this study, we aimed to clinically develop a PI questionnaire and to analyze the effectiveness of the four QBYY-Q scales as diagnostic tools for CF subtypes. We examined the correlations between CF and the QBYY-Q scales using KMD inter-rater agreement, the internal consistency and construct validity of the QBYY-Q, demographic characteristics, the convergent validity of the QBYY-Q, the least square means of the QBYY-Q scores with CF status, the associations between PIs and CF, and associations between PI and CF and QBYY-Q scores.

We compared the sociodemographic and clinical characteristics of CF patients with those of healthy subjects; however, it was difficult to delineate the clinical characteristics of CF in our study because of the small number of participants, i.e., 121 patients and 30 healthy subjects. In contrast to previous studies, the current study found no sex differences among groups, but it showed significant differences among groups for marital status and sex [33, 34].

Validation of the QBYY-Q and the Delphi methods were conducted using two different groups of clinicians, which strengthened the discriminant ability of the QBYY-Q [23, 28]. The revised QBYY-Q exhibited satisfactory internal consistency, with a Cronbach's α of 0.900 for the overall signs and symptoms, and the internal consistency of each pattern was satisfactory (0.717–0.826). The strong internal consistency reliability for each pattern suggested that the pattern constructs were homogenous or that the signs and symptoms were appropriate measures of these *deficiency* syndrome constructs.

Table 7 Associations between PI and QBYY-Q scores

		QD	BD	YnD	YgD
Crude	QD-Q score	Reference	0.05 (0.01, 0.26) ***	0.17 (0.02, 0.61) **	0.07 (0.01, 0.44) *
	BD-Q score	Reference	10.97 (2.10, 57.19) **	1.25 (0.25, 6.32)	4.99 (0.90, 27.60)
	YnD-Q score	Reference	1.32 (0.21, 8.18)	10.69 (1.72, 66.42) *	0.66 (0.10, 4.51)
	YgD-Q score	Reference	0.64 (0.17, 2.32)	0.28 (0.07, 1.13)	14.64 (3.80, 56.38) ***
Model 1	QD-Q score	Reference	0.04 (0.01, 0.24) ***	0.12 (0.02, 0.66) *	0.05 (0.01, 0.40) **
	BD-Q score	Reference	5.88 (1.04, 33.12)	1.07 (0.20, 5.79)	2.39 (0.38, 14.18)
	YnD-Q score	Reference	2.12 (0.32, 14.19)	12.57 (1.90, 83.07)**	1.22 (0.16, 9.20)
	YgD-Q score	Reference	0.53 (0.14, 2.01)	0.27 (0.07, 1.10)	13.56 (3.40, 53.99) ***

Odds ratio OR (95 % confidence interval) obtained from multinomial logistic regression, *qi deficiency* was used as a reference category, *Model 1* adjusted for sex and age, *QD qi deficiency, QD-Q qi deficiency* questionnaire, *BD blood deficiency, BD-Q blood deficiency* questionnaire, *YnD yin deficiency, YnD-Q yin deficiency* questionnaire, *YgD yang deficiency, YgD-Q yang deficiency* questionnaire, *FL* factor loading

* <0.05, ** <0.01, *** <0.001

The two QD factors were identified as weakness and shortage of *qi* or faint breathing. The two BD factors were identified as pale complexion and palpitations, i.e., a subjective sensation of rapid and forceful beating of the heart. *Yin* and *yang deficiencies* were divided into two factors each, as follows: (1) dry skin and mouth and heat vexation fever accompanied by uneasiness or restlessness for YnD and (2) and cold in the extremities up to the knees and elbows or beyond and diarrhea for YgD [35]. In summary, the QD, BD, YnD, and YgD scores might be beneficial for clarifying the characteristics of *deficiency* syndromes in clinical cases.

Convergent validity was assessed by investigating the relationships between the QBYY-Q scales and the CFS-K and FSS fatigue questionnaires. The convergent validity test showed that the QBYY-Q scales were significantly correlated with CFS-K and FSS scores ($0.29 < r < 0.72$).

Additionally, our study explored biochemical differences in the blood between the CF and control groups. The blood biochemistry and complete blood cell counts fell within the normal laboratory ranges [14, 35–37]. However, a CF diagnosis with YgD was significantly correlated with hemoglobin ($r = -0.28$) and red blood cell counts ($r = -0.29$), and a CF diagnosis with YnD was significantly correlated with chloride levels ($r = 0.28$). Statistically negative correlation coefficients of hematocrit ($r = -0.37$), hemoglobin ($r = -0.35$), red blood cells ($r = -0.32$), aspartate transaminase ($r = -0.29$), and alanine transaminase ($r = -0.28$) were observed in CF patients with BD. These data suggest that CF patients showed differences in physiological homeostasis.

YgD of the spleen and kidney is characterized by cold limbs, listlessness, cold and pain in the waist and knee joints, a pale tongue with a white coating, and a deep and thready pulse [9]. The cross-tabulation results of CF and the PIs showed that the YgD OR (4.68, CI 1.347–19.65) was significantly higher than the ORs of the other patterns (Table 6). The use of a questionnaire for *deficiency* syndromes might help to identify appropriate *qi, blood, yin,* and *yang* nourishing treatments for CF patients.

The YgD OR was significantly higher than the ORs of the other patterns (Table 7). However, the reliability of the YgD-Q ($\alpha = 0.717$) was lower than that of the other patterns, indicating that some of the YgD-Q items might not have accurately reflected the YgD pattern. In other words, the QBYY-Q did not distinguish YgD from QD because YgD simultaneously included QD. The ORs suggested that the QBYY-Q scores might be beneficial for clarifying the characteristics of *deficiency* syndromes in clinical cases.

The ORs derived from the multinomial logistic regression analysis demonstrated that each QD, BD, YnD, and YgD-Q score was positively associated with each corresponding *deficiency* pattern (adjusted ORs: qi score = 0.041, blood score = 5.877, yin score = 12.57, yang score = 13.56, reference category: QD). We constructed an algorithm for estimating the PI of a CF patient, including data on age, sex, and QBYY-Q scores, and tested its predictability (Fig. 3). We developed and validated this algorithm based on the diagnostic results and QBYY-Q scores to predict the PIs of patients with CF. To evaluate the distinction possibility of the four *deficiency* patterns, we developed and validated an algorithm based on diagnostic results and QBYY-Q scores. The algorithm was developed and validated based on bootstrap resampling (B = 500) using ordinary multinomial logistic regression (precision = 0.608) and subscales of each *deficiency* pattern questionnaire, based on EFA (precision = 0.530) [38]. The selected final model depended on the simulation results. Bootstrap validation with 500 resamples of the selected model produced moderate predictive performance, with Cox & Snell $R^2 = 0.346$, agreement = 0.523, $\kappa = 0.369$, area under the curve = 0.750, precision = 0.53, and recall = 0.535. The prevalence and severity of ICF and CFS varied according to ethnicity and psychosocial factors [39]. By validating the results, we confirmed the possibility of diagnosis using the QBYY-Q. Objective measurement of the subjective severity of fatigue is difficult, but it is essential in implementing therapy for unexplained CF [40, 41].

The study was limited by the small number of patients and the single-center design. Although CFS and ICF can be diagnosed using international guidelines, these standards are different from PI symptoms and signs, which are very difficult to standardize. However, we generated reference data that are applicable to future studies. Thus, the results of the present study could be used to improve the care of patients with CF and CF-related disorders and to facilitate research on anti-CF therapies. Large clinical trials in multiple centers on PI and the evaluation of the therapeutic effects on CF in randomized clinical trials are needed. Additional studies are required to assess the correlations between CF type and other demographic and clinical characteristics.

Conclusion

The QBYY-Q was a suitable instrument for estimating the influences of *qi, blood, yin,* and *yang deficiencies* in CF.

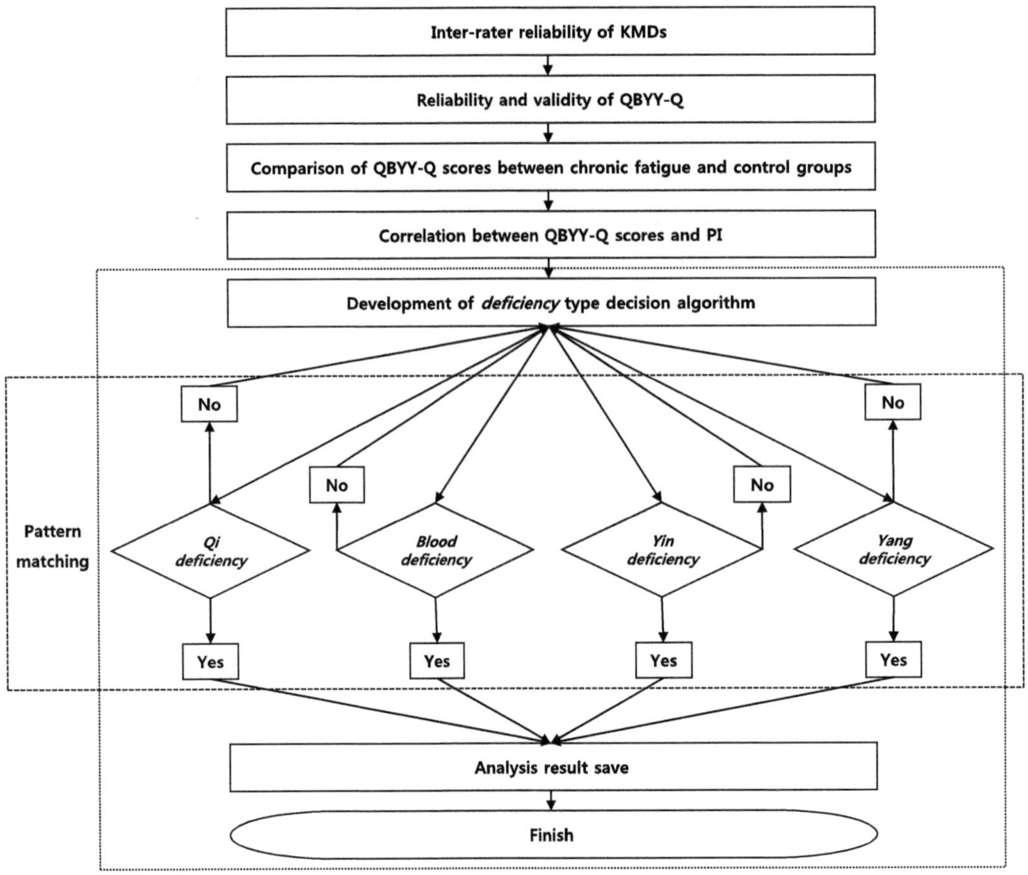

Fig. 3 Development of an algorithm for *deficiency*-type identification

Abbreviations

KM: Korean medicine; CFS: chronic fatigue syndrome; ICF: idiopathic chronic fatigue; CF: chronic fatigue; FSS: fatigue severity scale; CFS-K: Korean-translated Chalder fatigue scale; PSS: perceived stress scale; QBYY-Q: *qi blood yin yang deficiency* questionnaire; PI: pattern identification; KMD: Korean medical doctor; QD: *qi deficiency*; QD-Q: *qi deficiency* questionnaire; BD: *blood deficiency*; BD-Q: *blood deficiency* questionnaire; YnD: *yin deficiency*; YnD-Q: *yin deficiency* questionnaire; YgD: *yang deficiency*; YgD-Q: *yang deficiency* questionnaire; SBP: systolic blood pressure; DBP: diastolic blood pressure; KMO: Keiser Meyer Olkin; FL: factor loading; OR: odds ratio.

Authors' contributions

JH, BC and KH conceived and designed the clinical trials. JH and BC analyzed the data. JH wrote the manuscript. BC and KH reviewed the manuscript. All authors read and approved the final manuscript.

Acknowledgements

We thank all of the subjects who participated in this study and our colleagues. This study was supported by the Korea Institute of Oriental Medicine (K15011), Republic of Korea.

Competing interests

The authors declare that they have no competing interests.

References

1. Wong WS, Fielding R. Prevalence of chronic fatigue among Chinese adults in Hong Kong: a population-based study. J Affect Disord. 2010;127:248–56.
2. Jorgensen R. Chronic fatigue: an evolutionary concept analysis. J Adv Nurs. 2008;63:199–207.
3. Reeves WC, Jones JF, Maloney E, Heim C, Hoaglin DC, Boneva RS, Morrissey M, Devlin R. Prevalence of chronic fatigue syndrome in metropolitan, urban, and rural Georgia. Popul Health Metr. 2007;5:5.
4. Son CG. Review of the prevalence of chronic fatigue worldwide. J Korean Orien Med. 2012;33:25–33.
5. Wang YY, Li XX, Liu JP, Luo H, Ma LX, Alraek T. Traditional Chinese medicine for chronic fatigue syndrome: a systematic review of randomized clinical trials. Complem Ther Med. 2014;22:826–33.

6. Logan AC, Wong C. Chronic fatigue syndrome: oxidative stress and dietary modifications. Altern Med Rev. 2001;6:450–9.
7. Papadopoulos AS, Cleare AJ. Hypothalamic-pituitary-adrenal axis dysfunction in chronic fatigue syndrome. Nat Rev Endocrinol. 2011;8:22–32.
8. Rosenblum H, Shoenfeld Y, Amital H. The common immunogenic etiology of chronic fatigue syndrome: from infections to vaccines via adjuvants to the ASIA syndrome. Infect Dis Clin North Am. 2011;25:851–63.
9. Chen R, Moriya J, Yamakawa J, Takahashi T, Kanda T. Traditional Chinese medicine for chronic fatigue syndrome. Evid Based Complem Alternat Med. 2010;7:3–10.
10. Afari N, Buchwald D. Chronic fatigue syndrome: a review. Am J Psychiatr. 2003;160:221–36.
11. Lijue Z. Acupuncture and Chinese patent drugs for treatment of chronic fatigue syndrome. J Tradit Chin Med. 2005;25:99–101.
12. Kim JE, Hong KE, Kim HJ, Choi JB, Baek YH, Seo BK, Lee S, Kang KW, Lee MH, Kim JH, Lee S, Jung SY, Jung HJ, Shin MS, Choi SM. An open-label study of effects of acupuncture on chronic fatigue syndrome and idiopathic chronic fatigue: study protocol for a randomized controlled trial. Trials. 2013;14:147.
13. Kim JE, Seo BK, Choi JB, Kim HJ, Kim TH, Lee MH, Kang KW, Kim JH, Shin KM, Lee S, Jung SY, Kim AR, Shin MS, Jung HJ, Park HJ, Kim SP, Baek YH, Hong KE, Choi SM. Acupuncture for chronic fatigue syndrome and idiopathic chronic fatigue: a multicenter, nonblinded, randomized controlled trial. Trials. 2015;16:314.
14. Zaslawki C. Clinical reasoning in traditional Chinese medicine: implications for clinical research. Clin Acupunct Orien Med. 2003;4:94–101.
15. Jiang M, Lu C, Zhang C, Yang J, Tan Y, Lu A, Chan K. Syndrome differentiation in modern research of traditional Chinese medicine. J Ethnopharmacol. 2012;140:634–42.
16. Yiu YM, Qiu MY. A preliminary epidemiological study and discussion on traditional Chinese medicine pathogenesis of chronic fatigue syndrome in Hong Kong. Zhong Xi Yi Jie He Xue Bao. 2005;3:359–62.
17. Peng M, Ma HB, Si GM. A literature review on Chinese medicine syndrome and syndrome elements of chronic fatigue syndrome. Zhongguo Zhong Xi Yi Jie He Za Zhi. 2014;34:691–3.
18. Lee NH, Son CG. Fatigue severity of patients with idiopathic chronic fatigue compared to healthy subjects. J Tradit Chin Med. 2012;32:355–7.
19. Pacific WHO Regional Office for the Western. WHO international standard terminologies on traditional medicine in the western pacific region. Virginia: World Health Organization; 2007. p. 47–55.
20. Romero-Corral A, Somers VK, Sierra-Johnson J, Thomas RJ, Collazo-Clavell ML, Korinek J, Allison TG, Batsis JA, Sert-Kuniyoshi FH, Lopez-Jimenez F. Accuracy of body mass index in diagnosing obesity in the adult general population. Int J Obes (Lond). 2008;32:959–66.
21. Organization World Health. BMI classification: The WHO Global Database on BMI; 2014. [updated 12 May 2015]. http://apps.who.int/bmi/index.jsp?introPage=intro_3.html.
22. Fukuda K, Straus SE, Hickie I, Sharpe MC, Dobbins JG, Komaroff A. The chronic fatigue syndrome: a comprehensive approach to its definition and study. International chronic fatigue syndrome study group. Ann Intern Med. 1994;121:953–9.
23. Kim JH, Ku BC, Kim YS, Kim KH. Study on reliability and validity of the 'qi blood Yin Yang deficiency questionnaire. Korean J Orien Physiol Pathol. 2014;28:346–54.
24. Wang H, Liu X, Lv B, Yang F, Hong Y. Reliable multi-label learning via conformal predictor and random forest for syndrome differentiation of chronic fatigue in traditional Chinese medicine. PLoS ONE. 2014;9:e99565.
25. Park YJ, Cho SW, Lee BH, Park YB. Development and validation of the Yin deficiency scale. J Altern Complem Med. 2013;19:50–6.
26. Berle CA, Cobbin D, Smith N, Zaslawski C. A novel approach to evaluate Traditional Chinese Medicine treatment outcomes using pattern identification. J Altern Complem Med. 2010;16:357–67.
27. Feng Z, Pang Y, Ye FW. TCM non-medicinal therapy for regulation and treatment of chronic fatigue syndrome. J Acupun Tuina Sci. 2008;6:376–80.
28. Woo HJ, Kim SH, Lee SB, Choi MY, Kim YC, Lee JH. Development of Questionnaires for Differentiation of qì-xū, xuè-xū, yang-xū, yīn-xū analysis. Korean J Orient Int Med. 2008;29:856–70.
29. Krupp LB, LaRocca NG, Muir-Nash J, Steinberg AD. The fatigue severity scale. Application to patients with multiple sclerosis and systemic lupus erythematosus. Arch Neurol. 1989;46:1121–3.
30. Chalder T, Berelowitz G, Pawlikowska T, Watts L, Wessely S, Wright D, Wallace EP. Development of a fatigue scale. J Psychosom Res. 1993;37:147–53.
31. Ihaka R, Gentleman R. R: a language for data analysis and graphics. J Comput Graphic Stat. 1996;5:299–314.
32. Ferrari E, Veschi M, Guerzoni V, Bergamini L, Neviani F, Manni B, Pelosi A, Neri M. A scale evaluating the emotivity and well-being of elderly (Italian acronym: SVEBA): analysis of psychometric characteristics. Arch Gerontol Geriatr. 2009;49:77–81.
33. Kim CH, Shin HC, Won CW. Prevalence of chronic fatigue and chronic fatigue syndrome in Korea: community-based primary care study. J Korean Med Sci. 2005;20:529–34.
34. Buchwald D, Pearlman T, Kith P, Schmaling K. Gender differences in patients with chronic fatigue syndrome. J Gen Intern Med. 1994;9:397–401.
35. Lee BK, Kim TH, Park YB. Korean medicine diagnosis theory. 7th ed. Seoul: Seongbosa company press; 2009. p. 312–7.
36. Swanink CM, Vercoulen JH, Bleijenberg G, Fennis JF, Galama JM, van der Meer JW. Chronic fatigue syndrome: a clinical and laboratory study with a well matched control group. J Intern Med. 1995;237:499–506.
37. Niblett SH, King KE, Dunstan RH, Clifton-Bligh P, Hoskin LA, Roberts TK, Fulcher GR, McGregor NR, Dunsmore JC, Butt HL, Klineberg I, Rothkirch TB. Hematologic and urinary excretion anomalies in patients with chronic fatigue syndrome. Exp Biol Med (Maywood). 2007;232:1041–9.
38. Efron B, Tibshirani RJ. An introduction to the bootstrap. Boca Raton: CRC Press; 1994.
39. Mawle AC, Nisenbaum R, Dobbins JG, Gary HE Jr, Stewart JA, Reyes M, Steele L, Schmid DS, Reeves WC. Immune responses associated with chronic fatigue syndrome: a case-control study. J Infect Dis. 1997;175:136–41.
40. Dinos S, Khoshaba B, Ashby D, White PD, Nazroo J, Wessely S, Bhui KS. A systematic review of chronic fatigue, its syndromes and ethnicity: prevalence, severity, co-morbidity and coping. Int J Epidemiol. 2009;38:1554–70.
41. Whitehead L. The measurement of fatigue in chronic illness: a systematic review of unidimensional and multidimensional fatigue measures. J Pain Symptom Manag. 2009;37:107–28.

4

Antioxidant and physiological effects of *Si-Wu-Tang* on skin and liver: a randomized, double-blind, placebo-controlled clinical trial

Hui-Fang Chiu[1], Ying-Hua Wu[2], You-Cheng Shen[3], Shing-Jung Wang[4], Kamesh Venkatakrishnan[2] and Chin-Kun Wang[2*]

Abstract

Background: *Si-Wu-Tang* (SWT) is used to treat various gynecological disorders in Chinese medicine. This study investigated the antioxidant and physiological effects of SWT on the skin and liver in healthy adults.

Methods: This randomized, crossover, double-blind, placebo-controlled clinical trial was conducted at Chung Shan Medical University Hospital in December 2008. Participants with uncontrolled diabetes, heart disease, liver disease, kidney disease, cancer, and pregnancy were excluded. Sixty healthy volunteers taking no medications were recruited from the community based on the results of their medical history questionnaires and biochemical analyses to confirm their health status. The participants were assigned to two groups: one group drank 125 mL of placebo (n = 30) and the other drank SWT (n = 30) for six continuous days per month for 6 months. The placebo and SWT were then switched between the groups after a 1-month washout period. Anthropometric measurements (body weight, body fat, and body mass index) were performed and fasting blood samples were drawn for various biochemical assays at 1, 3, 6, 10 and 13 months. Abdominal ultrasound and skin examinations were performed at 1, 6 and 13 months. The skin examinations involved assessment of skin roughness, sebum content, hydration, surface water loss, erythema, melanin index, and elasticity on the face (sunlight-exposed sites: middle of ear and nose) and inner arm (sunlight-unexposed sites: center of wrist and elbow joint).

Results: Administration of SWT significantly increased the antioxidant index ($P = 0.001$) and antioxidant enzymes activities ($P = 0.001$) from baseline to month 6. SWT also suppressed the concentration of serum lipids (triglycerides, $P = 0.01$; high-density lipoprotein cholesterol, $P = 0.23$; low-density lipoprotein cholesterol, $P = 0.48$) and hepatic marker enzymes (glutamic pyruvic transaminase, $P = 0.76$; glutamic oxaloacetic transaminase, $P = 0.65$) when compared with the placebo group. Abdominal ultrasound in the SWT group revealed a positive impact of SWT on mild fatty liver, gallstones, and mild splenomegaly. Moreover, SWT intake concomitantly elevated erythema ($P = 0.011$) and markedly lowered skin surface water loss ($P = 0.016$), sebum content ($P = 0.021$), and wrinkles ($P = 0.024$).

Conclusions: Oral administration of SWT for 6 months improved the antioxidant level and positively regulated the lipid profile, liver function, and skin integrity and texture.

Background

The therapeutic essence of Chinese medicine (CM) can be attributed to multiple elements rather than just one in the product used [1]. *Si-Wu-Tang* (SWT) is a CM formula comprising four different medicinal herbs: *Radix Paeoniae Alba* (*bai shao yao*), *Rhizoma* Ligusticum *Chuanxiong* (*chuan xiong*), *Radix Angelica Sinensis* (*dang gui*), *and Radix Rehmanniae Preparata* (*shu di* huang) [2]. SWT is widely used for the treatment of gynecological disorders such as menstrual discomfort, climacteric syndrome, dysmenorrheic and other estrogen-related diseases [3], cutaneous diseases [4], and menstrual

*Correspondence: wck@csmu.edu.tw
[2] School of Nutrition, Chung Shan Medical University, Taichung, Taiwan
Full list of author information is available at the end of the article

discomfort [5]. Several preclinical (in vitro) studies of SWT have demonstrated antioxidative, anti-inflammatory, antiaging, antibacterial, and antipruritic activities [6, 7].

The major bioactive components in these four herbs include phenolics, phthalides, alkaloids, terpene glycosides, and iridoid glycosides. Some major constituents are gallic acid, paeoniflorin, senkyunolide A, ferulic acid, Z-ligustilide, butylphthalide, sodium ferulate, and catalpol [3]. Among these compounds, ferulic acid, paeoniflorin, and Z-ligustilide in SWT exhibited antioxidative, antimutagenic, anti-inflammatory, vasodilative, and antiallergic effects [8–10]. Sodium ferulate in *A. sinensis* and *Lignsticum chuangxiong* of SWT has lowered the oxidation process and lipid levels in various animal models [11, 12]. Additionally, SWT is rich in organic acids, amino acids, polysaccharides, vitamins, and minerals such as magnesium, calcium, phosphorus, and iron [13].

Liver cells (hepatocytes) metabolize toxins such as alcohol and drugs into their inactive metabolites. Hepatocytes are extremely prone to peroxide (free radical) formation because of their higher metabolic rate. These free radicals are effectively eliminated by antioxidants, especially glutathione peroxidase (GPx). GPx plays a major role in the reductive detoxification of peroxides in hepatocytes [14]. A decreased antioxidant level may lead to oxidative stress and eventual hepatic dysfunction. Several reports have proven that hepatic dysfunction might contribute to various dermal disorders such as dermatitis, eczema, psoriasis, acne, and boils or rashes secondary to decreased detoxification (excessive toxin buildup in skin) and elevated inflammation and oxidative stress [15, 16]. Hence, this study was designed to investigate the antioxidant and physiological effects of SWT on skin and liver in healthy adults.

Methods

Chemicals

Folin–Ciocalteu phenol reagent, sodium hydroxide, sodium nitrite, hydrochloric acid, 6-hydroxy-2,5,7,8-tetramethylchromane-2-carboxylic acid (Trolox), hydrogen peroxide, sodium dihydrogen phosphate, and trichloroacetic acid were purchased from Sigma (St. Louis, MO, USA).

SWT and placebo

Commercially available SWT and placebo as an oral suspension (glass vial) were provided by Standard Foods Corporation (Taipei, Taiwan). Each vial contained 125 mL of SWT (*Radix P. Alba, Rhizoma L. Chuanxiong, Radix A. Sinensis*, and *Radix R. Preparata* with cinnamon twig, rose hip extract, sucrose, vitamin C, malic acid, citric acid, and gelatin) or placebo (simulated SWT flavor with herb-rinsed water and sucrose solution). Both sample vials were indistinguishably packaged with a similar color, flavor, size, and shape.

Participants

This randomized, crossover, double-blind, placebo-controlled clinical trial was conducted in Chung Shan Medical University Hospital. The trial was carried out in accordance with the declaration of Helsinki and subsequent revisions and approved by the Institutional Review Board (IRB) of Chung Shan Medical University Hospital, Taichung, Taiwan (CSMUHCS08008) and registered with clinicaltrials.gov (NCT02634242) (Additional file 1). Written informed consent was received from all participants before enrollment (Additional file 2). Taking into account an expected dropout rate of approximately 25 % and the crossover design, the required sample size (95 % CI, $\alpha = 0.05$) was 60 participants (30 participants in each group) [17]. All participants (aged 20–80 years) were enrolled in the present experiment via advertisements displayed in public places.

The participants were requested to avoid using medications or supplements during the intervention. They could withdraw from the study at any time if desired. The exclusion criteria were a history of smoking, alcoholism, pregnancy or lactation, chronic diseases, and hepatic or renal dysfunction. A physical examination was performed in the 60 voluntary participants at the beginning of the study, and they were segregated into two groups of 30 participants in each (five male and 25 female): those who drank 125 mL of placebo and those who drank SWT for 6 days per month for 6 months. The placebo and SWT were switched between the two groups after a 1-month washout period. Anthropometric analyses of body weight, body fat, and body mass index were performed at 1, 3, 6, 10 and 13 months. The SWT and placebo vials were labeled with the participant number by an electrical randomization method [17]. The average percentage intake of SWT or placebo was 88.47 % at the end of the experiment based on the participants' records. During the crossover study, three and two female participants in the placebo and SWT groups, respectively, were excluded from the study because of an unwillingness to cooperate. Thus, the present study was performed with 27 and 28 participants in the placebo and SWT group, respectively ($n = 55$).

Blood sampling

At baseline (months 1 and 7), the middle time point (months 3 and 10), and the end of each intervention period (months 6 and 13), fasting blood samples were collected in an EDTA-coated vacuum tube, and plasma was separated by centrifugation (Supercentrifuge 1K15;

Sigma) at 1500×*g*. Blood samples were isolated after separating the intermediate film, and the settled portion was washed with isotonic saline and centrifuged at 1500×*g* to obtain the erythrocytes for assaying antioxidant enzymes. All samples were stored at −80 °C until analyses.

Abdominal ultrasonic examination was performed at month 1, 6 and 13 at Chung Shan Medical University Hospital, Taichung, Taiwan with the help of an experienced gastroenterology physician (Dr. Chen Ziyan).

Various oxidative indexes

The total antioxidant capacity (TEAC) [18, 19], total thiobarbituric acid reactive substances (TBARS) [20], and glutathione content [21] in plasma were determined by previously reported methods.

Antioxidative enzymes

Superoxide dismutase (SOD) activity was determined with the Ransod SD 125 kit (Randox Labs, Crumlin, UK), GPx and glutathione reductase (GR) activity were determined with the Ransel RS 504 kit (Randox Labs, Crumlin, UK), and catalase (CAT) activity was measured by Aebi [22]. The red blood cell protein content was determined based on the biuret reaction of the BCA kit from Thermo Fisher Scientific (MA, USA).

Serum lipids and hepatic markers

The serum concentrations of total cholesterol (TC), triglycerides (TG), and high-density lipoprotein cholesterol (HDL-c) were measured by commercially available lipid profile kits (CHODPAP for TC, GPO-PAP for TG, and a precipitation method for HDL-c; Roche Diagnostics, Mannheim, Germany) on a Hitachi 747 autoanalyzer. Low-density lipoprotein cholesterol (LDL-c) was calculated by the Friedewald equation. The plasma glutamic oxaloacetic transaminase (GOT) and glutamic pyruvic transaminase (GPT) concentrations were measured by AppliedBio assay kits (Hercules, CA, USA).

Skin examination

A multifunctional skin detector (MPA 580; Courage and Khazaka Electronic GmbH, Cologne, Germany) and skin roughness analyzer (VD 300; Courage and Khazaka Electronic GmbH) were used to detect the biophysical characteristics of skin in the face and arm regions. No skin care products were applied to the measured sites for at least 24 h prior to the measurements. The skin sebum content, hydration, surface water loss, erythema, melanin index, and elasticity were measured with the following respective probes: Sebumeter, Corneometer, TEWAmeter, Mexameter, and Cutometer (Courage and Khazaka Electronic GmbH).

The Sebumeter SM 815 utilizes the difference in light intensity via a plastic strip to indicate the quantity of absorbed sebum. The sebum level is expressed as $\mu g/cm^2$ [23]. Skin hydration was measured by Corneometer CM 825, which uses the high dielectric constant of water to evaluate the water-related changes in the electrical capacitance of the skin. It displays hydration measurements in system-specific arbitrary units [24]. A melanin index is calculated by the Mexameter MX 18 from the strength of the absorbed and reflected light at 660 and 880 nm, respectively. Erythema is processed similarly at 568 and 660 nm, respectively [25]. The measurement of cutaneous water loss by TEWAmeter TM 300 was analyzed based on the diffusion in an open chamber and is expressed as $g/m^2/h$ [26]. The Cutometer MPA 580 pulls the targeted skin into the probe with controlled vacuum pressure [27]. Skin wrinkles were measured using a Visioscan VC 98 (Courage and Khazaka Electronic GmbH). In brief, two points were measured: one at the middle of the nose and right ear, and the other at the middle of the wrist and inner elbow joint of right hand. All participants were instructed to wash and clean their face and arm, and then rested calmly for 30 min in a room kept at 20 ± 2 °C and a relative humidity of 50 ± 2 % before testing.

Statistical analysis

The results are expressed as a mean ± standard deviation. The paired t test was employed to compare differences within the same group (baseline vs. end of treatment), and Student's t test was used to compare differences between the experimental (SWT) and control (placebo) groups. All variables were analyzed via one-way analysis of variance with the *post doc* least-significant differences test. A $P < 0.05$ was considered statistically significant. The Statistical Package for the Social Sciences (SPSS) version 17.0 (Chicago, IL, USA) was used for analysis.

Results and discussion

A crossover design was chosen for the present investigation because of its numerous advantages such as decreased confounding covariants (because the same participants ingested both SWT and placebo) as well as statistically effective during chronic condition [28]. Based on our literature survey, a 1-month wash-out period was adopted for the present study to suppress the carry-over effect. A flowchart of the present study is illustrated in Fig. 1. The anthropometric parameters in the placebo and SWT groups are presented in Table 1. At baseline, the body weight, body fat, and body mass index were within the normal range in both the placebo and SWT groups. There were no significant differences in any of the anthropometric parameters between the placebo and SWT groups at the end of the intervention.

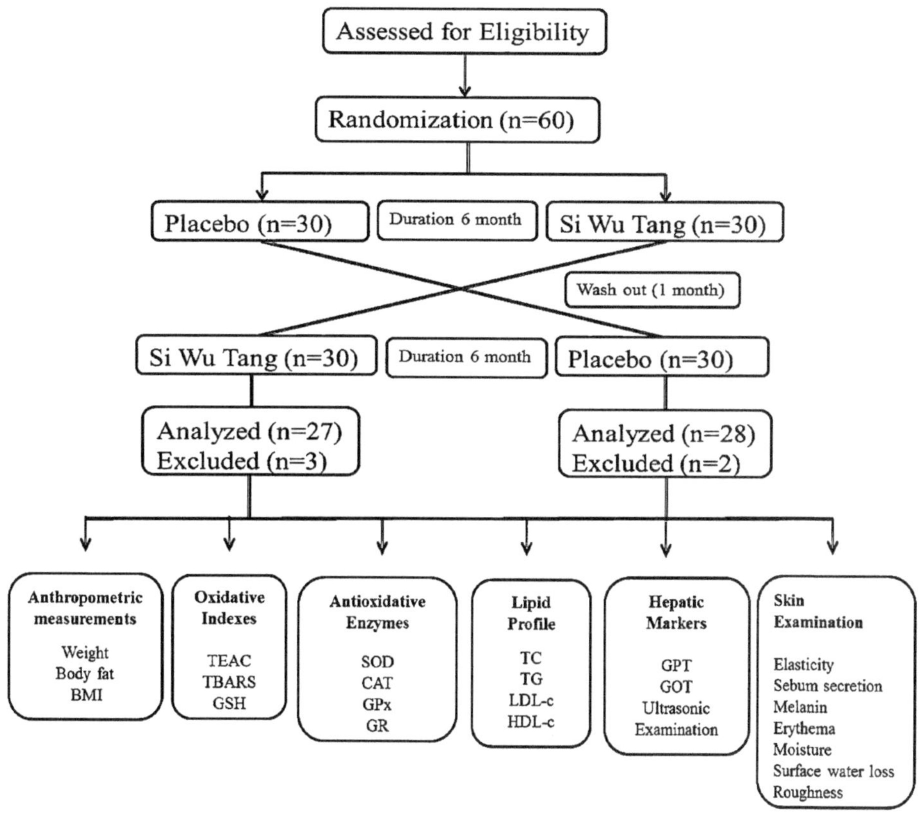

Fig. 1 Flow chart of present study

Table 1 The anthropometric parameters in placebo and SWT treated healthy subjects

Group	Weight (kg)	Body fat (%)	BMI (kg/m^2)
Baseline			
Placebo	57.46 ± 9.43^a	29.23 ± 5.82^a	22.29 ± 3.18^a
SWT	57.45 ± 9.58^a	29.27 ± 5.77^a	22.35 ± 3.19^a
3rd month			
Placebo	57.74 ± 9.80^a	29.47 ± 5.91^a	22.39 ± 3.28^a
SWT	57.70 ± 9.48^a	29.15 ± 5.70^a	22.44 ± 3.21^a
6th month			
Placebo	57.70 ± 9.28^a	29.32 ± 6.09^a	22.32 ± 3.46^a
SWT	57.41 ± 9.67^a	29.25 ± 5.77^a	22.07 ± 3.43^a

Values were expressed as mean ± SD ($n = 55$). Data within the same column of each group sharing different superscript letters were significantly different ($p < 0.05$)

BMI body mass index

Antioxidants interact with free radicals and stabilize by donating their electrons or protons. If untreated, these free radicals can cause various chronic diseases [29]. Table 2 shows the plasma oxidative indexes including, TEAC, glutathione (GSH) concentration, and TBARS in the placebo- and SWT-treated participants. The TEAC reflects the relative ability of hydrogen or electron-donating antioxidants to scavenge the 2,2′-azino-bis 3-ethylbenzothiazoline-6-sulphonic acid (ABTS) radical cation compared with that of Trolox. Treatment with SWT for 6 months substantially increased the levels of TEAC (0.35–0.59 μM; $P = 0.001$) and GSH (14.19–14.35 μM; $P = 0.88$), whereas the TBARS level (1.40–0.68 μM; $P = 0.001$) was lower than that in the baseline period; additionally, notable changes were found between the SWT and placebo groups. SWT comprises four medicinal plants with numerous active components including gallic acid, paeoniflorin, ferulic acid, and Z-ligustilide, which contain numerous OH groups that scavenge free radicals through electron delocalization [6]. Liu et al. [30] reported that polysaccharide from *A. sinensis* could directly scavenge oxygen-derived free radicals in colonic tissues of rats with colitis.

The antioxidant defense system consists of endogenous antioxidants SOD, CAT, GPx, and GR. SOD catalyzes the dismutation of superoxide into hydrogen peroxide and water molecules. After the decomposition of hydrogen peroxide by GPx at the expense of GSH, the GR-catalyzed

Table 2 Various plasma oxidative indexes in placebo and SWT treated healthy subjects

Group	TEAC (μM/mL)	*p* value*	TBARS (μM/L)	*p* value*	GSH (μM/L)	*p* value*
Baseline						
Placebo	0.34 ± 0.07[a]	0.82	1.43 ± 0.47[a]	0.87	14.18 ± 2.30[b]	0.67
SWT	0.35 ± 0.07[b]		1.40 ± 0.44[a]		14.19 ± 2.48[b]	
3rd month						
Placebo	0.34 ± 0.04[a]	0.001	1.42 ± 0.43[a]	0.001	14.19 ± 2.79[a]	0.83
SWT	0.40 ± 0.07[b]		0.83 ± 0.28[b]		14.31 ± 2.72[a]	
6th month						
Placebo	0.35 ± 0.03[a]	0.001	1.45 ± 0.32[a]	0.001	14.16 ± 2.85[a]	0.88
SWT	0.59 ± 0.06[a]		0.68 ± 0.23[c]		14.35 ± 2.94[b]	

Values were expressed as mean ± SD ($n = 55$). Data within the same column of each group bearing different superscript letters were significantly different ($p < 0.05$)

* Student's t test was used to assess statistical significance between placebo and Si Wu Tang (SWT)

regeneration of GSH from its oxidized form can sustain the GSH-dependent oxy-radical scavenging activity [31].

The antioxidant enzymes evaluated in this study (SOD, CAT, GPx, and GR in the erythrocytes of the placebo- and SWT-treated participants) are epitomized in Table 3. No notable changes were found from baseline to month 6 in the placebo-treated group. However, treatment with 125 mL of SWT showed a marked escalation in the levels of SOD (1478.12–1812.47 IU/g Hb; $P = 0.001$), CAT (565.82–803.32 IU/g Hb; $P = 0.001$), GPx (51.03–52.59 IU/g Hb; $P = 0.46$), and GR (10.51–11.93 IU/g Hb; $P = 0.02$) between baseline and the end of the treatment (month 6). Meanwhile, significant changes were also noted between the SWT and placebo groups at month 6.

Nuclear factor erythroid 2-related factor 2 (Nrf2) by Z-ligustilide was involved in the antioxidant activity in the SWT group. Activation of Nrf2 triggered the downstream antioxidant genes (SOD, CAT) and thereby enhanced antioxidant enzyme levels [32]. Additionally, the polyphenolics and numerous phytochemical constituents present in SWT might have elevated the levels of antioxidant enzymes by their free radical quenching ability [7]. Hou et al. [33] reported that treatment with *L. chuanxiong and A. sinensis* showed a better protection against hydrogen peroxide-induced endothelial damage by suppressing reactive oxygen species production. Furthermore, trace elements (calcium, magnesium, and selenium) in SWT act as cofactors to antioxidant enzymes [34].

Lipids are metabolized and regulated by hepatocytes. Any changes in the hepatic lipid status could directly reflect the serum lipid status. Although they are not major hepatic markers, lipids are still effective markers with which to determine whether SWT impacts physiological changes in hepatic tissue by estimating the lipid profile in serum. Table 4 shows the lipid profiles in the serum of the placebo and SWT groups. Supplementation with SWT for 6 months resulted in a significant decline in the levels of TG (102.12–85.89 mg/dL; $P = 0.01$) with a slight decrement in the level of LDL-c (113.05–112.84 mg/dL; $P = 0.48$), whereas the level of HDL-c was concomitantly improved when compared with the baseline value (57.52–59.13 mg/dL; $P = 0.23$). However, no marked changes were observed in the TC level. These

Table 3 Erythrocyte antioxidative enzymes in placebo and SWT treated healthy subjects

Group	SOD (IU/g Hb)	*p* value*	CAT (IU/g Hb)	*p* value*	GPx (IU/g Hb)	*p* value*	GR (IU/g Hb)	*p* value*
Baseline								
Placebo	1475.85 ± 155.91[a]	0.59	562.82 ± 91.86[a]	0.97	51.04 ± 8.61[a]	0.99	10.45 ± 1.69[a]	0.86
SWT	1478.86 ± 230.38[c]		565.13 ± 89.02[c]		51.02 ± 8.90[b]		10.54 ± 1.80[b]	
3rd month								
Placebo	1471.12 ± 183.53[a]	0.01	553.14 ± 66.28[a]	0.001	51.08 ± 6.99[a]	0.63	10.90 ± 1.98[a]	0.01
SWT	1572.01 ± 238.24[b]		677.61 ± 98.83[b]		51.82 ± 8.97[a]		11.94 ± 2.34[a]	
6th month								
Placebo	1475.67 ± 165.34[a]	0.001	569.36 ± 72.39[a]	0.001	51.61 ± 7.05[a]	0.46	10.86 ± 2.01[a]	0.02
SWT	1812.47 ± 343.74[a]		803.32 ± 93.10[a]		52.59 ± 6.86[ab]		11.93 ± 2.66[a]	

Values were expressed as mean ± SD ($n = 55$). Data within the same column of each group bearing different superscript letters were significantly different ($p < 0.05$)

* Student's t test was used to assess statistical significance between placebo and Si Wu Tang (SWT)

Table 4 The lipid profile in plasma of placebo and SWT treated healthy subjects

Group	TG (mg/dL)	*p* value*	TC (mg/dL)	*p* value*	HDL-c (mg/dL)	*p* value*	LDL-c (mg/dL)	*p* value*
Baseline								
Placebo	100.22 ± 25.60^a	0.81	192.85 ± 38.05^a	0.95	57.02 ± 11.21^a	0.87	114.98 ± 32.99^a	0.69
SWT	102.12 ± 28.60^a		192.05 ± 35.34^a		57.52 ± 10.25^b		113.05 ± 31.23^a	
3rd month								
Placebo	97.56 ± 14.96^a	0.01	191.71 ± 34.63^a	0.62	58.60 ± 12.88^a	0.45	113.60 ± 34.04^a	0.83
SWT	87.27 ± 14.64^b		192.20 ± 35.55^a		59.20 ± 13.41^a		113.13 ± 32.32^a	
6th month								
Placebo	97.64 ± 23.39^a	0.01	192.36 ± 32.85^a	0.88	57.51 ± 12.75^a	0.23	113.84 ± 32.21^a	0.48
SWT	85.89 ± 17.86^b		192.73 ± 36.25^a		59.13 ± 12.31^a		112.84 ± 33.68^a	

Values were expressed as mean ± SD ($n = 55$). Data within the same column of each group bearing different superscript letters were significantly different ($p < 0.05$)

* Student's t test was used to assess statistical significance between placebo and Si Wu Tang (SWT)

outcomes indicate that SWT did not change the cholesterol levels; instead, it substantially changed the TG levels, probably owing to the presence of paeoniflorin in SWT. Paeoniflorin works as an inhibitor of pancreatic lipase and thereby lowers TG levels [35]. Our results are consistent with those of Li et al. [36], who concluded that oral administration of polysaccharides from *A. sinensis* significantly reduced the TG and LDL-c levels and improved the HDL-c level in STZ-induced diabetic rats. Moreover, sodium ferulate in *A. sinensis* and *L. chuangxiong* lowered lipid levels in various animal models [11, 12].

The serum GOT and GPT activities are reliable indicators of liver injury [37]. The concentrations of these hepatic markers in the placebo and SWT groups of the present study are shown in Table 5. In a comparison of the baseline and end-of-intervention values in the SWT group, no significant changes were noted in the GOT concentration (20.67–20.33 U/L; $P = 0.65$), but a slight decrease was observed in the GPT concentration (19.00–18.51 U/L; $P = 0.76$). This indicates that SWT can improve hepatic function by lowering hepatic marker enzymes. Wang et al. [38] concluded that treatment with *Radix P. Rubra* and *Radix P. Alba* significantly attenuated CCl_4-induced acute liver injury in a rat model. *Angelica sinensis* exhibited a hepatoprotective effect against hepatotoxicity induced by CCl_4 attributing to its antioxidant activity [39].

The abdominal ultrasonic examination findings in the placebo- and SWT-treated participants are shown in Fig. 2. The examination findings revealed mild fatty liver (Fig. 2a), gallbladder stones (Fig. 2b), and splenomegaly (Fig. 2c) in participant nos. 3, 9 and 28, respectively, at baseline. Treatment with SWT for 6 months in these participants resulted in normal examination findings with no signs of fatty liver (Fig. 2d), gallbladder stones (Fig. 2e), or splenomegaly (Fig. 2f). SWT improved hepatic function by reducing reactive oxygen species, thereby lowering the lipid profile parameters and hepatic damage as well as normalizing various abnormal conditions such as fatty liver, gallbladder stones, and splenomegaly owing to its free radical quenching activity.

Table 5 The hepatic marker enzymes in plasma of placebo and SWT treated healthy subjects

Group	GPT (U/L)	*p* value*	GOT (U/L)	*p* value*
Baseline				
Placebo	19.05 ± 0.27^a	0.92	20.61 ± 6.37^a	0.91
SWT	19.00 ± 0.93^a		20.67 ± 6.46^a	
3rd month				
Placebo	19.27 ± 0.46^a	0.68	20.11 ± 6.63^a	0.72
SWT	19.44 ± 0.94^b		20.35 ± 7.74^a	
6th month				
Placebo	19.47 ± 0.79^a	0.76	21.42 ± 7.17^a	0.65
SWT	19.56 ± 15.11^b		21.16 ± 7.83^a	

Values were expressed as mean ± SD ($n = 55$). Data within the same column of each group bearing different superscript letters were significantly different ($p < 0.05$)

* Student's t test was used to assess statistical significance between placebo and Si Wu Tang (SWT)

The skin plays a crucial role in protecting the body from physical and chemical factors and moisture loss [40]. As discussed earlier, the liver is a major metabolic organ involved in detoxification with the help of GSH, GPx, GST, and GR. Decreases in the antioxidant levels in liver may lead to hepatic dysfunction. Several reports have proven that hepatic dysfunction can lead to various dermal disorders such as eczema, psoriasis, acne, boils, or rashes [15, 16]. The present study investigated the physiological correlation between hepatic and dermal organs with respect to antioxidation in healthy subjects.

Skin elasticity, moisture, surface water loss, sebum content, melanin, erythema, and wrinkles were analyzed to determine skin changes in the face and arm regions. Table 6 shows the results of the skin examination in the

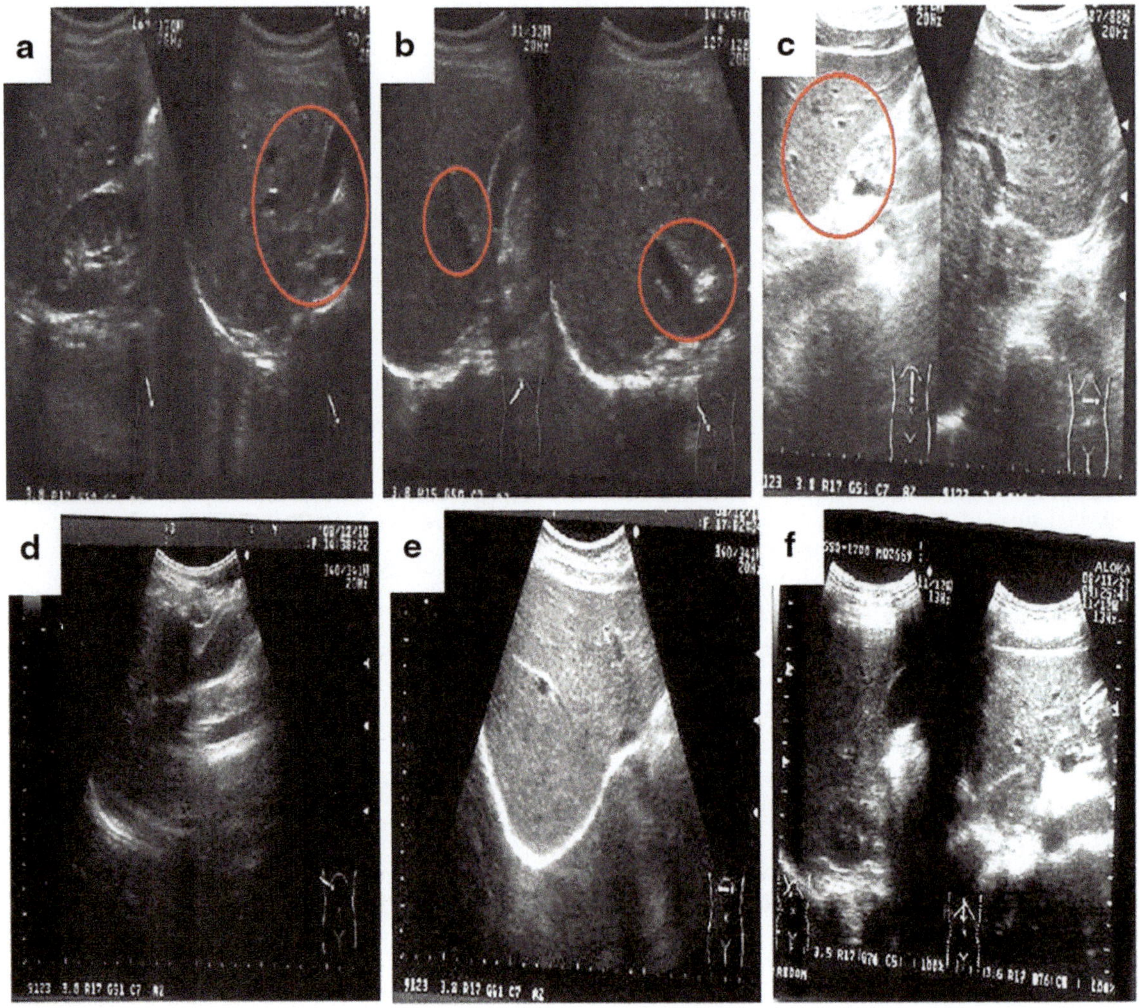

Fig. 2 The Abdominal ultrasonic image of SWT treated healthy participants. **a–c** represented participant no. 3, 9 and 28 at baseline with mild fatty liver, gall bladder stone and splenomegaly respectively (indicated with *arrow mark*). **d–f** represents participant no. 3, 9 and 28 at 6th month of SWT treatment with normal inference (no signs of fatty liver, gall bladder stone and splenomegaly)

placebo and SWT groups. In the placebo group, no significant changes were noted in any of the skin parameters. No marked changes in skin elasticity, moisture, or melanin content were observed between baseline and 6 months in the SWT group; however, a significant increment in erythema was noted in the facial skin (261.12–275.55), whereas the skin surface water loss (5.90–4.87 g/m^2/h), sebum content (163.86–144.96 μg/cm^2), and skin wrinkles (37.41–35.23) in the arm were substantially lower than those at baseline.

Table 7 shows the skin examination results in the placebo- and SWT-treated participants with and without a menstrual cycle. In the placebo group, no significant changes were noted in any of the skin parameters. No significant changes in skin elasticity, moisture, or melanin content from baseline to 6 months were observed in the SWT-treated group in either the face or arm region. A notable elevation in erythema was noted in the facial skin (295.57–303.66; $P = 0.031$) in participants without a menstrual cycle; however, participants with a menstrual cycle showed elevated erythema in both the facial (238.16–256.80; $P = 0.022$) and arm skin (206.65–222.97; $P = 0.021$). The skin surface water loss (5.97–5.06 g/m^2/h; $P = 0.025$), sebum content (164.91–138.00 μg/cm^2), and skin wrinkles (37.22–34.95; $P = 0.032$) in the arms of participants with a menstrual cycle were substantially lower than those of baseline.

SWT increased the blood circulation to maintain hemostasis via stimulation of hematopoietic stem cells [41] and thus increased the immune response and elevated the erythema condition. The elevation in the blood cell concentration may alter various hormone levels (e.g.,

Table 6 Skin examination in placebo and SWT treated all healthy subjects

Parameters	Duration	Placebo		SWT	
		Face	Arm/T-zone	Face	Arm/T-zone
Skin elasticity	Baseline	0.806 ± 0.09[a]	0.885 ± 0.08[a]	0.806 ± 0.09[a]	0.883 ± 0.05[a]
	6th month	0.805 ± 0.08[a]	0.874 ± 0.05[a]	0.814 ± 0.08[a]	0.805 ± 0.08[a]
Skin moisture	Baseline	45.18 ± 10.75[a]	49.45 ± 9.66[a]	45.18 ± 10.75[a]	49.45 ± 9.66[a]
	6th month	45.20 ± 9.86[a]	49.40 ± 10.83[a]	45.11 ± 8.62[a]	49.08 ± 9.49[a]
Surface water loss ($g/m^2/h$)	Baseline	9.43 ± 1.07[a]	5.90 ± 0.66[a]	9.43 ± 1.07[a]	5.90 ± 2.36[a]
	6th month	9.34 ± 1.54[a]	5.52 ± 1.79[a]	9.14 ± 3.73[a]	4.87 ± 1.61[b]
Sebum ($\mu g/cm^2$) content	Baseline	71.46 ± 6.42[a]	163.86 ± 26.46[a]	71.46 ± 6.42[a]	163.86 ± 26.46[a]
	6th month	64.02 ± 5.34[a]	152.76 ± 28.37[a]	62.06 ± 6.22[a]	144.96 ± 22.95[b]
Skin melanin index	Baseline	191.47 ± 40.59[a]	185.76 ± 28.02[a]	191.47 ± 40.59[a]	185.76 ± 31.02[a]
	6th month	193.68 ± 34.78[a]	185.22 ± 28.78[a]	190.95 ± 41.44[a]	184.91 ± 40.51[a]
Skin erythema index	Baseline	261.12 ± 49.07[a]	227.68 ± 35.96[a]	261.12 ± 79.07[a]	227.68 ± 55.96[a]
	6th month	266.37 ± 47.55[a]	229.40 ± 34.88[a]	275.55 ± 72.11[b]	239.06 ± 57.14[a]
Skin wrinkles	Baseline	34.84 ± 2.82[a]	37.41 ± 3.89[a]	34.84 ± 2.82[a]	37.41 ± 3.89[a]
	6th month	34.97 ± 3.42[a]	37.02 ± 3.04[a]	34.06 ± 5.70[a]	35.23 ± 3.20[b]

Values were expressed as mean ± SD ($n = 55$). Data within the same column of each group sharing different superscript letters ([a, b]) were significantly different ($p < 0.05$)

Table 7 Skin examination in placebo and SWT treated healthy subjects with and without menstrual cycle

Parameters	Duration	Placebo		Si Wu Tang (SWT)			
				Without menstrual cycle		With menstrual cycle	
		Face	Arm/T-zone	Face	Arm/T-zone	Face	Arm/T-zone
Skin elasticity	Baseline	0.806 ± 0.09[a]	0.883 ± 0.05[a]	0.774 ± 0.08[a]	0.856 ± 0.06[a]	0.827 ± 0.09[a]	0.901 ± 0.05[a]
	6th month	0.805 ± 0.08[a]	0.874 ± 0.05[a]	0.769 ± 0.08[a]	0.864 ± 0.06[a]	0.843 ± 0.06[a]	0.895 ± 0.06[a]
Skin moisture	Baseline	45.18 ± 10.75[a]	49.45 ± 9.66[a]	44.83 ± 10.75[a]	47.42 ± 9.20[a]	45.41 ± 10.40[a]	50.80 ± 9.86[a]
	6th month	45.20 ± 9.86[a]	49.40 ± 10.83[a]	48.11 ± 8.62[a]	51.08 ± 9.94[a]	43.11 ± 8.62[a]	47.45 ± 9.09[a]
Surface water loss ($g/m^2/h$)	Baseline	9.43 ± 1.07[a]	5.90 ± 0.66[a]	10.02 ± 1.90[a]	5.81 ± 0.98[a]	9.04 ± 1.07[a]	5.97 ± 1.89[a]
	6th month	9.34 ± 1.54[a]	5.52 ± 0.79[a]	9.83 ± 3.26[a]	4.59 ± 1.08[a]	9.34 ± 3.73[a]	5.06 ± 1.55[b]
Sebum ($\mu g/cm^2$) content	Baseline	71.46 ± 6.42[a]	152.86 ± 26.46[a]	68.82 ± 6.53[a]	162.27 ± 16.46[a]	73.24 ± 6.42[a]	164.91 ± 16.46[a]
	6th month	64.02 ± 5.34[a]	163.76 ± 28.37[a]	58.00 ± 6.96[a]	155.41 ± 30.47[a]	71.42 ± 6.22[a]	138.00 ± 22.95[b]
Skin melanin index	Baseline	191.47 ± 40.59[a]	185.76 ± 28.02[a]	201.02 ± 40.59[a]	204.27 ± 31.02[a]	185.10 ± 40.59[a]	173.41 ± 27.43[a]
	6th month	193.68 ± 34.78[a]	185.22 ± 28.78[a]	202.80 ± 41.44[a]	203.29 ± 40.51[a]	183.05 ± 41.44[a]	172.65 ± 30.51[a]
Skin erythema index	Baseline	261.12 ± 49.07[a]	227.68 ± 35.96[a]	295.57 ± 49.07[a]	259.23 ± 64.10[a]	238.16 ± 54.70[a]	206.65 ± 38.06[a]
	6th month	266.37 ± 47.55[a]	229.40 ± 34.88[a]	303.66 ± 41.17[b]	263.21 ± 64.58[a]	256.80 ± 59.54[b]	222.97 ± 45.88[b]
Skin wrinkles	Baseline	34.84 ± 2.82[a]	37.41 ± 3.89[a]	35.66 ± 3.15[a]	37.69 ± 4.96[a]	34.30 ± 2.48[a]	37.22 ± 3.05[a]
	6th month	34.97 ± 3.42[a]	37.02 ± 3.04[a]	34.83 ± 3.03[a]	36.66 ± 3.92[a]	34.54 ± 3.61[a]	34.95 ± 2.65[b]

Values were expressed as mean ± SD ($n = 55$). Data within the same column of each group sharing different superscript letters ([a, b]) were significantly different ($p < 0.05$)

antidiuretic hormone), which may decrease the skin surface water loss, control water retention, and stabilize collagen production, thus decreasing skin wrinkles with elevated antioxidation activity on the skin surface of SWT-treated participants. Because SWT eases menstrual cycle-related dysfunction, it may also boost blood circulation throughout the body and hence decrease skin-related dysfunctions by flushing out toxins in the skin. However, we also encountered a controversial result showing decreased sebum secretion in SWT-treated participants with a menstrual cycle. Ohta et al. [42] reported that the skin sebum content was reduced after menopause in women, but the exact mechanism remains unknown. *Lignsticum chuanxiong* exhibited skin regeneration effects in patients with eczema and psoriasis [43]. SWT inhibited mast cell activation and thus suppressed

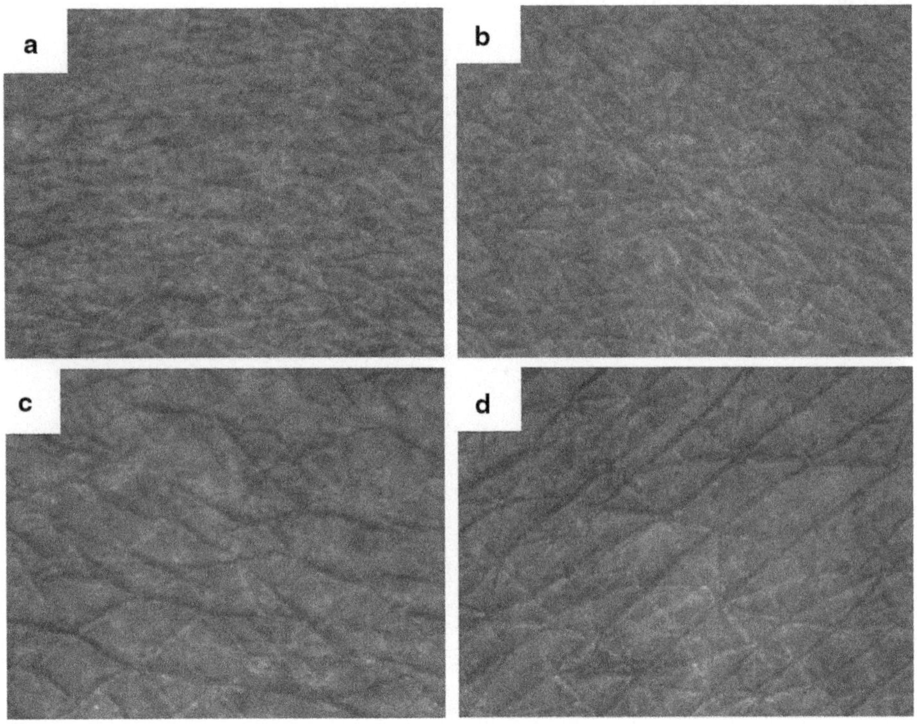

Fig. 3 Skin surface topography viewed under ultraviolet light (Visioscan VC 98). Examination of facial and arm skin of participant 23. **a**, **b** represents the facial and arm skin of placebo group, which indicate less skin integrity, whereas **c**, **d** represents the facial and arm skin of 6 month treated SWT group, which indicate *improved skin integrity* and *texture*

the inflammatory response, proving useful for alleviation of cutaneous pruritus [6].

Figure 3 depicts the skin surface topography of the facial and arm skin of Participant 23 as viewed under ultraviolet light. Figure 3a, b represents the facial and arm skin of patients in the placebo group, who displayed less skin integrity; Fig. 3c, d shows the facial and arm skin of patients in the SWT group at 6 months, showing improved skin integrity and texture. Elevated levels of free radicals are responsible for the weakening of elastin and collagen, skin wrinkles, fragility, dull appearance, and aging [44]. Because SWT is a good antioxidant, it can effectively scavenge free radicals and thus probably improve skin elasticity and texture. Moreover, cnidilide and ligustilide (*Rhizoma* L.) are present in SWT and may be primarily involved in the inhibition of the skin inflammatory reaction and stimulation of blood circulation by altering sebum secretion [5, 7].

Conclusions

Oral administration of SWT for 6 months significantly improved the antioxidant level and thereby positively regulated the lipid profile, liver function, and skin integrity and texture.

Authors' contributions

HFC, YHW and CKW conceived and designed the study protocol. YHW, HFC, KV and YCS conducted the clinical trial. CKW and KV collected data and wrote the manuscript. All authors read and approved the final manuscript.

Author details

[1] Department of Chinese Medicine, Taichung Hospital Ministry of Health and Well-being, Taichung, Taiwan. [2] School of Nutrition, Chung Shan Medical University, Taichung, Taiwan. [3] School of Health Diet and Industry Management, Chung Shan Medical University, Taichung, Taiwan. [4] Division of Research and Development, Standard Foods Corporation, Taipei, Taiwan.

Acknowledgements

Thanks to the cooperation and support rendered by Dr. Chen Ziyan, Chung Shan Medical University Hospital, Taichung, Taiwan, ROC for conducting ultrasonic examination.

Competing interests

The authors declare that they have no competing interests.

References

1. Xue T, Roy R. Studying traditional Chinese medicine. Science. 2003;300(5620):740–1.
2. Zhang H, Shen P, Cheng Y. Identification and determination of the major constituents in traditional Chinese medicine Si-Wu-Tang by HPLC coupled with DAD and ESI–MS. J Pharm Biomed Anal. 2004;34(3):705–13.
3. Wang ZJ, Wo SK, Wang L, Lau C, Lee VH, Chow MS, Zuo Z. Simultaneous quantification of active components in the herbs and products of Si-Wu-Tang by high performance liquid chromatography–mass spectrometry. J Pharm Biomed Anal. 2009;50(2):232–44.
4. Liang QD, Lu XQ, Ma ZC, Tan HL, Ma BP, Gao Y, Wang SQ. Preliminary study on hematopoietic constituents of si-wu-tang. Zhongguo Zhong Yao Za Zhi. 2004;29(6):546–9.
5. Cheng JF, Lu ZYJ, Su YC, Chiang LC, Wang RY. A traditional Chinese herbal medicine used to treat dysmenorrhoea among Taiwanese women. J Clin Nurs. 2008;17(19):2588–95.
6. Dai Y, But PPH, Chan YP, Matsuda H, Kubo M. Antipruritic and antiinflammatory effects of aqueous extract from Si-Wu-Tang. Biol Pharm Bull. 2002;25(9):1175–8.
7. Tahara E, Satoh T, Toriizuka K, Nagai H, Nunome S, Shimada Y, Saiki I. Effect of Shimotsu-to (a Kampo medicine, Si-Wu-Tang) and its constituents on triphasic skin reaction in passively sensitized mice. J Ethnopharmacol. 1999;68(1):219–28.
8. Ou S, Kwok KC. Ferulic acid: pharmaceutical functions, preparation and applications in foods. J Sci Food Agric. 2004;84(11):1261–9.
9. Zheng YQ, Wei W, Zhu L, Liu JX. Effects and mechanisms of Paeoniflorin, a bioactive glucoside from paeony root, on adjuvant arthritis in rats. Inflam Res. 2007;56(5):182–8.
10. Du J, Yu Y, Ke Y, Wang C, Zhu L, Qian ZM. Ligustilide attenuates pain behavior induced by acetic acid or formalin. J Ethnopharmacol. 2007;112(1):211–4.
11. Liao ZX, Wang H, Peng RX, Kong R. Antagonistic effect of sodium ferulate on glycerol-induced renal oxidative injury in mice. Yao Xue Xue Bao. 2003;38:900–3 **(in Chinese)**.
12. Wang BH, Ouyang JP, Liu M, Yang J, Wei L, Li K, Yang H. Sodium ferulate inhibits atherosclerogenesis in hyperlipidemia rabbits. J Cardiovasc Pharmacol. 2004;43:549–54.
13. Millikan M, Xu H, Trevean H. Metal analysis of Si Wu Tang'in relation to its clinical application. Aust J Acupunt Chin Med. 2011;6(2):12–7.
14. Handy DE, Lubos E, Yang Y, Galbraith JD, Kelly N, Zhang YY, Loscalzo J. Glutathione peroxidase-1 regulates mitochondrial function to modulate redox-dependent cellular responses. J Biol Chem. 2009;284(18):11913–21.
15. Kazakevich N, Moody MN, Landau JM, Goldberg LH. Alcohol and skin disorders: with a focus on psoriasis. Skin Therapy Lett. 2011;16(4):5–6.
16. Emre S, Metin A, Demirseren DD, Akoglu G, Oztekin A, Neselioglu S, Erel O. The association of oxidative stress and disease activity in seborrheic dermatitis. Arch Dermatol Res. 2012;304(9):683–7.
17. Gargari BP, Mobasseri M, Valizadeh H, Asghari-Jafarabadi M. Effects of *Silybum marianum* (L.) Gaertn. (silymarin) extract supplementation on antioxidant status and hs-CRP in patients with type 2 diabetes mellitus: a randomized, triple-blind, placebo-controlled clinical trial. Phytomedicine. 2015;22(2):290–6.
18. Arnao MB, Casas JL, Del Rio JA, Acosta M, Garcia-Canovas F. An enzymatic colorimetric method for measuring naringin using 2,20-azino-bis-(3-ethylbenzthiazoline-6-sulfonic acid) (ABTS) in the presence of peroxidase. Anal Biochem. 1990;185:335–8.
19. Miller NJ, Rice-Evans C, Davies MJ, Gopinathan V, Milner A. A novel method for measuring antioxidant capacity and its application to monitoring the antioxidant status in premature neonates. Clin Sci (Lond). 1993;84:407–12.
20. Draper HH, Hadley M. Malondialdehyde determination as index of lipid peroxidation. Methods Enzymol. 1990;186:421–31.
21. Halliwell B, Gutteridge JM. The antioxidants of human extracellular fluids. Arch Biochem Biophys. 1990;280:1–8.
22. Aebi H. Catalase in vitro. Methods Enzymol. 1984;105:121–6.
23. Pande SY, Misri R. Sebumeter. Indian J Dermatol Venereol Leprol. 2005;71(6):444–6.
24. Gerhardt LC, Strässle V, Lenz A, Spencer ND, Derler S. Influence of epidermal hydration on the friction of human skin against textiles. J R Soc Interface. 2008;5(28):1317–28.
25. Yamamoto T, Takiwaki H, Arase S, Ohshima H. Derivation and clinical application of special imaging by means of digital cameras and Image J freeware for quantification of erythema and pigmentation. Skin Res Technol. 2008;14(1):26–34.
26. Shah JH, Zhai H, Maibach HI. Comparative evaporimetry in man. Skin Res Technol. 2005;11(3):205–8.
27. Ryu HS, Joo YH, Kim SO, Park KC, Youn SW. Influence of age and regional differences on skin elasticity as measured by the Cutometer®. Skin Res Technol. 2008;14(3):354–8.
28. Mills EJ, Chan AW, Wu P, Vail A, Guyatt GH, Altman DG. Design, analysis, and presentation of crossover trials. Trials. 2009;10(1):27.
29. Hamid AA, Aiyelaagbe OO, Usman LA, Ameen OM, Lawal A. Antioxidants: its medicinal and pharmacological applications. Afr J Pure Appl Chem. 2010;4(8):142–51.
30. Liu SP, Dong WG, Wu DF, Luo HS, Yu JP. Protective effect of angelica sinensis polysaccharide on experimental immunological colon injury in rats. World J Gastroenterol. 2003;9(12):2786–90.
31. Kamesh V, Sumathi T. Nephroprotective potential of Bacopa monniera on hypercholesterolemia induced nephropathy via the NO signaling pathway. Pharm Biol. 2014;52:1327–34.
32. Liu M, Ravula R, Wang Z, Zuo Z, Chow MS, Thakkar A, Huang Y. Traditional Chinese medicinal formula Si-Wu-Tang prevents oxidative damage by activating Nrf2-mediated detoxifying/antioxidant genes. Cell Biosci. 2014;4(1):1–8.
33. Hou YZ, Zhao GR, Yang J, Yuan YJ, Zhu GG, Hiltunen R. Protective effect of Ligusticum chuanxiong and Angelica sinensis on endothelial cell damage induced by hydrogen peroxide. Life Sci. 2004;75(14):1775–86.
34. Iranzo O. Manganese complexes displaying superoxide dismutase activity: a balance between different factors. Bioorg Chem. 2011;39:73–87.
35. Lin HR. Paeoniflorin acts as a liver X receptor agonist. J Asian Nat Prod Res. 2013;15(1):35–45.
36. Li CJ, Zhang YZ, Meng WF. The hypoglycemic mechanism of Angelica polysaccharide in type-2 diabetic rats. J Qiqihar Med Coll. 2007;28:1422–4.
37. Holt MP, Ju C. Mechanisms of drug-induced liver injury. AAPS J. 2006;8:E48–54.
38. Wang R, Xiong AZ, Teng ZQ, Yang QW, Shi YH, Yang L. Radix paeoniae rubra and radix paeoniae alba attenuate CCl_4-induced acute liver injury: an ultra-performance liquid chromatography-mass spectrometry (UPLC-MS) based metabolomic approach for the pharmacodynamic study of traditional Chinese medicines (TCMs). Int J Mol Sci. 2012;13(11):14634–47.
39. Yu F, Li H, Meng Y, Yang D. Extraction optimization of Angelica sinensis polysaccharides and its antioxidant activity in vivo. Carbohydr Polym. 2013;94(1):114–9.
40. Song EJ, Lee JA, Park JJ, Kim HJ, Kim NS, Byun KS, Moon TK. A study on seasonal variation of skin parameters in Korean males. Int J Cosmet Sci. 2014;37(1):92–7.
41. Sarker SD, Nahar L. Natural medicine: the genus Angelica. Curr Med Chem. 2004;11:1479–500.
42. Nam GW, Baek JH, Koh JS, Hwang JK. The seasonal variation in skin hydration, sebum, scaliness, brightness and elasticity in Korean females. Skin Res Technol. 2014;21(1):1–8.
43. Meepagala K, Sturtz G, Wedgem CE, Schraderm KK, Duke SO. Phytotoxic and antifungal compounds from two apiaceae species, Lomatium clifornicum and Ligusicum hultenii, rich sources of z-ligustilide and apiol, respectively. J Chem Ecol. 2005;31:1567–78.
44. Palmer DM, Kitchin JS. Oxidative damage, skin aging, antioxidants and a novel antioxidant rating system. J Drugs Dermatol. 2010;9(1):11–5.

5

Adjunctive use of modified *Yunu-Jian* in the non-surgical treatment of male smokers with chronic periodontitis: a randomized double-blind, placebo-controlled clinical trial

Kwan-Yat Zee†, Pui Sze Chan†, Johnson Chun Sing Ho†, Stanley Man Lung Lai, Esmonde Francis Corbet and Wai Keung Leung*

Abstract

Background: *Yunu-Jian* (YJ) is a Chinese medicine (CM) *heat* purging formula, which is used to reduce *wei huo* (*stomach-heat*, SH) and enrich *shen yin* (*kidney-yin*, KY). This formula is also commonly used to manage diabetes mellitus and gum/oral inflammation. The activity of YJ can be modified or refined by the addition of other CM herbs and/or minor changes to one of its five key ingredients. The aim of this study was to evaluate the adjunctive use of modified YJ (mYJ) or YJ containing additional osteoblast-stimulating and inflammation-modulating CM herbs in the non-surgical periodontal treatment of smokers with chronic periodontitis in a randomized, double-blind, prospective, placebo-controlled study.

Methods: Healthy adult male smokers with untreated chronic periodontitis who showed CM syndrome of SH and KY deficiency (KYD) whilst attending a dental teaching hospital from October to December, 2005, were invited to participate in a randomized double-blind, placebo-controlled clinical trial. The trial itself involved the once-daily oral administration of a placebo or mYJ for 3 months as an adjunct to non-surgical periodontal therapy. Several periodontal parameters, including radiographic alveolar bone density, were measured by computer-assisted densitometric image analysis (CADIA) on selected sites, and CM signs of SH and KYD were followed from their baseline values to various time points up to 12 months or the end of study.

Results: Twenty-five smokers (consumed 25.0 ± 15.3 smoking-pack years, ranged 7.5–80; aged 46.3 ± 6.8 years) with periodontitis and SH and KYD were recruited (Placebo, n = 14; mYJ, n = 11). All of the participants showed good tolerance towards the CM recipe. All of the periodontal parameters had improved after 12-month follow-up, and no statistically significant differences were detected between the control group and test group, except for the higher CADIA values observed compared with the baseline at 12 months for test sites ($P = 0.025$). 4/3/3 test vs 14/13/13 control participants had persisting SH and KYD at 6, 9 and 12 months ($P < 0.001$), respectively.

Conclusions: The adjunctive use of mYJ preserved the post-treatment increases in the radiographic alveolar bone density at the study sites and led to an overall improvement in SH and KYD compared with the controls.

Trial registration HKU Clinical Trial Register, HKCTR-1848 (www.hkuctr.com/Study/Show/3acbf983831244d29d50b543540bf6e9)

*Correspondence: ewkleung@hkucc.hku.hk
†Kwan-Yat Zee, Pui Sze Chan and Johnson Chun Sing Ho contributed equally to this work
Faculty of Dentistry, The University of Hong Kong, Hong Kong, SAR, China

Background

Periodontal disease is an infectious disease that affects the periodontium of susceptible hosts, and is characterized by the inflammation and destruction of the surrounding tooth-supporting tissues [1]. Approximately 20 % of the adult population of Hong Kong has a probing pocket depth (PPD) ≥6 mm [2]. Although bacteria play a critical role in the life cycle of this disease, they are not solely responsible for the onset of this disease, with host factors playing an important role in the outcome of this disease [3]. Smoking is one of the greatest risk factors for periodontitis [4, 5], and is associated with an increased risk of periodontal attachment loss [2, 6]. Although routine non-surgical periodontal therapy has been shown to be effective for the treatment of chronic periodontitis in smokers, smokers tend to exhibit more residual periodontal pockets [7–9] than non-smokers. Smokers also show a greater tendency towards progressive radiographic alveolar bone loss despite post-treatment periodontal maintenance care [10].

In the conceptual context of Chinese medicine (CM), periodontal disease is mainly categorized as *ya xuan* (gaping gums), *ya lou* (leaking gums) and *ya nu* (bleeding gums) [11, 12]. The recommended treatment for this disease involves the mechanical removal of deposits from the affected teeth [13, 14]. The use of herbal medicine recipes has also been suggested to rectify the disease-associated imbalance in the human body along the four major philosophical frameworks, including attention to poor oral hygiene, *wei huo* (*stomach-heat*, SH), *shen yin xu* (*kidney-yin deficiency*, KYD) and weakness in *qi* and *xue* (*blood*) [15]. The concept of CM dictates that the *kidney* dominates the *gu* (*bone*) and *sheng sui* (*create marrow*) and that the *kidney* therefore also dominates the teeth, whereas the *pi* (*spleen*) and *stomach meridians* pass through the teeth and gum. Accordingly, periodontal disease could therefore be a problem associated with unwanted changes to the homeostasis in the *spleen* and *stomach* or *kidney* [14]. From the perspective of CM, smoking would not only affect the lungs and airways, but would also fire up the *qi*, destroy blood and consume *yin* fluids [16].

Several CM formula have been used to treat *ya xuan*, *ya lou* and *ya nu*, including *Radix Achyranthis bidentatae* (*Huai Ni Xi*), *Rhizoma Drynariae* (*Gu Su Bu*), *Radix Ophiopogonis* (*Mai Men Dong*), *Cortex Phellodendri* (*Huang Bai*) and *Radix et Rhizoma Rehmanniae* (*Sheng Di Huang*). All of these recipes have been reported to attenuate in vivo inflammation, enhance immune function and/or modulate bone homeostasis [17, 18]. *Rhizoma Drynariae* and *Rehmannia glutinosa* (*Shu Di Huang*) has also been reported to exhibit therapeutic effects towards bone fracture healing, including the induction of proliferation and osteogenic differentiation of human bone mesenchymal stem cells [19, 20]. *Rhizoma Drynariae*, which contains naringin as its main effective component, is one of the most widely investigated of all of these herbal preparations [20].

Yunu-Jian (YJ), which is also known as Jade maiden/women decoction, Fair maiden decoction or *Rehmannia* and *gypsum* combination, is a CM *heat* purging formula used to reduce *stomach-heat* (SH) and enrich *kidney-yin* (KY) [13]. This formula is also commonly used to manage diabetes mellitus and gum/oral inflammation. In terms of the different concepts of CM, the regular smoking of cigarettes leads to the *burning* of the *stomach* and *fei* (*lung*) [21], placing the affected individual at a higher risk of experiencing *ya xuan* due to SH. The activity of YJ can be modified or refined by the addition of CM herbs and/or minor changes to one of its five key ingredients. The aim of this study was to explore the adjunctive effect of using a specifically modified YJ (mYJ) formulation (Table 1) to target SH and KYD in male smokers with chronic periodontitis. In terms of its modification, *Rhizoma Drynariae, Cortex Phellodendri* and *Radix Puerariae* (*Ge Gen*; to promote circulation and increase blood flow) were added to YJ, whereas *Rehmannia glutinosa* was replaced with *Radix et Rhizoma Rehmanniae*. Overall, this study applied the CM *ya xuan* treatment philosophy to achieve host modulation in contemporary periodontal therapy [18].

In recent years, over-the-counter CM preparations such as *Guchi-Jianzhou* granules, *Guchi* pills (or *Guchi Wan*), *Guchi* extract and *Yazhou Baidu* powders have been developed to aid in the management of chronic periodontitis [18]. Despite the increasing availability of potential adjunctive agents, there have been very few properly designed CM-periodontal clinical trials or reports pertaining to the correct clinical usage of these preparations or formulae.

Non-surgical mechanical therapy can be effective for the treatment of periodontitis [22]. Smokers, however, have been repeatedly shown to experience inferior healing responses following non-surgical periodontal therapy [7, 9]. Clinicians have attempted a variety of approaches, including adjunctive antibiotics [23], toothpastes containing triclosan/copolymers in an un-blinded fashion [24], and Er:YAG lasers, in place of regular mechanical therapy [25] to enhance or augment non-surgical periodontal healing in smokers. Unfortunately, however, none of these efforts have produced satisfactory results.

This study aimed to evaluate the adjunctive use of mYJ (Table 1) for the non-surgical periodontal treatment of male smokers with chronic periodontitis in a randomized, double blind, prospective, placebo-controlled study. Middle-aged male smokers who had been diagnosed with CM syndrome of SH and/or KYD, but

Table 1 Composition of modified *Yunu-Jian* (mYJ) and placebo

Chinese name *Yunu-Jian*	Pharmaceutical name *Rehmannia* and *gypsum* combination	g/day[a]
Shi Gao[b]	*Gypsum Fibrosum*	25
Sheng Di Huang	*Radix et Rhizoma Rehmanniae*	20
Mai Men Dong[b]	*Radix Ophiopogonis*	18
Zhi Mu[b]	*Rhizoma Anemarrhenae*	15
Huai Niu Xi[b]	*Radix Achyranthis Bidentatae*	15
Gu Sui Bu	*Rhizoma Drynariae*	15
Huang Bo	*Cortex Phellodendri*	10
Ge Gen	*Radix Puerariae*	15
Placebo		
Ku Gua	*Momordica Charantia*	20

[a] Weight equivalent of the raw ingredient per preparation

[b] Together with *Rehmannia glutinosa (Gaetn.) Libosch. Ex Fisch. Et Mey.* (20 g raw ingredient per preparation) constituted the original *Yunu-Jian* recipe

were otherwise healthy, were recruited into this trial. Full-mouth clinical treatment responses were measured, together with radiographic treatment outcomes at selected sites, which were measured by computer-assisted densitometric image analysis (CADIA) and gingival crevicular fluid (GCF) volume. Digital subtraction radiography (DSR) was used to supplement the periodontal healing response assessment as described before [26], which is considered as a sensitive follow-up protocol for alveolar bone healing after periodontal treatment [27, 28]. General CM signs of SH and KYD were recorded over a 12-month study period. Standard clinical and radiographical periodontal parameters were followed throughout the clinical trial to provide an indication of the reduction in the periodontal inflammation (reduction of bleeding on probing or BOP), resolution/remodeling of the diseased periodontium (reduction of PPD) and bony repair (increase in radiographic periodontal bone density) [29]. As the monitoring of changes in the key CM syndrome of participants during a CM clinical trial was deemed necessary [30], and the current study was conducted accordingly.

Methods

Ethics

The research protocol was approved by the Ethics Committee, Faculty of Dentistry, The University of Hong Kong (HKU) (1/8/12d) (Additional file 1). Interested individuals were verbally briefed about the nature and details of the study with the aid of written explanatory notes covering for any potential risks or benefits from participating. They were given 1 week to think about the project and were advised to discuss participation with family members, referring doctors or dentists before returning to the Periodontology Clinic, HKU and expressing whether to part-take the study or not. On both occasions they were invited to ask as many questions as they liked and the person responsible (PSC) took as long as needed to answer all issues raised. Written informed consent (Additional file 1) was obtained from all participants.

Study design

This study was conducted as a prospective, randomized, double-blinded, placebo-controlled clinical trial. Participants were randomized into control and test groups as follows. All enrolled individuals diagnosed with SH and/or KYD received non-surgical periodontal therapy over four appointments (i.e., four times, each time a quadrant or upper/lower, left/right quarter of mouth treated) completed in a 3-week period. All of the participants received an oral once-daily dose of mYJ or placebo for 3 months, followed by regular post-treatment recalls for up to 12 months (i.e., the end of study or 11 months post-periodontal treatment completion) (Fig. 1). A placebo powder (total 25 g) with a similar physical appearance and taste to mYJ was prepared using several inactive components, including starch, glucose and *Momordica charantia* or *Ku Gua* (2 g), which was used as a naturally bitter component.

CM formula preparation

A mYJ, which contained eight Chinese medicinal ingredients, was used (Table 1). The mYJ or placebo were produced in dissolvable powder form by a registered CM manufacturer in Hong Kong (Eu Yan Sang [Hong Kong] Limited). In brief, correct amounts of all raw materials were boiled together in water to extract their ingredients. The aqueous extract was then concentrated, dried, and crushed into fine powder. The correct amount of powder was then packed into an individually sealed plain aluminum sachet (25 g). A placebo powder (total 25 g) was packed in the similar aluminum sachets as the active recipe. The placebo or active sachet was coded as PH001 or PH002, respectively by the manufacturer. The identity of the sachets was kept by one of the authors (KYZ) who did not participate in the collection and analysis of the data. Contamination screening against heavy metals, pesticides, and aflatoxins in both the active and placebo sachets was performed by an independent laboratory to ensure safety before human consumption. All CM agent preparation and toxicity testing were completed by September 2004.

Sample size determination

This clinical study targeted males with chronic periodontitis, who were otherwise healthy (self-assessment),

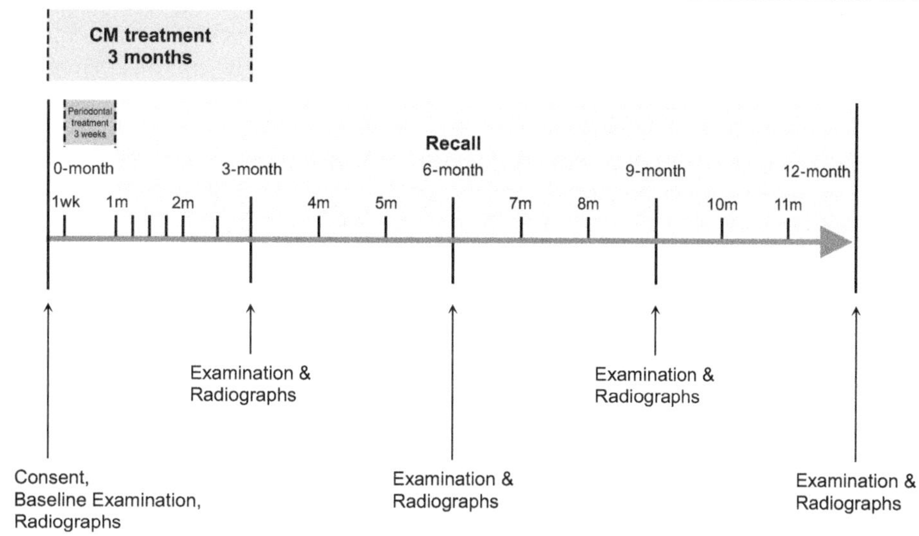

Fig. 1 Study design

except for the fact that they had been diagnosed with SH and/or KYD syndrome. Changes in the CADIA value were considered as the primary dependent variable. The sample size for this study was computed according to the following formula [31]:

$$n = \left[2\sigma^2 (Z_{\alpha/2} + Z_\beta)^2\right] / \delta^2$$

where n = sample size, σ^2 = variance, δ = expected difference, $Z_{\alpha/2} = 1.96$ if $\alpha = 0.05$, $Z_\beta = 0.842$ if power = 80 %.

In a study involving non-smokers from the same local population, participants with chronic periodontitis showed changes of 60 ± 25 in their CADIA values at 12 months after non-surgical therapy [26]. We assumed that the SD would be the same for smokers as it was for the non-smokers in this previous study. We also assumed that there would be an increase of 30 units (expected difference or δ) in the CADIA value at the diseased sites between smokers taking the placebo compared with those taking mYJ. Based on these assumptions, the above formula indicated that 10.9 or 11 participants would be required in each group to enable a difference of 30 units in the CADIA values to be detected.

Participant selection and screening

New male participants attending the Reception Clinic, Prince Philip Dental Hospital (PPDH), Faculty of Dentistry, The University of Hong Kong and satisfying the inclusion criteria were recruited to participate in the study. The target sample size was at least 14 participants each for control and treatment group, to allow for retention of 11 individuals in each group at 12 months. For inclusion, participants had to be reportedly free of systemic disease, and displaying the following features: (1) 36- to 64-years-old ethnic Chinese with untreated chronic periodontitis; (2) smokers with a current consumption of ≥10 cigarettes per day for at least 10 years and expressing no interest in quitting smoking in the coming 12 months; (3) at least 16 standing teeth, with at least 1 tooth having PPD ≥5 mm in each quadrant, excluding the third molars; (4) radiographic evidence of alveolar bone loss at a proximal site up to one-third of root length in at least two teeth per quadrant; and (5) diagnosed as showing signs of SH and/or KYD CM syndrome (Additional file 2: Table S1). Participants were excluded if the initial interview revealed: (1) systemic disease history; (2) history of taking systemic antibiotics in the preceding 30 days; (3) history of any dental treatment, other than oral hygiene instructions, in the preceding 30 days; (4) known hypersensitivity to any Chinese medicine in particular to any ingredients of mYJ or control recipe used in this study; (5) history of rheumatic fever or other conditions for which antibiotic prophylaxis prior to periodontal examination or invasive dental treatment might be advisable; (6) undergoing concurrent dental therapy such as orthodontic treatment.

Thirty two individuals satisfying the inclusion criteria were recruited by the end of a 3-month period (October to December 2005) while the whole study was finished approximately 12 months later.

Participant management and non-surgical mechanical periodontal treatment

This clinical study was carried out at the Periodontology Clinic, PPDH, Faculty of Dentistry, HKU, China. A member of the research team (JCSH) evaluated the dental eligibility of male smokers presenting at the clinic with untreated chronic periodontitis. Male smokers satisfying the eligibility requirements were asked whether they would like to participate in this study, and the CM eligibility of those who accepted the invitation was confirmed by PSC. Eligible participants were then assigned a numerical personal identification code (study number) as a personal identifier to be used throughout the study (Fig. 2). JCSH then followed up with all of the eligible participants to ensure that all of the necessary pre-treatment processes had been conducted. Emergency treatments such as extractions, caries stabilization and initial endodontic therapy were completed prior to the commencement of the non-surgical periodontal treatment trial.

After the required number of participants had been secured, receptionists at the Periodontology Clinic, PPDH, were instructed by KYZ via a concealed envelope, which was prepared prior to the recruitment process, to arrange appointments with all of the participants. Each envelope also included a predetermined table with a study number against randomized blocks indicating sachet allocation. Critically, the attending receptionists were completely unaware of the contents of the different sachets. All of the participants signed an informed consent form at their first appointment and were subsequently presented with seven designated sachets with specific instruction to take one sachet per day for the week prior to the commencement of the non-surgical periodontal therapy. On the first day of the non-surgical periodontal therapy, each participant was presented with 23 identical sachets to those that they had already received. The participants were subsequently presented with 30 more of the same sachets at onw and 2 months after the commencement of the non-surgical periodontal therapy. KYZ was responsible for concealing the details of each participant's allocation, whilst simultaneously refrained from contact with any of the participants, receptionists or clinicians involved in the study until it reached completion.

Each participant was instructed to start consuming the content of the allocated sachets 1 week before starting the non-surgical periodontal therapy process. The participants were instructed to dissolve the powder in each sachet in 200 mL of hot water and drink the resulting solution while it was still warm at the beginning of each day. Each participant was issued with a total of 90 sachets. Self-completion compliance sheets were given to each participant, when CM sachets were issued, to be completed at predefined intervals, including (1) within the 1 week pre-periodontal treatment period; (2) from day 8–day 30 after commencement of the periodontal treatment; and (3) over the second and third month study period. These forms were provided to encourage proper CM medication consumption and to monitor self-reported compliance. Participants had to sign the

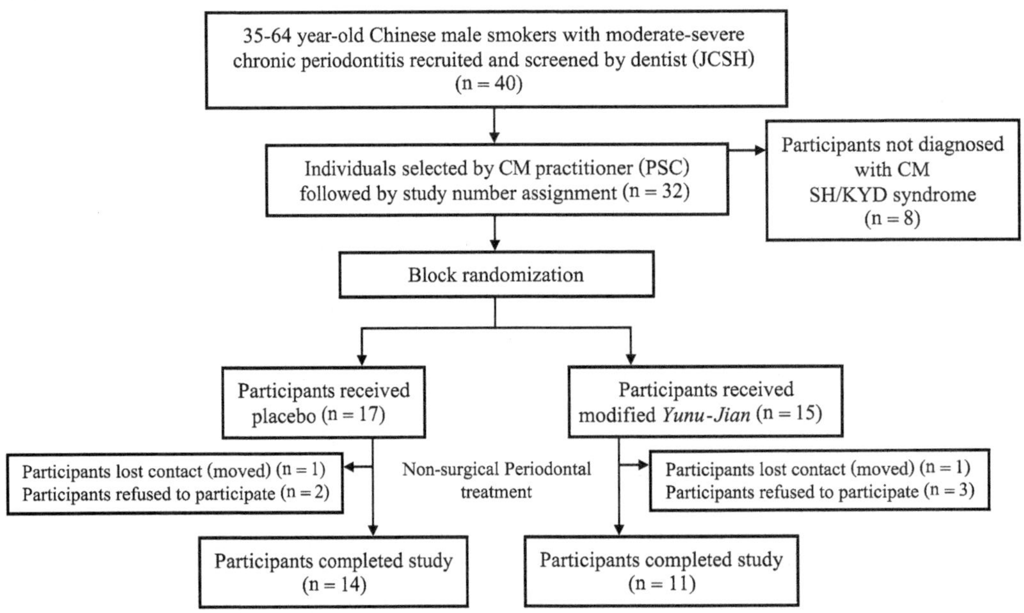

Fig. 2 Flow of participants through each stage of the randomized trial

compliance sheets to confirm their medication consumption and return the sheet, together with any untaken CM medication, according to the schedule set. On each compliance sheet, there was a section for participants to fill in the date, time and type of any suspected adverse effect experienced. Two phone numbers (accessible to PSC or JCSH anytime during the study period concerned) were written on the compliance sheet in case any participant wanted to contact the investigation team.

The receptionists at the Periodontology Clinic were instructed to arrange the non-surgical periodontal treatment appointments (4 visits) within a 3-week period for all of the participants. The appointments were subsequently delivered by JCSH, who was not involved in the clinical data collection. All of the participants received the same non-surgical periodontal treatment, together with the same oral hygiene instructions regarding brushing and interdental cleaning, followed by quadrant-wise scaling and root surface debridement under local anesthesia.

Recall appointments were scheduled once every week for the first month after the periodontal treatment, with reduced frequencies thereafter (i.e., once a week at month 2; once every 2 weeks for month 3, and once every month until the end of study). Oral hygiene reinforcement and motivation were provided as necessary. Supra- and subgingival debridement was performed if needed during the recall appointments. Clinical and radiographic examinations were carried out at the 3-, 6-, 9- and 12-month recall visits.

Any residual periodontal problems detected at the conclusion of the study at the 12-month recall, namely any sites with residual PPD >5 mm, were followed-up with an appropriate periodontal treatment process (e.g., re-root planing or access surgery), which was arranged and delivered without delay. All of the participants were again reminded of the deleterious effects resulting from their continued smoking and were advised to quit smoking at all of the recall appointments and at the end of the clinical trial.

Clinical examination

Several clinical parameters were recorded at the baseline, as well as being recorded at 3, 6, 9 and 12 months after enrollment. All of the clinical examinations were performed by one calibrated examiner (SMLL).

The PPD and probing attachment level (PAL) measurements were recorded at six different sites for each tooth, excluding the third molars (i.e., the mesio-buccal, mid-buccal, disto-buccal, mesio-lingual, mid-lingual and disto-lingual sites). Custom-made poly-ethylene occlusal stents were fabricated for each participant as reference guides to ensure the reproducibility of the probing sites and for measuring the probing attachment level throughout the study using a manual periodontal probe (PCP-UNC 15, Hu-Friedy probe®, Chicago, IL, USA). The presence of any plaque was recorded dichotomously as the presence or absence of plaque according to the detection of plaque deposits determined by running the tip of the periodontal probe along the tooth surface at the gingival margin of each site. BOP was designated as positive if bleeding occurred within 10 s of periodontal probing.

Radiographic examinations were carried out at the two deepest proximal single-root tooth-sites in each participant. The two deepest non-neighboring sites (PPD $\geq$ 5 mm) of the mouth on two individual teeth with well-defined angular defects were selected as described previously [26]. The sites were selected initially from the panoramic oral radiograph taken as part of the PPDH admission screening procedure and subsequently confirmed by paralleling periapical radiographs. The gingival crevicular fluid volumes of these sites were also recorded (last paragraph of this section).

Radiographic examinations for following up any changes in alveolar bone by standardized DSR were carried out as described by Woo et al. [29] and Lai et al. [26]. Briefly, after selecting suitable sites for follow up, a custom-made acrylic bite block attached to a Rinn XCP film holder (Rinn Corporation, Elgin, IL, USA) was constructed for each of the selected sites to produce standardized reproducible periapical radiographs for digital subtraction [32]. Rectangular and long cone techniques were used with a radiographic film requiring a short exposure time (Kodak Insight, Eastman Kodak Co., Rochester, NY, USA) to minimize the level of radiographic exposure to the participant. The X-ray cone was also modified to allow for the rigid attachment of the bite block to the cone. As a consequence, the angulations between the X-ray source, the object and the film were reproducible. All periapical radiographs were taken using the paralleling technique with the same X-ray machine (GE 700, General Electric Co., Fairfield, CT, USA) using the same settings (70 kV, 15 mA). The size-1 radiographic films were used for the anterior regions, where size-2 radiographic films were used for the posterior regions to minimize the distortion of the films. All of the films were developed in a batch with an automatic developing machine (Periomat, Dürr Dental, Bietigheim-Bissingen, Germany) to reduce variability during the developing process.

All of the radiographs were subsequently scanned into a computer at 600 dpi with a flatbed scanner equipped with a transparency module (Agfa Studiostar, Agfa Gaevert, Mortsel, Belgium). The images were imported into software based on the Linux system. Selected sites were defined as regions of interest (ROI) on the radiographs, and the CADIA values were calculated for each ROI according to a previously reported formula [27]. The CADIA values were used to quantify changes in the alveolar bone and were presented as the net values of two standardized radiographic images, which were recorded at different time points [26].

GCF sampling was conducted according to the procedure reported by Jin et al. [33]. Briefly, for a subject tooth (same sites as the DSR study), after isolation with a cotton roll and the removal of the supragingival plaque, a standard filter GCF strip (Periopaper® GCF strips, IDE Interstate, Amityville, NY, USA) was inserted into the gingival crevice or pockets until mild resistance was felt. The GCF strip was then left in place for 30 s. The amount of GCF collected was represented by the electric conductance, which was measured immediately using a GCF meter (Periotron 8000, IDE Interstate). The electrode jaws of the GCF meter were cleaned and dried after each measurement with the machine reading set to zero. The GCF volumes of two periodontitis-free sites were also followed in each participant, preferably from the same tooth type as the diseased tooth of interest. The GCF volumes from each sample site were calculated based on their electric conductance readings, which were measured using a Periotron 8000 GFC meter, as described previously [33]. Clinical data collection for the last participant was completed in December 2006.

Data analysis

Data analysis was carried out using the statistics software: SPSS (SPSS 16.0, Chicago, IL, USA). Simple descriptive statistics were used to summarize the variables studied. Variations in demographic data and smoking habits between control and test groups were assessed by unpaired t tests. Variations in CM signs between control and test groups were assessed by Fisher's exact test. Change of participants' CM syndrome over time was assessed by Chi square test for trend.

As the normality (Kolmogorow-Smirnoff test) and homoscedasticity assumptions (Levene test) of the following data appeared to be valid, clinical parameters, including changes in CADIA, PAL, PPD, Pl % and BOP % were analyzed by repeated measures analysis of variance (ANOVA) with Dunnett's post-test. Significance level was set as $\alpha < 0.05$.

Results

Eight of the 40 participants were considered ineligible by the CM practitioner because their CM signs and symptoms did not fit with the inclusion criteria. A total of 40 male smokers with chronic periodontitis were screened, and 32 met the inclusion criteria and were arbitrarily allocated (Fig. 2). Seventeen participants were assigned to receive PH001 (placebo), with the remaining 15 being assigned to receive PH002 (mYJ). A total of 7 (21.9 %) participants dropped out from the trial during the study period: 2 (11.8 %) and 3 (20.0 %) participants withdrew from the placebo and CM groups, respectively, because they believed that they had recovered already, while 1 participant from each group did not complete the trial because they left Hong Kong (Fig. 2).

The baseline characteristics of the participants are summarized in Table 2. No significant differences were observed between the two groups. The full-mouth periodontal parameters collected for all of the participants over the entire study period are shown in Fig. 3a–d. The results revealed that both groups showed improved plaque control and gingival inflammation (reflected by BOP % reduction) at 3 and 6 months post treatment commencement. However, the levels of plaque and the clinical signs of periodontal tissue inflammation appeared to increase beyond this point in both groups. The mean PPD and PAL values improved and became stable at 6–9 months, although the mean PPD value showed a tendency towards the baseline level at 12 months. No differences were observed in the mean Pl %, BOP % and PPD values between the test and control groups at any of the follow-up time points. Furthermore, the changes observed in the mean PAL over time were not significant for either of the groups compared with the baseline, except at 12 months, where we observed a significant improvement in PAL compared with the baseline in the control participants (Fig. 3d).

All of the participants exhibited good tolerance to the study medicines, with none of the participants reporting any adverse effects. The overall compliance with the dose regimen was also good. According to the compliance sheets, all of the participants completed their course of herbal medicine, except for one participant who failed to attend the scheduled appointment and was therefore unable to collect the prepared medicine on time. In this particular case, the participant missed 2 weeks of CM medication during the third month. This participant was subsequently determined to be a control group participant, and was allowed to remain in the study.

The efficacy of the CM was noted (Fig. 4). The determination of SH syndrome can be subjective because of variations in the severity of the swelling and gum pain, thirst, halitosis, apatite, constipation and *long bi* (*short urine*) or dribbling urination [34]. The determination of KYD syndrome can also be subjective because of variations in the severity of the soreness of waist, backache, hot flushes and night sweating (*gu zheng* or *steaming bone)*, mobile teeth, hair loss, dryness of the mouth and throat, dizziness, tinnitus and deafness, wasting, insomnia, forgetfulness, while CM tongue and pulse signs are objectively

Table 2 Demography, pre-treatment clinical and CADIA sites profiles of participants

Characteristic	Categories	Placebo (n = 14)	mYJ (n = 11)	Test	Statistics	*P* value
Age	mean ± SD	43.6 ± 7.6	49.0 ± 5.0	*t*	2.0317	0.0539
Smoking habit (self-reported)						
Baseline	Smoked years	22.4 ± 7.7	25.0 ± 8.1	*t*	0.8193	0.4210
	Cigarettes/day	20.0 ± 9.2	22.3 ± 8.2	*t*	0.6502	0.5220
	Pack-years	22.2 ± 11.0	30.2 ± 21.4	*t*	1.2140	0.2371
End of study	Cigarettes/day	18.6 ± 7.6	21.4 ± 7.8	*t*	0.9040	0.3754
Full-mouth parameter						
Standing teeth	mean ± SD	23.1 ± 3.5	21.4 ± 3.2	*t*	1.272	0.2166
Plaque %	mean ± SD	89.4 ± 4.4	88.3 ± 7.1	*t*	0.3991	0.6954
BOP %	mean ± SD	83.7 ± 11.9	86.8 ± 13.2	*t*	0.6085	0.5497
% PPD ≥ 5 mm	mean ± SD	42.7 ± 19.4	44.6 ± 20.1	*t*	0.2382	0.8140
% PAL ≥ 7 mm	mean ± SD	80.6 ± 13.1	73.3 ± 21.0	*t*	1.009	0.3290
CADIA sites (2/participant)						
Tooth type	Incisor	8/0 (8)[a]	6/1 (7)	χ^2	2.487	0.2884
	Canine	7/5 (12)	3/2 (5)			
	Premolar	4/4 (8)	5/5 (10)			
Plaque %		100	100			
BOP %		90.8	96.1	χ^2	1.255	0.2626
PPD	mean ± SD	6.17 ± 1.68	6.33 ± 1.23	*t*	0.592	0.5598
PAL	mean ± SD	9.86 ± 2.23	9.02 ± 1.53	*t*	1.066	0.2977

BOP bleeding on probing, *PAL* probing attachment level, *PPD* probing pocket depth

[a] Upper/lower teeth (total)

accessed (Additional file 2: Table S1). The administration of a placebo during the non-surgical periodontal therapy led to the remission of KYD or SH syndrome in no more than half of the control group participants as early as 2 or 9 months after the commencement of the therapy, respectively. However, the use of mYJ as an adjunctive therapy for the treatment of non-surgical periodontal led to the remission of KYD and SH syndrome in approximately 80 % of the participants evaluated in this trial (Fig. 4). These effects were particularly prominent at 6 and 9 months post-treatment commencement for KYD and SH syndrome, respectively, and remained low at 12 months. Notably, only 1 out of the 14 participants in the control group showed total remission for the CM syndrome of SH/KYD at the end of the study, whereas complete CM syndrome resolutions were observed in 8 out of the 11 participant in the mYJ treatment group (Fig. 4c).

Data pertaining to the selected periodontitis sites evaluated throughout this study are summarized in Fig. 5. Plaque control improved considerably at these periodontitis sites after the therapy, although the reoccurrence of some plaque was observed at the end of the study (i.e., at 12 months). A similar outcome was also observed for the percentage of sites with BOP and PAL. It is noteworthy that the mean depth of selected pockets sites in the mYJ group appeared significantly greater than that of the placebo group ($P = 0.02$, unpaired *t* test, Fig. 5a, b). The GCF volumes (μL/30 s paper strip sampling) of the selected sites remained low after the treatment process (Fig. 5c), with the corresponding GCF volumes of the periodontitis-free sites from the reference teeth on the same participant remained at a low level of 0.018–0.074 μL at every time point. Significant improvements were observed in the changes in the mean CADIA values at selected sites in the mYJ group participants at 12 months (Fig. 5d). Similar improvements were not observed in the control group.

Discussion

Research towards the use of CM as adjunctive therapies in contemporary periodontal treatment appears to progressing slowly [17]. The symptoms of CM syndrome in patients suffering with periodontitis include *stomach-heat, kidney-yin* deficiency and weakness in the *qi* and *blood* [15, 35, 36]. Of the male smokers diagnosed with chronic periodontitis prior to this study, 80 % were also diagnosed with SH and KYD syndrome and were consequently invited to participate in our clinical trial (Fig. 2). Zhang et al. [37] reported that 27.8 % of the participants in their cohort study of 26 mild, 41 moderate and 23 severe conveniently recruited periodontitis participants

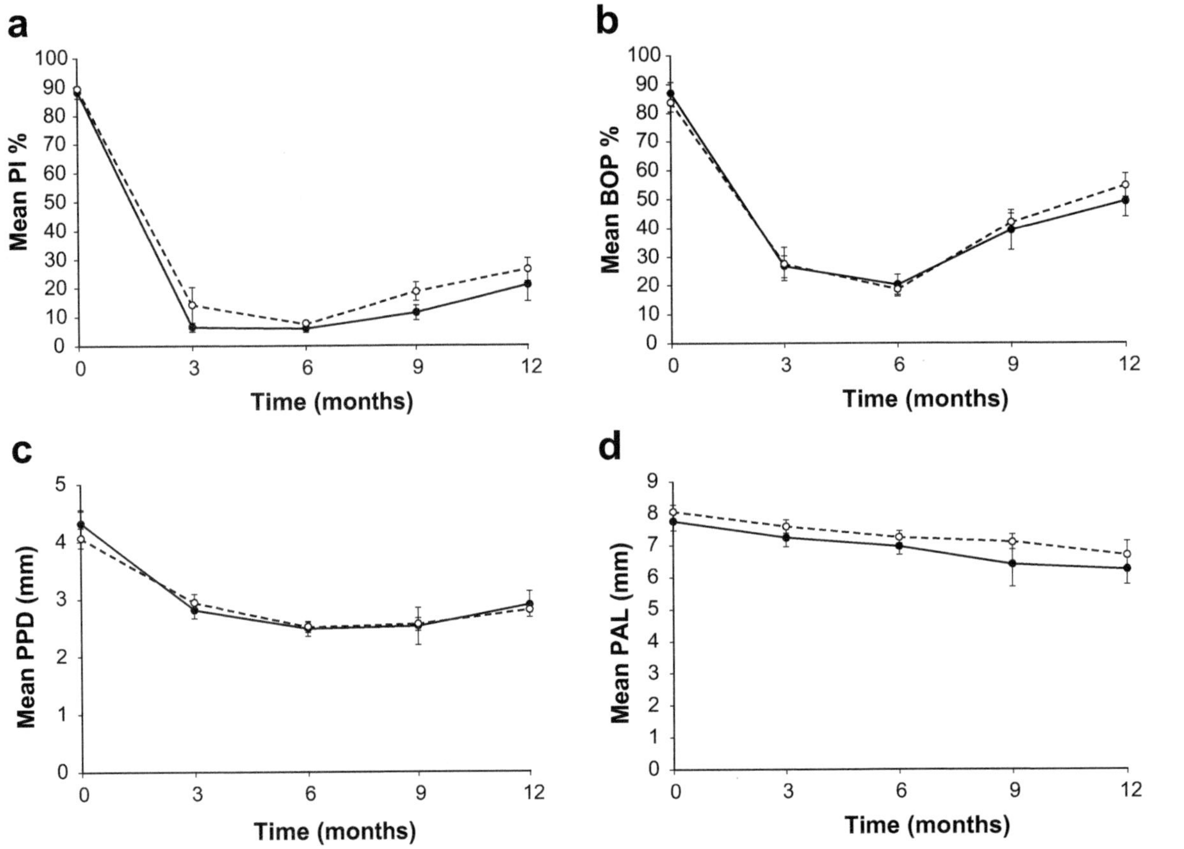

Fig. 3 Mean (±SD) full-mouth periodontal parameters of participants from baseline to 12 months following periodontal treatment commencement. **a** PI %, **b** BOP %, **c** PPD, **d** PAL, *Dashed line* placebo group; *solid line* mYJ group. No difference observable regarding mean PI %, BOP % and PPD between test and control groups at any follow up time point while significant reduction was discernible regarding these three clinical parameters from base-line to all follow ups (**a–c**, $P < 0.01$, repeated measures ANOVA with Dunnett's post-test). No difference observable in mean PAL between test and control groups at any time point and between baseline and all four time points for the test group, or up to 9 months for control group, while significant reduction of mean PAL from baseline was observable at month-12 in control group ($P < 0.01$, repeated measures ANOVA with Dunnett's post-test)

(50 % female, unknown smoking habit) were diagnosed to have SH and KYD. The results of a subsequent study by the same group based on a similar group of conveniently recruited periodontitis patients (52.5 % female, unknown smoking habit) revealed that half of the participants experienced *kidney deficiency* syndrome [35]. Both of these studies showed a lower prevalence of SH and KYD than our current cohort. This difference was attributed to the fact that it was relatively easy to recruit and secure our trial sample size, especially male smokers with severe chronic periodontitis. However, a more in depth population study would be required to fully establish the relationship between severe chronic periodontitis and SH and/or KYD.

This study was therefore deigned to evaluate the effects of mYJ on the proximal periodontal radiographic alveolar bone density using the CADIA values as the primary dependent variable following therapy. In line with results from previous trials involving smokers treated periodontally according to a variety of different approaches [9, 23, 25], we did not expect to see significant differences in the non-radiographic periodontal clinical parameters like PPD reduction or PAL gain in the current small sample of smokers followed, instead CADIA was chosen as the dependent variable.

In general, despite having severe periodontitis, the smokers in the current study exhibited favorable initial periodontal healing in response to non-surgical periodontal therapy, as exemplified by the reduction in their PPD and PAL, which were similar to those reported previously [9]. The favorable clinical responses observed in this case were comparable with those reported in previous studies regarding non-surgical therapy in smokers [9, 38, 39].

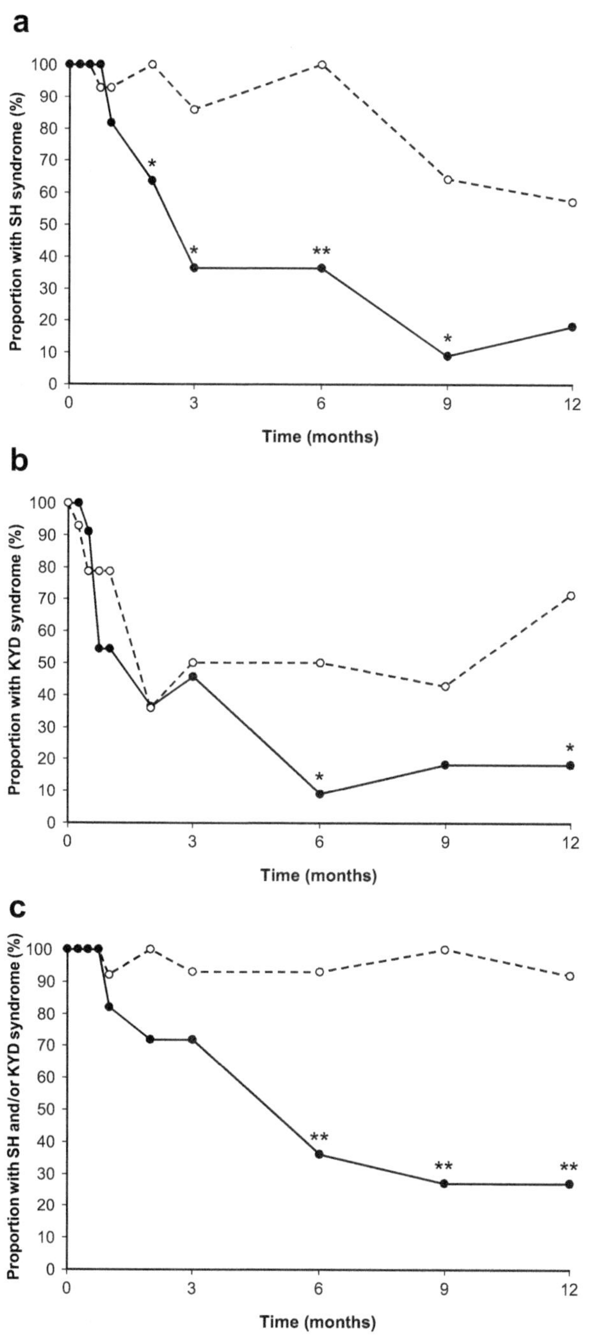

Fig. 4 Proportion of participants with CM *stomach-heat* syndrome and/or *kidney-yin deficiency* over the study period. **a** *Stomach-heat* (SH) syndrome, **b** *Kidney-yin deficiency* (KYD), **c** combined *stomach-heat* and *kidney-yin deficiency*, *Dashed line* placebo group; *solid line* mYJ group. *$P < 0.05$, **$P < 0.001$, control vs. test group at corresponding time point, Fisher exact test. Significant improvement of *stomach-heat*, *kidney-yin deficiency* alone in test or placebo group or *stomach-heat* and/or *kidney-yin deficiency* in test group over time was observed (Chi square test for trend, $P < 0.001$); no such improvement could be observed in control group when combined *stomach-heat* and/or *kidney-yin deficiency* was followed over time (**c**)

Similar to the results of an earlier report [40], our control group of smokers exhibited only minor changes in their amount of radiographic bone density at 12 months after the commencement of non-surgical periodontal therapy compared with the baseline. In contrast, the test participants appeared to maintain the initial bone density gained after the non-surgical periodontal therapy (Fig. 5d). mYJ could therefore maintain the radiographic bone density gained after the non-surgical periodontal therapy for up to 12 month after the commencement of treatment. The control medication, however, did not maintain the radiographic bone density of the smokers 11 months after the periodontal therapy.

An un-blinded study by Luo et al. [41] used a 1 month, twice-daily CM recipe containing 12 different ingredients, including *gypsum fibrosum, Radix et Rhizoma Rehmanniae, Rhizoma Anemarrhenae* and *Cortex Phellodendri* as an adjunctive therapy in a 3-month clinical trial involving non-surgical periodontal therapy on twenty 40–50-year-old females (test group). The control group received non-surgical periodontal therapy without any placebo agent. The authors did not profile the CM status of their participants before and after the study period. Except for a lower BOP % value in the test group at 3 months, the changes in the PAL and PPD values between the two groups were not significant over the study period. One earlier study compared the twice-daily oral administration of a 4 mg dose of *Guchi* pills over 3 months ($n = 50$) with the four-times daily administration of an oral 200 mg dose of spiramycin over 5 days ($n = 40$) as adjunctive agents to non-surgical periodontal therapy [37]. *Guchi* pill contains 18 different ingredients, including *Radix et Rhizoma Rehmanniae, Radix Achyranthis Bidentatae* and *Rhizoma Drynariae,* which are three of the eight active ingredients of mYJ. The study monitored the participants for 24 months after the initiation of the study (i.e., the baseline). The authors reported that participants in the *Guchi* pills and spiramycin groups improved considerably. The 90 participants in this study consisted of a mixture of aggressive and chronic periodontitis patients with mild-to-severe disease at presentation and varied CM syndromes at baseline, including 28 % with SH and KYD. Unfortunately the authors presented limited clinical information, making it difficult to establish the true efficacy of the CM preparation or the spiramycin as adjunctive agents in non-surgical periodontal treatment.

With reference to the literature, purified or enriched extracts from the ingredients of the mYJ preparation used in this study have been independently reported to positively affect bone density in laboratory animals and cell cultures. For example, *Rehmanniae* has been reported to

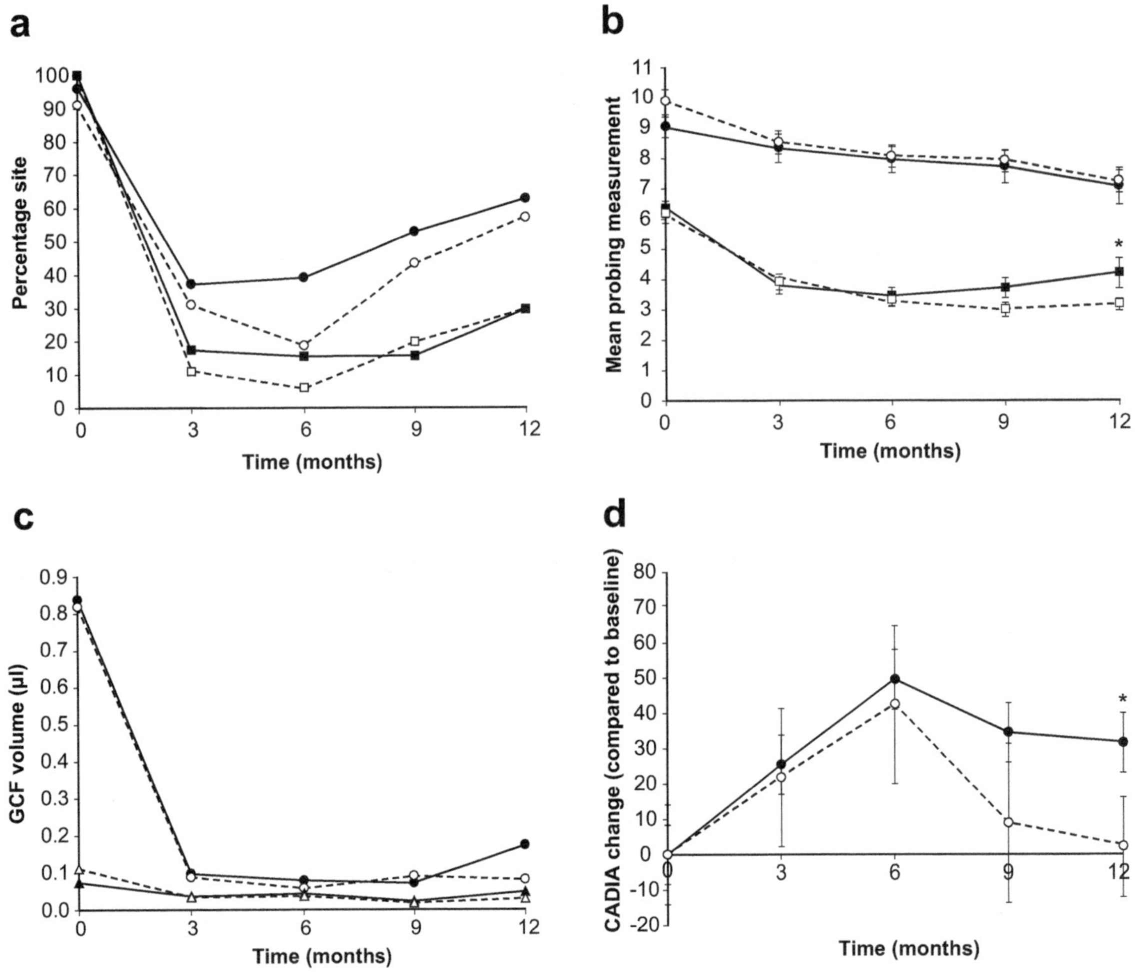

Fig. 5 Mean (±SD) periodontal profiles of periodontitis sites of interest. **a** PI % (*squares*) and BOP % (*circles*), **b** PPD (*squares*) and PAL (*circles*), **c** Gingival crevicular fluid (GCF) volume (μL/30 s) of periodontitis-free (*triangles*) or periodontits (*circles*) sites, and **d** change in CADIA values over the study period. *Dashed line* placebo group; *solid line* mYJ group. Significant difference in CADIA value changes between periodontitis sites in placebo group compared with mYJ group at 12 months (*$P = 0.025$, repeated measures ANOVA with Dunnett's post-test)

stimulate the proliferation of osteoblasts [42]; *Rhizoma Anemarhenae* [43] and *Drynariae Rhizoma* [44] have been reported to promote bone formation; and *Achyranthis bidentatae* [45] and *Puerariae radix* [46] have been reported inhibit bone loss. The remaining ingredients of mYJ including *Phellodendri cortex* and *Ophiopogonis* root have been reported to attenuate bacterial lipopolysaccharide-induced inflammation [47] and protect frog palatal epithelial cells against sodium metabisulphite induced damage [48], respectively. The major alkaloid component of *Phellodendri cortex*, berberine, has been reported to modulate the post-transcriptional regulatory mechanism of the iNOS gene, inhibit the activity of COX-2 and reduce the production of PGE_2 in LPS-stimulated mouse macrophages [49]. *Cortex Phellodendri* and rhizome *Rehmanniae* have been shown to inhibit *Porphyromonas gingivalis* in vitro [50]. The major ingredients in mYJ could potentially attenuate periodontal inflammation and promote bone healing.

The control flavoring agent: *Momordica Charantia* despite having CM *heat* clearing alleviation of dental pain plus hypoglycemic effects [51], was not reported to possess bone cell stimulation functions. The dose and duration use of *Momordica Charantia* administered could not clear the SH of all the periodontitis-affected male smokers.

The fact that 64–73 % of the mYJ group participants remained free from SH and/or KYD syndromes after the 6-month recall in the study indicated that mYJ was effective in alleviating the corresponding syndrome in these smoking periodontitis individuals. The reason why 3-to-4 mYJ group participants continued exhibiting SH and/or KYD syndrome, remains to be elucidated.

The mYJ formula might maintain the improved alveolar bone density from the immediate post-treatment stage up to 12 months, while the positive hard tissue effects detectable on radiographs at selected sites with placebo adjunctive to non-surgical periodontal therapy could only be maintained over the first 6 months. By 9 months, radiographic bone densities of control sites had reverted to the pre-treatment levels.

Conclusions

The adjunctive use of mYJ preserved the post-treatment increases in the radiographic alveolar bone density at the study sites and led to an overall improvement in SH and KYD compared with the controls.

Abbreviations

BOP: bleeding on probing; CADIA: computer-assisted densitometric image analysis; CM: Chinese medicine; DSR: digital subtraction radiography; GCF: gingival crevicular fluid; KYD: *kidney-yin deficiency*; mYJ: modified *Yunu-Jian*; PI %: plaque percentage; PPD: probing pocket depth; PAL: probing attachment level; ROI: regions of interest; SH: *stomach-heat*.

Authors' contributions

KYZ, PSC and JCSH designed the study. KYZ took charge of the randomization and concealment. PSC, JCSH and SMLL collected the data. PSC, JCSH, KYZ and WKL performed the data analysis. PSC, KYZ, EFC and WKL wrote the manuscript. All authors read and approved the final manuscript.

Acknowledgements

The work described in this paper was fully and partially supported by grants from the Chinese Medicine Research Fund, Managing Board, Hong Kong Baptist Hospital (to KYZ), and the Research Grants Council of the Hong Kong Special Administrative Region, China (HKU 772110M, to WKL), respectively. We thank Eu Yan Sang (Hong Kong) Limited for providing and preparing the test (modified *Yunu-Jian*) and placebo CM sachets, and further acknowledge Mr. Shadow K.W. Yeung's assistance in the data analysis.

Competing interests

The authors declare that they have no competing interests.

References

1. Williams RC. Understanding and managing periodontal diseases: a notable past, a promising future. J Periodontol. 2008;79(8 Suppl):1552–9.
2. Ng SKS, Leung WK. A community study on the relationship between stress, coping, affective dispositions and periodontal attachment loss. Community Dent Oral Epidemiol. 2006;34:252–66.
3. Page RC, Kornman KS. The pathogenesis of human periodontitis: an introduction. Periodontol. 2000;1997(14):9–11.
4. Johnson GK, Hill M. Cigarette smoking and the periodontal patient. J Periodontol. 2004;75:196–209.
5. Zee KY. Smoking and periodontal disease. Aust Dent J. 2009;54:44–50.
6. Grossi SG, Zambon JJ, Ho AW, Koch G, Dunfort RG, Machtei EE, Norderyd OM, Genco R. Assessment of risk for periodontal disease. I. Risk indicators for attachment loss. J Periodontol. 1994;65:260–7.
7. Jin L, Wong KY, Leung WK, Corbet EF. Comparison of treatment response patterns following scaling and root planing in smokers and non-smokers with untreated adult periodontitis. J Clin Dent. 2000;11:35–41.
8. Darby I, Hodge PJ, Riggio MP, Kinane DF. Clinical and microbiological effect of scaling and root planing in smoker and non-smoker chronic and aggressive periodontitis patients. J Clin Periodontol. 2005;32:200–6.
9. Wan CP, Leung WK, Wong MC, Wong RM, Wan P, Lo EC, Corbet EF. Effects of smoking on healing response to non-surgical periodontal therapy: a multilevel modelling analysis. J Clin Periodontol. 2009;36:229–39.
10. Machtei EE, Hausmann E, Schmidt M, Grossi SG, Dunford R, Schifferle R, Munoz K, Davies G, Chandler J, Genco RJ. Radiographic and clinical responses to periodontal therapy. J Periodontol. 1998;69:590–5.
11. Flaws B, Sionneau P. The treatment of modern western diseases with Chinese Medicine: a textbook and clinical manual. 2nd ed. Boulder: Blue Poppy Press; 2005. p. 429–34.
12. Gold SI. Periodontics. The past. Part (I). Early sources. J Clin Periodontol. 1985;12:79–97.
13. Wang T. Waitai Miyao. Beijing: People's Medical Publishing House; 752. (Reprinted 1955) (**In Chinese**).
14. Zhao W, Zhao Q. The overview of the prevention and treatment of dental disease in ancient China. Zhonghua Yi Shi Za Zhi. 2009;39:90–2 (**In Chinese**).
15. Zhang J: Jingyue Quan Shu. Beijing: People's Medical Publishing House; 1624. (Reprinted 1991) (**In Chinese**).
16. Wu Y: Bencao Congxin. Shanghai: Shanghai scientific and Technical Publishers; 1886. (Reprinted 2002) (**In Chinese**).
17. Cao CF, Sun XP. Herbal medicine for periodontal diseases. Int Dent J. 1998;48(3 Suppl 1):316–22.
18. Xu ZH. Current status and prospect of prevention and treatment of oral diseases by integrative medicine. Chin J Integr Med. 2006;12:241–3.
19. Wong RWK, Rabie ABM. Traditional Chinese medicines and bone formation—a review. J Oral Maxillofac Surg. 2006;64:828–37.
20. Zhang P, Dai KR, Yan SG, Yan WQ, Zhang C, Chen DQ, Xu B, Xu ZW. Effects of naringin on the proliferation and osteogenic differentiation of human bone mesenchymal stem cell. Eur J Pharmacol. 2009;607(1–3):1–5.
21. Liu ZW. Essentials of Chinese Medicine. London: Springer; 2007.
22. Badersten A, Nilveus R, Egelberg J. Effect of nonsurgical periodontal therapy. II. Severely advanced periodontitis. J Clin Periodontol. 1984;11:63–76.
23. Angaji M, Gelskey S, Nogueira-Filho G, Brothwell D. A systematic review of clinical efficacy of adjunctive antibiotics in the treatment of smokers with periodontitis. J Periodontol. 2010;81:1518–28.
24. Kerdvongbundit V, Wikesjö UME. Effect of triclosan on healing following non-surgical periodontal therapy in smokers. J Clin Periodontol. 2003;30:1024–30.
25. Krohn-Dale I, Bøe OE, Enersen M, Leknes KN. Er:YAG laser in the treatment of periodontal sites with recurring chronic inflammation: a 12-month randomized, controlled clinical trial. J Clin Periodontol. 2012;39:745–52.
26. Lai SML, Zee K-Y, Lai MK, Corbet EF. Clinical and radiographic investigation of the adjunctive effects of a low-power He-Ne laser in the treatment of moderate to advanced periodontal disease: a pilot study. Photomed Laser Surg. 2009;27:287–93.
27. Brägger U, Pasquali L, Rylander H, Carnes D, Kornman KS. Computer-assisted densitometric image analysis in periodontal radiography. A methodological study. J Clin Periodontol. 1988;15:27–37.
28. Hausmann E. Radiographic and digital imaging in periodontal practice. J Periodontol. 2000;71:497–503.
29. Woo BM, Zee KY, Chan FH, Corbet EF. In vitro calibration and validation of a digital subtraction radiography system using scanned images. J Clin Periodontol. 2003;30:114–8.
30. Jiang HL, She B, Liu W, Mao B, Zhang JY. Efficacy and safety of Qi-Wei-Qing-Yan aerosol in treatment of acute pharyngitis (*lung-stomach* excess-heat syndrome): study protocol for a randomized controlled trial. Trials. 2016;17:99.
31. Kadam P, Bhalerao S. Sample size calculation. Int J Ayurveda Res. 2010;1:55–7.
32. Janssen PTM, van Palenstein Helderman WH, van Aken J. The effect of in vivo-occurring errors in the reproducibility of radiographs on the use of the subtraction technique. J Clin Periodontol. 1989;16:53–8.

33. Jin L, Yu C, Corbet EF. Granulocyte elastase activity in static and flow gingival crevicular fluid. J Periodontal Res. 2003;38:303–10.
34. Zhu W, Fan Z, Liu G, Yan J, Zhong T, Zheng W, Wang R, Wang C. Symptom clustering in chronic gastritis based on spectral clustering. J Tradit Chin Med. 2014;34:504–10.
35. Ma Z-J, Zhang J-Z. Changes of serum zinc level of periodontitis patients with kidney deficiency. Chin J Integr Med. 1993;13:606–7.
36. Xu ZX, Peng XZ, Ma HM, Wang X, Liu GX. Relationship between kidney insufficiency and some endocrine hormones in periodontitis patients. Zhonghua Kou Qiang Yi Xue Za Zhi. 1995;30:301–3.
37. Zhang J-Z, Yang X-X, Tong Y-H. Clinical study of combined Gu Chi Wan and spiramycin in the treatment of periodontal disease. Zhongguo Zhong Xi Yi Jie He Za Zhi. 1992;12:83–5 (**In Chinese**).
38. Renvert S, Dahlén G, Wikström M. The clinical and microbiological effects of non-surgical periodontal therapy in smokers and non-smokers. J Clin Periodontol. 1998;25:153–7.
39. Palmer RM, Matthews JP, Wilson RF. Non-surgical periodontal treatment with and without adjunctive metronidazole in smokers and non-smokers. J Clin Periodontol. 1999;26:158–63.
40. Preshaw PM, Heasman PA. Periodontal maintenance in a specialist periodontal clinic and in general dental practice. J Clin Periodontol. 2005;32:280–6.
41. Luo LJ, Gu JJ, Liu XF, Yu J, Shu R. Treatment of chronic periodontitis with traditional Chinese medicine. J Pract Stomatol. 2004;20:737–9 (**in Chinese**).
42. Oh KO, Kim SW, Kim JY, Ko SY, Kim HM, Baek JH, Ryoo HM, Kim JK. Effect of *Rehmannia glutinosa Libosch* extracts on bone metabolism. Clin Chim Acta. 2003;334:185–95.
43. Nian H, Qin LP, Chen WS, Zhang QY, Zheng HC, Wang Y. Protective effect of steroidal saponins from rhizome of *Anemarrhena asphodeloides* on ovariectomy-induced bone loss in rats. Acta Pharmacol Sin. 2006;27:728–34.
44. Wong RW, Rabie B, Bendeus M, Hägg U. The effects of *Rhizoma Curculiginis* and *Rhizoma Drynariae* extracts on bones. Chin Med. 2007;2:13.
45. He CC, Hui RR, Tezuka Y, Kadota S, Li JX. Osteoprotective effect of extract from *Achyranthes bidentata* in ovariectomized rats. J Ethnopharmacol. 2010;127:229–34.
46. Wang X, Wu J, Chiba H, Yamada K, Ishimi Y. *Puerariae radix* prevents bone loss in castrated male mice. Metabolism. 2005;54:1536–41.
47. Mao YF, Li YQ, Zong L, You XM, Lin FQ, Jiang L. Methanol extract of *Phellodendri cortex* alleviates lipopolysaccharide-induced acute airway inflammation in mice. Immunopharmacol Immunotoxicol. 2010;32:110–5.
48. O'Brien DW, Morris MI, Lee MS, Tai S, King M. *Ophiopogon* root (*Radix Ophiopogonis*) prevents ultra-structural damage by SO_2 in an epithelial injury model for studies of mucociliary transport. Life Sci. 2004;74:2413–22.
49. Lee DU, Kang YJ, Park MK, Lee YS, Seo HG, Kim TS, Kim CH, Chang KC. Effects of 13-alkyl-substituted berberine alkaloids on the expression of COX-II, TNF-α, iNOS, and IL-12 production in LPS-stimulated macrophages. Life Sci. 2003;73:1401–12.
50. Wong RW, Hägg U, Samaranayake LP, Yuen MKZ, Seneviratne CJ, Kao R. Antimicrobial activity of Chinese medicine herbs against common bacteria in oral biofilm. A pilot study. Int J Oral Maxillofac Surg. 2010;39:599–605.
51. Basch E, Gabardi S, Ulbricht C. Bitter melon (*Momordica charantia*): a review of efficacy and safety. Am J Health Syst Pharm. 2003;60:356–9.

6

Apoptosis-inducing effects of jujube (*Zǎo*) seed extracts on human Jurkat leukemia T cells

Natthanan Taechakulwanijya[1], Natthida Weerapreeyakul[2*], Sahapat Barusrux[3] and Sirithorn Siriamornpun[4]

Abstract

Background: Jujube (*Zǎo*) seeds exhibited anticancer effects and used in Chinese medicine for many years. This study aims to investigate the apoptosis-inducing effects of seed extracts from eight different cultivated species ('Apple', 'Bombay', 'Jumbo', 'Kaew', 'Nomsod', 'Rianthong', 'Samros', and 'Taiwan') on human Jurkat leukemia T cells.

Methods: We evaluated the effects of seed extracts from eight jujube cultivated species on human Jurkat leukemia T cells. The crude seed extracts were prepared sequentially by using water, 95 % ethanol, dichloromethane, ethyl acetate, chloroform or hexane. The antiproliferative effects of the jujube seed extracts relative to that of melphalan were evaluated by neutral red assays. Apoptotic cell death induced by the ethanolic extracts at 1 × IC_{50} and 2 × IC_{50} concentrations was demonstrated by DAPI staining, gel electrophoresis, flow cytometry with Annexin V/propidium iodide staining, and caspase-3, -8, and -9 enzyme activities.

Results: Ethanolic extracts of 'Taiwan', 'Jumbo', 'Nomsod', 'Rianthong', 'Samros', and 'Bombay', significantly inhibited the proliferation of Jurkat cells compared with untreated cells (all $P < 0.001$), while the extracts of 'Kaew' and 'Apple' were inactive. The six active extracts preferentially induced apoptotic cell death in a concentration-dependent manner with DNA fragmentation (2 × IC_{50}). Increased caspase-3 activity was detected after treatment with the six extracts. The 'Taiwan', 'Nomsod', 'Jumbo', and 'Rianthong' extracts (2 × IC_{50}) induced both the extrinsic and intrinsic apoptosis pathways by increasing caspase-8 and caspase-9 activity, respectively. Alkaloids (Dragendorff's method) and reducing sugars (Fehling's test) were mainly identified in the apoptosis-inducing extracts.

Conclusions: The tested of six active extracts ('Taiwan', 'Jumbo', 'Nomsod', 'Rianthong', 'Samros' and 'Bombay') contained alkaloids or reducing sugars, and induced caspase-dependent apoptosis in human Jurkat leukemia T cells.

Keywords: Jujube, Apoptosis, Jurkat leukemia T cells, Cancer

Background

Complementary and alternative medicines have been evaluated in addition to chemotherapy, radiation, and surgery in treating cancer. The development of an effective strategy for cancer drug discovery has been outlined [1]. Apoptosis is a major target for chemoprevention and chemotherapy [2].

Jujube (*Zǎo*) is a functional food with nutritional value that is consumed in Asia, the Mediterranean and the United States [3–6]. The two extant species include Indian jujube (*Ziziphus mauritiana* Lam.) and Chinese jujube (*Ziziphus jujuba* Mill.) [4], and were reported to exhibit sedative, anodyne, pectoral, stomachic, styptic, and tonic effects [7], as well as anticancer, antianxiolytic, antifungal, and antispastic effects [8].

Different parts of *Z. mauritiana* and *Z. jujuba* exhibit various medicinal effects. *Z. jujuba* has long been used as a crude drug in Chinese medicine [5]. The seeds of *Z. jujuba* enhanced cell membrane permeability for drugs [9] and exhibited sedative effects [10]. Linoleic and stearic acids from seed extracts of *Z. jujuba* significantly inhibited cyclooxygenase (COX)-1 and COX-2 activity

*Correspondence: natthida@kku.ac.th
[2] Faculty of Pharmaceutical Sciences, Khon Kaen University, Khon Kaen 40002, Thailand
Full list of author information is available at the end of the article

[11]. The fruits of *Z. jujuba* activated choline acetyltransferase and increased acetylcholine synthesis [12], through both antioxidant [13, 14] and anti-allergenic [15] effects. Triterpenoids from the leaves of *Z. jujuba* were sweetness inhibitors [16]. The leaves of *Z. mauritiana* protected the liver from alcohol damage [17]. The bark of *Z. mauritiana* possessed both antiulcer [18] and antifertility [19] activities. The roots of *Z. mauritiana* exhibited antifungal [20] and antidiarrheal [21] activities. The functional constituents of jujube possessed anticancer activity [22]. *Z. jujuba* fruits induced apoptosis in liver (HepG2) and breast (MCF-7 and KBR3) cancer cell lines [7, 23]. The seeds of *Z. mauritiana* induced apoptosis in promyelocytic leukemia cells (HL-60) [24].

New jujube hybrids are crossbred from the two varieties (*Z. jujuba* and *Z. mauritiana*). Presently, many new cultivated varieties are available in Thailand and independently exhibit various biological functions [25–27]. Evidence of changes in phytoconstituents between the wild-type plants and new cultivars has been reported [28, 29]. The metabolites found in the leaves of new carrot cultivars possessed higher contents of feruloyl acid, quinic acid, malic acid, and leucine, but lower contents of glucose and sucrose than the wild-type (*Z. mauritiana*) [28]. A new peanut cultivar possessed higher 4α-monomethylsterol contents, but lower 4-desmethylsterol and triterpene alcohol contents than the wild-type plant [29].

This study aims to investigate the apoptosis-inducing effects of seed extracts from eight different jujube cultivated species ('Apple', 'Bombay', 'Jumbo', 'Kaew', 'Nomsod', 'Rianthong', 'Samros', and 'Taiwan') on human Jurkat leukemia T cells. The anticancer activities were evaluated based on the cytotoxicity and apoptosis-inducing effects on human Jurkat leukemia T cells, relative to melphalan as a positive control. Nuclear morphological changes and caspase-mediated apoptosis were determined. Phytochemical groups in the seed extracts were identified.

Methods

Chemicals and reagents

Methanol, isopropanol, dichloromethane, ethyl acetate, chloroform, and hexane were purchased from RCI Labscan Ltd., Thailand, and 95 % ethanol from J.T. Baker® (Center Valley, PA, USA). Sodium hydroxide, citric acid and hydrochloric acid were obtained from BDH Prolabo chemicals (Poole, UK) Neutral red and 4-(p-nitrobenzyl) pyridine (NBP) and acetonitrile were obtained from Sigma-Aldrich® (St. Louis, MO, USA). Melphalan, 4,6-diamidino-2-phenylindole (DAPI), copper (II) sulfate were from Sigma-Aldrich Chemie GmbH (Munich, Germany). Dulbecco's modified Eagle medium (DMEM), RPMI Media 1640, fetal bovine serum and penicillin streptomycin were from GIBCO, Invitrogen Corp. (Grand Island, NY, USA). Sodium chloride and boric acid were from Vivantis Inc., (Oceanside, CA, USA). Dimethylsullfoxide (DMSO) (molecular grade) was from Sigma-Aldrich Chemie GmbH (Saint-Quentin Fallavier, France). Trypan blue was from Fluka Chemika (Buchs, Switzerland) and potassium sodium tartrate was from Loba Chemie (Mumbai, India). Agarose molecular grade was purchased from Bio-Rad (Hercules, CA, USA). A 100 bp DNA ladder marker was purchased from Invitrogen (Carlsbad, CA, USA). Caspase-Glo® 3/7, 8 and 9 were purchased from Promega (Madison, WI, USA).

Preparation of crude extracts

Eight jujube cultivated species ('Apple', 'Bombay', 'Jumbo', 'Kaew', 'Nomsod', 'Rianthong', 'Samros' and 'Taiwan') were commercially cultivated and authenticated based on fruit and seed morphological characters by Assistant Professor Thaweesak Thitimetharoch, Division of Pharmacognosy and Toxicology, Faculty of Pharmaceutical Sciences, Khon Kaen University. The jujubes were collected from the local market in Amphoe Muang, Khon Kaen, Thailand, in 2012. The picture vouchers of the specimens (NW-55-2012–NW-62-2012) were deposited at the herbarium of the Faculty of Pharmaceutical Sciences, Khon Kaen University, Khon Kaen province, Thailand. The seed characteristics of each jujube cultivated species (five samples for each) are presented in Fig. 1. The seed was separated and dried at ≤ 55 °C. The seeds were macerated in deionized water (1 g:3 mL) overnight. The water crude extract was collected after being freeze-dried. The remaining residue from water extraction was dried at 55 °C and further macerated with 95 % ethanol, dichloromethane, ethyl acetate, chloroform or hexane, respectively. Each round of solvent extraction lasted 72 h, using different dry residue to solvent ratios (1 g:3 mL). Solvent was removed by a rotary evaporator (IKA®, Staufen, Germany), resulting in a dry residue. Six types of crude extract were obtained for each cultivars. The crude extracts were stored at −20 °C. The concentrations of 10, 25, 50, 100, 250 and 500 μg/mL were used in the antiproliferation study.

Cell culture

The human Jurkat leukemia T cells were cultured in RPMI 1640 media while the normal African green monkey kidney epithelial cell line (Vero) was cultured in DMEM. Both cell lines were provided by Associate Professor Sahapat Barusrux. Both media were maintained with 10 % fetal bovine serum and 1 % penicillin–streptomycin. Cells were incubated at 37 °C and 5 % CO_2.

Cultivated species	Seeds characteristics (n=5)	
'Samros'	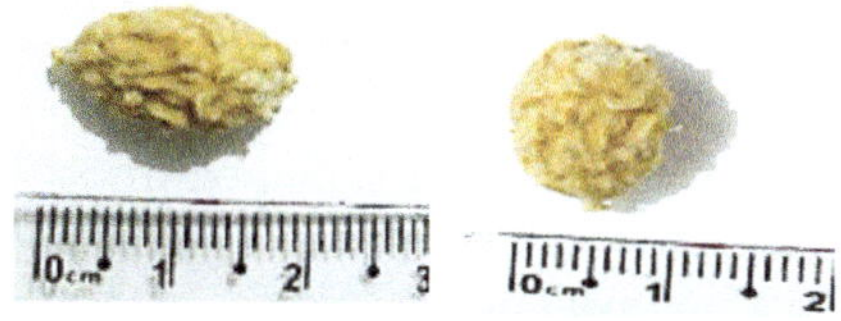	0.86 ±0.18 cm wide × 1.58 ±0.19 cm long, round shape, light brown
'Bombay'	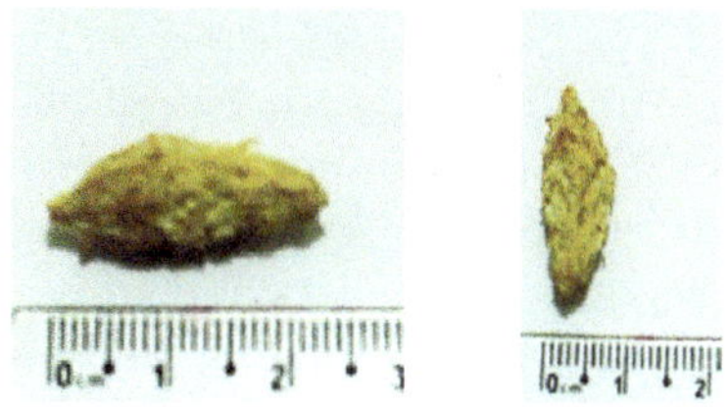	0.66±0.11 cm wide × 2.4±0.12 cm long, ovate, tapered at both ends, pale yellow
'Apple'	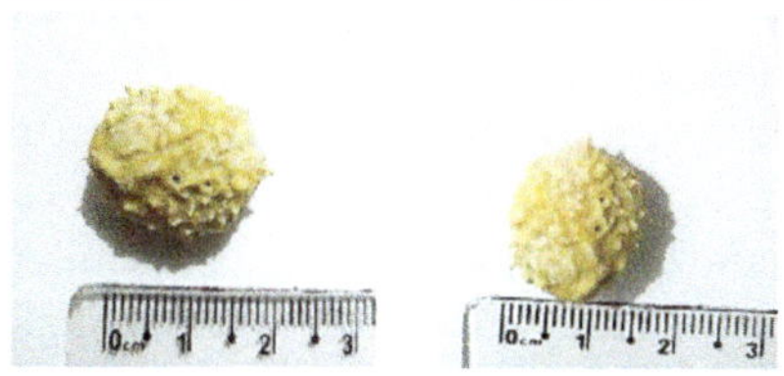	1.1±0.11 cm wide × 1.5±0.18 cm long, round shape, rough surface with tiny spines, off-white
'Taiwan'	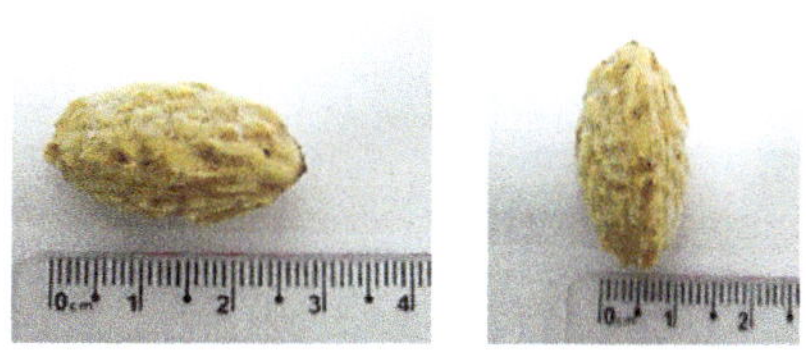	1.04 ±0.11 cm wide × 2.94 ±0.19 cm long, ovate, pale yellow
'Nomsod'	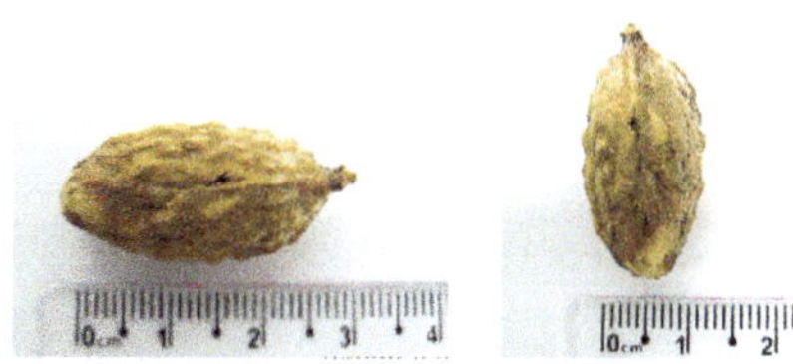	1.12±0.21 cm wide × 2.6±0.21 cm long, ovate, light brown
'Jumbo'	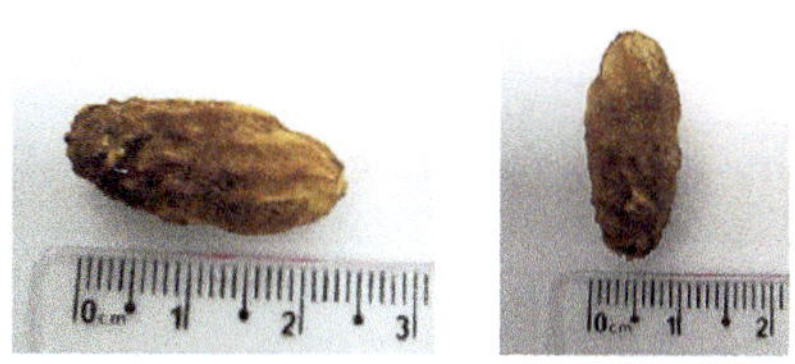	1.1±0.15 cm wide × 2.52±0.16 cm long, ovate, brown
'Kaew'	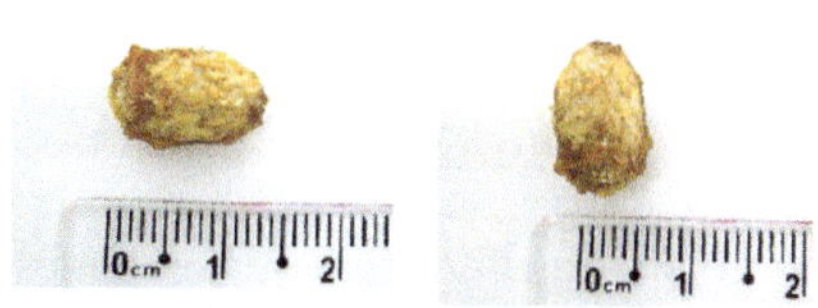	0.54 ±0.11 cm wide × 1.16±0.21 cm long, ovate, light brown
'Rianthong'	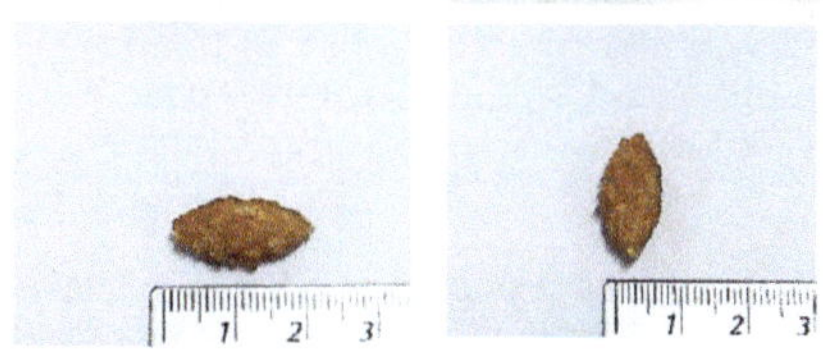	0.6±0,12 cm wide × 1.7±0,16 cm long, ovate, brown

Fig. 1 Characteristics of jujube seeds

Antiproliferation assay

The antiproliferation test was determined based on modified neutral red assay [30]. A Jurkat cell density of 5×10^5 cells/mL and Vero 3×10^5 cells/mL were seeded in 96-well plates and maintained at 37 °C for 24 h in humidified 5 % CO_2. The extracts dissolved in DMSO were pipetted into each well to generate various final concentrations ranging between 10 and 500 µg/mL. The final concentration of DMSO did not exceed 1 % v/v to minimize the cytotoxic effect of DMSO [30]. After treatment with the extracts for 24 h, cells were re-suspended. Neutral red dyes (50 µg/mL) were added to each well. Cells were incubated for another 2 h, then washed with 1 × PBS (pH 7.4) and lysed with 0.33 % HCl in isopropanol. The absorbance of viable cells and dye solution was measured at 537 nm (650 nm reference wavelength) by a microplate reader (TECAN, Grödig, Austria). The untreated cells comprised the control group and cells treated with alkylating drug melphalan are the positive control. A plot of %cell viability and various extract concentrations was used to calculate the IC_{50}—which represents the concentration possessing 50 % antiproliferation. The selectivity index (SI) was calculated from the IC_{50} of the extracts in normal Vero cells over the Jurkat cancer cells to indicate the cytotoxic selectivity (i.e., safety) of the crude extracts [31].

Detection of apoptosis

Nuclear morphological alteration

Morphological changes in cell nuclei undergoing apoptosis was determined by DAPI staining [32]. The stained nuclei were then detected by a fluorescent microscope (Nikon Eclipse 80i, Kanagawa, Japan). Cells were seeded in 24-well plates at a density of 3×10^5 cells/mL per well and incubated for 24 h. Cells were treated with 500 µg/mL extracts and incubated for another 24 h. Then cells were washed with PBS and collected by centrifugation (Daihan Scientific, Seoul, Korea) at 1677*g* for 5 min. Cells were fixed in ice-cold methanol for 15 min. After the methanol was removed, the cells were incubated for 30 min, at room temperature, in the dark, with 0.3 µg/mL DAPI. The mixture of PBS to glycerin (at a 1:1 ratio) was added to achieve a 20-µL volume. Cells were wet-mounted on a glass slide and observed under a fluorescent microscope by fluorescence filters with an excitation band of 358 nm and an emission of 461 nm. The images of stained nuclei were captured by the NIS-Element AR 3.2 imaging software (Nikon Instruments Inc, NY, USA).

Mode of cell death

Flow cytometry was used to determine various types of cell death including early and late stage apoptosis as well as necrosis. Annexin V-FITC and propidium iodide (Annexin V-FITC apoptosis detection kit, eBiosciences, Inc., San Diego, CA, USA) [33]. Cells were seeded in 24-well plates at a density of 5×10^5 cells/ml per well and incubated for 24 h. Cells were treated with the crude extracts at a concentration of $1 \times IC_{50}$ and $2 \times IC_{50}$, obtained from the antiproliferation study at 12 and 24 h. Afterward, cells were harvested by centrifugation (Wisds' Laboratory Instruments, Korea) at 1677*g* for 5 min then the supernatant was removed. The cells were washed with 200 µL of 1x binding buffer. After removal of the supernatant, 95 µL of binding buffer and 5 µL Annexin V-FITC were added and the mixture incubated in the dark for 15 min at room temperature. Then 95 µL of binding buffer and 5 µL of propidium iodide (final concentration of 2 µg/mL per cell sample) were pipetted into an Eppendrof tube and the mixture incubated for 15 min in the dark at the room temperature. Cells were re-suspended in 200 µL of binding buffer. The stained cells were analyzed immediately by flow cytometry (BD FACSCanto II, Franklin Lakes, NJ, USA) by FACSDiva software version 6.1.3 (BD Biosciences, San Jose, CA, USA).

Caspases activity

The activity of caspase-3/7, -8 and -9 were evaluated to confirm whether apoptosis was induced by the jujube seed extract(s) and to determine the apoptosis induction pathway. Jurkat cells (1.3×10^4 cells/well) were seeded into 96-well white plates (Costar™, Corning, NY, USA). Cells were incubated at 37 °C for 24 h and extracts added to each well for a final concentration of $2 \times IC_{50}$. Treated cells were incubated at various intervals. Supernatant (50 mL) was pipetted out of each well and 50 µL of caspase reagent mixture added and incubated in the dark for 40 min [34]. The relative luminescence units (RLU) were measured at 562 nm by a Multifunction Microplate Reader (Varioskan™ Flash Multimode Reader, Thermo Scientific, USA) equipped with SkanIt Software 2.4.3 DDE's program (Thermo Scientific, Waltham, MA USA).

DNA fragmentation

Late stage apoptotic death mode was confirmed by a DNA fragment assay. Cells (2×10^6 cells/mL density) were seeded in 24-well plates and incubated for 24 h. Cells were treated with the jujube seed extracts as described above in the cell death mode assay. Cells were harvested and washed with PBS. After PBS was removed, 300 µL of lysis buffer (FlexiGenen DNA kit; Qiagen, Germany) was added to each well and mixed thoroughly. After that 150 µL of denaturation buffer and 20 µL of Protease K (10 mg/mL) were added to the reaction mixture. Cells were incubated at 65 °C for 15 min and 600 µL of absolute isopropanol added and thoroughly mixed until the DNA became visible. DNA was collected after centrifugation (Daihan Scientific, Seoul, Korea) at 10,000*g* for 5 min. The supernatant was discarded and the pellet washed with 70 % ethanol. After the liquid was removed by inverting the Eppendrof tube onto a clean piece of paper, 15 μL of hydration buffer was added to dissolve the DNA for 15 min at 65 °C. The resulting 300 ng/μL of DNA (DNA counting by GE healthcare Life Sciences, United Kingdom) was analyzed by electrophoresis on 1.8 % agarose gels containing 0.75 % ethidium bromide. The DNA was mixed with 6× loading dye and the gel was electrophoresed in 0.5xTBE buffer at 90 V for 1 min and 50 V for 1 h. DNA fragmentation was visualized by a UV transilluminator (Vilberlourmat, Germany) and the image was captured.

Alkylating reaction in vitro

An alkylation reaction of the jujube seed extract was performed to understand the interaction of the extract with DNA resulting DNA damage. The alkylation assay was conducted following the method modified by Machana et al. [30]. NBP (final concentration 20 mM) was prepared in acetonitrile. The buffer solution (pH 4) comprised 0.5 μM of citric acid, 1 μM of boric acid, 4.9 μM of sodium chloride, and 1 M sodium hydroxide adjusted to a volume of 10 mL with deionized water. The mixture of 180 μL NBP and 420 μL buffer solution was prepared and heated to 70 °C for 30 min. The extracts at 2 × IC_{50} concentrations dissolved in acetonitrile were pipetted into the NBP mixture. Then, 120 μL of solution mixture was pipetted and added into a 160 μL ethanol–acetonitrile mixture at a ratio of 1:3. The wavelength of NBP adduct was measured at 580 nm at different time points (5, 15, 30, 45, 60 and 75 min).

Phytochemicals screening

Phytochemical screening was performed to identify the presence of the main phytoconstituents in 0.025 g of jujube seed extract of each cultivar. Identification of alkaloids, saponins and carbohydrates were tested as per Anandanayaki [35], while identification of flavonoids was conducted as per Bello et al. [36].

Alkaloids identification

Jujube seed extracts were dissolved in 500 μL of methanol and centrifuged (Daihan Scientific, Seoul, Korea) at 268.3*g* for 10 min. HCl (1 %, 1 mL) and 1 drop of Dragendorff's reagent (potassium bismuth iodide) was added to the supernatant. An orange or reddish-brown precipitate indicated a positive test.

Flavonoids identification

Methanol (2.5 mL) and 0.5 mL of 10 % NaOH were added to the extracts. A few drop of 1 % HCl was added to 0.5 ml of supernatant. The disappearance of the yellow color indicated the presence of flavonoids.

Saponins identification

The extracts were diluted with deionized water to a final volume of 1.5 mL and shaken for 30 min. Permanent foamation indicated the presence of saponins.

Reducing sugar identification

Fehling's solution A was prepared by dissolving 3.5 g of copper II sulfate in deionized water and adjusted to 50 mL. Fehling's solution B was prepared by dissolving 17.5 g potassium sodium tartrate with 5 g sodium hydroxide in 50 mL of deionized water. The extracts were diluted in 1.5 mL of deionized water, heated with Fehling's A and B solution (mixture 1:1) for 10 min. An orange-red precipitate indicated a positive result and the presence of reducing sugar.

Statistical analysis

The results from multiple independent experiments were expressed as mean ± standard deviation. One-way ANOVA was used to test for significant differences between means. $P < 0.05$ was considered statistically significant. The variation between groups was tested by the Tukey range test with IBM SPSS software version 19.0 (SPSS Inc., USA). The concentration- and time-dependence shown in the graphs was visually determined.

Results and discussion

Characteristics of seeds

The eight jujube cultivars had diverse seed characteristics (Fig. 1). Generally, the cultivars had different shapes, sizes, and gnarled seed surfaces, with the average width and length being 0.5 cm and 1.6 cm, respectively. The 'Nomsod' and 'Taiwan' cultivars had the largest seed sizes, while the 'Kaew' cultivar had the smallest.

Antiproliferative effects

The antiproliferative effects of seed extracts from the eight jujube cultivars were evaluated on the leukemic Jurkat cell line, in comparison with the non-cancer Vero cell line, by neutral red assays (Table 1). The cationic neutral red dye can penetrate through cell membranes and lysosomal membranes to attach to anionic charges in the lysosomal matrix of living cells [37].

The antiproliferative effects were represented as IC_{50} values calculated from linear plots between the concentrations and the %cell viability. Extracts with the maximum concentration (500 μg/mL) that inhibited cell viability by <50 % were classified as inactive extracts [30]. Seeds extracted using water, dichloromethane, ethyl acetate, or hexane inhibited Jurkat cell viability by <50 %

Table 1 Antiproliferative activity of different jujube seed extracts on non-cancer Vero cell line and T cell leukemic Jurkat cell line evaluated by the NR assay for 24 h incubation

Sample	IC_{50} (μg/mL)												Selectivity index
	Vero cell line						Jurkat cell line						
	Water	Ethanol	Dichloro-methane	Ethyl acetate	Chloroform	Hexane	Water	Ethanol	Dichloro-methane	Ethyl acetate	Chloroform	Hexane	
'Samros'	Inactive	Inactive	Inactive	nd	nd	nd	Inactive	417.7 ± 10.4^{b}	Inactive	nd	nd	nd	1.0
'Bombay'	Inactive	Inactive	Inactive	Inactive	Inactive	Inactive	Inactive	487.9 ± 17.5^{a}	Inactive	Inactive	Inactive	Inactive	1.0
'Apple'	Inactive	Inactive	Inactive	Inactive	Inactive	Inactive	Inactive	Inactive	Inactive	Inactive	Inactive	Inactive	nd
'Taiwan'	Inactive	Inactive	Inactive	Inactive	nd	inactive	Inactive	232.4 ± 7.8^{d}	Inactive	Inactive	nd	Inactive	2.1
'Nomsod'	Inactive	Inactive	Inactive	Inactive	nd	Inactive	Inactive	333.4 ± 2.8^{c}	Inactive	Inactive	nd	Inactive	1.0
'Jumbo'	Inactive	Inactive	Inactive	Inactive	nd	Inactive	Inactive	312.0 ± 18.3^{c}	Inactive	Inactive	nd	Inactive	1.6
'Kaew'	Inactive	Inactive	Inactive	Inactive	Inactive	Inactive	Inactive	Inactive	Inactive	Inactive	Inactive	Inactive	nd
'Rianthong'	Inactive	Inactive	Inactive	Inactive	nd	Inactive	Inactive	401.6 ± 9.9^{b}	Inactive	Inactive	nd	Inactive	1.2
Melphalan	75.0 ± 2.3							119.1 ± 10.4^{e}					0.6

Data presented as IC_{50} values and selectivity index in Jurkat cell line ($n = 3$)

Means in the same column with different superscript letter(s) are significantly different, $P < 0.05$ (one-way ANOVA). Inactive means at the extract caused <50 % cytotoxicity even using the maximum concentration at 500 μg/mL

nd not determined due to their low yield

even when the maximum concentration of 500 μg/mL was used. Therefore, these solvent extracts were defined as inactive against both Jurkat and Vero cell lines. The ethanolic extract of 'Taiwan' (232.4 ± 7.8 μg/mL) exhibited the highest antiproliferative effect, followed by the ethanolic extracts of 'Jumbo' (312.2 ± 18.3 μg/mL), 'Nomsod' (333.4 ± 2.8 μg/mL), 'Rianthong' (401.6 ± 9.9 μg/mL), 'Samros' (417.7 ± 10.4 μg/mL), and 'Bombay' (487.9 ± 17.5 μg/mL). These six ethanolic extracts showed significant antiproliferative effects compared with the untreated cells (all $P < 0.001$). The antiproliferative effects of individual pairs of 'Jumbo' vs. 'Nomsod' ($P = 0.322$) and 'Samros' vs. 'Rianthong' ($P = 0.841$) did not differ significantly. The chemotherapeutic drug melphalan, used as the positive control, showed nonselective antiproliferative effects on Jurkat cells over Vero cells with IC_{50} values of 119.1 ± 10.4 μg/mL vs. 75.0 ± 2.3 μg/mL, respectively. Although the IC_{50} values of the ethanolic extracts were higher than those of melphalan (i.e., lesser antiproliferative effects) (all $P < 0.001$), the selectivity index of the ethanolic extracts toward Jurkat cells was higher than that of melphalan.

The antiproliferative effects of the ethanolic extracts of the jujube seeds on normal cells were in agreement with previous studies [23, 24, 38]. Ethanolic extracts of *Z. mauritiana* seeds showed antiproliferative effects on HL-60, HeLa, and Molt-4 cell lines without affecting the normal HGF cell line [24], and exerted no cytotoxicity on normal rat liver cells [38]. A chloroform extract of *Z. jujuba* fruit pulp showed antiproliferative effects on MCF-7 and SKBR3 cells without toxicity on normal cells [23]. The present study documented the nonselective cytotoxicity of chloroform seed extracts on Jurkat cells. Owing to the low yields of some chloroform extracts, their cytotoxicity was not determined. Six of the eight ethanolic extracts (i.e., 'Samros', 'Bombay', 'Taiwan', 'Nomsod', 'Jumbo', and 'Rianthong') were selected to determine the mode of cell death.

Apoptosis morphological changes

As shown in Fig. 2a, the normal nuclei of untreated cells had an intact round morphology, whereas the apoptotic nuclei of cells treated with 500 μg/mL melphalan showed chromatin condensation with heterogeneous staining (Fig. 2b, c) and apoptotic body formation (Fig. 2d). The nuclear morphologies of Jurkat cells treated with the ethanolic seed extracts (500 μg/mL) for 24 h were shown in Fig. 2e. The six ethanolic jujube seed extracts induced apoptosis with nuclear morphological changes reminiscent of apoptotic characteristics (i.e., cell shrinkage, chromatin condensation, membrane blebbing, and apoptotic body formation).

Mode of cell death

The stages of apoptosis can be differentiated from necrotic cell death by flow cytometry using Annexin V-FITC/propidium iodide (PI) staining of cells. Apoptotic lymphocytes are identified by their externalized phosphatidylserine (PS) bound with Annexin V-FITC (green), while necrotic cells are identified by their DNA intercalation of PI (red) [39]. During the early stages of apoptosis, the PS comprising the cell membrane flip to the outside and bind with Annexin V-FITC, showing a cell dot plot in quadrant 4. Damaged or injured cells lose their membrane integrity, including nuclear membrane integrity, such that PI can pass through the nuclear membrane and appear in quadrant 1 (necrotic cells). In the late stages of apoptosis, cells are double-stained and appear in quadrant 2. Normal cells are not stained and appear in quadrant 3.

The ethanolic jujube seed extracts induced cell death in a concentration- and time-dependent manner through diverse modes of cell death (Fig. 3). In general, the extracts induced relatively high late-stage apoptosis and low necrosis compared with melphalan, which induced more early-stage apoptosis. After incubation for 12 h, the 2 × IC_{50} concentrations of 'Bombay' (99.2 ± 0.4 %), 'Samros' (95.1 ± 1.8 %), and 'Nomsod' (90.2 ± 2.7 %) were the first three extracts to induce high total apoptosis (>90 %) in Jurkat cells. The total apoptosis inductions for 'Bombay' vs. 'Samros' ($P = 0.988$), 'Bombay' vs. 'Nomsod' ($P = 0.928$), and 'Samros' vs. 'Nomsod' ($P = 0.050$) did not differ significantly. Under the same conditions (12 h, 2 × IC_{50}), only 'Samros' (29.9 ± 2.6 %) ($P = 0.004$) and 'Bombay' (20.9 ± 1.4 %) ($P < 0.001$) significantly induced higher %early-stage apoptosis than melphalan (10.7 ± 0.4 %). By contrast, the 2 × IC_{50} concentrations of 'Nomsod' (79.2 ± 3.0 %) ($P < 0.001$), 'Bombay' (78.3 ± 1.6 %) ($P < 0.001$), and 'Samros' (65.2 ± 1.2 %) ($P < 0.001$) caused more significant late-stage apoptosis than melphalan (3.5 ± 0.3 %) and the other extracts.

At 24 h, the 2 × IC_{50} concentration of 'Bombay' showed the highest %total apoptosis (97.3 ± 2.9 %) followed by those of 'Jumbo' (93.7 ± 2.4 %), 'Nomsod' (86.0 ± 1.9 %), 'Samros' (80.1 ± 3.2 %), 'Rianthong' (53.9 ± 2.6 %), melphalan (51.6 ± 1.1 %), and 'Taiwan' (45.8 ± 3.0 %). Only the 2 × IC_{50} concentration of 'Bombay' (46.1 ± 2.5 %) ($P < 0.001$) was found to induce early-stage apoptosis significantly more than melphalan (35.0 ± 2.2 %). Furthermore, the first three jujube seed extracts that induced high %late-stage apoptosis were 'Jumbo' (80.8 ± 0.8 %), 'Nomsod' (75.8 ± 2.3 %), and 'Bombay' (51.2 ± 3.7). The %late-stage apoptosis for 'Jumbo' vs. 'Nomsod' did not differ significantly ($P = 0.599$, one-way ANOVA), while the %late-stage apoptosis of 'Jumbo' and 'Nomsod'

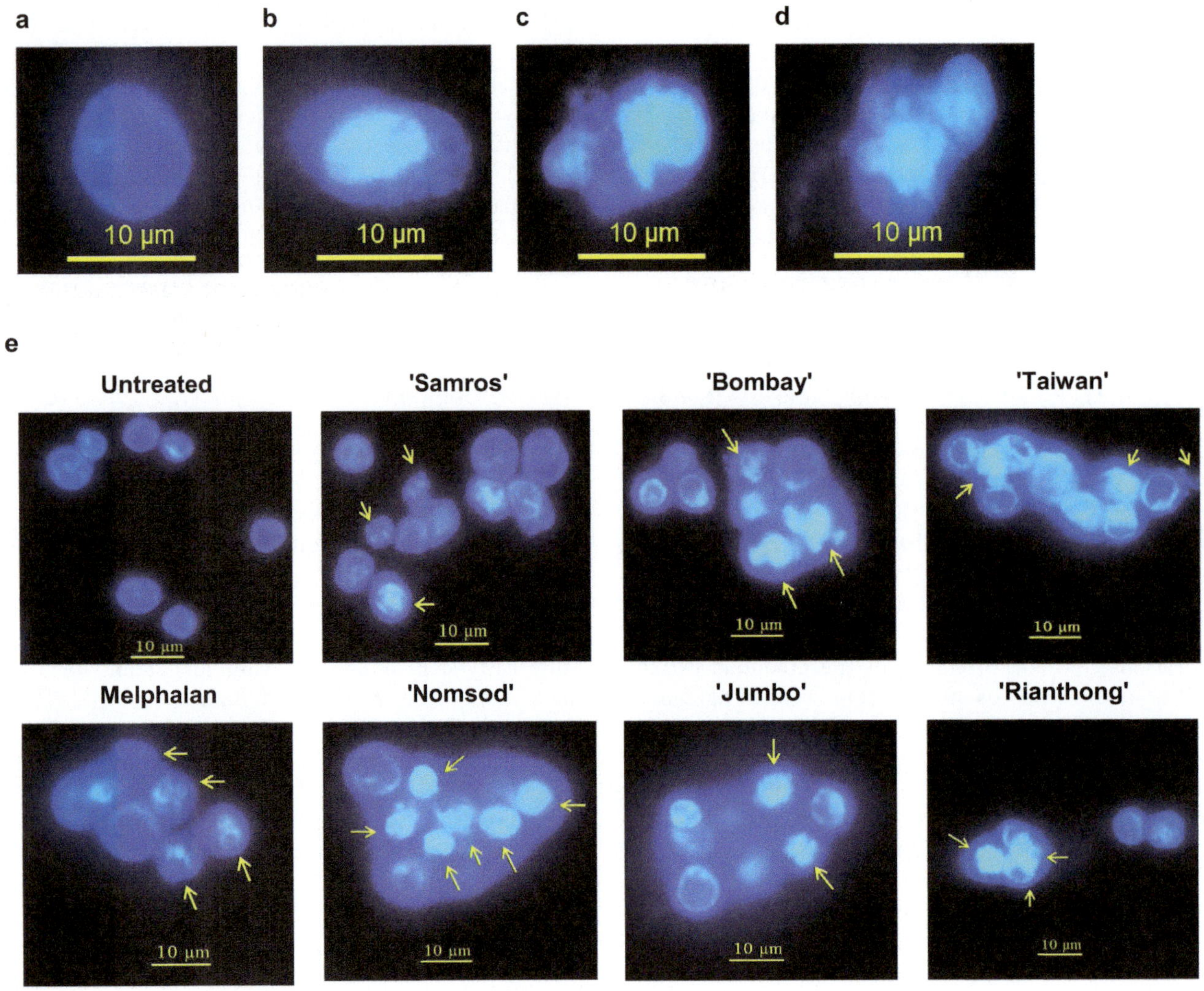

Fig. 2 Nuclear morphological changes of apoptotic Jurkat cells stained with DAPI after being treated with 500 μg/mL melphalan (**a**–**d**) and ethanolic jujube seed extracts (**e**) for 24 h and observed under fluorescent microscope at ×100 magnification: (**a**) normal Jurkat nuclei, (**b**) and (**c**) chromatin condensation, and (**d**) apoptotic body formation. Apoptotic nuclei indicated by *arrows*

vs. 'Bombay' did differ significantly ($P < 0.001$ and $P < 0.0.001$, one-way ANOVA).

The six ethanolic seed extracts induced apoptosis in a concentration-dependent manner. The ranks of the %total apoptosis-inducing effects at the 2 × IC_{50} concentrations after 24 h of incubation were in the descending order: 'Bombay', 'Jumbo', 'Nomsod', 'Samros', 'Rianthong', melphalan, and 'Taiwan'. Apoptosis in the HL-60 cell line was induced by the ethanolic jujube seed extracts in a concentration-dependent manner, and our findings were in agreement with a previous report [24].

The extracts needed to cause less necrotic cell death to achieve effectiveness of their anticancer action. After incubation for 12 h, the 2 × IC_{50} concentrations of 'Jumbo' (13.0 ± 1.5 %), 'Taiwan' (12.6 ± 4.9 %), and 'Nomsod' (6.8 ± 2.4 %) induced relatively high necrotic cell death compared with the other extracts and melphalan (0.5 ± 0.3 %). At 24 h, the 2 × IC_{50} concentrations of the extracts increased necrotic cell death in the descending order: 'Taiwan' (19.8 ± 2.0 %), 'Nomsod' (7.6 ± 0.8 %), 'Samros' (4.2 ± 0.5 %), and 'Jumbo' (2.3 ± 0.8 %).

Caspase activity

Apoptosis can be triggered through both extrinsic and intrinsic pathways, involving caspase cascades that act through initiator caspases and executioner caspases [40, 41]. The initiators are caspase-8 for the extrinsic pathway and caspase-9 for the intrinsic pathway. When the initiator caspases are activated by apoptotic stimuli, the

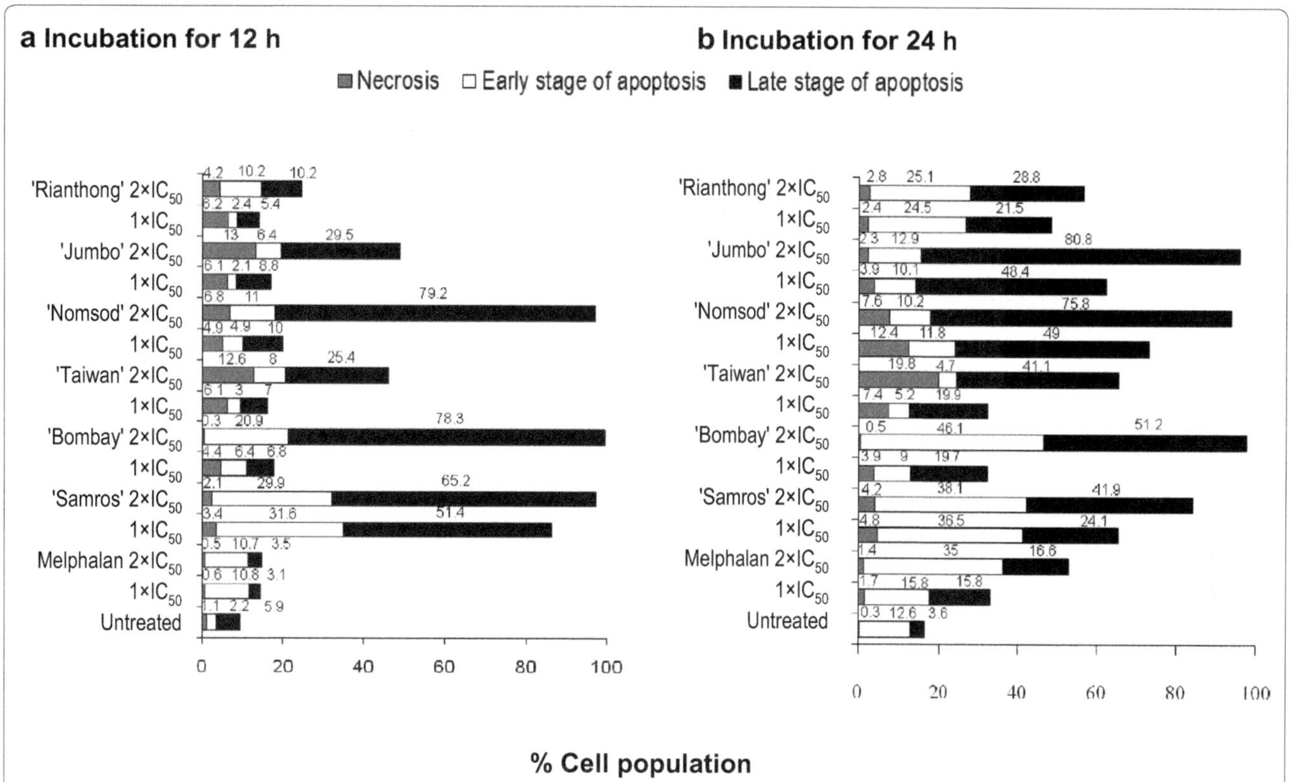

Fig. 3 Different modes of cell death determined by flow cytometry. Jurkat cells induced by the ethanolic jujube seed extract and melphalan at $1 \times IC_{50}$ and $2 \times IC_{50}$ at (**a**) 12 and (**b**) 24 h. *Bar graph* represents %cell population at each stage of apoptosis: (*Filled square*) late, (*open square*) early and (*grey coloured square*) necrosis, respectively. Results are representative of three separate experiments

function of the executioner caspase-3 is triggered, which culminates in DNA fragmentation and apoptotic body formation [2, 39, 41]. The present study assessed the activity of both initiator caspases, caspase-8 and caspase-9, to distinguish the extrinsic pathway from the intrinsic apoptotic pathway. Executioner caspase-3 activity was also determined.

Increased caspase-3 activity was detected at 30 min in Jurkat cells (Fig. 4), suggesting that apoptosis induction by the jujube seed extracts was mediated through the caspase-mediated pathways. 'Taiwan', 'Nomsod', 'Jumbo', 'Rianthong', and melphalan all significantly increased caspase-8 and caspase-9 activity compared with untreated cells at different time points (all $P < 0.001$). The increases in caspase-8 activity for 'Taiwan' vs. melphalan differed significantly ($P = 0.006$). However, there were no significant differences in the increases in caspase-8 activity for 'Rianthong' vs. melphalan ($P = 0.344$), 'Jumbo' vs. melphalan ($P = 0.402$), 'Taiwan' vs. 'Rianthong' ($P = 0.064$), 'Taiwan' vs. 'Jumbo' ($P = 0.053$), and 'Rianthong' vs. 'Jumbo' ($P = 0.999$). The increases in caspase-9 activity for 'Nomsod' vs. 'Taiwan' ($P = 0.018$), 'Nomsod' vs. melphalan ($P = 0.009$), 'Taiwan' *vs.* 'Jumbo' ($P = 0.019$), 'Taiwan' vs. 'Rianthong' ($P = 0.003$), 'Taiwan' vs. melphalan ($P < 0.001$), and 'Jumbo' vs. melphalan ($P = 0.009$) all differed significantly. In contrast, the increases in caspase-9 activity for 'Nomsod' vs. 'Taiwan' ($P = 0.018$), 'Nomsod' vs. 'Jumbo' ($P = 1.000$), 'Nomsod' vs. 'Rianthong' ($P = 0.773$), 'Nomsod' vs. melphalan ($P = 0.009$), and 'Jumbo' vs. 'Rianthong' ($P = 0.771$) did not differ significantly.

'Samros' and 'Bombay' did not increase the caspase-8 and -9 activities, although they did activate caspase-3 activity. While activation of caspase-9 was not evident, the 'Samros' and 'Bombay' extracts were postulated to cleave the caspase-8 substrate earlier than 15 min because of the high activity at 15 min and lower activities at later time points. Activation of caspase-9 and -3 in a concentration-dependent manner in melanoma cells was previously reported for polysaccharides extracted from the fruit part of *Z. jujuba* [42]. The ethanolic extracts of 'Taiwan', 'Jumbo', 'Nomsod', 'Rianthong', 'Samros', and 'Bombay' induced apoptosis via a caspase-mediated pathway in a similar manner to melphalan, but to different extents. The ethanolic extracts of 'Taiwan', 'Nomsod', 'Jumbo', and 'Rianthong' and melphalan evidently induced apoptosis via the intrinsic and extrinsic pathways.

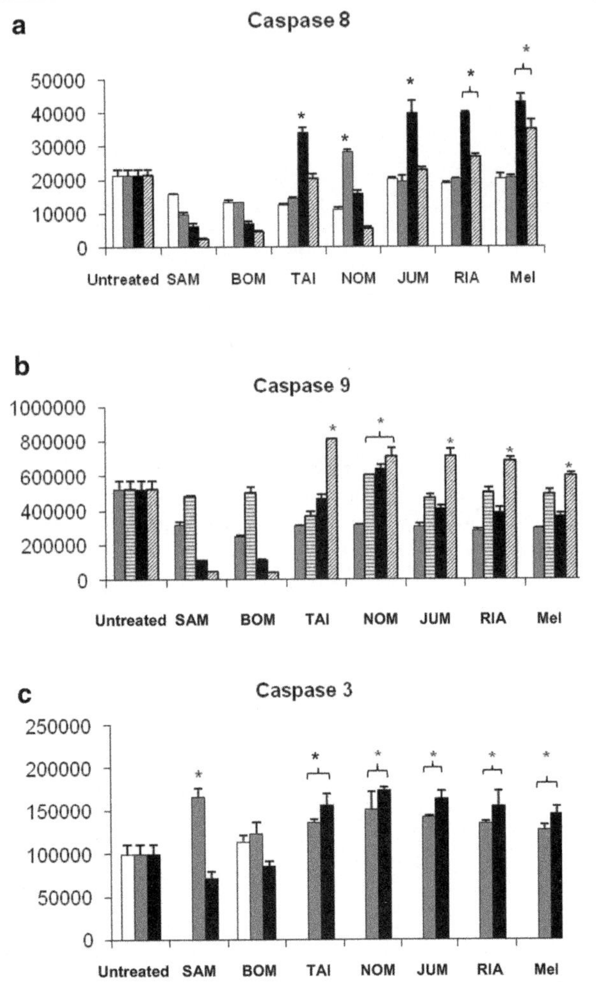

Fig. 4 Activity of caspases of the respective ethanolic jujube seed extracts in Jurkat cell line at various times. (**a**), (**b**) and (**c**) represent activity of caspases 3, 8 and 9 after Jurkat cells treated with 2 × IC_{50} of jujube seed extracts at (open square) 15 min, (*grey coloured square*) 30 min, (*lined square*) 60 min, (*filled square*) 180 min, and (*cross lined square*) 360 min (*$P < 0.05$ compared to untreated cells)

DNA fragmentation

DNA fragmentation occurs through the activation of endogenous endonucleases with subsequent cleavage of chromatin DNA into internucleosomal fragments of 180 bp and multiples thereof. Similar to the case for melphalan, all six ethanolic jujube seed extracts at 2 × IC_{50} concentrations clearly exhibited the characteristic DNA ladder formation (Fig. 5).

Alkylation effects of the selected crude extracts compared with melphalan

An alkylation reaction of the jujube seed extracts was performed to understand the interactions of the extracts with DNA resulting in DNA damage, by testing their alkylating activity. The nitrobenzylpyridine (NBP) assay was used as a model for nucleophilic DNA bases [43–45]. This reaction depends on high temperature and low acidic media to catalyze NBP, which is converted into a blue/violet chromophore product. This specific reaction is positively detected in the presence of electrophilic functional groups or alkylating agents. Only the alkylating drug melphalan led to NBP product formation, suggesting that the DNA damage induced by the jujube seed extracts did not arise from an alkylation reaction. The findings also implied that no electrophilic functional groups were present in the constituents of the jujube seed extracts.

Phytochemical constituents of the extracts

The phytochemical identification of the ethanolic jujube seed extracts showed that alkaloids predominated in all jujube cultivated species followed by reducing sugars (Table 2). Neither saponins nor flavonoids were found in the cultivars tested. The 'Apple', 'Taiwan', and 'Nomsod' extracts had relatively high amounts of alkaloids, followed by the 'Samros', 'Bombay', 'Jumbo', 'Kaew', and 'Rianthong' extracts. The 'Nomsod' and 'Rianthong' extracts had relatively high amounts of reducing sugars.

Ethanolic extracts of *Z. mauritiana* seeds contained alkaloids, terpenes, flavonoids, saponins, and tannins [46]. The alkaloids exhibited anticancer activity [47]. Alkaloids from *Z. jujuba* seeds (i.e., sanjoine K, zizyphusine, and amphibine) processed a sedative action [48, 49]. The fruit pulp of *Z. jujuba* induced apoptosis in various cancer cells, including breast cancer, liver cancer, and leukemia cells [7, 23]. The bioactive compounds in jujube with the anticancer effects (through induction of apoptotic cell death) were triterpene and betulinic acid [23, 24, 46, 50, 51].

The ethanolic extracts of jujube seeds from different cultivars exhibited diverse inhibition of leukemic Jurkat cell viability. The chloroform extracts and melphalan were toxic toward both Jurkat and Vero cells. The ethanolic extracts selectively caused death in Jurkat cells, but not in normal Vero cells. The 'Taiwan' extract exhibited the highest cytotoxicity followed by the 'Jumbo', 'Nomsod', 'Rianthong', 'Samros', and 'Bombay' extracts. The modes of cell death induced by these six jujube extracts were distinguished and confirmed by different methods. The Jurkat cells treated with these six ethanolic extracts exhibited various stages of apoptotic nuclear morphological alterations similar to those found in Jurkat cells treated with melphalan. The analyses for mode of cell death at 12 h, detected by flow cytometry, revealed that the 'Bombay' extract at 2 × IC_{50} induced significantly more apoptosis than the other extracts and melphalan (99.2 ± 0.4 %; $P < 0.001$). At 24 h, the 'Bombay', 'Jumbo', and 'Nomsod' extracts induced apoptotic cell death at

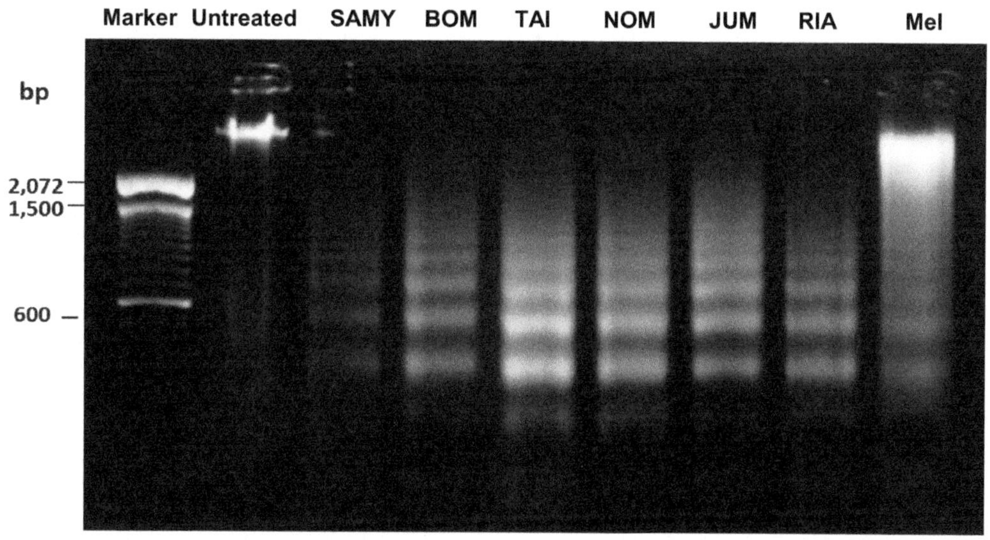

Fig. 5 DNA laddering based on gel electrophoresis after the cells were treated with 2 × IC_{50} of ethanolic jujube seed extracts and melphalan for 24 h

Table 2 Phytochemicals screening of the ethanolic seed extracts of eight jujube cultivars

Phyto-chemicals	Presence of phyto-chemical	Jujube cultivars							
		'Samros'	'Bombay'	'Apple'	'Taiwan'	'Nomsod'	'Jumbo'	'Kaew'	'Rianthong'
Alkaloids	Orange or reddish brown precipitate	++	++	+++	+++	+++	++	++	+
Flavonoids	Colorless	–	–	–	–	–	–	–	–
Saponins	Permanent foam	–	–	–	–	–	–	–	–
Reducing sugar	Orange red precipitate	–	–	–	–	+++	–	++	+++

–, absence of phytochemicals; +, presence of phytochemicals; +++, indicates the highest level; +, indicates the lowest level of phytochemical in positive results

97.3 ± 2.9 %, 93.7 ± 2.4 %, and 86.0 ± 1.9 %, respectively. Although 'Taiwan' and 'Jumbo' were the first two cultivars possessing high cytotoxicity, they also caused higher degrees of undesirable necrotic cell death. DNA damage was detected in the Jurkat cells treated with the 'Taiwan', 'Jumbo', 'Nomsod', 'Rianthong', 'Samros', and 'Bombay' extracts. This DNA damage did not occur via an alkylation reaction between the extracts and the nucleophilic DNA model, as confirmed by the NBP assays. The Jurkat cellular changes, reflecting apoptosis induced by the seed extracts of the six jujube cultivars, were mediated by caspases. Increased caspase-3 activity was detected after all six extract treatments. The 'Taiwan', 'Nomsod', 'Jumbo', and 'Rianthong' extracts induced apoptosis through both extrinsic and intrinsic apoptosis pathways, based on increases in caspase-8 and -9 activities, respectively. The 'Samros' and 'Bombay' extracts seemed to augment the initiator caspase-8 activity at an earlier time point, but did not induce the intrinsic apoptosis pathway.

Conclusions

The six active extracts ('Taiwan', 'Jumbo', 'Nomsod', 'Rianthong', 'Samros' and 'Bombay') contained alkaloids and reducing sugars, and induced caspase-dependent apoptosis in human Jurkat leukemia T cells.

Abbreviations

APP: 'Apple' cultivar; BOM: 'Bombay' cultivar; JUM: 'Jumbo' cultivar; KAE: 'Kaew' cultivar; Mel: chemotherapeutic drug melphalan; NOM: 'Nomsod' cultivar; RIA: 'Rianthong' cultivar; SAM: 'Samros' cultivar; TAI: 'Taiwan' cultivar.

Authors' contributions

NW designed the study. NT performed the experiment, collected, and analyzed the data. NW and NT wrote the manuscript. NW, SB and SS revised the manuscript. All authors read and approved the final manuscript.

Author details

[1] Graduate School, Faculty of Pharmaceutical Sciences, Khon Kaen University, Khon Kaen 40002, Thailand. [2] Faculty of Pharmaceutical Sciences, Khon Kaen University, Khon Kaen 40002, Thailand. [3] Faculty of Associate Medical Sciences, Khon Kaen University, Khon Kaen 40002, Thailand. [4] Department of Food Technology and Nutrition, Mahasarakham University, Mahasarakham 44000, Thailand.

Acknowledgements

NT was grateful to the Faculty of Pharmaceutical Sciences for the Master degree scholarship in the second semester of 2013. The Thai Research Fund (RDG5420072) financially supported this research. The authors thank Mr. Bryan Roderick Hamman and Mrs. Janice Loewen-Hamman for assistance with the English-language presentation.

Competing interests

The authors declare that they have no competing interests.

References

1. Khazir J, Mir BA, Pilcher L, Riley DL. Role of plants in anticancer drug discovery. Phytochemistry Lett. 2014;7:173–81.
2. Brunelle JK, Zhang B. Apoptosis assays for quantifying the bioactivity of anticancer drug products. Drug Resist Updat. 2010;13:172–9.
3. Yan YH, Gao ZP. Industrialization of Chinese jujube. J Northwest Sci Tech Univ Agri For. 2002;30:95–8.
4. Williams JT. From introduction, taxonomy, and history. In: Smith RW, Haq N, Dunsiger Z, editors. Fruits for the future 2 (revised edition): ber and other jujubes. Southampton: Int Cen Underutil Crops; 2006. p. 1–17.
5. Li JW, Fan LP, Ding SD, Ding XL. Nutritional composition of five cultivars of Chinese jujube. Food Chem. 2007;103:454–60.
6. Saha D, Srivastava SC, Ramani R. Genetic relationships among fruit cultivars and host plants of Indian lac insect in ber (*Ziziphus mauritiana* Lam.) revealed by RAPD and ISSR markers. Indian. J Biotechnol. 2012;12:170–7.
7. Huang X, Kojima-Yuasa A, Norikura T, Kennedy DO, Hasuma T, Matsui-Yuasa I. Mechanism of the anti-cancer activity of *Zizyphus jujuba* in HepG2 cells. Am J Chin Med. 2007;35:517–32.
8. Kumar S, Jawaid T, Dubey SD. Therapeutic plants of Ayurveda; a review on anticancer. Pharm J. 2011;3:1–11.
9. Eley JG, Dovlatabadi H. Permeability enhancement activity from *Ziziphus jujuba*. Pharm Biol. 2002;40:149–53.
10. Peng WH, Hsieh MT, Lee YS, Lin YC, Liao J. Anxiolytic effect of seed of *Ziziphus jujuba* in mouse models of anxiety. J Ethnopharmacol. 2000;72:435–41.
11. Su BN, Cuendet M, Farnsworth NR, Fong HH, Pezzuto JM, Kinghorn AD. Activity-guided fractionation of the seeds of *Ziziphus jujuba* using a cyclooxygenase-2 inhibitory assay. Planta Med. 2002;68:1125–8.
12. Heo HJ, Park YJ, Suh YM, Choi SJ, Kim MJ, Cho HY, Shin DH. Effects of oleamide on choline acetyltransferase and cognitive activities. Biosci Biotechnol Biochem. 2003;67:1284–91.
13. Lamien-Meda A, Lamien CE, Compaoré MMY, Meda RNT, Kiendrebeogo M, Zeba B, Nacoulma OG. Polyphenol content and antioxidant activity of fourteen wild edible fruits from Burkina Faso. Molecules. 2008;13:581–94.
14. Memarpoor-Yazdi M, Mahaki H, Zare-Zardini H. Antioxidant activity of protein hydrolysates and purified peptides from *Zizyphus jujuba* fruits. J Funct Foods. 2013;5:62–70.
15. Su XS, Chen ZD, Jiao BL, Huang QM, Li WY. Studies on anti-allergic activity of common foodstuffs in China and their constituents. J Southwest Agri Univ. 2000;21:77–80.
16. Suttisri R, Lee IS, Kinghorn AD. Plant-derived triterpenoid sweetness inhibitors. J Ethnopharmacol. 1995;47:9–26.
17. Dahiru D, Obidoa O. Pretreatment of albino rats with aqueous leaf extract of *Ziziphus mauritiana* protects against alcohol-induced liver damage. Trop J Pharm Res. 2007;6:705–10.
18. Siddharth P, Kailash P, Niraj V, Karuna M, Vimal P, Bharadia P, Pundarikakshudu K. Antiulcer activity of methanolic extract of *Ziziphus mauritiana* Stem Bark. Int J Pharm Phytochem Res. 2010;2:6–11.
19. Gupta M, Mazumder UK, Vamsi MLM, Sivakumar T, Kandar CC. Antisteroidogenic activity of the two Indian medicinal plants in mice. J Ethnopharmacol. 2004;90:21–5.
20. Adamu HM, Abayeh OJ, Ibok NU, Kafu SE. Antifungal activity of extracts of some *Cassia*, *Detarium* and *Ziziphus* species against dermatophytes. Nat Prod Radiance. 2006;5:357–60.
21. Dahiru D, Sini JM, John-Africa L. Antidiarrhoeal activity of *Ziziphus mauritiana* root extract in rodents. Afr J Biotechnol. 2006;5:941–5.
22. Mahajan R, Chopda M. Phyto-Pharmacology of *Ziziphus jujuba* Mill-A plant review. Pharmacogn Rev. 2009;3:320–9.
23. Plastina P, Bonofiglio D, Vizza D, Fazio A, Rovito D, Giordano C, Gabriele B. Identification of bioactive constituents of *Ziziphus* jujube fruit extracts exerting antiproliferative and apoptotic effects in human breast cancer cells. J Ethnopharmacol. 2012;140:325–32.
24. Mishra T, Khullar M, Bhatia A. Anticancer potential of aqueous ethanol seed extract of *Ziziphus mauritiana* against cancer cell lines and Ehrlich ascites carcinoma. Evid Based Complement Alternat Med. 2011;2011:1–11.
25. Buanong M, Techavuttiporn C, Boonyaritthongchai P, Lichanporn I. Analysis of bioactive compound contents in commercial fruits locally cultivated in Thailand. 2009. http://elibrary.trf.or.th/fullP/RDG5220054//RDG5220054_abstract.pdf.
26. Taechakulwanijya N, Weerapreeyakul N, Barusrux S, Siriamornpun S. Apoptosis induction effect of three jujube cultivars in HepG2 and Jurkat cell lines. Int J Biosci Biochem Bioinforma (IJBBB). 2013;3:540–4.
27. Siriamornpun S, Weerapreeyakul N, Barusrux S. Bioactive compounds and health implications are better for green jujube fruit than for ripe fruit. J Funct Foods. 2015;12:246–55.
28. Grebenstein C, Choi YH, Rong J, De Jong TJ, Tamis WLM. Metabolic fingerprinting reveals differences between shoots of wild and cultivated carrot (*Daucus carota* L.) and suggests maternal inheritance or wild trait dominance in hybrids. Phytochemistry. 2011;72:1341–7.
29. Cherif AO, Messaouda MB, Kaabi B, Pellerin I, Boukhchina S, Kallel H, Pepe C. Characteristics and pathways of bioactive 4-desmethylsterols, triterpene alcohols and 4a-monomethylsterols, from developing Tunisian cultivars and wild peanut (*Arachis hypogaea* L.). Plant Physiol Bioch. 2011;49:774–81.
30. Machana S, Weerapreeyakul N, Barusrux S, Nonpunya A, Sripanidkulchai B, Thitimetharoch T. Cytotoxic and apoptotic effects of six herbal plants against the human hepatocarcinoma (HepG2) cell line. Chinese Med. 2011;6:39.
31. Bézivin C, Tomasi S, Lohézic-Le Dévéhat F, Boustie J. Cytotoxic activity of some lichen extracts on murine and human cancer cell lines. Phytomedicine. 2003;10:499–503.
32. De Castro LFP, Zacharias M. DAPI binding to the DNA minor groove: a continuum solvent analysis. J Mol Recognit. 2002;15:209–20.
33. Nasri T, Bosch RR, Voorde S, Fink-Gremmels J. Differential induction of apoptosis by type A and B trichothecenes in Jurkat T-lymphocytes. Toxicol In Vitro. 2006;20:832–40.
34. Hickey TE, Majam G, Guerry P. Intracellular survival of *Campylobacter jejuni* in human monocytic cells and induction of apoptotic death by cytholethaldistending toxin. Infect Immun. 2005;73:5194–7.
35. Anandanayaki S. Comparative pharmacognostical studies on selected plants (*Pedalium murex* Roen ex. L. and *Martynia annua* L.). Ph.D. thesis. Tamil University, Department of Environmental and Herbal Science; 2010.
36. Bello IA, Ndukwe GI, Audu OT, Habila JD. A bioactive flavonoid from *Pavetta crassipes* K. Schum. Org Med Chem Lett. 2011;1:14.
37. Shirazi FH, Ahmadi N, Kamalinejad M. Evaluation of northern Iran *Mentha pulegium* L. cytotoxicity. DARU. 2004;12:106–10.
38. Suriyavadhana M, Pakutharivu T. Evaluation of acute and sub-acute toxicity of ethanol extracts of *Entada pursaetha*, *Toddalia aculeata*, and *Ziziphus mauritiana*. World J Life Sci Med Res. 2011;1:43–7.
39. Dai ZJ, Gao J, Ji ZZ, Wang XJ, Ren HT, Liu XX, Wu WY, Kang HF, Guan HT. Matrine induces apoptosis in gastric carcinoma cells via alteration of Fas/FasL and activation of caspase-3. J Ethnopharmacol. 2009;123:91–6.
40. Budihardjo I, Oliver H, Lutter M, Luo X, Wang X. Biochemical pathways of caspase activation during apoptosis. Annu Rev Cell Dev Biol. 1999;15:269–90.
41. McIlwain DR, Berger T, Mak TW. Caspase functions in cell death and disease. Cold Spring Harb Perspect Biol. 2013;5:a008656.
42. Hung CF, Hsu BY, Chang SC, Chen BH. Antiproliferation of melanoma cells by polysaccharide isolated from *Zizyphus jujuba*. Nutrition. 2012;28:98–105.
43. Meier I, Shephard SE, Lutz WK. Nitrosation of aspartic acid, aspartame, and glycine ethylester. Alkylation of 4-(p-nitrobenzyl) pyridine (NBP) in vitro and binding to DNA in the rat. Mutat Res. 1990;238:193–201.

44. Dierickx KME, Journé F, Gerbaux P, Morandini R, Kauffmann JM, Ghanem GE. Improving the spectrophotometric determination of the alkylating activity of anticancer agents: a new insight into the mechanism of the NBP method. Talanta. 2009;77:1370–5.
45. Gómez-Bombarelli R, González-Pérez M, Calle E, Casado J. Potential of the NBP method for the study of alkylation mechanisms: NBP as a DNA-model. Chem Res Toxicol. 2012;25:1176–91.
46. Mishra T, Bhatia A. Augmentation of expression of immunocytes' functions by seed extract of *Ziziphus mauritiana* (Lamk.). J Ethnopharmacol. 2010;127:341–5.
47. Saxena M, Saxena J, Nema R, Singh D, Gupta A. Phytochemistry of medicinal plants. J Pharmacogn Phytochem. 2013;1:168–82.
48. Liu J, Chen B, Yao S. Simultaneous analysis and identification of main bioactive constituents in extract of *Zizyphus jujuba* var. *sapinosa* (Zizyphispinosi semen) by high performance liquid chromatography-photodiode array detection-electrospray mass spectrometry. Talanta. 2007;71:668–75.
49. Han BH, Park MH, Park JH. Chemical and pharmacological studies on sedative cyclopeptide alkaloids in some Rhamnaceae plants. Pure Appl Chem. 2009;61:443–8.
50. Pisha E, Chai H, Lee IS, Chagwedera TE, Farnsworth NR, Cordell GA, Brown DM. Discovery of betulinic acid as a selective inhibitor of human melanoma that functions by induction of apoptosis. Nat Med. 1995;1:1046–51.
51. Lee SM, Min BS, Lee CG, Kim KS, Kho YH. Cytotoxic triterpenoids from the fruits of *Zizyphus jujuba*. Planta Med. 2003;69:1051–4.

7

Anti-cancer effects of *Gynostemma pentaphyllum* (Thunb.) Makino (*Jiaogulan*)

Yantao Li, Wanjun Lin, Jiajun Huang, Ying Xie and Wenzhe Ma*

Abstract

Gynostemma pentaphyllum (Thunb.) Makino (GpM) (*Jiaogulan*) has been widely used in Chinese medicine for the treatment of several diseases, including hepatitis, diabetes and cardiovascular disease. Furthermore, GpM has recently been shown to exhibit potent anti-cancer activities. In this review, we have summarized recent research progress on the anti-cancer activities and mechanisms of action of GpM, as well as determining the material basis for the anti-cancer effects of GpM by searching the PubMed, Web of Science and China National Knowledge Infrastructure databases. The content of this review is based on studies reported in the literature pertaining to the chemical components or anti-cancer effects of GpM up until the beginning of August, 2016. This search of the literature revealed that more than 230 compounds have been isolated from GpM, and that most of these compounds (189) were saponins, which are also known as gypenosides. All of the remaining compounds were classified as sterols, flavonoids or polysaccharides. Various extracts and fractions of GpM, as well as numerous pure compounds isolated from this herb exhibited inhibitory activity towards the proliferation of cancer cells in vitro and in vivo. Furthermore, the results of several clinical studies have shown that GpM formula could have potential curative effects on cancer. Multiple mechanisms of action have been proposed regarding the anti-cancer activities of GpM, including cell cycle arrest, apoptosis, inhibition of invasion and metastasis, inhibition of glycolysis and immunomodulating activities.

Background

Cancer is the world's leading cause of death, accounting for 8.2 million deaths in 2012, and it is expected that the annual number of global cancer cases will rise from 14 million in 2012 to 22 million within the next two decades [1]. The isolation and evaluation of anti-cancer agents and lead compounds from natural resources represents a traditional and effective approach for the development of new drugs for the treatment of cancer [2, 3], as exemplified by Paclitaxel, which was derived from *Taxus brevifolia* [3, 4].

Gynostemma pentaphyllum (Thunb.) Makino (GpM) (*Jiaogulan*) has been widely used in Chinese medicine for the treatment of various diseases, including hepatitis, diabetes and cardiovascular disease. Modern medical research has shown that GpM exhibits a variety of pharmacological properties, including anti-inflammatory [5–8], antioxidative [9–13], lipid metabolism regulatory [14–18], antiproliferative [19–22], neuroprotective [23, 24] and anxiolytic activities [25–27]. GpM has consequently been widely used for the treatment of hepatitis [15, 28–30], diabetes [11, 30–32], cardiovascular disease [33–35] and cancer [20, 23, 36, 37]. GpM is also widely used as a health supplement in beverages, biscuits, noodles, face washes and bath oils [38–41].

We have conducted a comprehensive review of the literature associated with GpM to provide a summary of recent research towards the anti-cancer activities and mechanisms of action of GpM. We have also searched the PubMed, Web of Science and China National Knowledge Infrastructure (CNKI) databases to identify the material basis for the anti-cancer effects of GpM.

Literature search strategy and exclusion criteria

Our literature search covered all of the records in the PubMed, Web of Science Core Collection and CNKI databases up until the beginning of August, 2016. All of the studies included in this review reported on either the chemical components or the anti-cancer effects of GpM. The following search strategy was used to search PubMed

*Correspondence: wzma@must.edu.mo
State Key Laboratory of Quality Research in Chinese Medicine, Macau University of Science and Technology, Taipa, Macao, China

with the "All Fields" option and the Web of Science Core Collection in the "Topic" field (Table 1). Studies were excluded if they were: (a) duplicated; (b) not pertinent to the chemical components or the anti-cancer effects of GpM; or (c) not full-text journal articles.

Clinical studies were not excluded from the searches conducted using the PubMed and Web of Science database; however, no records involving clinical trials were found in either of these databases. For this reason, we searched the CNKI database for clinical studies pertaining to the use of GpM for the treatment of cancer. The following search strategy was used to search the CNKI database using the "Abstract" field (Table 2). Studies were excluded from the results if they were: (a) not pertinent to the clinical anti-cancer effects of GpM; (b) review articles; or (c) not full-text journal articles.

Two reviewers independently searched the databases and screened all of the articles for their eligibility. The search strategies and selection processes used by the reviewers are shown in Fig. 1. In this way, we identified 108 articles, which have been included in this review.

Chemical components of GpM

Over 230 compounds have been identified as being derived from GpM and can be grouped according to their chemical structures into saponins, sterols, flavonoids, polysaccharides and several other compound classes.

Saponins

One hundred and eighty-nice saponins, which are also known as gypenosides (Gyps), have been isolated from GpM and fully characterized using spectroscopic methods [42–45]. At the 23rd meeting of the Japanese society of pharmacognosy, Nagai et al. [46] reported the isolation of two dammarane-type saponins, including panoxadiol and 2α-OH-panoxadiol, from the hydrolysate of Gyps. The research groups of Takemotoet [47–50] and Yoshikawa [51, 52] subsequently reported the isolation and characterization of many other Gyps from GpM. Gyps are the major components of GpM, and mainly consist of triterpenoid saponins, which can be purified from ethyl acetate or n-butanol extracts [53]. One hundred and sixty-five of the 189 Gyps reported to date have been grouped into 12 classes based on the nature of their aglycone moiety [43]. However, the remaining 24 Gyps [44, 45, 54–60] do not belong to any of these classes. The general structure of Gyps is shown in Table 3, and shows that these compounds consist of a hydrophobic sapogenin moiety (where R_1 = hydrocarbon chain with or without double bond(s), cyclopentane, oxacyclopentane or some other group) and a hydrophilic sugar group (where R_4 = glucose, rhamnose or xylose).

Table 1 Strategy in searching PubMed and Web of Science

Step	Search terms	Citations reviewed	
		PubMed	Web of Science
1	*Gynostemma pentaphyllum*	280	314
2	Jiaogulan	284	22
3	Gypenoside	137	96
4	Constituents	58,058	137,552
5	Composition	328,924	780,071
6	Components	471,244	1,371,871
7	Tumor	3,285,652	983,570
8	Cancer	3,336,622	1,467,455
9	Carcinoma	797,702	521,059
10	1 or 2 or 3	322	364
11	4 or 5 or 6	821,820	2,163,770
12	7 or 8 or 9	3,699,522	2,049,723
13	10 and 11	66	109
14	10 and 12	81	83
15	13 or 14	130	162

Table 2 Strategy in searching CNKI

Step	Search terms	Citations reviewed
1	Jiaogulan	2876
2	Zhongliu	767,939
3	Linchuang	3,366,530
4	1, 2 and 3	43

Sterols

Sterols are composed of 17 carbon atoms across four rings, i.e., three 6-carbon rings and a single 5-carbon ring, with a side chain extending from C17 containing nine or ten carbon atoms (Additional file 1: Table S1). Eighteen sterols were isolated from GpM and fully characterized using a unique method from 1986 to 1990 [61–67]. Briefly, GpM was extracted with CH_2Cl_2, and the extracted lipids were saponified with 5 % KOH in MeOH. After purification by column chromatography over silica gel, the sterol mixture was acetylated, crystallized and characterized using spectroscopic methods. This process resulted in the isolation of sterols with ergostane, cholestane and stigmastane skeletons. The structures of these 18 sterols are shown in Additional file 1: Table S1. These compounds contained one double bond between C5–C6, C7–C8 or C9–C11, with R_2 = H or CH_3 and R_1 = hydrocarbon chain with 10 carbons, and one double bond or one alkynyl group.

Polysaccharides

Polysaccharides are major components of GpM, where they are typically conjugated with proteins [68]. The

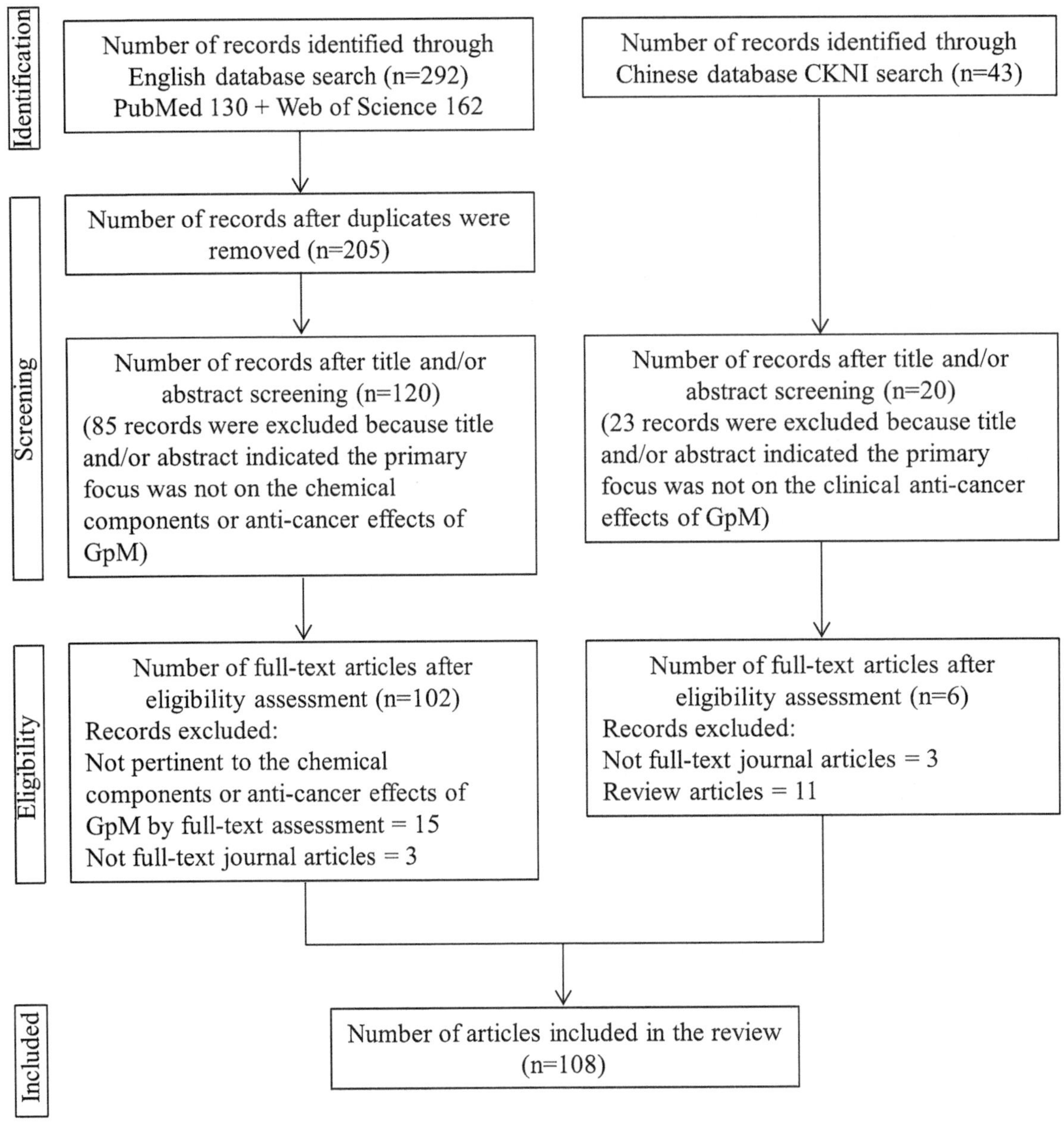

Fig. 1 Flowchart indicating the search strategies and processes used in this study

molecular weight of the polysaccharides found in GpM varies from 9000 to 33,000 Da [69]. Several different kinds of polysaccharides have been found in GpM, and the molar ratios of the monosaccharide components of these systems have been reported to vary considerably. For instance, the neutral polysaccharide fraction CGPP mainly consists of mannose, glucose, arabinose, rhamnose, galactose and glucuronic acid with molar ratios of 2.0:2.2:1.3:2.2:1.2:2.5 [20]. Another polysaccharide fraction (NaCl eluted fraction of crude polysaccharides from GpM by DEAE-Sepharose CL-6B chromatography, GMC) consisted of glucose, galactose, mannose and fructose with the molar ratios of 1:2.17:1.25:1.02 [70]. Furthermore, the water-soluble GpM polysaccharide fraction GP-I contains glucose, galactose, mannose, rhamnose and arabinose with molar ratios of 5.3:4.2:3.0:0.7:0.8 [69]. Based on the differences in the possible arrangements of the monosaccharides, various polysaccharides have been isolated from GpM [71].

Table 3 Structures and in vitro anti-cancer activity of identified GpM components

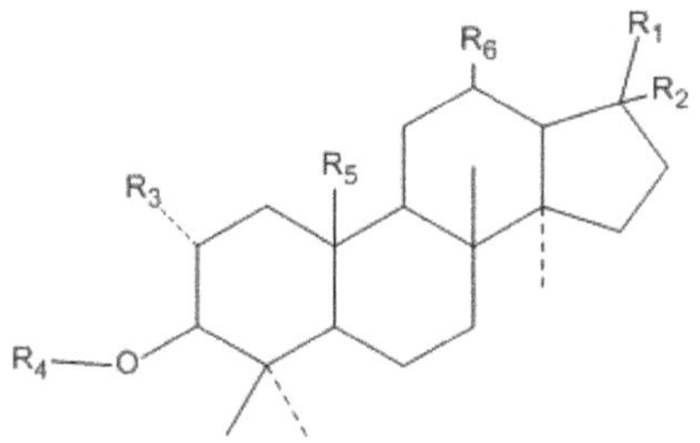

Compd	R_1	R_2	R_3	R_4	R_5	R_6	Anti-cancer activity[a]	Reference
1	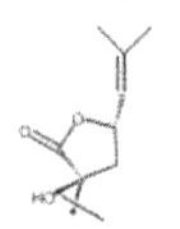	H	H	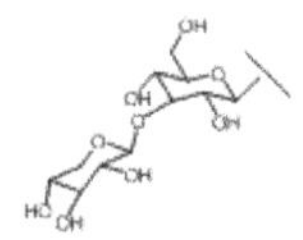	CH_3	H	47.12 (HL-60)	[122]
2	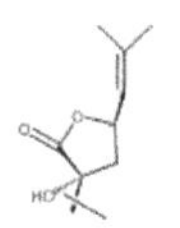	H	H	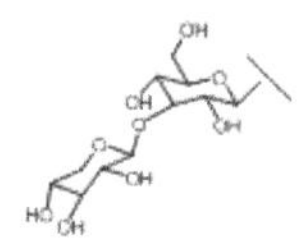	CH_3	H	45.50 (HL-60)	[122]
3	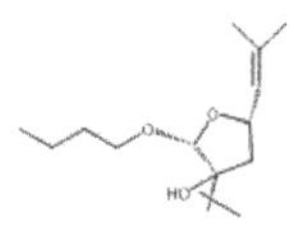	H	H	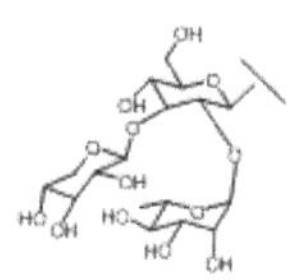	CH_3	H	HL-60, Colon 205, Du145, GC-7901, BEL-7402	[85, 86]
4	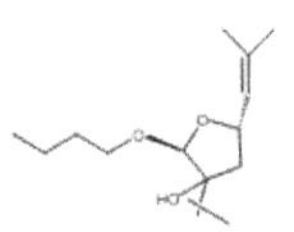	H	H	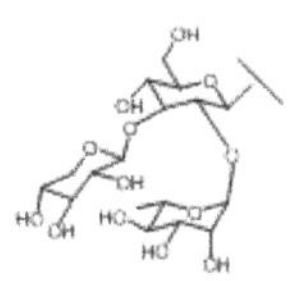	CH_3	H	HL-60, Colon 205, Du145, GC-7901, BEL-7402	[85, 86]
5	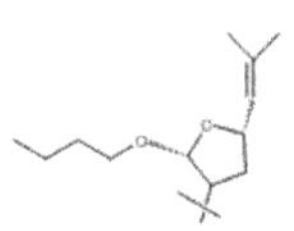	H	H	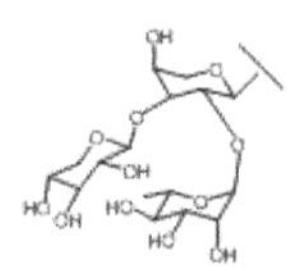	CHO	H	HL-60, Colon 205, Du145, GC-7901, BEL-7402	[85, 86]
6	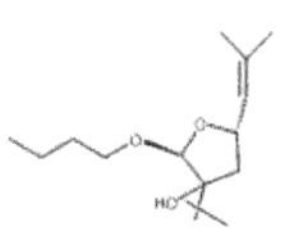	H	H	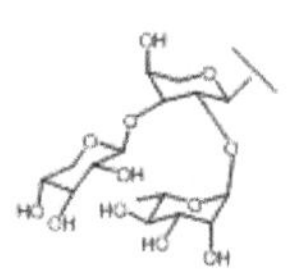	CHO	H	HL-60, Colon 205, Du145, GC-7901, BEL-7402	[85, 86]
7	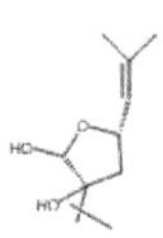	CH_3	H	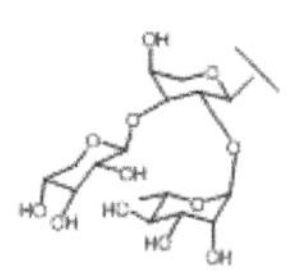	CHO	H	HL-60, Colon 205, Du145, GC-7901, BEL-7402	[85, 86]
8	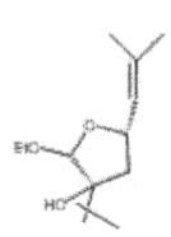	CH_3	H	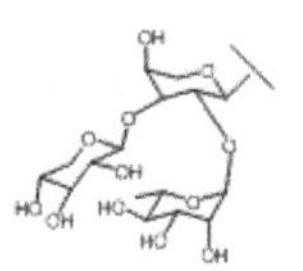	CHO	H	HL-60, Colon 205, Du145, GC-7901, BEL-7402	[85, 86]
9	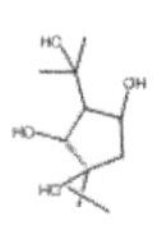	CH_3	H	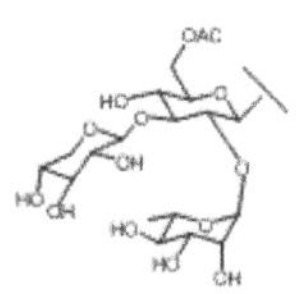	CH_3	H	HL-60, Colon 205, Du145, GC-7901, BEL-7402	[85, 86]

Table 3 continued

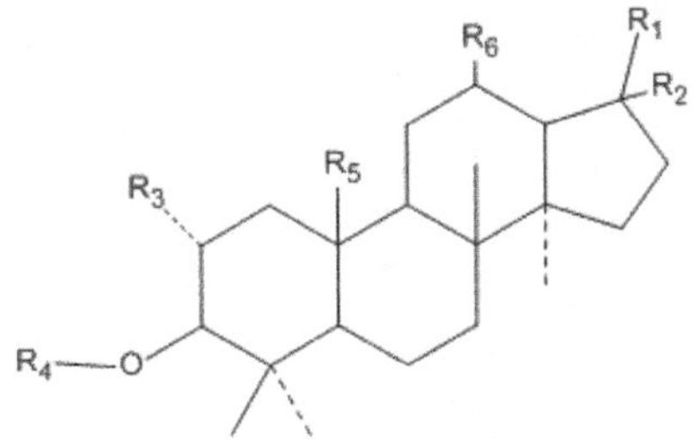

Compd	R1	R2	R3	R4	R5	R6	Anti-cancer activity[a]	Reference
10	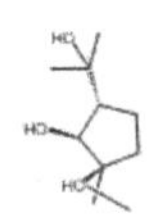	CH_3	H	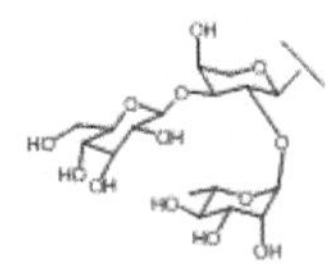	CH_3	OH	67.66 ± 3.36 (HL-60), 18.45 ± 0.93 (MCF-7), 34.95 ± 0.93(HT-29), 20.97 ± 1.49 (A549), 27.68 ± 1.58 (SK-OV-3)	[53]
11	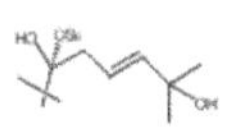	CH_3	H	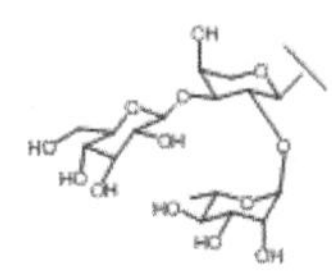	CH_3	=O	>109.2 (HL-60), 42.81 ± 3.60 (MCF-7), 22.06 ± 2.18 (HT-29), 31.45 ± 2.62 (A549), 30.25 ± 1.53 (SK-OV-3)	[53]
12	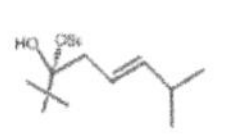	CH_3	H	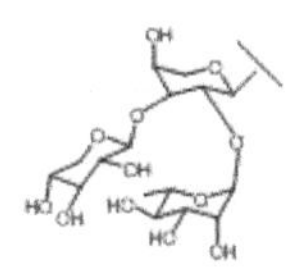	CH_3	=O	>107.6 (HL-60), 23.03 ± 1.40 (MCF-7), 46.30 ± 1.08 (HT-29), 21.09 ± 1.18 (A549), 35.62 ± 0.97 (SK-OV-3)	[53]
13	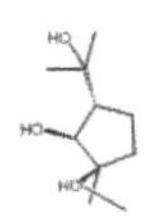	CH_3	H	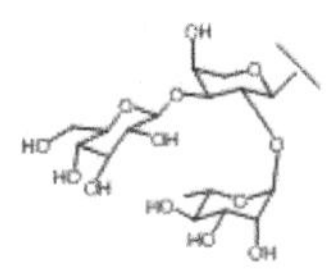	CH_3	=O	76.63 ± 2.98 (HL-60), 23.62 ± 1.02 (MCF-7), 39.34 ± 1.02 (HT-29), 19.90 ± 1.40 (A549), 19.90 ± 1.49 (SK-OV-3)	[53]
14	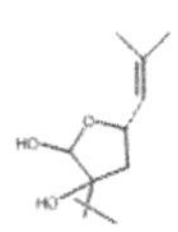	H	H	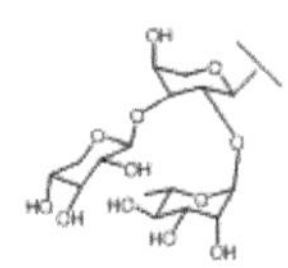	CH_3	H	7.44 (HL-60), 27.80 (Colon 205), 24.12 (Du145)	[127]
15	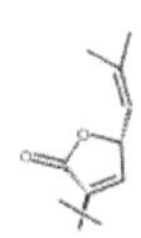	H	H	H	CH_3	H	3.90 (MDA-MB-435)	[128]
16	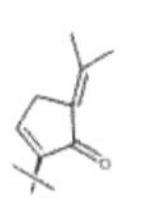	H	H	H	CH_3	H	0.05 ± 0.01 (A549), 0.25 ± 0.07 (U87)	[129]
17	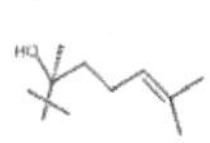	H	OH	H	CH_3	OH	12.54 ± 0.53 (A549)	[130]
18	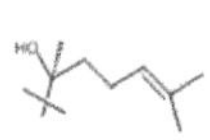	H	OH	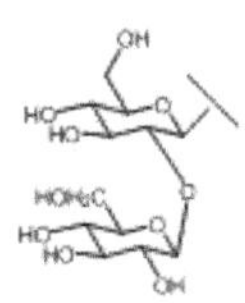	CH_3	OH	34.94 ± 4.23 (A549)	[130]
19	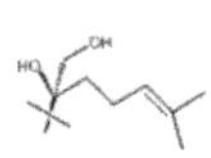	H	H	H	CH_3	H	40 ± 0.7 (HepG2)	[44]
20	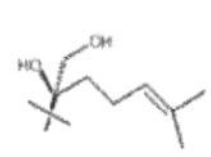	H	H	H	CH_3	OH	38 ± 0.5 (HepG2)	[44]

Table 3 continued

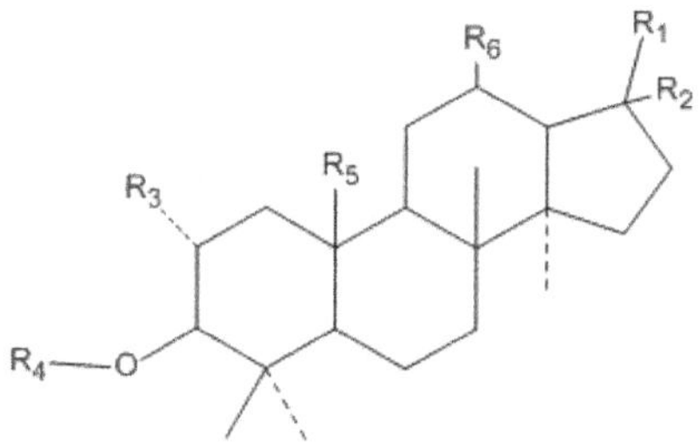

Compd	R_1	R_2	R_3	R_4	R_5	R_6	Anti-cancer activity[a]	Reference
21	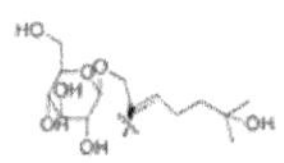	H	H	H	CH_3	H	41.89 (HCT116), 20.94 (HT-29), 32.61 (MCF-7)	[55]
22	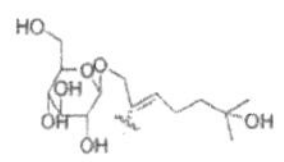	H	H	H	CH_3	H	41.40 (HCT116), 19.00 (HT-29), 28.82 (MCF-7)	[55]
23	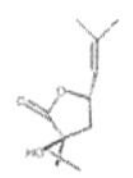	H	H	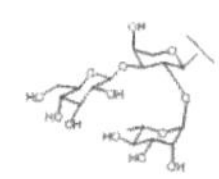	CHO	H	32.00 ± 1.24 (HepG2)	[56]
24	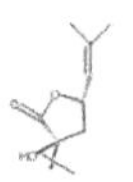	H	H	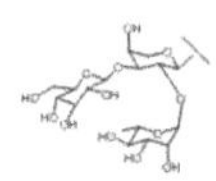	CH_3	H	21.38 ± 1.06 (HepG2)	[56]
25	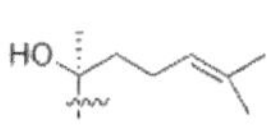	H	OH	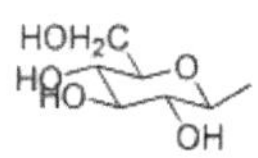	CH_3	OH	74.3 ± 1.9 (A549)	[59]
26	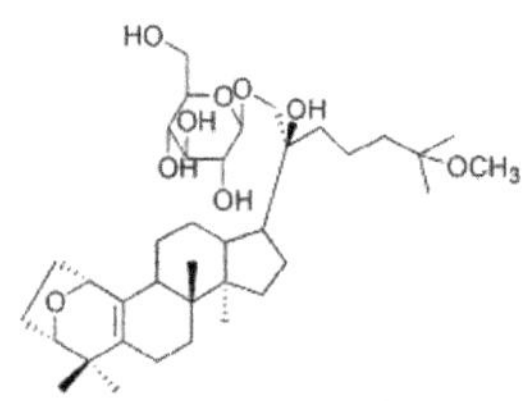						18.41 (HT-29), 4.46 (MCF-7), 9.39 ± 0.9 (DI145), 6.93 ± 0.5 (22RV-1)	[54, 55]
27	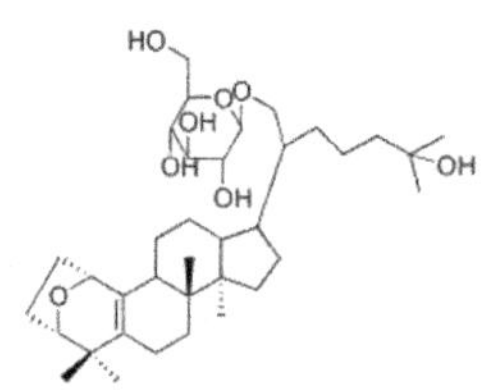						20.38 (HT-29), 13.51 (MCF-7)	[55]
28	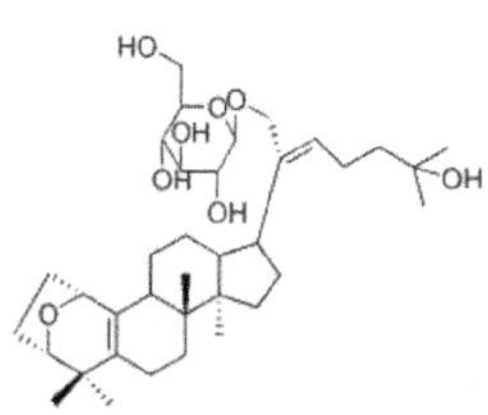						16.14 (HT-29), 8.84 (MCF-7)	[55]
Flavonoid fraction							33.3 (PC-3)	[21]
Carotenoid fraction							1.6 (Hep3B)	[84]
Chlorophyll fraction							57.5 (Hep3B)	[84]
Nonpolar fraction							38.02 ± 2.98 (MDA-MB-453), 31.62 ± 1.76 (HCT116), 35.48 ± 3.81 (LNCaP), 35.48 ± 6.45 (MCF7)	[22]

Table 3 continued

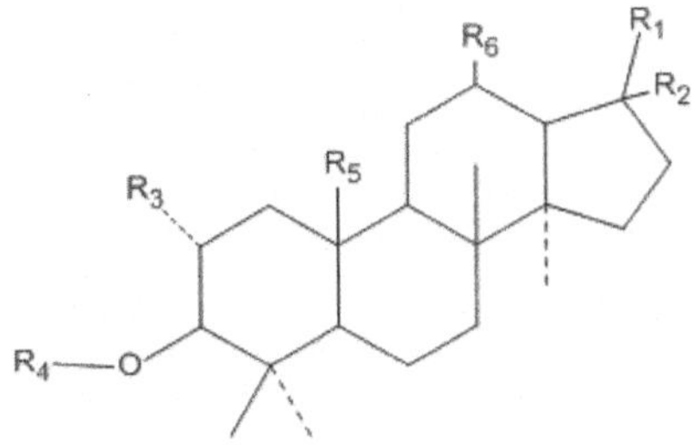

Compd	R_1	R_2	R_3	R_4	R_5	R_6	Anti-cancer activity[a]	Reference
Gypenosides							47.6 (Hep3B), 39.3 (PC-3), 30.6 (A549) HL-60, MCF-7, HT-29, Colon 205, Du145, MDA-MB-435, U87, A549, SK-OV-3, HepG2, SGC-7901, BEL-7402, Huh-7, HA22T, SW620, Eca-109, SAS, L1210, WEHI-3, SW-480, KB/VCR, MCF-7/ADR	[19, 21, 36, 44, 85–87, 89–91, 105–109, 111, 112, 114, 115, 119, 121, 131, 132]
Polysaccharide							65.4 (B16), HT-29, B16, Hela, SW-1116, HepG2	[44, 87, 88, 119]
Ethanolic extract							C6, HT-59	[113, 133]

[a] The anti-cancer activities, IC_{50} (μg/ml), of components of GpM are expressed as mean ± SD following cell line names in bracket. Only the mean value is listed if there is no SD value available and only cancer cell line name is listed if no IC_{50} data is available. The unit of compound 10, 11, 12, 13, 16, 21, 22, 26, 27 and 28 are transformed based on molecular weight. This table also presents 30 cancer cell lines whose proliferation could be inhibited by GpM, which indicates that GpM exerts broad spectrum anti-cancer activities

Flavonoids

Flavonoids are an important class of polyphenol compounds that are widely distributed in fruits and vegetables, where they usually exist in their glycosidic form [72]. In terms of their general structure, flavonoids consist of a 15-carbon skeleton, containing two phenyl rings (A and B) and a heterocyclic ring (C). The carbon structure of these compounds is usually abbreviated as C6–C3–C6. Several flavonoids have been isolated from GpM, including quercetin, rutin, ombuoside [73], ombuin [74], isorhamnetin-3-*O*-rutinoside, isorhamnetin [75], quercetin-di-(rhamno)-hexoside, quercetin-rhamno-hexoside, kaempferol-rhamno-hexoside and kaempferol-3-*O*-rutinoside [76], and the structures of these flavonoids are shown in Additional file 1: Table S2.

Other components of GpM

GpM contains various trace elements (e.g., Cu, Fe, Zn, Mn, Co, Ni, Se, Mo and Sr) [77], 18 amino acids [78] (including eight essential amino acids) and various vitamins and proteins, but the relative amounts of these components vary considerably across the different parts of the GpM plant (i.e., leaf, stem and subterranean stem) [78]. Malonic acid [74], benzyl-*O*-β-D-glucopyranoside [79], lutein, vomifoliol, palmitic acid [80], linolenic acids [81, 82] and carrot glycosides [83] have also been isolated from GpM. Furthermore, Tsai et al. [84] reported the isolation of numerous carotenoids and chlorophylls from the carotenoid and chlorophyll fractions of GpM, respectively.

Anti-cancer activities of GpM

In vitro anti-cancer activities of GpM

The in vitro antiproliferative activities of some of the pure compounds and extracts isolated from GpM have been widely reported and the details of these materials are summarized in Table 3. Shi et al. [85] obtained four dammarane-type triterpene saponins (compounds **3–6**) from the aerial parts of GpM, which exhibited moderate cytotoxic activities in vitro against several human cancer cell lines, including HL-60 (human promyelocytic leukemia cells), Colon 205 (human colon cancer cells) and Du145 (human prostate carcinoma cells) cells. Yin et al. [86] isolated nine dammarane saponins from the methanol extract of the aerial part of GpM, and found that compounds **7**, **8** and **9** exhibited inhibitory activities towards the growth of SGC-7901 (stomach cancer cells) and BEL-74020 (hepatocellular carcinoma cells) at a concentration of 100 μM with percentage inhibition values of 21, 93 and 8 %, and 77, 92 and 40 %, respectively.

Almost all of the compounds and extracts isolated from GpM to date have be reported to exhibit noticeable antiproliferative activities with IC_{50} values ranging from 0.05 to 74.3 μg/mL (Table 3). Compound **16** exhibited potent antiproliferative activities against A549 human lung cancer cells and U87 glioblastoma cells with IC_{50} values of 0.05 and 0.25 μg/mL, respectively. Compound **15** showed antiproliferative activity against MDA-MB-435 human breast cancer cells with an IC_{50} value of 3.90 μg/mL, whereas the carotenoid fraction of GpM exhibited the strongest activities of all of the reported extracts with an

IC_{50} value of 1.6 μg/mL against Hep3B human hepatocellular carcinoma cells.

The hydrolysates of the extracts of GpM have also been reported to exhibit anti-cancer activities, together with several other derivatives of the natural products found in GpM. For example, Chen et al. [87] reported the synthesis of four sulfated derivatives of GPP2, which is a native polysaccharide isolated from GpM. One of the sulfated derivatives prepared by Chen (GPP2-s4) inhibited the growth of HepG2 human hepatocellular carcinoma cells by 46.4 ± 2.8 % at a concentration of 2000 μg/mL. Compared with GPP2, all four sulfated derivatives exhibited stronger antiproliferative activities against HeLa cervical cancer cells at concentrations as low as 100 μg/mL. GP-B1, which is an acidic polysaccharide derived from GpM, significantly inhibited the growth of B16 melanoma cells with an IC_{50} of 65.4 μg/mL with very little cytotoxicity against normal cells [88]. Moreover, GP-B1 not only significantly inhibited the growth of cancer cells, but also improved cellular immune response by increasing levels of tumor necrosis factor-α (TNF-α), interferon-γ (IFN-γ), interleukin-10 (IL-10) and interleukin-12 (IL-12) observed in the serum of melanoma-B16-bearing mice [88].

In vivo anti-cancer activities of GpM

The in vivo anti-cancer activities of GpM are summarized in Table 4. Gyps led to significant reductions in the size of solid tumors in nude mice injected with SAS oral cancer cells [89]. Gyps also promoted the survival of mice xenografted with WEHI-3 leukemia cells, which was accompanied by an increase in the number of megakaryocytes and reduced spleen weight in these animals, indicating an enhanced immune response [90]. Similar anti-cancer activities have also been reported for Gyps in another leukemia mouse model [91]. The intraperitoneal treatment of tumor-bearing mice with Gyps (5 or 20 mg/kg/day) for 4 weeks led to considerable decreases in the size and weight of their tumors without altering their body weight. Gyps also strongly suppressed tumor growth in mice bearing advanced S180 sarcoma, which was associated with an increase in the ratio of tumor necrosis area to tumor total area and lymphocyte/macrophage infiltration into the peripheral areas of tumors. This effect also led to an increase in the weight of the spleens of these animals, as well as increases in the quantity and size of their splenic white pulp [92]. Gyps enhanced the anti-cancer effects of 5-fluorouracil in colorectal cancer cells and xenografts [93]. Gyps have also been reported to inhibit tumorigenesis in a transgenic mouse models of cancer, such as the $Apc^{Min/+}$ mouse model of intestinal neoplasia [94, 95]. Moreover, rats fed with a standardized extract of GpM did not show any mortal or toxic effects, highlighting the good safety profile of this material [96].

A polysaccharide from GpM inhibited the development of transplanted S180 sarcoma in a dose-dependent manner and increased the phagocytosis of macrophages, as well as increasing the production of NO, IL-1β and TNF-α from the peritoneal macrophages [97]. The neutral polysaccharide fraction CGPP inhibited the growth of H22 hepatocarcinoma cells transplanted into ICR mice [20]. CGPP treatment also led to improvements in the body weight, spleen/thymus index and degree of splenocyte proliferation in tumor-bearing mice [20]. Furthermore, CGPP treatment led to considerable increases in the levels of cytokines, such as IL-2, TNF-α and IFN-γ in tumor-bearing mice, as well as increases in the activity of natural killer (NK) cells and cytotoxic T lymphocytes (CTL) [20]. The tumor inhibitory and immunoregulatory effects of CGPP greatly increased the life span of H22 ascites in tumor-bearing mice [20].

Clinical anti-cancer studies on GpM

A clinical study was conducted in 1993 involving 59 patients with advanced malignant tumors to assess the effects of GpM [98]. The results revealed that patient treated with a GpM formula showed cancer relapse and metastasis rates of 11.9 and 8.5 %, respectively, compared with values of 72.4 and 55.2 % in the control group. The results of this study also revealed that the T lymphocyte transformation rate and acid α-naphthyl acetate esterase (ANAE+) activity increased by 8.2 % following GpM treatment [98]. The results of a separate 5-year observational study also showed that the treatment of cancer patients with GpM formula led to significant reductions in cancer relapse and metastasis rates, as well as reduced mortality and improved immune function in these patients [99]. GpM has also been reported to enhance NK cell activity in breast cancer patients [100], and improve the immune function of cancer patients after chemotherapy, as demonstrated by increased T lymphocyte transformation rate and decreased IgG and IgM levels [101]. Furthermore, GpM enhanced the immunological function of lung cancer patients after chemotherapy [102]. The results of a recent study [103] demonstrated that GpM formula can work in synergy with chemotherapy reagents. The clinical uses of GpM are summarized in Table 5.

Mechanisms of action

Multiple mechanisms of action have been proposed regarding the anti-cancer activities of GpM, including cell cycle arrest, apoptosis induction, inhibition of invasion and metastasis, glycolysis inhibition and immunomodulation (Fig. 2).

Cell cycle arrest

Gyps induced cell cycle arrest at the G0/G1 phase SAS human oral cancer cells [89], WEHI-3 leukemia cells [90], A549 human lung adenocarcinoma cells [104], HL-60 human myeloid leukemia cells [91] and Colo 205 human colon cancer cells [105]. Gyps also induced cell cycle arrest by modulating the expression of several cell cycle regulatory proteins, including cyclin-dependent kinase 2 (CDK2), cyclin-dependent kinase 4 (CDK4) and cyclin-dependent kinase 6 (CDK6) [21, 106]. The treatment of SCC-4 human tongue cancer cells with Gyps induced checkpoint kinase 2 (Chk2) expression. This effect subsequently led to the upregulation of p53 and its targets p21 and p16, which led to decreased levels of cyclin D and cyclin E and G0/G1 cell cycle arrest [106]. The treatment of PC-3 human prostate carcinoma cells with flavonoids and saponins isolated from GpM led to cell cycle arrest in the S and G2/M phases in both cases by modulating the expression of cyclins [21]. Furthermore, A549 cells treated with flavonoids from GpM went into cell cycle arrest in the S and G2/M phases, and showed upregulated levels of Cyclin A, Cyclin B, p21 and p53 [24].

Induction of apoptosis

A large number of studies have shown that GpM exerts its anti-cancer activities by inducing cellular apoptosis through various signaling pathways. Gyps downregulated the anti-apoptotic proteins Bcl-2 and Bcl-xL, and upregulated the pro-apoptotic proteins Bax, Bad and Bak, thereby activating the formation of Bax/Bak pores on the outer mitochondrial membrane [89–91, 107, 108]. Bax/Bak pores allow for the release of cytochrome c and other pro-apoptotic proteins into the cytosol, leading to the activation of initiator caspases-8 and -9, followed by the cleavage of effector caspase-3, which ultimately triggers apoptosis [104–106]. The formation of Bax/Bak pores following Gyps treatment also led to the release of apoptosis inducing factor (AIF) and endonuclease G (EndoG) from the mitochondria [89, 106], following DNA fragmentation and chromatin condensation.

Gyps also induced the production of reactive oxygen species (ROS) [36, 89, 105, 106, 108, 109] and led to increased intracellular Ca^{2+} concentrations [89–91, 105, 106, 108]. ROS and Ca^{2+} are both well-studied modulators of the permeability transition pores located on the inner mitochondrial membrane. The opening of these pores leads to an influx of solutes and water into the mitochondrial matrix, causing the outer mitochondrial matrix to swell and rupture, which leads to the release of cytochrome c and apoptosis [89–91, 105–107]. Gyps treatment led to increased levels of DNA-damage-inducible transcript 3 (GADD153), glucose-regulated protein (GRP78), activating transcription factor 6 alpha (ATF6-α) and activating transcription factor 4 alpha (ATF4-α). These increases resulted in endoplasmic reticulum (ER) stress, which could result in the release of Ca^{2+} from the ER [89–91, 106]. Moreover, Sun et al. [110] reported increased store-operated Ca^{2+} entry as another mechanism of action for the activity of Gyps.

Furthermore, Gyps induced dose-dependent DNA damage in SAS cells and reduced the expression of several DNA repair genes, including ataxia telangiectasia mutated, ataxia-telangiectasia and Rad3-related, breast cancer gene 1, 14-3-3σ, DNA-dependent serine/threonine protein kinase and p53, in a time-dependent manner. In this way, Gyps treatment stalled the DNA damage repair process, forcing the cells to undergo apoptosis [109, 111].

Several other components and fractions of GpM have also been reported to induce apoptosis. For instance, flavonoids [21] and a water extract [112] from GpM induced apoptosis in tumor cells via the regulation of the Bcl-2 protein family. Furthermore, an ethanolic extract from GpM selectively shifted the intracellular H_2O_2 concentration to toxic levels in tumor cells because of the increased superoxide dismutase activity of these cells compared with healthy cells [113].

Inhibition of invasion and metastasis

Gyps suppressed the invasion and migration of SCC4 human tongue cancer cells in a dose- and time-dependent manner by downregulating nuclear factor kappa B (NF-κB) and matrix metalloproteinase-9 (MMP-9) [114]. Gyps also inhibited the invasion and migration of SAS cells, as demonstrated by the results of in vitro wound-healing and Boyden Chamber assays. Treatment with Gyps led to decreases in the levels of several migration- and invasion-associated proteins, including NF-κB, cyclooxygenase-2, extracellular signal-regulated kinase 1/2 (ERK1/2), matrix metalloproteinase-2 (MMP-2), MMP-9, sevenless homolog, Ras, urokinase-type plasminogen activator, focal adhesion kinase and alpha serine/threonine protein kinase [115]. Furthermore, Gyps exhibited anti-migration activities towards SW620 human colon adenocarcinoma cells and Eca-109 human esophageal squamous carcinoma cells [19]. Gyps also inhibited the migration of SW-480 human colon adenocarcinoma cells in vitro at a concentration of 100 μg/mL [36]. This effect was observed in clinical studies. For example, patients with advanced malignant tumors that were treated with GpM formula showed a reduced cancer metastasis rate of 8.5 % compared with 55.2 % in the control group [36].

Table 4 In vivo anti-cancer activity of identified GpM components

Component	Animal model	Anti-cancer activity[a]	Reference
Gypenosides	Nude mice: xenografted with human oral cancer SAS cells	65.76 % (tumor size, 20 mg/kg for 28 days)	[89]
Gypenosides	BALB/c mice: injected with human leukemia WEHI-3 cells	150 % (survival rate, 2 mg/kg for 2 weeks) 175 % (survival rate, 4 mg/kg for 2 weeks)	[90]
Gypenosides	Nude mice: xenografted with human leukemia HL-60 cells	44 % (tumor size, 20 mg/kg for 28 days)	[91]
Gypenosides	BALB/c mice: xenografted with murine S180 sarcoma cells	39.57 % (tumor size, 30 mg/kg for 4 days)	[92]
Gypenosides	BALB/c mice: xenografted with murine colorectal cancer CT-26 cells	75 % (tumor size, 25 mg/kg for 19 days) 55 % (tumor size, 50 mg/kg for 19 days) 26 % (tumor size, 50 mg/kg + 5 mg/kg 5-Fu for 19 days)	[93]
Gypenosides	$Apc^{Min/+}$ mice: intestinal neoplasia model	66.06 % (polyps number, 500 mg/kg for 4 weeks) 59.92 % (polyps number, 750 mg/kg for 4 weeks)	[94]
Gypenosides	$Apc^{Min/+}$ mice: intestinal neoplasia model	59.32 % (polyps number, 500 mg/kg for 8 weeks)	[95]
Polysaccharide	BALB/c mice: xenografted with murine S180 sarcoma cells	62.77 % (tumor size, 100 mg/kg for 14 days) 59.24 % (tumor size, 200 mg/kg for 14 days)	[97]
Polysaccharide	ICR mice: xenografted with mouse hepatoma H22 cells	62.89 % (tumor size, 50 mg/kg for 10 days) 49.22 % (tumor size, 200 mg/kg for 10 days)	[20]

[a] The anti-cancer activities of components of GpM are expressed as the percentage of control (readout, dose)

Glycolysis inhibition

One of the hallmarks of cancer cells is deregulated energy metabolism, which can lead to a state known as "aerobic glycolysis" [116]. Targeting glucose metabolism has therefore proven to be a promising avenue for the development of new cancer treatments [117]. GpMix, which is a mixture of triterpenoid saponins from GpM, effectively inhibited the growth of cancer cells in the presence of co-cultivated normal cells [118]. Furthermore, GpMix exhibited both chemopreventive and therapeutic effects towards the formation of intestinal polyps in $Apc^{min/+}$ mice (a mouse model of colon cancer). Several key enzymes along the glycolysis pathway, including pyruvate kinase (PK), α-enolase, glyceraldehyde 3-phosphate dehydrogenase (GAPDH), mitochondrial aconitase and ATP synthase-α and -β were found to be downregulated in R6 cells treated with GpMix by proteomic analysis [118]. These findings therefore implied that the inhibition of the glycolysis pathway was involved in the suppression of cell proliferation by GpMix.

Immune modulation

GpM also exhibited anti-cancer effects indirectly through its immunomodulating activities. For example, Yang et al. [119] found that a water-soluble polysaccharide from *G. pentaphyllum* herb tea (PSGP) indirectly exerted anti-cancer activity against SW-1116 human colorectal adenocarcinoma cells and HT-29 by enhancing the immune response of macrophages with increased TNF-α secretion in a dose-dependent manner. Moreover, GP-B1, the acidic polysaccharide obtained from GpM, not only significantly inhibited the growth of cancer cells, but also improved cellular immune response with increased levels of TNF-α, IFN-γ, IL-10 and IL-12 in the serum of melanoma-B16-bearing mice [88]. The anti-cancer activity of Gyps was attributed to the elevated immune systems of the xenografted mice [120]. Gyps significantly suppressed tumor growth in mice transplanted with Lewis lung cancer cells with tumor weight inhibition rates of 29.8 ± 1.3, 51.4 ± 2.2 and 50.0 ± 1.6 % following intraperitoneal Gyps injections of 10, 20 and 40 mg/kg, respectively. Notably, the immune responses of these mice improved considerably, as demonstrated by increases in their total splenic cell number and the enhanced biological activities of the NK and splenic cells [120]. Clinical studies have also shown that GpM enhanced the activity of NK cells in breast cancer patients [100], improved the immune function of cancer patients after chemotherapy, increased the T lymphocyte transformation rate and decreased the IgG and IgM levels [101].

Perspectives

Numerous studies have been published during the last four decades regarding the anti-cancer effects of GpM, including reports focused on (i) the isolation and characterization of its chemical components [121, 122]; (ii) the evaluation of its anti-cancer activities and mechanisms of action [107, 115]; and (iii) studies on its toxicity [96]. Taken together, the results of these reports have demonstrated that GpM has a broad anti-cancer spectrum (against 30 cancer cell lines, Table 3) without any obvious inhibitory effect on normal cell proliferation. However, there are limitations associated with most of these studies.

Table 5 Clinical uses of GpM

Component	Patient tumor type	Anti-cancer activity[a]	Reference
GpM formula	Multiple types	16.44 % (relapse rate) 15.40 % (metastasis rate)	[98]
GpM formula	Multiple types	14.23 % (relapse and metastasis rate)	[99]
GpM formula	Breast cancer	129.56 % (NK cell activity)	[100]
GpM formula	Multiple types	157 % (T lymphocyte transformation rate) 78.4 % (IgG levels) 75.1 % (IgA levels) 59.9 % (IgM levels)	[101]
GpM formula	Lung cancer	128 % (curative rate)	[102]
GpM formula	Middle-late gastric cancer	163 % (short term curative rate) 140 % (quality of life)	[103]

[a] The anti-cancer activities of components of GpM are expressed as the percentage of control (readout)

The standard preparation of Gyps needs to be unified

Gyps consist of a mixture of approximately 189 dammarane-type saponin glycosides. Most of the studies reported to date on GpM have focused exclusively on the use of its fractions, such as Gyps, as well as the use of its extracts. In contrast, there have been very few reports pertaining to the use of single compounds isolated from GpM. For example, in all of the papers published during the last 15 years regarding the anti-cancer mechanisms of GpM there has only been one study involving the use of single compounds. Based on to the lack of chemical consistency in the fractions and extracts of GpM, greater efforts should be taken to explore the anti-cancer activities of single compounds derived from GpM in future studies, where possible. Moreover, none of the Gyps tested in any of the studies reported to date were prepared using a unified procedure, which could have led to completely different chemical component profiles amongst the different samples. Most of these studies also failed to provide essential chemical composition information for their Gyps, such as the exact molecular structure of each saponin, the number of saponins in the mixture, the relative contents of the different saponins in Gyps and a standard HPLC fingerprint [19, 89, 90, 106, 107, 109, 111, 115]. Studies on the chemical structures of the saponins in Gyps are therefore urgently needed, as well as further studies towards the chemical composition and the quantitative analysis of Gyps. These data would allow researchers to develop a deeper understanding of the anti-cancer activities and mechanisms of action of Gyps and facilitate further studies.

Experimental systems need to be closer to the clinical settings

Most of the studies reported to date concerning the anti-cancer activities and mechanisms of action of GpM have been conducted using in vitro cellular systems. This trend could therefore explain why non-specific cell cycle arrest and the induction of apoptosis have been cited, in the majority of cases, as the principal mechanisms of action of GpM [89, 104, 106], with very few reports citing specific molecular targets or enzymatic pathways. In contrast, most of the in vivo studies conducted on GpM, have focused on the use of cancer cell lines implanted into immunodeficient mice [20, 90, 91]. According to this model, cancer cell lines are selected to survive in culture, and tumor-resident cells and proteins that interact with the cancer cells are eliminated to give a phenotypically homogeneous culture [123]. Patient-derived tumor xenograft (PDTX) models have several advantages over cell line xenograft models, such as maintaining the heterogeneity of the tumor and mimicking the microenvironment of human tumors [124]. Humanized-xenograft models can also be created by co-engrafting a sample of a patient-derived tumor together with peripheral blood or bone marrow cells into an immunodeficient mouse, followed by the reconstitution of the murine immune system. Advanced tumor models of this type can be used to study the interactions between xenogenic human stroma and tumor environments in cancer progression and metastasis [125]. Genetically engineered mouse models represent an interesting alternative for evaluating the effects of anti-cancer agents because these animals maintain a competent immune system, allowing for changes in the tumor microenvironment and the tumor itself to be thoroughly evaluated from an early stage [126]. Based on our review of the literature, we believe that further experiments should be performed in a PDTX, humanized-xenograft or genetically engineered mouse model to evaluate the effects of GpM on tumor development with greater clinical accuracy. The latter of these two models would be especially interesting in terms of evaluating the potential immunomodulatory activity of GpM.

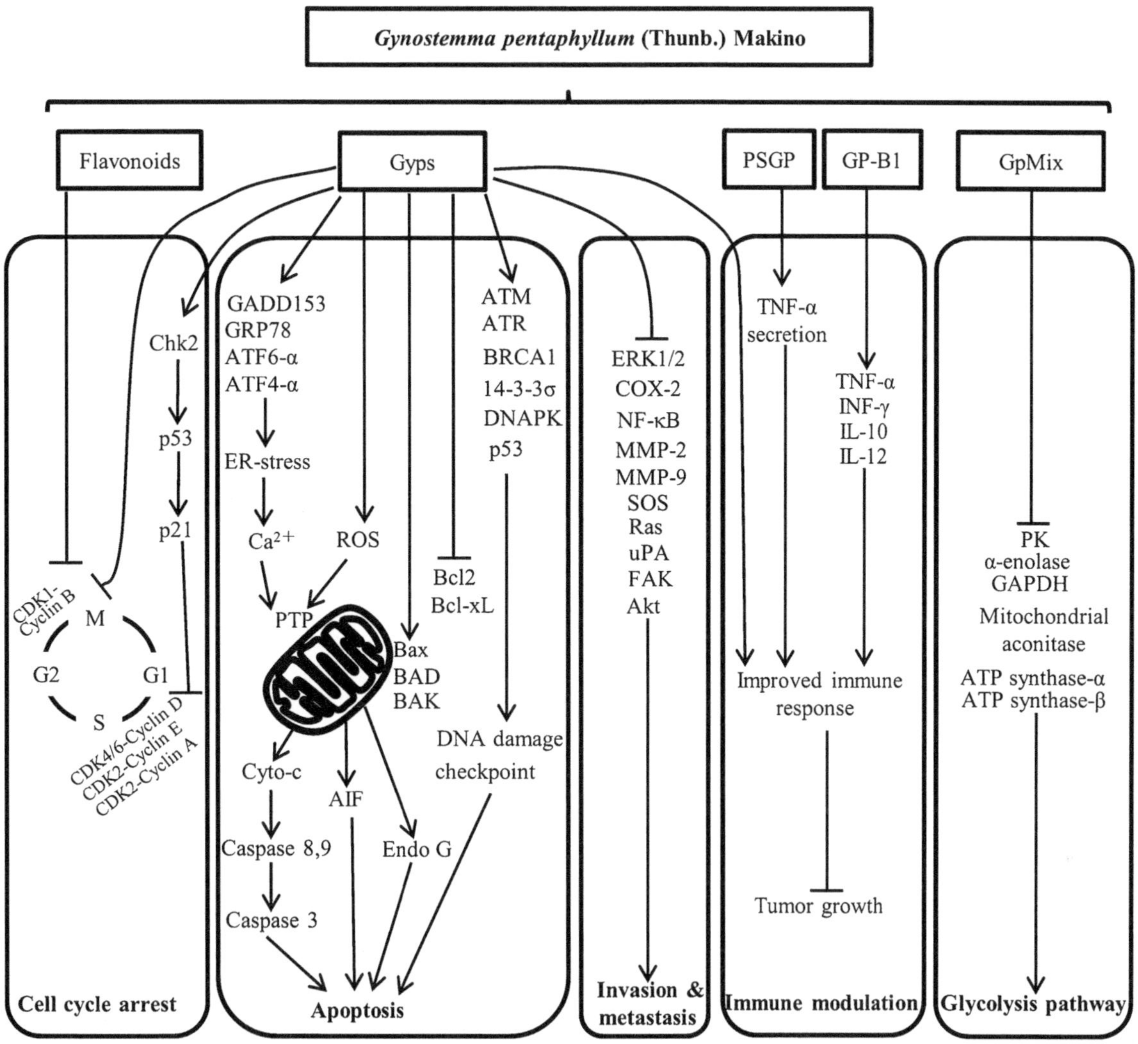

Fig. 2 Mechanisms of action for the anti-cancer activities of GpM

Conclusion

In summary, GpM has been investigated extensively as a potent anti-cancer agent against many types of cancers both in vitro and in vivo. The general consensus from the literature is that GpM exerts its anti-cancer activities through multiple mechanisms, including cell cycle arrest, the induction of apoptosis, inhibition of invasion and metastasis, glycolysis inhibition and immunomodulation.

Abbreviations

AIF: apoptosis inducing factor; Akt: alpha serine/threonine protein kinase; ANAE+: acid α-naphthyl acetate esterase; ATF4-α: activating transcription factor 4 alpha; ATF6-α: activating transcription factor 6 alpha; ATM: ataxia telangiectasia mutated; ATR: ataxia-telangiectasia and Rad3-related; CDK2: cyclin-dependent kinase 2; CDK4: cyclin-dependent kinase 4; CDK6: cyclin-dependent kinase 6; Chk2: checkpoint kinase 2; CM: Chinese medicine; COX-2: cyclooxygenase-2; DNAPK: DNA-dependent serine/threonine protein kinase; EndoG: endonuclease G; ER: endoplasmic reticulum; ERK1/2: extracellular signal-regulated kinase ½; FAK: focal adhesion kinase; GADD153: growth arrest and DNA damage-inducible gene 153; GpM: *Gynostemma pentaphyllum* (Thunb.) Makino; GAPDH: glyceraldehydes 3-phosphate dehydrogenase; GRP78: glucose-regulated protein 78; Gyps: gypenosides; IFN-γ: interferon-γ; IL-10: interleukin-10; IL-12: interleukin-12; MMP-2: matrix metalloproteinase-2; MMP-9: matrix metalloproteinase-9; NF-kB: nuclear factor kappa B; NK: natural killer; CTL: cytotoxic T lymphocytes; PK: pyruvate kinase; SOD: superoxide dismutase; SOS: sevenless homolog; TNA: tumor necrosis area; TNF-α: tumor necrosis factor-α; TTA: tumor total area; uPA: urokinase-type plasminogen activator.

Authors' contributions

YL, WL, JH, XY and WM conceived and designed the review. YL, WL, JH, XY and WM wrote the manuscript. All authors read and approved the final manuscript.

Acknowledgements
This work was supported by Grants from the Science and Technology Development Fund (FDCT) of Macau (Project codes: 034/2015/A1 and 088/2012/A3).

Competing interests
The authors declare that they have no competing interests.

References

1. Cancer IARC. World cancer report 2014. Geneva: World Health Organization; 2014.
2. Carter GT. Natural products and pharma 2011: Strategic changes spur new opportunities. Nat Prod Rep. 2011;28:1783–9.
3. Pezzuto JM. Plant-derived anticancer agents. Biochem Pharmacol. 1997;53:121–33.
4. Lilenbaum RC, Green MR. Novel chemotherapeutic agents in the treatment of non-small-cell lung cancer. J Clin Oncol. 1993;11:1391–402.
5. Quan Y, Qian M. Effect and mechanism of gypenoside on the inflammatory molecular expression in high-fat induced atherosclerosis rats. Zhongguo Zhong Xi Yi Jie He Za Zhi. 2010;30:403–6.
6. Cai H, Liang Q, Ge G. Gypenoside attenuates beta amyloid-induced inflammation in n9 microglial cells via SOCS1 signaling. Neural Plast. 2016;2016:6362707.
7. Liou CJ, Huang WC, Kuo ML, Yang RC, Shen JJ. Long-term oral administration of *Gynostemma pentaphyllum* extract attenuates airway inflammation and Th2 cell activities in ovalbumin-sensitized mice. Food Chem Toxicol. 2010;48:2592–8.
8. Yang F, Shi H, Zhang X, Yang H, Zhou Q, Yu LL. Two new saponins from tetraploid jiaogulan (*Gynostemma pentaphyllum*), and their anti-inflammatory and α-glucosidase inhibitory activities. Food Chem. 2013;141:3606–13.
9. Zhao J, Ming Y, Wan Q, Ye S, Xie S, Zhu Y, Wang Y, Zhong Z, Li L, Ye Q. Gypenoside attenuates hepatic ischemia/reperfusion injury in mice via anti-oxidative and anti-apoptotic bioactivities. Exp Ther Med. 2014;7:1388–92.
10. Yu H, Guan Q, Guo L, Zhang H, Pang X, Cheng Y, Zhang X, Sun Y. Gypenosides alleviate myocardial ischemia-reperfusion injury via attenuation of oxidative stress and preservation of mitochondrial function in rat heart. Cell Stress Chaperones. 2016;21:429–37.
11. Gao D, Zhao M, Qi X, Liu Y, Li N, Liu Z, Bian Y. Hypoglycemic effect of *Gynostemma pentaphyllum* saponins by enhancing the nrf2 signaling pathway in stz-inducing diabetic rats. Arch Pharm Res. 2016;39:221–30.
12. Schild L, Cotte T, Keilhoff G, Brodemann R. Preconditioning of brain slices against hypoxia induced injury by a *Gynostemma pentaphyllum* extract–stimulation of anti-oxidative enzyme expression. Phytomedicine. 2012;19:812–8.
13. Li B, Zhang XY, Wang MZ, Jiao LL. Characterization and antioxidant activities of acidic polysaccharides from *Gynostemma pentaphyllum* (Thunb.) Markino. Carbohydr Polym. 2015;127:209–14.
14. la Cour B, Molgaard P, Yi Z. Traditional chinese medicine in treatment of hyperlipidaemia. J Ethnopharmacol. 1995;46:125–9.
15. Gou SH, Huang HF, Chen XY, Liu J, He M, Ma YY, Zhao XN, Zhang Y, Ni JM. Lipid-lowering, hepatoprotective, and atheroprotective effects of the mixture Hong-Qu and gypenosides in hyperlipidemia with NAFLD rats. J Chin Med Assoc. 2016;79:111–21.
16. Wang M, Wang F, Wang Y, Ma X, Zhao M, Zhao C. Metabonomics study of the therapeutic mechanism of *Gynostemma pentaphyllum* and atorvastatin for hyperlipidemia in rats. PLoS One. 2013;8:e78731.
17. Muller C, Gardemann A, Keilhoff G, Peter D, Wiswedel I, Schild L. Prevention of free fatty acid-induced lipid accumulation, oxidative stress, and cell death in primary hepatocyte cultures by a *Gynostemma pentaphyllum* extract. Phytomedicine. 2012;19:395–401.
18. Qin R, Zhang J, Li C, Zhang X, Xiong A, Huang F, Yin Z, Li K, Qin W, Chen M, Zhang S, Liang L, Zhang H, Nie H, Ye W. Protective effects of gypenosides against fatty liver disease induced by high fat and cholesterol diet and alcohol in rats. Arch Pharm Res. 2012;35:1241–50.
19. Yan H, Wang X, Wang Y, Wang P, Xiao Y. Antiproliferation and anti-migration induced by gypenosides in human colon cancer SW620 and esophageal cancer Eca-109 cells. Hum Exp Toxicol. 2014;33:522–33.
20. Liu J, Zhang L, Ren Y, Gao Y, Kang L, Qiao Q. Anticancer and immunoregulatory activity of *Gynostemma pentaphyllum* polysaccharides in H22 tumor-bearing mice. Int J Biol Macromol. 2014;69:1–4.
21. Cheng TC, Lu JF, Wang JS, Lin LJ, Kuo HI, Chen BH. Antiproliferation effect and apoptosis mechanism of prostate cancer cell PC-3 by flavonoids and saponins prepared from *Gynostemma pentaphyllum*. J Agric Food Chem. 2011;59:11319–29.
22. Li Y, Huang J, Lin W, Yuan Z, Feng S, Xie Y, Ma W. In vitro anticancer activity of a nonpolar fraction from *Gynostemma pentaphyllum* (Thunb.) Makino. Evid Based Complement Altern Med. 2016;2016:6308649.
23. Hou J, Liu S, Ma Z, Lang X, Wang J, Liang Z. Effects of *Gynostemma pentaphyllum* Makino on the immunological function of cancer patients. J Tradit Chin Med. 1991;11:47–52.
24. Tsui K-C, Chiang T-H, Wang J-S, Lin L-J, Chao W-C, Chen B-H, Lu J-F. Flavonoids from *Gynostemma pentaphyllum* exhibit differential induction of cell cycle arrest in H460 and A549 cancer cells. Molecules. 2014;19:17663–81.
25. Choi HS, Zhao TT, Shin KS, Kim SH, Hwang BY, Lee CK, Lee MK. Anxiolytic effects of herbal ethanol extract from *Gynostemma pentaphyllum* in mice after exposure to chronic stress. Molecules. 2013;18:4342–56.
26. Zhao TT, Shin KS, Choi HS, Lee MK. Ameliorating effects of gypenosides on chronic stress-induced anxiety disorders in mice. BMC Complement Altern Med. 2015;15:323.
27. Shin KS, Zhao TT, Choi HS, Hwang BY, Lee CK, Lee MK. Effects of gypenosides on anxiety disorders in MPTP-lesioned mouse model of Parkinson's disease. Brain Res. 2014;1567:57–65.
28. Lin C-C, Huang P-C, Lin J-M. Antioxidant and hepatoprotective effects of *Anoectochilus formosanus* and *Gynostemma pentaphyllum*. Am J Chin Med. 2000;28:87–96.
29. Liu ZL, Xie LZ, Zhu J, Li GQ, Grant SJ, Liu JP. Herbal medicines for fatty liver diseases. Cochrane Database Syst Rev. 2013;(8):CD009059. doi:10.1002/14651858.CD009059.pub2.
30. He Q, Li JK, Li F, Li RG, Zhan GQ, Li G, Du WX, Tan HB. Mechanism of action of gypenosides on type 2 diabetes and non-alcoholic fatty liver disease in rats. World J Gastroenterol. 2015;21:2058–66.
31. Megalli S, Davies NM, Roufogalis BD. Anti-hyperlipidemic and hypoglycemic effects of *Gynostemma pentaphyllum* in the zucker fatty rat. J Pharm Pharm Sci. 2006;9:281–91.
32. Lokman EF, Gu HF, Wan Mohamud WN, Ostenson CG. Evaluation of antidiabetic effects of the traditional medicinal plant *Gynostemma pentaphyllum* and the possible mechanisms of insulin release. Evid Based Complement Altern Med. 2015;2015:120572.
33. Circosta C, De Pasquale R, Occhiuto F. Cardiovascular effects of the aqueous extract of *Gynostemma pentaphyllum* Makino. Phytomedicine. 2005;12:638–43.
34. Purmova J, Opletal L. Phytotherapeutic aspects of diseases of the cardiovascular system. 5. Saponins and possibilities of their use in prevention and therapy. Ceska Slov Farm. 1995;44:246–51.
35. Tanner MA, Bu X, Steimle JA, Myers PR. The direct release of nitric oxide by gypenosides derived from the herb *Gynostemma pentaphyllum*. Nitric Oxide. 1999;3:359–65.
36. Yan H, Wang X, Niu J, Wang Y, Wang P, Liu Q. Anti-cancer effect and the underlying mechanisms of gypenosides on human colorectal cancer SW-480 cells. PLoS One. 2014;9:e95609.
37. Wu PK, Liu X, Hsiao WWL. The assessment of anti-cancer activities and saponin profiles of *Gynostemma pentaphyllum* saponins obtained from different regions of China. J Biotechnol. 2008;136:S85.
38. Juchi S. Preparation of a tea-like beverage containing *Gynostemma pentaphyllum* saponins. Osaka Yakuhin Kenkyusho KK Patent-Japan Kokai Tokkyo Koho-61. 1986;104:772.
39. Kenkyusho K. Saponins from *Gynostemma pentaphyllum* as health food supplements. Osaka Yakuhin assignee Jpn Kokai Tokkyo Koho JP. 60:85.
40. KK OYK. Rice vinegar containing saponins as health food supplement. Osaka Yakuhin Kenkyusho KK Patent-Japan Kokai Tokkyo Koho-60. 1985.
41. Guo W, Wang W, editor. Cultivation and utilisation of Gynostemma pentaphyllum. Beijing: Publishing house of electronics; 1993.
42. Cui J, Eneroth P, Bruhn JG. *Gynostemma pentaphyllum*: identification of major sapogenins and differentiation from Panax species. Eur J Pharm Sci. 1999;8:187–91.

43. Shi L, Song D, Pan M, Liu D. Research advances on the saponins of *Gynostemma pentaphyllum*. Drug Eval Res. 2011;34:456–64.
44. Piao XL, Xing SF, Lou CX, Chen DJ. Novel dammarane saponins from *Gynostemma pentaphyllum* and their cytotoxic activities against HepG2 cells. Bioorg Med Chem Lett. 2014;24:4831–3.
45. Yang F, Shi H, Zhang X, Yu LL. Two novel anti-inflammatory 21-nordammarane saponins from tetraploid jiaogulan (*Gynostemma pentaphyllum*). J Agric Food Chem. 2013;61:12646–52.
46. Nagai M. ea. Abstracts. In: The 23rd meeting of the Japanese Society of Pharmacognosy. 1976:37.
47. Takemoto T, Arihara S, Nakajima T, Okuhira M. Studies on the constituents of *Gynostemma pentaphyllum* Makino. II. Structures of gypenoside xv–xxi. Yakugaku Zasshi. 1983;103:1015–23.
48. Takemoto T, Arihara S, Yoshikawa K, Kusumoto K, Yano I, Hayashi T. Studies on the constituents of Cucurbitaceae plants. VI. On the saponin constituents of Luffa cylindrica Roem. Yakugaku Zasshi. 1984;104:246–55.
49. Takemoto T, Arihara S, Yoshikawa K. Studies on the constituents of Cucurbitaceae plants on the saponin constituents of *Gynostemma pentaphyllum* Makino. Yakugaku Zasshi. 1986;106:664–70.
50. Takemoto T, Arihara S, Nakajima T, Okuhira M. Studies on the constituents of *Gynostemma pentaphyllum* Makino structures of gypenoside ixiv. Yakugaku Zasshi. 1983;103:173–85.
51. Yoshikawa K, Arimitsu M, Kishi K, Takemoto T, Arihara S. Studies on the constituents of Cucurbitaceae plants on the saponin constituents of *Gynostemma pentaphyllum* Makino. Yakugaku Zasshi. 1987;107:361–6.
52. Yoshikawa K, Takemoto T, Arihara S. Studies on the constituents of Cucurbitaceae plants on the saponin constituents of *Gynostemma pentaphyllum* Makino. Yakugaku Zasshi. 1987;107:262–7.
53. Kim JH, Han YN. Dammarane-type saponins from *Gynostemma pentaphyllum*. Phytochemistry. 2011;72:1453–9.
54. Zhang XS, Zhao C, Tang WZ, Wu XJ, Zhao YQ. Gypensapogenin H, a novel dammarane-type triterpene induces cell cycle arrest and apoptosis on prostate cancer cells. Steroids. 2015;104:276–83.
55. Zhang XS, Cao JQ, Zhao C, Wang XD, Wu XJ, Zhao YQ. Novel dammarane-type triterpenes isolated from hydrolyzate of total *Gynostemma pentaphyllum* saponins. Bioorg Med Chem Lett. 2015;25:3095–9.
56. Shi L, Pi Y, Luo C, Zhang C, Tan D, Meng X. In vitro inhibitory activities of six gypenosides on human liver cancer cell line HepG2 and possible role of HIf-1α pathway in them. Chem Biol Interact. 2015;238:48–54.
57. Liu J, Yang PY, Shi HM, Sun XJ, Lee SH, Yu LL. A novel *Gynostemma pentaphyllum* saponin and its adipogenesis inhibitory effect through modulating Wnt/β-catenin pathway and cell cycle in mitotic clonal expansion. J Funct Foods. 2015;17:552–62.
58. Lee C, Lee JW, Jin Q, Jang H, Jang HJ, Rho MC, Lee MK, Lee CK, Lee MK, Hwang BY. Isolation and characterization of dammarane-type saponins from *Gynostemma pentaphyllum* and their inhibitory effects on IL-6-induced STAT3 activation. J Nat Prod. 2015;78:971–6.
59. Xing SF, Jang M, Wang YR, Piao XL. A new dammarane-type saponin from *Gynostemma pentaphyllum* induces apoptosis in A549 human lung carcinoma cells. Bioorg Med Chem Lett. 2016;26:1754–9.
60. Liu J, Li YF, Shi HM, Wang T, Wu XL, Sun XJ, Yu LL. Components characterization of total tetraploid jiaogulan (*Gynostemma pentaphyllum*) saponin and its cholesterol-lowering properties. J Funct Foods. 2016;23:542–55.
61. Akihisa T, Tamura T, Matsumoto T. 14α-methyl-5α-ergosta-9 (11) 24 (28)-dien-3β-ol a sterol from *Gynostemma pentaphyllum*. Phytochemistry. 1987;26:2412–3.
62. Akihisa T, Kanari M, Tamura T, Matsumoto T. (24r)-and (24s)-14α-methyl-5α-ergost-9 (11)-en-3β-ols from *Gynostemma pentaphyllum*. Phytochemistry. 1989;28:1271–3.
63. Akihisa T, Mihara H, Fujikawa T, Tamura T, Matsumoto T. 24, 24-dimethyl-5α-cholestan-3β-ol, a sterol from *Gynostemma pentaphyllum*. Phytochemistry. 1988;27:2931–3.
64. Akihisa T, Kokke W, Yokota T, Tamura T, Matsumoto T. 4α, 14α-dimethyl-5α-ergosta-7, 9 (11), 24 (28)-trien-3β-ol from *Phaseolus vulgaris* and *Gynostemma pentaphyllum*. Phytochemistry. 1990;29:1647–51.
65. Akihisa T, Tamura T, Matsumoto T, Kokke W, Yokota T. Isolation of acetylenic sterols from a higher plant. Further evidence that marine sterols are not unique. J Org Chem. 1989;54(606–10):0022–3263.
66. Akihisa T, Thakur S, Rosenstein FU, Matsumoto T. Sterols of cucurbitaceae: the configurations at c-24 of 24-alkyl-δ5-, δ7-and δ8-sterols. Lipids. 1986;21(39–47):0024–4201.
67. Akihisa T, Shimizu N, Tamura T, Matsumoto T. Structures of three new 24, 24-dimethyl-δ7-sterols *fromGynostemma pentaphyllumfromGynostemma pentaphyllum*. Lipids. 1986;21(515–7):0024–4201.
68. Song S-l, Ji A-g, Liang H, Wang W-L. Purification and structure analysis of polysaccharides from *Gynostemma pentaphyllum* (Thunb.) Makino. Zhong Yao Cai. 2008.
69. Li X-L, Wang Z-H, Zhao Y-X, Luo S-J, Zhang D-W, Xiao S-X, Peng Z-H. Purification of a polysaccharide from *Gynostemma pentaphyllum* Makino and its therapeutic advantages for psoriasis. Carbohydr Polym. 2012;89:1232–7.
70. Wang Z, Luo D. Antioxidant activities of different fractions of polysaccharide purified from *Gynostemma pentaphyllum* Makino. Carbohydr Polym. 2007;68:54–8.
71. Chi A-P, Chen J-P, Wang Z-Z, Xiong Z-Y, Li Q-X. Morphological and structural characterization of a polysaccharide from *Gynostemma pentaphyllum* Makino and its anti-exercise fatigue activity. Carbohydr Polym. 2008;74:868–74.
72. Tsai YC, Lin CL, Chen BH. Preparative chromatography of flavonoids and saponins in *Gynostemma pentaphyllum* and their antiproliferation effect on hepatoma cell. Phytomedicine. 2010;18:2–10.
73. Yin F, Hu L, Lou F, Pan R. Dammarane-type glycosides from *Gynostemma pentaphyllum*. J Nat Prod. 2004;67:942–52.
74. Fang Z-P, Zeng X-Y. Isolation and identification of flavonoid glycosides and organic acid from *Gynostemma pentaphyllum* (Thunb.) Makino. Zhongguo Zhong Yao Za Zhi. 1989;14:36.
75. Chang Q, Chen D, Shen L, Si J, Zhang J, Li X. Studies on the chemical constituents of *Gynostemma pubescens* (Gagnep.) C.Y. Wu i. Flavonoids. Nat Prod Res Dev. 1991;4:16–8.
76. Kao T, Huang S, Inbaraj BS, Chen B. Determination of flavonoids and saponins in *Gynostemma pentaphyllum* (Thunb.) Makino by liquid chromatography–mass spectrometry. Anal Chim Acta. 2008;626:200–11.
77. Nookabkaew S, Rangkadilok N, Prachoom N, Satayavivad J. Concentrations of trace elements in organic fertilizers and animal manures and feeds and cadmium contamination in herbal tea (*Gynostemma pentaphyllum* Makino). J Agric Food Chem. 2016;64:3119–26.
78. Deng S, Li X, Chen B, Deng F, Zhou X. Analysis of amino acids, vitamins and chemical elements in *Gynostemma pentaphyllum* (Thunb.) Makino. Hunan Yi Ke Da Xue Xue Bao. 1994;19:487–90.
79. Chen Y-G, Zhang Y. Isolation and characterization of benzyl-o-β-D-glucopyranoside from *Gynostemma pentaphyllum*. Yunnan Shi Fan Da Xue Xue Bao. 2001;21:58–9.
80. Z-l XU, F-q YANG, Z-n XIA. Chemical constituents of *Gynostemma pentaphyllum*. Nat Prod Res Dev. 2013;8:1067–9.
81. Zou C, Shi HM, Liu X, Sheng YQ, Ding TT, Yan J, Gao BY, Liu J, Lu WY, Yu LL. Conjugated linolenic acids and nutraceutical components in jiaogulan (*Gynostemma pentaphyllum*) seeds. LWT Food Sci Technol. 2016;68:111–8.
82. Wang L, Wang XB, Wang P, Xiao YP, Liu QH. Optimization of supercritical carbon dioxide extraction, physicochemical and cytotoxicity properties of *Gynostemma pentaphyllum* seed oil: a potential source of conjugated linolenic acids. Sep Purif Technol. 2016;159:147–56.
83. Lin S. Research on the chemical constituents of *Gynostemma pentaphyllum* (Thunb.) Makino: Shenyang Pharmaceutical University; 2010.
84. Tsai YC, Wu WB, Chen BH. Preparation of carotenoids and chlorophylls from *Gynostemma pentaphyllum* (Thunb.) Makino and their antiproliferation effect on hepatoma cell. J Med Food. 2010;13:1431–42.
85. Shi L, Cao JQ, Shi SM, Zhao YQ. Triterpenoid saponins from *Gynostemma pentaphyllum*. J Asian Nat Prod Res. 2011;13:168–77.
86. Yin F, Zhang YN, Yang ZY, Hu LH. Nine new dammarane saponins from *Gynostemma pentaphyllum*. Chem Biodivers. 2006;3:771–82.
87. Chen T, Li B, Li Y, Zhao CD, Shen JM, Zhang HX. Catalytic synthesis and antitumor activities of sulfated polysaccharide from *Gynostemma pentaphyllum* Makino. Carbohydr Polym. 2011;83:554–60.
88. Li XL, Wang ZH, Zhao YX, Luo SJ, Zhang DW, Xiao SX, Peng ZH. Isolation and antitumor activities of acidic polysaccharide from *Gynostemma pentaphyllum* Makino. Carbohydr Polym. 2012;89:942–7.

89. Lu KW, Chen JC, Lai TY, Yang JS, Weng SW, Ma YS, Lin HY, Wu RS, Wu KC, Wood WG, Chung JG. Gypenosides suppress growth of human oral cancer SAS cells in vitro and in a murine xenograft model: the role of apoptosis mediated by caspase-dependent and caspase-independent pathways. Integr Cancer Ther. 2012;11:129–40.
90. Hsu HY, Yang JS, Lu KW, Yu CS, Chou ST, Lin JJ, Chen YY, Lin ML, Chueh FS, Chen SS, Chung JG. An experimental study on the antileukemia effects of gypenosides in vitro and in vivo. Integr Cancer Ther. 2011;10:101–12.
91. Lin J-J, Hsu H-Y, Yang J-S, Lu K-W, Wu RS-C, Wu K-C, Lai T-Y, Chen P-Y, Ma C-Y, Wood WG. Molecular evidence of anti-leukemia activity of gypenosides on human myeloid leukemia HL-60 cells in vitro and invivo using a HL-60 cells murine xenograft model. Phytomedicine. 2011;18:1075–85.
92. Xu C, Wang B, Ren S. The suppressive effect of gypenosides on murine s_ (180) sarcoma and cultured erythroleukemia cell line k_ (562). Xi'an Yi Ke Da Xue Xue Bao. 2002;23:217–9.
93. Kong L, Wang X, Zhang K, Yuan W, Yang Q, Fan J, Wang P, Liu Q. Gypenosides synergistically enhances the anti-tumor effect of 5-fluorouracil on colorectal cancer in vitro and in vivo: a role for oxidative stress-mediated DNA damage and p53 activation. PLoS One. 2015;10:e0137888.
94. Tai WC, Wong WY, Lee MM, Chan BD, Lu C, Hsiao WL. Mechanistic study of the anti-cancer effect of *Gynostemma pentaphyllum* saponins in the apc(min/+) mouse model. Proteomics. 2016;16:1557–69.
95. Chen L, Brar MS, Leung FC, Hsiao WL. Triterpenoid herbal saponins enhance beneficial bacteria, decrease sulfate-reducing bacteria, modulate inflammatory intestinal microenvironment and exert cancer preventive effects in ApcMin/+ mice. Oncotarget. 2016.
96. Chiranthanut N, Teekachunhatean S, Panthong A, Khonsung P, Kanjanapothi D, Lertprasertsuk N. Toxicity evaluation of standardized extract of *Gynostemma pentaphyllum* Makino. J Ethnopharmacol. 2013;149:228–34.
97. Du X-Y, Hou Y, Tan H, Han Y, Fan H. Studies on the anti-tumor activity of polysaccharide from *Gynostemma pentaphyllum* and its mechanism. Sci Technol Eng. 2009;20:5968–72.
98. Wang J-R, Zhao J-B. The effect of preventing recurrence of cancer metastasis on jiaogulan soup in clinical study. Zhejiang Zhong Yi Za Zhii. 1993;28:529–30.
99. Wang J-M, Wang J-R, Bi H-G, Fu G-X, Zhao J-B. Jiaogulan soup prevent recurrence of cancer metastasis on cancer patients after chemotherapy. Hebei Zhong Yi. 1997;19:23–4.
100. Yu S-Q, Wang J-R. Jiaogulan formula increase NK cell activity in breast cancer patients. Zhong Yi Yao Yan Jiu. 1997;13:7–8.
101. Wang J, Cao B. Immunological effects of jiaogulan granule in 19 cancer patients. Zhejiang Zhong Yi Za Zhi. 1989;24:449.
102. Liu S-X, Wang J-R. Experimental and clinical study on treatment of cancer with *Gynostemma pentaphyllum* Makin. Zhongguo Zhong Xi Yi Jie He Wai Ke Za Zhi 1996:110–1.
103. Zhou K, Bai S. The quality of randomized parallel controlled study of chemotherapy in advanced gastric cancer and improve survival of yiqi jianpi qingre huoxue method. Shiyong Zhongyi Neike Zazhi. 2015;29:42–4.
104. Lu HF, Chen YS, Yang JS, Chen JC, Lu KW, Chiu TH, Liu KC, Yeh CC, Chen GW, Lin HJ, Chung JG. Gypenosides induced G0/G1 arrest via inhibition of cyclin e and induction of apoptosis via activation of caspases-3 and -9 in human lung cancer A-549 cells. In Vivo. 2008;22:215–21.
105. Chen J-C, Lu K-W, Lee J-H, Yeh C-C, Chung J-G. Gypenosides induced apoptosis in human colon cancer cells through the mitochondria-dependent pathways and activation of caspase-3. Anticancer Res. 2006;26:4313–26.
106. Chen J-C, Lu K-W, Tsai M-L, Hsu S-C, Kuo C-L, Yang J-S, Hsia T-C, Yu C-S, Chou S-T, Kao M-C. Gypenosides induced G0/G1 arrest via CHk2 and apoptosis through endoplasmic reticulum stress and mitochondria-dependent pathways in human tongue cancer scc-4 cells. Oral Oncol. 2009;45:273–83.
107. Wang QF, Chen JC, Hsieh SJ, Cheng CC, Hsu SL. Regulation of Bcl-2 family molecules and activation of caspase cascade involved in gypenosides-induced apoptosis in human hepatoma cells. Cancer Lett. 2002;183:169–78.
108. Wang QF, Chiang CW, Wu CC, Cheng CC, Hsieh SJ, Chen JC, Hsieh YC, Hsu SL. Gypenosides induce apoptosis in human hepatoma Huh-7 cells through a calcium/reactive oxygen species-dependent mitochondrial pathway. Planta Med. 2007;73:535–44.
109. Yang L, Wang P, Cheng XX, Zhang MY, Xiao YP. Suppressive effect of gypenosides on murine leukemia l1210 cell lines. Zhong Yao Cai. 2010;33:1588–92.
110. Sun D-P, Li X-X, Liu X-L, Zhao D, Qiu F-Q, Li Y, Ma P. Gypenosides induce apoptosis by Ca^{2+} overload mediated by endoplasmic-reticulum and store-operated Ca^{2+} channels in human hepatoma cells. Cancer Biother Radiopharm. 2013;28:320–6.
111. Lu KW, Chen JC, Lai TY, Yang JS, Weng SW, Ma YS, Tang NY, Lu PJ, Weng JR, Chung JG. Gypenosides causes DNA damage and inhibits expression of DNA repair genes of human oral cancer SAS cells. In Vivo. 2010;24:287–91.
112. Yuan G, Wei J, Zhou J, Guo X, Yang M. Apoptosis of human hepatoma cells induced by *Gynostemma pentaphyllum* Makino. Chin German J Clin Oncol. 2006;5:173–7.
113. Schild L, Chen BH, Makarov P, Kattengell K, Heinitz K, Keilhoff G. Selective induction of apoptosis in glioma tumour cells by a *Gynostemma pentaphyllum* extract. Phytomedicine. 2010;17:589–97.
114. Lu KW, Tsai ML, Chen JC, Hsu SCH, Hsia TC, Lin MW, Huang AC, Chang YH, Ip SW, Lu HF, Chung JG. Gypenosides inhibited invasion and migration of human tongue cancer SCC4 cells through down-regulation of NFκB and matrix metalloproteinase-9. Anticancer Res. 2008;28:1093–9.
115. Lu KW, Chen JC, Lai TY, Yang JS, Weng SW, Ma YS, Lu PJ, Weng JR, Chueh FS, Wood WG, Chung JG. Gypenosides inhibits migration and invasion of human oral cancer SAS cells through the inhibition of matrix metalloproteinase-2-9 and urokinase-plasminogen by ERK1/2 and NFκB signaling pathways. Hum Exp Toxicol. 2011;30:406–15.
116. Hanahan D, Weinberg RA. Hallmarks of cancer: the next generation. Cell. 2011;144:646–74.
117. Hamanaka RB, Chandel NS. Targeting glucose metabolism for cancer therapy. J Exp Med. 2012;209:211–5.
118. Hsiao W, Tai WCS, Mo Z, Wu PK. The assessment of anti-cancer activities and saponin profiles of *Gynostemma pentaphyllum* saponins obtained from different regions of china. J Biotechnol. 2008;136:S22–3.
119. Yang XB, Zhao Y, Yang Y, Ruan Y. Isolation and characterization of immunostimulatory polysaccharide from an herb tea, *Gynostemma pentaphyllum* Makino. J Agric Food Chem. 2008;56:6905–9.
120. Liu X, Wang P-J, Xu F-X. Study on gypenosides inhibiting neoplasm growth and elevating immunological function in lewis lung cancer of mice. Anhui Zhong Yi Xue Yuan Xue Bao. 2001;1:21.
121. Ky PT, Huong PT, My TK, Anh PT, Kiem PV, Minh CV, Cuong NX, Thao NP, Nhiem NX, Hyun JH, Kang HK, Kim YH. Dammarane-type saponins from *Gynostemma pentaphyllum*. Phytochemistry. 2010;71:994–1001.
122. Shi L, Lu F, Zhao H, Zhao YQ. Two new triterpene saponins from *Gynostemma pentaphyllum*. J Asian Nat Prod Res. 2012;14:856–61.
123. Williams SA, Anderson WC, Santaguida MT, Dylla SJ. Patient-derived xenografts, the cancer stem cell paradigm, and cancer pathobiology in the 21st century. Lab Invest. 2013;93:970–82.
124. Tentler JJ, Tan AC, Weekes CD, Jimeno A, Leong S, Pitts TM, Arcaroli JJ, Messersmith WA, Eckhardt SG. Patient-derived tumour xenografts as models for oncology drug development. Nat Rev Clin Oncol. 2012;9:338–50.
125. Siolas D, Hannon GJ. Patient-derived tumor xenografts: transforming clinical samples into mouse models. Cancer Res. 2013;73:5315–9.
126. Richmond A, Su Y. Mouse xenograft models vs gem models for human cancer therapeutics. Dis Model Mech. 2008;1:78–82.
127. Lin S, Jia-qing C, Hong Z, Yu-qing Z. A new triterpene saponin from *Gynostemma pentaphyllum*. Chin Herb Med. 2010;2:317.
128. Bai MS, Gao JM, Fan C, Yang SX, Zhang G, Zheng CD. Bioactive dammarane-type triterpenoids derived from the acid hydrolysate of *Gynostemma pentaphyllum* saponins. Food Chem. 2010;119:306–10.
129. Li N, Wu CF, Xu XY, Liu ZY, Li X, Zhao YQ. Triterpenes possessing an unprecedented skeleton isolated from hydrolyzate of total saponins from *Gynostemma pentaphyllum*. Eur J Med Chem. 2012;50:173–8.
130. Chen DJ, Liu HM, Xing SF, Piao XL. Cytotoxic activity of gypenosides and gynogenin against non-small cell lung carcinoma A549 cells. Bioorg Med Chem Lett. 2014;24:186–91.
131. Zhu H, Liu Z, Tang L, Liu J, Zhou M, Xie F, Wang Z, Wang Y, Shen S, Hu L, Yu L. Reversal of P-gp and MRP1-mediated multidrug resistance

by H6, a gypenoside aglycon *from Gynostemma pentaphyllum*, in vincristine-resistant human oral cancer (kb/vcr) cells. Eur J Pharmacol. 2012;696:43–53.
132. Liu JS, Chiang TH, Wang JS, Lin LJ, Chao WC, Inbaraj BS, Lu JF, Chen BH. Induction of p53-independent growth inhibition in lung carcinoma cell a549 by gypenosides. J Cell Mol Med. 2015;19:1697–709.
133. Xie Z, Liu W, Huang H, Slavin M, Zhao Y, Whent M, Blackford J, Lutterodt H, Zhou H, Chen P. Chemical composition of five commercial *Gynostemma pentaphyllum* samples and their radical scavenging, antiproliferative, and anti-inflammatory properties. J Agric Food Chem. 2010;58:11243–9.

8

Chi-Ju-Di-Huang-Wan protects rats against retinal ischemia by downregulating matrix metalloproteinase-9 and inhibiting p38 mitogen-activated protein kinase

Ji-Min Cheng[1], Xiao-Qian Liu[2], Jorn-Hon Liu[3], Wynn Hwai-Tzong Pan[4], Xiu-Mei Zhang[2], Lei Hu[1*†] and Hsiao-Ming Chao[3,4,5*†]

Abstract

Background: Retinal ischemia is a retinal disorder related to retinal vascular occlusion, glaucoma, diabetic retinopathy and age-related macular degeneration. The study aimed to evaluate the protective effects and underlying mechanisms of Chi-Ju-Di-Huang-Wan (CJDHW) against retinal ischemia in rats.

Methods: High intraocular pressure (HIOP)-induced retinal ischemia was established in Wistar rats by raising their intraocular pressure to 120 mmHg for 60 min with in an eye whose anterior chamber was cannulated with a 30-guage needle adapted to a normal saline bottle through an intravenous line. This ischemic insult was followed by 1 or 7 days of reperfusion. The effects of CJDHW were studied by (i) electroretinogram (ERG); (ii) real-time polymerase chain reaction to determine the retinal mRNA levels of Thy-1 and matrix metalloproteinase-9 (MMP-9); (iii) Western blot analysis to determine the retinal protein levels of B cell lymphoma 2 (Bcl-2), heme oxygenase-1 (HO-1), phosphorylated-p38 mitogen-activated protein kinase (P-p38 MAPK) and MMP-9; (iv) hematoxylin and eosin (HE) staining; (v) fluorogold retrograde labeling; and (vi) terminal deoxynucleotidyl-transferase (TdT)-mediated dUTP nick end-labeling (TUNEL) apoptosis assay. Moreover, after fixation with 4 % paraformaldehyde and 30 % sucrose, the isolated retinas were sectioned and immunolabeled with goat anti-choline acetyltransferase (ChAT) polyclonal antibody, mouse anti-vimentin monoclonal antibody and rabbit anti-glial fibrillary acidic protein (GFAP) polyclonal antibody. The retinal sections were then incubated with rhodamine-conjugated rabbit anti-goat antibody, fluorescein isothiocyanate (FITC)-conjugated goat anti-mouse IgG or FITC-conjugated goat anti-rabbit IgG. A daily oral intake of 3 mL of water (vehicle; Group 2) or CJDHW (2.8 or 4.2 g/kg/day; CJDHW2.8 or CJDHW4.2; Group 3 or 4) was given for 7 consecutive days either before (preischemic drug administration) or after HIOP-induced retinal ischemic injury (postischemic drug administration). In Group 5, an intravitreal injection of 4 μL of 0.5 mM SB203580 (p38 MAPK inhibitor) was performed on the ischemic eye 15 min before retinal ischemia. The control rats received a sham procedure (Group 1) where the saline reservoir was not raised.

Results: The ischemia-induced changes (Group 2) were significantly modulated by pretreating the rats with 4.2 g/kg/day of CJDHW (Group 4; ERG: $P < 0.001$ on I/R day 7; HE stain: $P < 0.001$ on I/R day 7; TUNEL: $P = 0.05$ on I/R day 7; retrograde labeling: $P = 0.007$ on I/R day 7; Thy-1 mRNA: $P = 0.02$; MMP-9 mRNA: $P < 0.001$; Bcl-2 protein: $P = 0.02$; HO-1 protein: $P = 0.03$; P-p38 MAPK protein: $P < 0.001$; MMP-9 protein: $P = 0.02$). These modulations included the following

*Correspondence: misshulei@126.com; hsiaoming.chao@gmail.com
†Hsiao-Ming Chao and Lei Hu contributed equally to this work
[1] Department of Ophthalmology, Affiliated Hospital of Taishan Medical University, Shandong, China
[3] Department of Ophthalmology, Cheng Hsin General Hospital, Taipei, Taiwan
Full list of author information is available at the end of the article

features (Group 2 vs. 4), increased ERG b-wave amplitudes (0.38 ± 0.04 vs. 0.81 ± 0.03), increased inner retinal thickness (45.08 ± 2.85 vs. 67.98 ± 5.48 μm), increased ChAT immunolabeling, decreased vimentin/GFAP immunoreactivity, less numerous apoptotic cells in the ganglion cell layer (1.40 ± 0.55 vs. 0.60 ± 0.55), and more numerous retinal ganglion cells (887.73 ± 158.18 vs. 1389.02 ± 53.20). Moreover, increased Thy-1 (0.31 ± 0.15 vs. 0.78 ± 0.32) and decreased MMP-9 mRNA levels were found (4.44 ± 0.84 vs. 1.13 ± 0.34), respectively. Furthermore, the Bcl-2 protein level (0.78 ± 0.08 vs. 1.80 ± 0.34) was increased while the HO-1 (0.99 ± 0.20 vs. 4.15 ± 2.08), P-p38 MAPK (1.12 ± 0.18 vs. 0.57 ± 0.18) and MMP-9 levels were decreased (0.70 ± 0.23 vs. 0.39 ± 0.10). The ischemia-associated increases in P-p38 and MMP-9 protein levels were also attenuated by 0.5 mM SB203580 (P-p38 MAPK: 1.12 ± 0.18 vs. 0.18 ± 0.07, $P < 0.001$; MMP-9: 0.70 ± 0.23 vs. 0.21 ± 0.07, $P = 0.002$). This was also the case to the MMP_enzyme activity (Group 2 vs. 4: 5.03 ± 1.57 vs. 1.59 ± 0.47, $P = 0.002$; Group 2 vs. 5: 5.03 ± 1.57 vs. 1.35 ± 0.41, $P = 0.001$).

Conclusion: Treatment of the rats suffering from retinal ischemia with CJDHW inhibited apoptosis, increased antioxidative activity, downregulated MMP-9 and inhibited p38 MAPK.

Background

Retinal vascular occlusion, glaucoma, diabetic retinopathy and age-related macular degeneration (AMD) are related to retinal ischemia [1–3]. The incidences of these diseases are 0.0018 % for central retinal artery occlusion (CRAO) [4], 4 % for primary open angle glaucoma (in urban areas) [5], 2.9 % for sight-threatening diabetic retinopathy (type 2 diabetes) [6] and 0.36 % for AMD (age ≥40) [7]. Amacrines and their neuronal processes were susceptible to ischemia plus reperfusion (I/R) [1–3, 8, 9]. I/R led to an increase in the immunolabeling of vimentin/glial fibrillary acidic protein (GFAP) in Müller cells [1, 8, 9]. Ischemia-induced retinal ganglion cell (RGC) death was correlated positively to a significant increase in MMP-9 activity [10]. Heme oxygenase-1 (HO-1) is involved in the cellular response to oxidative stress and hypoxia, and elevated levels of HO-1 can protect against retinal ischemia and/or AMD via its antioxidative activity [11, 12]. Mitogen-activated protein kinases (MAPKs) are involved in signal transduction pathways, and several members of the MAPK subfamily (e.g., JNK, p38 and ERK1/2) were implicated in neuronal injury and several diseases [13, 14]. The MAPK protein, p38, which is stimulated by various stresses, including ischemia and oxidative stress, is involved in apoptosis [13, 14].

Chi-Ju-Di-Huang-Wan (CJDHW) consists of several components, including Fructus lycii (Gou qi zi), Chrysanthemi flos (Ju hua) and Liu Wei Di Huang Wan, Rehmanniae Radix Preparata (Shu di huang), Corni fructus (Shan zhu yu), Rhizoma Diocoreae (Shan yao), Poria (Fu ling), Cortex Moutan radicis (Mu dan pi) and Alismatis Rhizoma (Ze xie) [15]. Several active compounds have been identified in this mixture, including the antioxidants zeaxanthin and lutein from F. lycii and C. flos [16], and trehalose from R. radix preparata [17]. CJDHW has been reported to stabilize tear film, as well as decreasing abnormalities of the corneal epithelium to treat dry eyes [15]. However, the molecular mechanisms responsible for the effects of CJDHW remain unknown.

The study aimed to evaluate the protective effects and underlying mechanisms of Chi-Ju-Di-Huang-Wan (CJDHW) against retinal ischemia in rats. The effects and mechanisms of CJDHW were assessed by electrophysiology, retinal thickness, choline acetyltransferase (ChAT) immunochemistry, vimentin/GFAP immunochemistry (indexing Müller cells), fluorogold retrograde RGC labeling, TUNEL staining (for apoptotic cells), Bcl-2/HO-1/phosphorylated-p38 (P-p38)/MMP-9 protein level analysis and MMP-9 activity (as measured by zymography), as well as by measuring the mRNA expression levels of Thy-1 and MMP-9.

Methods

Animals

The Institutional Animal Care and Use Committee at Cheng Hsin General Hospital (CHGH; Taipei, Taiwan; Animal Experiment Approval No: CHIACUC 102-08 approved all the animal experiments, which complied with the Association for Research in Vision and Ophthalmology Statement for the Use of Animals in Ophthalmology and Vision Research. Six-week old sex-matched Wistar rats (250–300 g; n = 136; BioLasco, Taipei, Taiwan) were raised in a large plastic cage (Shineteh Instruments Co., Ltd., Taipei, Taiwan) of maximal six companions with the 40–60 % humidity and at 19–23 °C. They were maintained on a 12-h light/dark period with 12–15 air exchanges/h. They were fed with food and water at liberty. The animal studies were performed following the ARRIVE guideline (Additional file 1).

Anesthesia was carried out by intraperitoneal administration of ketamine (Pfizer, Taipei, Taiwan) (100 mg/kg) and xylazine (Sigma-Aldrich, St. Louis, USA) (5 mg/kg). Sodium pentobarbitone (SCI Pharmtech, Inc., Taiwan) (>140 mg/kg) was intraperitoneally administered to sacrifice the animals (Scientific Procedures Acts 1986) [18].

Induction of retinal ischemia

After anesthesia, the rats were kept in a stereotaxic frame. A 120 mmHg high intraocular pressure (HIOP) was induced and maintained for 60 min by cannulating an eye's anterior chamber with adapting a 30-gauge needle to a normal saline bottle, which was raised [19]. The induction of an ischemic insult was confirmed by the detection of a pale eye fundus [1–3]. Sixty minutes of retinal ischemia was subsequently followed by the removal of the 30-gauge needle from the rat's anterior chamber for the return of the blood supply, namely reperfusion. The control rats' eyes received a sham procedure where the saline reservoir was not raised [3].

Drug administration

The rats were arbitrarily allocated into various Groups. A daily oral intake 3 mL of water (vehicle; Group 2), a low intake of CJDHW (Sun Ten Pharmaceutical Co., Taipei, Taiwan; 2.8 g/kg/day; CJDHW2.8; Group 3) or a high intake of CJDHW (4.2 g/kg/day; CJDHW4.2; Group 4) was given for 7 consecutive days either before (preischemic drug administration) or after HIOP-induce retinal ischemic injury (postischemic drug administration). The control rats' eyes received a sham procedure (Group 1) as mentioned above. Intravitreal injections were performed by a 30-gauge needle attached to a 25 μL syringe after pupil dilation with 1 % tropicamide (Alcon, Inc., Puurs, Belgium) and 2.5 % phenylephrine (Akorn, Inc., IL, USA). In Group 5, intravitreal injections of 4 μL of 0.5 mM SB203580 (p38 MAPK inhibitor; Calbiochem, San Diego, CA, USA) were performed on ischemic eyes 15 min before pressure-induced retinal ischemia.

Flash ERG measurement

We recorded ERG data on all the animals pre-ischemia (day 0) followed by at 1, 3, 5, and 7 days post-ischemia and administration of the appropriate compounds. Dark adaptation for at least 8 h, anesthesia during the ERG recordings and pupil dilation with 1 % tropicamide and 2.5 % phenylephrine were performed on the rats [1, 2]. A stimulus of 0.5 Hz was induced by placing a strobe 2 cm before the eye of each rat. We recorded 15 consecutive responses at 2-s intervals as well as 10 kHz; these responses were amplified and averaged as described previously [1, 2]. The b-wave reflects the function of the bipolar cells and the inner layers of the retina [20]. The b-wave ratio was calculated, which was the treated ischemic retina's b-wave amplitude divided by the untreated contralateral normal retina's b-wave amplitude [1, 2].

Hematoxylin and eosin staining

Following retinal ischemia plus 1 or 7 days of reperfusion, the eyeballs were marked at the 12 o'clock position of the cornea with silk suture; they were then enucleated and fixed in 4 % paraformaldehyde at 4°C for 24 h. After fixation, the anterior segment was removed, and the posterior eyeball containing the optic disc was dehydrated in a graded ethanol series and embedded in paraffin. For hematoxylin and eosin (HE) stain [21, 22], 5 μm thick sections were taken along the vertical meridian and observed under a light microscope (Leica, Heidelberg, Germany).

To quantify the retinal ischemic injury, we measured various layer thicknesses. Mounted sections were microscopically observed and photographed at the same magnification (Ilford Pan-F plus film, 50 ASA) and the thickness of the various areas of the retina was measured from the photographs.

The overall retinal thicknesses (from the inner limiting membrane to the RPE layer), the inner retinal thickness [(from the inner limiting membrane to the inner nuclear layer (INL)], and the thickness of the inner plexiform layer (IPL) were measured. All measurements were carried out approximately 1000 μm from the optic disc. Three sections per eye were averaged. The various thicknesses were measured by research staff blinded to the source of the tissue to investigate any differences in the thickness between the four Groups (Groups 1, 2, 3 and 4).

Immunofluorescence analysis

After sacrifice, intracardial perfusion with normal saline (w/v) was given to the rats; the retinal sections were retrieved, soaked with 4 % (w/v) paraformaldehyde (Sigma-Aldrich, St. Louis, USA) for 45 min fixation and immersed in 30 % sucrose (Sigma-Aldrich, St. Louis, USA) for cryosection [1, 2]. Retinal sections were collected 1 and 7 days following retinal ischemia with pre-administration of CJDHW or vehicle, or following the sham procedure. Overnight, the retinal samples were incubated with primary antibodies: goat anti-ChAT polyclonal antibody, mouse anti-vimentin monoclonal antibody and rabbit anti-GFAP polyclonal antibody as described previously [1, 2]. Afterwards, the retinal samples were incubated with secondary antibody: rhodamine-conjugated rabbit anti-goat antibody, fluorescein isothiocyanate-conjugated goat anti-mouse IgG or FITC-conjugated goat anti-rabbit IgG as described previously. In parallel, the cellular nuclei were stained with 4,6-diamidine-2-phenylindole dihydrochloride as described previously. We utilized a fluorescence microscope (Olympus BX-51, Olympus, Tokyo, Japan) to evaluate the retinal samples as described previously [1, 2]. When it is was necessary to compare the immunoreactivity in retinal tissues treated in different ways an independent scientist of the laboratory was asked to grade any changes by relating to the immunoreactivity in Group 1. In this way bias was avoided as far as possible.

For example, the enhanced vimentin/GFAP immunoreactivity in Group 2 was alleviated by high dose of CJDHW as shown in Group 4.

Terminal deoxynucleotidyl-transferase (TdT)-mediated dUTP nick end-labeling (TUNEL) assay

After I/R, the rats were sacrificed one and 7 days later and their eyes were removed for TUNEL staining (In situ Cell Death Detection Kit, Fluorescein; Roche; Mannheim, Germany) to investigate cell apoptosis [3]. The retinal samples were fixed with 10 % formaldehyde for 24 h afterwards. The retinal samples were soaked with proteinase K (Sigma-Aldrich, St. Louis, USA) (25 μg/mL) followed by incubation in H_2O_2/methanol for 5 min at 25°C to inactivate endogenous peroxidases. Negative and positive controls were measured as described previously [3]. After washing with Tris buffered saline, the retinal samples were soaked with a TdT enzyme/labeling reaction mix at 37 °C for 90 min. This reaction was initialized on the binding of digoxigenin-dUTP to the 3′-OH end of DNA by TdT, followed by incubation in an anti-digoxigenin antibody conjugated with peroxidase. Upon termination of the labeling reaction in stop buffer with 2× SSC (300 mM NaCl, 30 mM sodium citrate; GeneCopoeia, MD, USA), the retinal sections were processed in a standard streptavidin-horseradish peroxidase (HRP) reaction with 3,3′ diaminobenzidine (Sigma-Aldrich, St. Louis, USA) as the chromogenic peroxidase substrate, and counterstained with methyl green (Sigma-Aldrich, St. Louis, USA). The average number of TUNEL positive cells per field was counted as described previously [3].

Retrograde labeling of RGCs

After anesthesia, the rats were made a 2-cm incision in the scalp, and drilled two small holes into the skull as described previously [3]. Next, 2 μL of 5 % fluorogold (Sigma-Aldrich, St. Louis, USA) were injected by a micropipette at depths of 3.8, 4.0, and 4.2 mm below the skull. Three days after retrograde immunolabeling of RGCs, HIOP was carried out on the right eyes of the animals whose fellow eyes served as the sham. The retina was gently retrieved, fixated, dissected and processed as described previously [3] The average RGC density was defined as the ratio of the total RGC number to the total retinal area evaluated [3].

Measurement of the concentrations of various retinal mRNAs

The retinal mRNA concentrations of Thy-1 and MMP-9 were investigated by a real-time polymerase chain reaction (PCR) technique [1, 23]. One day following retinal ischemia with either preadministration of mentioned compounds or following a sham procedure, the animals were sacrificed and the retinal samples were processed as described previously [1, 23]. Retinal RNA was extracted and first strand complementary DNA (cDNA) synthesis was carried out on 2 μg deoxyribonuclease (DNase)-treated RNA [1, 23]. The first-strand cDNA subsequently went on real-time PCR [1, 23]. The PCR and cycling were performed as instructed previously [1, 23]. Relative quantitation was carried out utilizing β-actin as the internal control. This procedure normalized the measurement of the mRNA target (Ct) and took into consideration the alterations in the quantity of total RNA applied to each reaction (Ct). The relative Thy-1/MMP-9 amount differences were measured as fold alterations correspondent to the control in regards to the calibrator (Ct). Relative measurement of mRNA level was based on the formula of 2^{-Ct} as stated [1, 23]. The PCR reagents, software and machine were bought from AB Applied Biosystems. The results collected were compared for each management, and a total percentage alteration correspondent to the control was measured. As outlined in Table 1, the following PCR oligonucleotide primers (β-actin, Thy-1 and MMP-9) were purchased at Mission Biotech Co., Ltd. (Taipei, Taiwan).

Western blotting assay

One day after treatment of retinal ischemia with preadministration of relevant compounds or following a sham procedure, the animals were sacrificed. Retinal samples were retrieved and sonicated by a sonicator (Misonix XL-2000, Misonix, NY, USA) in a lysis buffer (25 mM bicine, 150 mM sodium chloride; pH 7.6), mammalian protein extraction reagent (Thermo Scientific, Rockford, IL 61105 USA). Equal amounts of denatured proteins (30 μg/20 μL/well) were processed on a sodium dodecyl sulfate polyacrylamide gel electrophoresis (SDS-PAGE; Bio-Rad, Hercules, CA, USA) as described previously [23, 24]. The nitrocellulose blots (NC) were next soaked 12 h at 4 °C with various primary antibodies: mouse monoclonal [AC-15] anti-β-actin antibody (1:5000; Abcam Inc., Cambridge, UK), rabbit monoclonal antibody Bcl-2 (50E3; 1:1000; Cell Signaling, Danvers, MA 01923, USA), mouse monoclonal antibody HO-1 (ab 13248) (1:1000; Abcam Inc., Cambridge, UK), mouse monoclonal antibody P-p38 MAPK (1:1000; Cell Signaling, Danvers, MA 01923, USA), rabbit monoclonal antibody p38 MAPK (1:1000; Cell Signaling, Danvers, MA 01923, USA) and rabbit monoclonal antibody MMP-9 (EP1255Y; 1:1000; Abcam Inc., Cambridge, UK). The blots were soaked with relevant secondary antibody, HRP-conjugated goat anti-rabbit or anti-mouse IgG (1:5000 or 1:2000; Amersham, UK) at 37 °C for 1 h. Finally, the membranes were then developed, and exposed as described previously [23, 24], and then scanning densitometry was utilized to evaluate the level of each protein.

Table 1 Sequences of oligonucleotide primers and details of polymerase chain reactions

mRNA	Primers (5′→3′)	Bases in base pairs	Product size	Cycles profile Denaturation/annealing/ extension (temperature and time in seconds)	Cycles number
β-actin	F: AGGGAAATCGTGCGTGACAT	694–713	150	95/95/60 °C (20/3/30 s)	40
	R: GAACCGCTCATTGCCGATAG	824–843			
Thy-1	F: ACCAAGGATGAGGGCGACTA	380–399	120	95/95/60 °C (20/3/30 s)	40
	R: CAGGCTTATGCCACCACACTT	479–499			
MMP-9	F: TGCGCTGGGCTTAGATCATT	1218–1237	105	95/95/60 °C (20/3/30)	40
	R: TGGATGCCTTTTATGTCGTCTTC	1300–1322			

F forward; *R* reverse

Gel zymography

Protein samples were prepared in a similar manner to that described for the Western blotting analysis; these samples were then loaded onto and separated by 10 % Tris–glycine gel [1.5 M Tris–Cl 2.5 mL, pH 8.8 (Sigma-Aldrich, St. Louis, USA); 10 % (w/v) sodium dodecyl sulfate 0.1 ml (Sigma-Aldrich, St. Louis, USA); 40 % polyacryamide. 2.475 mL (Merck KGaA, Darmstadt, Germany); 10 % (w/v) ammonium persulfate 0.1 mL (Sigma-Aldrich, St. Louis, USA); *N,N,N′,N′* tetramethylethylenediamine 0.01 mL (J.T.Baker Inc., Phillipsburg, NJ, USA); Sterile deionised water 4.625 mL)] with 0.1 % gelatin (Sigma-Aldrich, St. Louis, USA) as protease substrate [25]. After separation by electrophoresis, the gel was incubated in renaturation buffer (2.7 % Triton X-100 in distilled water) at room temperature with gentle shaking for 30 min. The renaturation buffer was discarded and replaced with developing buffer (50 mmol/L Tris Base, 40 mmol/L HCl, 200 mmol/L NaCl, 5 mmol/L $CaCl_2$, 0.2 % Brij 35). After 30 min equilibration by the developing buffer, the gel was incubated with fresh developing buffer at 37 °C for 48 h. After being developed, the gel was stained with 0.5 % Coomassie Blue R-250 (J.T.Baker Inc., Phillipsburg, NJ, USA) for 30 min and then destained appropriately. The visualized bands were then analyzed by scanning densitometry (software: ImageJ Version 1.48, NIH, USA).

Statistical analysis

Three or more Groups were compared by one-way analysis of variance (ANOVA; SigmaPlot Version 12.5, Systat Software Inc., California, USA). The Tukey multiple-comparison test was performed to compare the control column (i.e., vehicle-treated ischemic retinas) to other columns (i.e., CJDHW-treated ischemic retinas). The results were represented as mean ± SD. *P* values less than 0.05 were considered statistically significant. The dose–response relationship was determined visually.

Results

The effect of CJDHW on the amplitude or the ratio of the b-wave

In the sham retina (Fig. 1a), the ERG b-wave was determined to be 0.98 mV. However, retinal ischemia plus 1 day of reperfusion led to a considerable decrease in the amplitude of the b-wave to 0.11 mV. Notably, pretreating rats with CJDHW (Groups 3 and 4) counteracted this ischemia-induced decrease in the amplitude of the b-wave in a dose-dependent manner, with the amplitude of the b-wave increasing to 0.26 and 0.39 mV, respectively, 1 day after I/R. As shown in Fig. 1b (n = 5), administering I/R following the rats' pretreatment with the vehicle (Group 1) led to a significant ($P < 0.001$) decrease in the b-wave ratio on I/R days 1, 3, 5 and 7 compared with the preischemic b-wave ratio (day 0: 0.95 ± 0.05; day 1: 0.44 ± 0.07; day 3: 0.44 ± 0.05; day 5: 0.38 ± 0.04; day 7: 0.38 ± 0.04). Pretreating rats with CJDHW (Group 3 vs. 4) led to a significant ($P < 0.001$; at 2.8 and 4.2 g/kg/day) dose-dependent decrease in the ischemia-induced b-wave ratio on I/R day 1 (0.66 ± 0.07 vs. 0.72 ± 0.07), day 3 (0.70 ± 0.05 vs. 0.78 ± 0.04), day 5 (0.70 ± 0.03 vs. 0.80 ± 0.04) and day 7 (0.69 ± 0.07 vs. 0.81 ± 0.03) after ischemia. Moreover, the preischemic b-wave ratio (day 0) was recorded at 0.99 ± 0.12 vs. 0.93 ± 0.10 ($P = 0.391$; Group 3 vs. 4).

Furthermore, there was a significant ($P = 0.003$; n = 5) decrease in the b-wave ratio (0.43 ± 0.02) compared with the preischemic b-wave ratio (baseline at day 0: 1.04 ± 0.07) 7 days after I/R and the postischemic administration of vehicle (Group 2). In contrast, there was a significant dose-dependent improvement in the ischemia-induced b-wave ratio reduction (0.56 ± 0.23 vs. 0.63 ± 0.09; $P < 0.001$) 7 days after I/R and the postischemic administration of CJDHW (Group 3 vs. 4). Notably, in Group 1, comparing the ERG b-wave ratios (the sham eye's b-wave amplitude divided by the untreated fellow normal eye's one) revealed that there were no significant differences between the pre-sham ERG b-wave ratio (day 0) and the post-sham values (day 1, 3, 5 or 7).

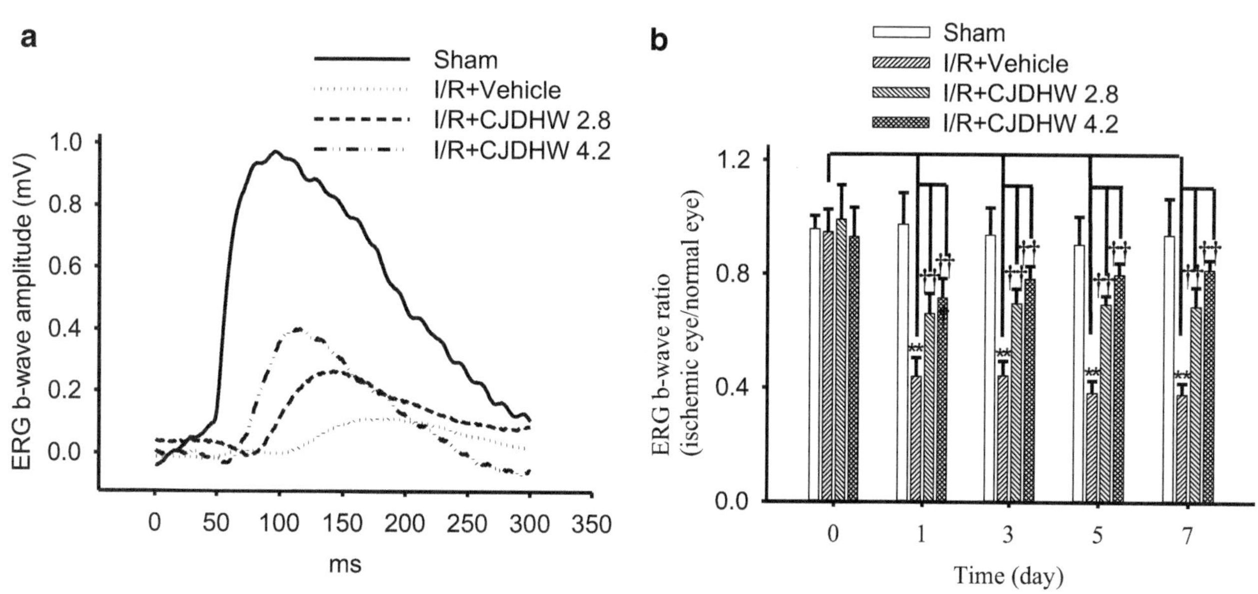

Fig. 1 Electroretinogram (ERG): The effect of CJDHW on retinal ischemia plus reperfusion (I/R). **a** There was a considerable reduction in the amplitude of the ERG b-wave following pressure-induced retinal ischemia plus reperfusion (I/R) and pretreatment with vehicle in a representative animal of the I/R + Vehicle (Group 2) compared with the sham procedure retina (Group 1). Pretreatment with CJDHW (at 2.8 g/kg/day, I/R + CJDHW2.8, Group 3; at 4.2 g/kg/day, I/R + CJDHW4.2, Group 4) led to a dose-dependent attenuation in this reduction in one rat from each defined Group. **b** In contrast with the Group 1, there was a significant (**$P < 0.01$) decrease in the b-wave ratio in the Group 2 1, 3, 5 and 7 days following ischemia. Dose-dependent and significant ($^{††}P < 0.01$) attenuation of this ischemia-induced decrease was achieved after pretreating rats with 2.8 g/kg/day (Group 3) and 4.2 g/kg/day of CJDHW (Group 4). These results are expressed as the mean ± SD (n = 5). *CJDHW* Chi-Ju-Di-Huang-Wan

The effect of CJDHW on the thickness of the various retinal layers stained by HE

Figure 2 and Table 2 show details of the retinal sections collected from a similar eccentricity (1 mm from disc) for the four different Groups (n = 4–6). Compared with the samples collected from the Group 1 (sham 1 day, Fig. 2a, e: 174.12 ± 3.64 μm for whole retina, 41.68 ± 2.69 μm for INL, 41.93 ± 1.58 μm for IPL; sham 7 days, Fig. 2f, j: 180.25 ± 4.35 μm for whole retina, 38.10 ± 1.39 μm for INL, 38.38 ± 1.43 for IPL) following ischemia plus 1 and 7 days of reperfusion (I/R) and pretreating rats with vehicle [Group 2 on I/R day 1 (Fig. 2b, e) vs. day 7 (Fig. 2g, j)], the INL ($P = 0.0483$ vs. $P = 0.004$; 37.13 ± 5.04 vs. 24.74 ± 3.60 μm), IPL ($P = 0.003$ vs. $P < 0.001$; 36.81 ± 2.21 vs. 20.34 ± 1.79 μm) and whole retina ($P = 0.005$ vs. $P = 0.03$; 165.43 ± 4.44 vs. 141.02 ± 9.47 μm) samples showed a significant reduction in their thickness. Treating animals with 2.8 g/kg/day of CJDHW resulted in a small dose-dependent effect against retinal ischemia following 1 day (Group 3, Fig. 2c, e: 168.45 ± 12.89 μm for the whole retina with $P = 0.67$, 37.52 ± 2.09 for the INL with $P = 0.89$, 37.16 ± 4.55 for the IPL with $P = 0.89$) or 7 days of reperfusion (Group 3, Fig. 2h, j: 156.18 ± 7.92 μm for the whole retina with $P = 0.04$, 29.23 ± 5.43 for the INL with $P = 0.18$, 26.20 ± 3.60 for the IPL with $P = 0.01$). In contrast, the use of a larger dose of 4.2 g/kg/day of CJDHW led to a significant reduction in the effect of ischemia plus 1 day (Group 4, Fig. 2d, e: 172.00 ± 1.57 μm for whole retina with $P = 0.045$, 39.74 ± 3.13 for INL with $P = 0.047$, 40.39 ± 0.86 for IPL with $P = 0.042$) or 7 days of reperfusion (Group 4, Fig. 2i, j: 171.78 ± 10.38 μm for whole retina with $P = 0.002$, 34.45 ± 4.02 for INL with $P = 0.007$, 33.53 ± 1.85 for IPL with $P < 0.001$). Ischemia pretreated with vehicle (Group 2) led to a significant reduction in the thickness of the inner retinal layers (INL + IPL; 45.08 ± 2.85 μm; $P < 0.001$) compared with the sham (Group 1; 76.48 ± 1.72 μm) on day 7 after ischemia. Notably, this reduction in the thickness was attenuated in a dose-dependent manner by CJDHW ($P = 0.03$, 55.38 ± 7.57 μm in Group 3; $P < 0.001$, 67.98 ± 5.48 μm in Group 4).

The effect of CJDHW on ChAT immunolabeling

Figure 3 and Table 3 (n = 6) showed the relationships between the ChAT (*red*) immunolabeling and the amacrine cell bodies (short arrows; sham 1 day, Fig. 3a, e: 34.33 ± 6.59 cells/field; sham 7 days, Fig. 3f, j: 36.83 ± 6.68 cells/field) in the inner nuclear layer (INL) and the ganglion cell layer on days 1 and 7 after the sham procedure (Group 1). Moreover, the neuronal processes in these animals demonstrated two well-delineated

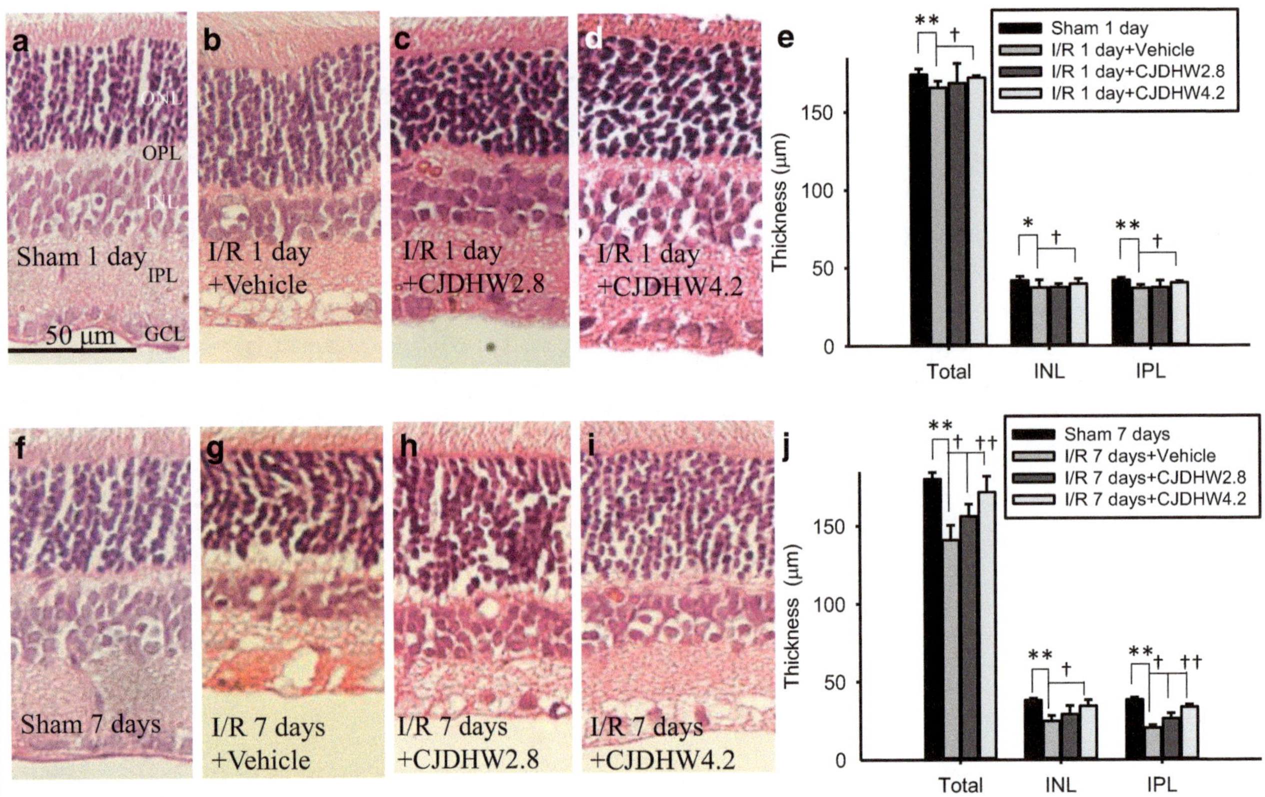

Fig. 2 The thicknesses of various retinal layers. This figure shows sections of retina from approximately the same eccentricity. (**a** sham 1 day) and (**f** sham 7 days) show sections of Group 1 1 day and 7 days following the sham procedure, respectively. Pictures **b** and **g** respectively show retinas that received ischemia plus reperfusion (I/R) for 1 day (I/R 1 day + Vehicle) or 7 days and pretreatment of vehicle (I/R 7 days + vehicle; Group 2). Compared with the Group 1 (**a, f**), the thickness of the inner retina [*INL* inner nuclear layer, *IPL* inner plexiform layer and ganglion cell layer] in the ischemic retina pretreated with vehicle (Group 2; **b, g**) was reduced considerably. This reduction in the thickness of the inner retinal layers was attenuated in animals given I/R for 1 or 7 days and pretreated with 2.8 g/kg/day [Group 3; on I/R day 1, (**c**) on I/R day 7, (**h**)] and 4.2 g/kg/day of CJDHW [Group 4; on I/R day 1, (**d**) on I/R day 7, (**i**)]. *Scale bar* = 50 μm. Morphometric analysis of the thicknesses of various retinal layers from sections of similar eccentricity (**e, j**). Compared with the Group 1 (sham 1 day; sham 7 days), the thicknesses of the whole retinal layer, INL and IPL were significantly reduced in the vehicle-treated ischemic retinas (Group 2). Moreover, these reductions were attenuated in a dose-dependent manner when the ischemic retinas were pretreated with 2.8 (Group 3) and 4.2 g/kg/day of CJDHW (Group 4). Results are the mean ± SD of the number of experiments (n = 4–6). *or **significantly different ($P < 0.05$ or $P < 0.01$) from the Group 1. † or ††significantly different ($P < 0.05$ or $P < 0.01$) from the Group 2 on I/R day 1 or 7. *Total* whole retina, *CJDHW* Chi-Ju-Di-Huang-Wan

Table 2 Hematoxylin and eosin staining

Group	1	2	3	4
Retinal thickness on day 1				
Whole	174.12 ± 3.64	165.43 ± 4.44**	168.45 ± 12.89	172.00 ± 1.57†
INL	41.68 ± 2.69	37.13 ± 5.04*	37.52 ± 2.09	39.74 ± 3.13†
IPL	41.93 ± 1.58	36.81 ± 2.21**	37.16 ± 4.55	40.39 ± 0.86†
Retinal thickness on day 7				
Whole	180.25 ± 4.35	141.02 ± 9.47**	156.18 ± 7.92†	171.78 ± 10.38††
INL	38.10 ± 1.39	24.74 ± 3.60**	29.23 ± 5.43	34.45 ± 4.02†
IPL	38.38 ± 1.43	20.34 ± 1.79**	26.20 ± 3.60†	33.53 ± 1.85†

In comparison of the control retina, 1 or 7 days following sham procedure (Group 1; Sham 1 day, n = 6; Sham 7 days, n = 6), after retinal ischemia plus 1 or 7 days of reperfusion and pretreatment with vehicle (Group 2; I/R 1 day + vehicle, n = 4; I/R 7 days + vehicle, n = 5), there was a significant decrease (* $P < 0.05$; ** $P < 0.01$) in the thickness of the whole retina, the INL and the IPL. In contrast, this significant decrease was dose-dependently (with a less effect at 2.8 g/kg/day, I/R + CJDHW2.8, Group 3, n = 4) and significantly († $P < 0.05$; †† $P < 0.01$; Group 3; I/R + CJDHW4.2, Group 4, n = 4) inhibited by pretreatment with CJDHW. The results are the mean ± SD (μm)

CJDHW4.2 Chi-Ju-Di-Huang-Wan at 4.2 g/kg/day, *INL* inner nuclear layer, *IPL* inner plexiform layer bands in the inner plexiform layer (IPL; long arrows), which was consistent with previous reports [1, 23]. In the ischemic retina pretreated with the vehicle, the immunolabeled amacrine cell bodies (Group 2 on I/R 1 day, Fig. 3b, e: 12.67 ± 2.80 cells/field; Group 2 on I/R 7 day, Fig. 3g, j: 13.17 ± 4.07 cells/field) were significantly less numerous ($P < 0.001$) following retinal ischemia plus 1 and 7 days of reperfusion. Furthermore, there was a significant decrease in the IPL immunoreactivity of these cells. The ischemic activity was therefore inhibited in a dose-dependent manner after pretreating rats with a low (Group 3 on I/R day 1, Fig. 3c, e: 28.33 ± 2.16 cells/field with $P < 0.001$; Group 3 on I/R day 7, Fig. 3h, j: 23.50 ± 3.45 cells/field with $P < 0.001$) or high dose of CJDHW (Group 4 on I/R day 1, Fig. 3d, e: 31.67 ± 3.88 cells/field with $P < 0.001$; Group 4 on I/R day 7, Fig. 3i, j: 28.50 ± 4.59 cells/field with $P < 0.001$).

The effect of CJDHW on vimentin or GFAP immunoreactivity

As shown in Fig. 4, the immunolabeling of the vimentin found in the Müller cell processes extended from the end foot of these cells to the IPL, as well as progressing into the INL and the outer nuclear layer, which was consistent with previous reports [1, 16]. Anti-vimentin immunolabeling was found to be enhanced 1 and 7 days after I/R and pretreating rats with the vehicle (Group 2 on I/R day 1, Fig. 4c; Group 2 on I/R day 7, Fig. 4l). Nevertheless, the ischemic effect was alleviated after pretreating rats with a low (Group 3 on I/R day 1,

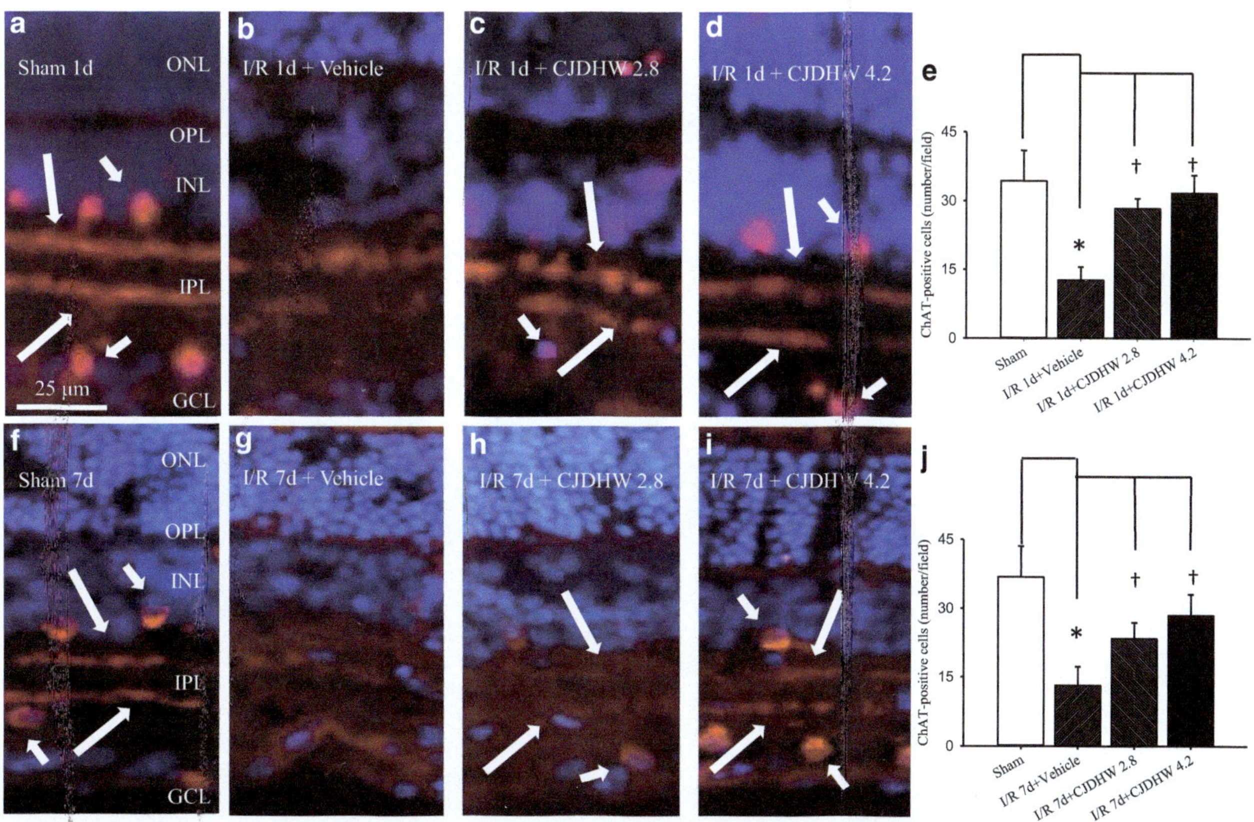

Fig. 3 Choline acetyltransferase (ChAT; *red*) immunohistochemistry. Amacrine cell bodies (*short arrows*) were located in the INLs and ganglion cell layers of the retinas subjected to the sham procedure (Group 1) for 1 day (**a**; sham 1 day) and 7 days (**f**; sham 7 day); the neuronal processes displayed two well-delineated bands (*long arrows*) in the inner plexiform layer (*IPL*). Retinal ischemia plus reperfusion (I/R) for 1 or 7 days led to a considerable reduction in the ChAT immunolabeling of the IPLs as well as the number of ChAT immunolabeled amacrine cell bodies; the pretreatment with the vehicle had no influence on the defined ischemic changes [Group 2; on I/R day 1, (**b**) on I/R day 7, (**g**)]. However, these ischemic alterations were clearly alleviated after pretreating the rats with 2.8 g/kg/day [Group 3; on I/R day 1, (**c**); on I/R day 7, (**h**)] and 4.2 g/kg/day of CJDHW [Group 4; on I/R day 1, (**d**); on I/R day 7, (**i**)]. The ChAT immunolabeled images were merged with those obtained for 4,6-diamidine-2-phenylindole dihydrochloride staining [DAPI *blue*; (**a–d**, **f–i**)]. Each bar represents the mean ± SD (n = 6) 1 day (**e**) and 7 days following the sham procedure or I/R (**j**). *represents significance ($P < 0.05$; Group 1 vs. 2 on I/R day 1 or 7). †represents significance ($P < 0.05$; Group 2 vs. 3 or Group 4 on I/R day 1 or 7). *CJDHW* Chi-Ju-Di-Huang-Wan. *Scale bar* = 35 μm

Table 3 Choline acetyltransferase (ChAT) immunolabelling

Group	1	2	3	4
Cholinergic amacrines (number/field) on day 1	34.33 ± 6.59	12.67 ± 2.80*	28.33 ± 2.16†	31.67 ± 3.88†
Cholinergic amacrines (number/field) on day 7	36.83 ± 6.68	13.17 ± 4.07*	23.50 ± 3.45†	28.50 ± 4.59†

In comparison of the control retina, 1 or 7 days following sham procedure (Sham; Group 1), after retinal ischemia plus 1 or 7 days of reperfusion and pretreatment with vehicle (I/R + vehicle; Group 2), the number of CHAT-immunolabeling amacrine cells per field was significantly decreased (* $P < 0.05$) in the inner nuclear layer and the ganglion cell layer. In contrast, this significant decrease was dose-dependently (with a less effect at 2.8 g/kg/day, I/R + CJDHW2.8, Group 3) and significantly († $P < 0.05$; Group 3; I/R + CJDHW4.2, Group 4) inhibited by pretreatment with CJDHW. The results are the mean ± SD (n = 6)

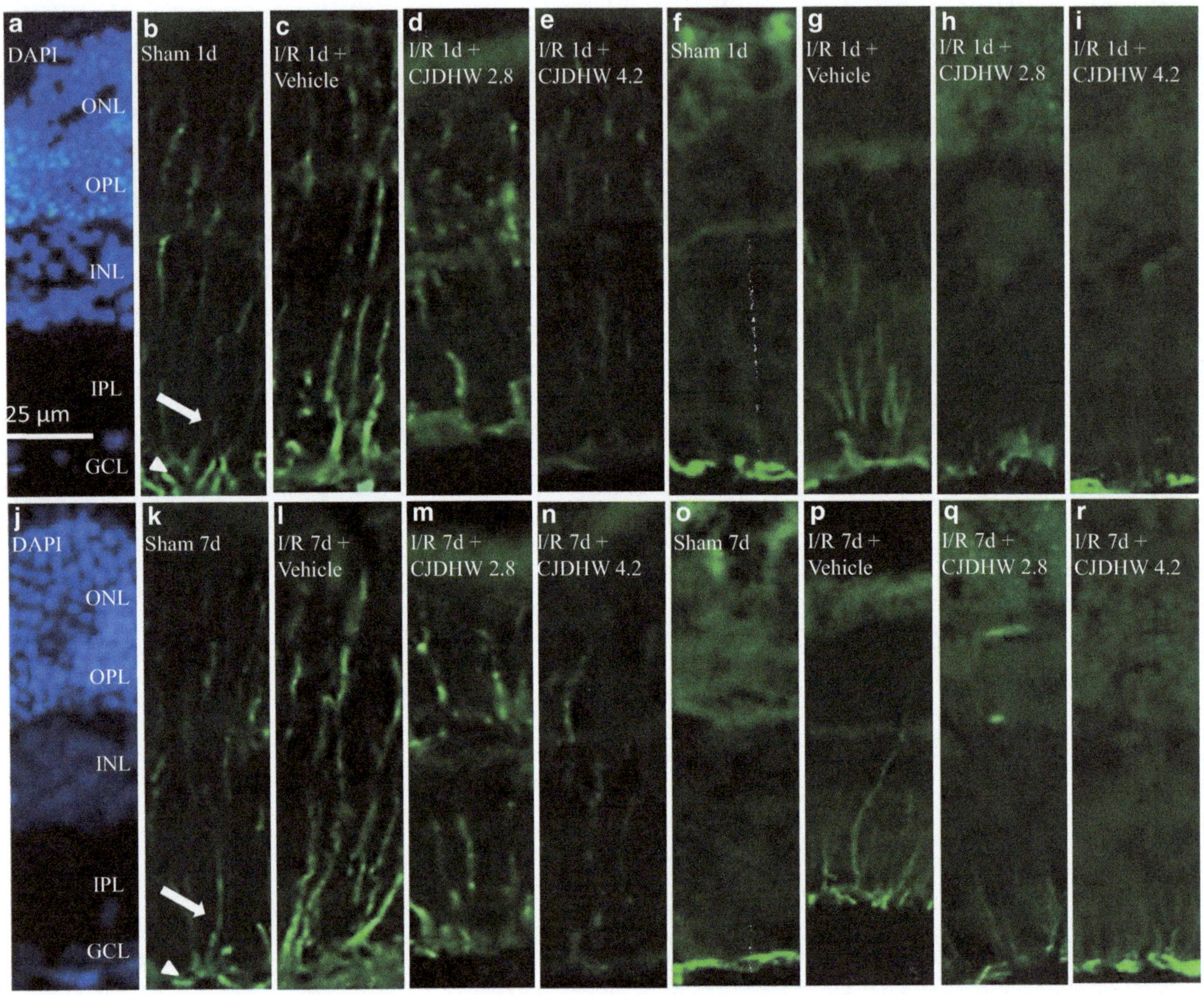

Fig. 4 Vimentin immunohistochemistry. One (**b**) or 7 days following the sham procedure (**k**; Group 1), the Müller cells were demonstrated with vimentin (*green*) immunolabeling at the end feet (*arrow heads*) in the ganglion cell layer (GCL) and at the processes in the *IPL* inner plexiform layer (*arrows*), *INL* inner nuclear layer and *ONL* outer nuclear layer. In contrast with the Group 1, anti-vimentin immunolabeling was increased one or 7 days after ischemia plus reperfusion (I/R) with preadministration of vehicle [Group 2; on I/R day 1, (**c**); on I/R day 7, (**l**)]. This enhancement was attenuated by pretreatment with 2.8 g/kg/day [Group 3; on I/R day 1, (**d**) on I/R day 7, (**m**)] or 4.2 g/Kg/day of CJDHW [Group 4; on I/R day 1, (**e**); on I/R day 7, (**n**)]. The cellular nuclei of the Group 1 (**a**, **j**) were immunolabeled with 4,6-diamidine-2-phenylindole dihydrochloride (DAPI; *blue*). GFAP immunohistochemistry. In contrast with the Group 1, one (**f**) or 7 days following the sham procedure (**o**), anti-GFAP immunolabeling was also increased 1 (**g**) or 7 days day after ischemia plus reperfusion (I/R) with preadministered vehicle (**p**, Group 2). This enhancement was blunted by pretreatment with 2.8 g/kg/day (Group 3; on I/R day 1, H; on I/R day 7, **q**) or 4.2 g/kg/day of CJDHW (Group 4; on I/R day 1, **I**; on I/R day 7, **r**). GFAP, glial fibrillary acidic protein; *CJDHW* Chi-Ju-Di-Huang-Wan. *Scale bar* = 25 μm

Fig. 4d; Group 3 on I/R day 7, Fig. 4m) or high dose of CJDHW (Group 4 on I/R day 1, Fig. 4e; Group 4 on I/R day 7, Fig. 4n). DAPI (blue; Fig. 4a, j) was used to stain the nuclei in the normal control cells.

Anti-GFAP immunoreactivity was also enhanced 1 and 7 days after retinal ischemia in the rats pretreated with vehicle (Group 2 on I/R day 1, Fig. 4g; Group 2 on I/R day 7, Fig. 4p) compared with those in the control retina Group (sham 1 day, Fig. 4f; sham 7 days, Fig. 4o). However, this enhancement was nullified by pretreating the rats with a low (Group 3 on I/R day 1, Fig. 4h; Group 3 on I/R day 7, Fig. 4q) or high dose of CJDHW (Group 4 on I/R day 1, Fig. 4i; Group 4 on I/R day 7, Fig. 4r).

The effect of CJDHW on the presence of apoptotic cells in the RGC layer

In contrast to the control retina 1 or 7 days after the sham procedure (Group 1 on days 1 and 7: no TUNEL-positive cells), ischemic rats pretreated with vehicle showed a significant ($P = 0.008$ on I/R days 1 and 7) increase in the number of TUNEL-positive cells in the RGC layer (Group 2; on I/R day 1: 1.40 ± 0.55 cells/field; on I/R day 7: 1.40 ± 0.55 cells/field), as shown in Table 4 (n = 5). This increase in the number of TUNEL-positive cells was alleviated in a dose-dependent (with a small effect at 2.8 g/kg/day; Group 3; on I/R day 1: 0.80 ± 0.45 cells/field, $P = 0.09$; on I/R day 7: 0.80 ± 0.84 cells/field, $P = 0.2$) and significant (at 4.2 g/kg/day) manner 1 or 7 days after ischemia after pretreating the rats with CJDHW (Group 4; on I/R day 1: 0.40 ± 0.55 cells/field, $P = 0.02$; on I/R day 7: 0.60 ± 0.55 cells/field, $P = 0.0497$).

Retrograde fluorogold immunolabeling of RGCs

As shown in Fig. 5 and Table 5 (n = 3), the RGC densities were 1952.16 ± 125.29 (sham 1 day) and 1737.23 ± 151.94 cells/mm^2 (sham 7 day) 1 and 7 days after the sham procedure (Group 1). In contrast, the RGC densities 1 and 7 days after retinal ischemia pretreated with vehicle decreased significantly to 929.01 ± 135.00 (Group 2 on I/R day 1; $P < 0.001$) and 887.73 ± 158.18 (Group 2 on I/R day 7; $P = 0.003$), respectively. Notably, this decrease was alleviated in a dose-dependent manner (with a small effect at 2.8 g/kg/day; Group 3 on I/R day 1: 1112.65 ± 164.10 cells/mm^2, $P = 0.21$; Group 3 on I/R day 7: 941.89 ± 38.91, $P = 0.60$). The extent of this alleviation effect was significantly and much more pronounced after pretreating rats with a high dose of CJDHW (Group 4 on I/R day 1: 1691.36 ± 237.57, $P = 0.008$; Group 4 on I/R day 7: 1389.02 ± 53.20, $P = 0.007$).

Table 4 Terminal deoxynucleotidyl-transferase dUTP nick end-labeling (TUNEL)

Group	1	2	3	4
Apoptotic cell No. on day 1	0	1.40 ± 0.55**	0.80 ± 0.45	0.40 ± 0.55†
Apoptotic cell No. on day 7	0	1.40 ± 0.55**	0.80 ± 0.84	0.60 ± 0.55†

No TUNEL-positive apoptotic cell was observed 1 or 7 days after the sham procedure (Sham; Group 1). After retinal ischemia plus 1 or 7 days of reperfusion and pretreatment with vehicle (I/R + vehicle; Group 2), the number of apoptotic cells was significantly (** $P < 0.01$) increased in the retinal ganglion cell layer. In contrast, this significant increase was dose-dependently (with a less effect at 2.8 g/kg/day, I/R + CJDHW2.8; Group 3) and significantly († $P < 0.05$; at 4.2 g/kg/day, I/R + CJDHW4.2; Group 4) inhibited by pretreatment with CJDHW. The results are the mean ± SD (n = 5)

The effect of CJDHW on the retinal mRNA concentrations of Thy-1 and MMP-9

As shown in Fig. 6 and Table 6 (n = 5 for Thy-1; n = 3–4 for MMP-9), there were significant differences in the ratios of Thy-1 (0.31 ± 0.15; $P = 0.006$) and MMP-9 (4.44 ± 0.84; $P = 0.003$) in the vehicle-pretreated ischemic retina samples 24 h after retinal ischemia compared with the control sham retina (Group 1; Thy-1: 0.99 ± 0.38; MMP-9: 0.75 ± 0.55). Compared with the vehicle-pretreated ischemic retina samples (Group 2), the ischemic rats pretreated with CJDHW showed a dose-dependent (Group 3; with a small effect at 2.8 g/kg/day; Thy-1: 0.45±0.20; MMP-9: 3.01±1.90) and significant (Group 4; at 4.2 g/kg/day) decrease in the overexpression of MMP-9 (1.13 ± 0.34; $P = 0.03$). This effect was also coupled by a significant (Group 4; at 4.2 g/kg/day) counteraction in the underexpression of Thy-1 (0.78 ± 0.32; $P = 0.02$).

The effect of CJDHW on the levels of in vivo retinal proteins

As shown in Fig. 7 and Table 7 (n = 4–9 for Bcl-2; n = 4 for HO-1; n = 4–9 for P-p38 MAPK; n = 4–5 for MMP-9), retinal ischemia plus 24 h of reperfusion and pretreatment with vehicle (Group 2) led to a significant decrease in the Bcl-2 ratio (0.78 ± 0.08; $P = 0.03$) or increase in HO-1 (0.99 ± 0.20; $P = 0.008$), P-p38 MAPK (1.12 ± 0.18; $P = 0.03$) and MMP-9 (0.70 ± 0.23; $P = 0.02$) ratios compared with the control sham retina (Group 1; Bcl-2: 1.06 ± 0.25; HO-1: 0.27 ± 0.12; P-p38 MAPK: 0.15 ± 0.06; MMP-9: 0.25 ± 0.26) 24 h after the sham procedure. However, these changes underwent dose-dependent (with a small effect at 2.8 g/Kg/day of CJDHW; Group 3; Bcl-2: 0.83±0.11; HO-1: 1.46 ± 0.99; P-p-38 MAPK: 0.83 ± 0.21; MMP-9: 0.44 ± 0.15) and significant changes after pretreating rats with 4.2 g/kg/day of CJDHW (Group 4; Bcl-2: 1.80 ± 0.34, $P = 0.001$; P-p38 MAPK: 0.57 ± 0.18, $P < 0.001$; MMP-9: 0.39 ± 0.10, $P = 0.02$) and/or a 2 nmole solution of SB203580 (Group 5; p38 MAPK inhibitor; MMP-9: 0.21 ± 0.07, $P = 0.002$; P-p38 MAPK: 0.18 ± 0.07, $P < 0.001$), as well as a significant increase in the expression of HO-1 (4.15 ± 2.08;

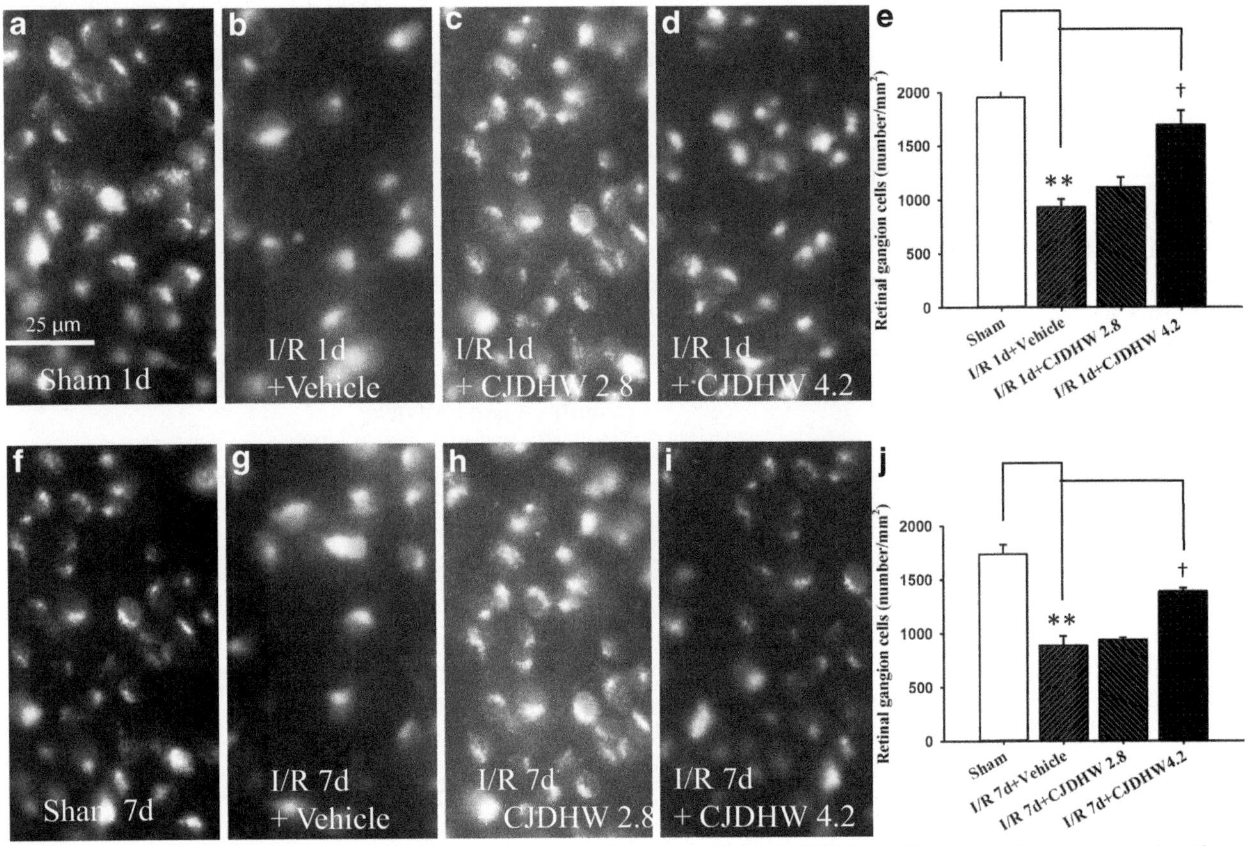

Fig. 5 Fluorogold-labeling. The microscopic images show the density of retinal ganglion cells (RGCs) **a** and 7 days after the sham-procedure (**f**; Group 1), or **b** and 7 days of reperfusion following ischemia (I/R) with preadministered vehicle (**g**; Group 2) or Chi-Ju-Di-Huang-Wan at 2.8 g/kg/day (Group 3; on I/R day 1, **c**; on I/R day 7, **h**) and at 4.2 g/kg/day (Group 4; on I/R day 1, **d**; on I/R day 7, **i**). Each bar indicates the mean ± SD (**e**; **j**; n = 3). **indicates significant difference ($P < 0.01$; Group 1 vs. 2 on I/R day 1 or 7); †indicates significant difference ($P < 0.05$; Group 2 vs. 4 on I/R day 1 or 7). *Scale bars* = 25 μm

Table 5 Fluorogold immunolabeling

Group	1	2	3	4
RGCs (number/mm²) On day 1	1952.16 ± 125.29	929.01 ± 135.00**	1112.65 ± 164.10	1691.36 ± 237.57††
RGCs (number/mm²) On day 7	1737.23 ± 151.94	887.73 ± 158.18**	941.89 ± 38.91	1389.02 ± 53.20††

In comparison of the control retina, 1 or 7 days following sham procedure (Sham; Group 1), after retinal ischemia plus 1 or 7 days of reperfusion and pretreatment with vehicle (I/R + Vehicle; Group 2), the number of fluorogold-immunolabeling retinal ganglion cells (RGCs) per field was significantly decreased (** $P < 0.01$). In contrast, this significant decrease was dose-dependently (with a less effect at 2.8 g/kg/day, I/R + CJDHW2.8; Group 3) and significantly (†† $P < 0.01$; at 4.2 g/kg/day, I/R + CJDHW4.2; Group 4) inhibited by pretreatment with CJDHW. The results are the mean ± SD (μm; n = 3)

$P = 0.03$) in Group 4. Notwithstanding the changes listed above, the total p38 protein levels in the retina were unchanged across all of the different Groups.

The MMP-9 activities in the retina samples collected from the different Groups were detected by zymography (Fig. 8; Table 8; n = 4–5). The results revealed that there was a significant ($P < 0.001$; 5.03 ± 1.57) increase in the MMP-9 activity in the vehicle-pretreated ischemic retina samples (Group 2) 24 h after ischemia compared with the sham procedure control retina (Group 1). However, the ischemic rats pretreated with CJDHW or SB203580 (p38 MAPK inhibitor) demonstrated a dose-dependent (with a significant but smaller effect at Group 3; 3.05 ± 0.88; $P = 0.03$) and significant (Group 4: 1.59 ± 0.47; $P = 0.002$; Group 5: 1. 35 ± 0.41; $P = 0.001$) decrease in MMP-9 activity compared with the retina samples of Group 2.

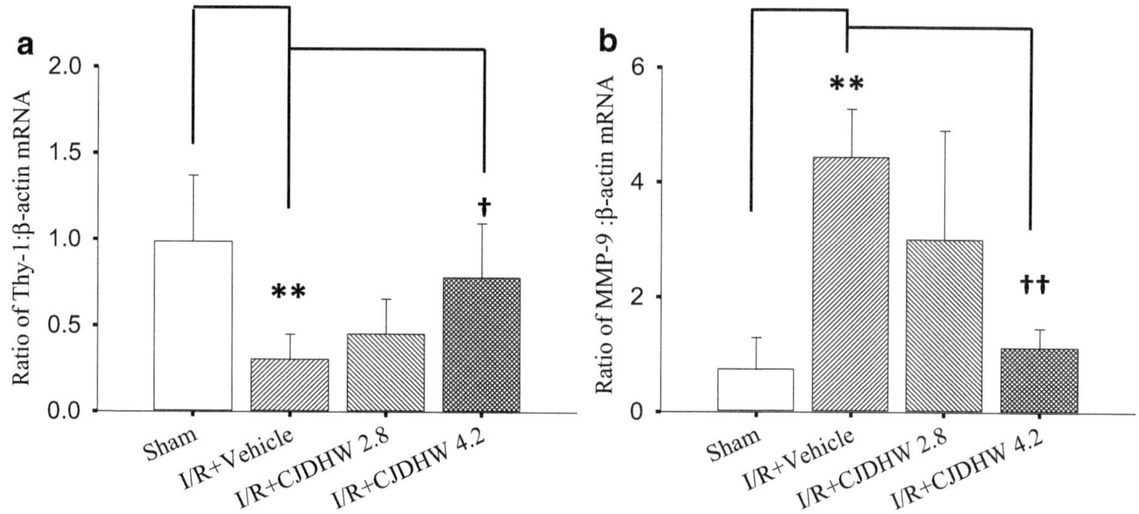

Fig. 6 The mRNA expression levels of Thy-1 (**a**), MMP-9 (**b**) and β-actin. Total mRNA was extracted and isolated from the sham procedure retinas (Group 1) or the ischemic retinas preadministered with vehicle (Group 2), or low (2.8 g/Kg/day; Group 3)/high dose (4.2 g/kg/day) of CJDHW (Group 4). We evaluated the effect of each defined compound on the mRNA concentrations of Thy-1 or MMP-9 divided by the mRNA levels of β-actin. **represents significance ($P < 0.01$; Group 1 vs. 2). † or ††represents significance for Thy-1 ($P < 0.05$; Group 2 vs. 4) or MMP-9 ($P < 0.01$; Group 2 vs. 4), respectively. The findings are presented as the mean ± SD (Thy-1, n = 5; MMP-9, n = 3–4)

Table 6 The ratios of mRNA expression levels of Thy-1 or MMP-9 to that of β-actin

Group	1	2	3	4
Thy-1/β-actin (n = 5)	0.99 ± 0.38	0.31 ± 0.15**	0.45 ± 0.20	0.78 ± 0.32†
MMP-9/β-actin (n = 3–4)	0.75 ± 0.55	4.44 ± 0.84**	3.01 ± 1.90	1.13 ± 0.34††

In retinal ischemia plus 24 h of reperfusion (I/R), total mRNA was extracted and isolated from the sham procedure retinas (Group 1) or the ischemic retinas preadministered with vehicle (Group 2), or low (2.8 g/kg/day; Group 3)/high dose (4.2 g/kg/day) of CJDHW (Group 4)

CJDHW Chi-Ju-Di-Huang-Wan

** represents significance ($P < 0.01$; Group 1 vs. 2)

† or †† represents significance for Thy-1 ($P < 0.05$) or significance for MMP-9 ($P < 0.01$; Group 2 vs. 4), respectively. The findings are presented as the mean ± SD (Thy-1, n = 5; MMP-9, n = 3–4)

Discussion

Vimentin and GFAP immunoreactivity were enhanced in Müller cells 1 and 7 days after I/R [1, 23], and this result was confirmed in the current study (Fig. 4c/g, l/p). Functionally compromised Müller cells exhibited a pronounced effect on the normal ERG b-wave [1, 2, 23], as shown in the current study (Fig. 1). In the ischemic retinas pretreated with vehicle, the observed increase in vimentin/GFAP immunolabeling coincided with a decrease in the amplitude of the b-wave. Notably, these ischemic changes were alleviated after pretreating the rats with CJDHW.

After retinal ischemia/reperfusion, the glutamatergic neurons (i.e., RGCs and amacrines) in the inner retina become susceptible to damage [1, 2, 9, 23], as shown in the current study. The number of cholinergic amacrines decreased following ischemia plus 1 or 7 days of reperfusion and pretreating the rats with the vehicle (Fig. 3b/e or g/j). The RGCs became dysfunctional following the disruption of the cholinergic signaling pathways in laser ablated retina [9]. The ischemic insult provided in the current study led to pronounced changes in the RGCs and amacrine cells, as evidenced by changes in the Thy-1 mRNA levels (Fig. 6; Table 6), RGC fluorogold retrograde labeling (Fig. 5) and ChAT immunoreactivity (Fig. 3). The synapses between starburst amacrine cells and direction-selective RGCs are essential to their functionality [26]. The ischemia induced reductions in ChAT immunoreactivity (Fig. 3d/e, i/j), the number of the fluorogold immunolabeled RGCs (Fig. 5d/e, i/j; Table 5) and the expression level of Thy-1 mRNA (Fig. 6a; Table 6) therefore provide clear and significant evidence of the blunting effect of pretreating ischemic rats with CJDHW.

After I/R, the ischemic retinas pretreated with the vehicle contained fewer RGCs (indexed by Thy-1 mRNA) in the RGC layer (Fig. 6a; Table 6) compared with the sham retinas (Fig. 6; Table 4), along with numerous apoptotic cells in the RGC layer (Table 4). The ischemic retinas pretreated with CJDHW contained significantly more RGCs (Fig. 6a; Table 6) and significantly fewer apoptotic cells in their RGC layer than the ischemic retinas pretreated with the vehicle (Table 4). The protective effect of CJDHW on retinal cells could therefore involve its ability to modulate the activity of

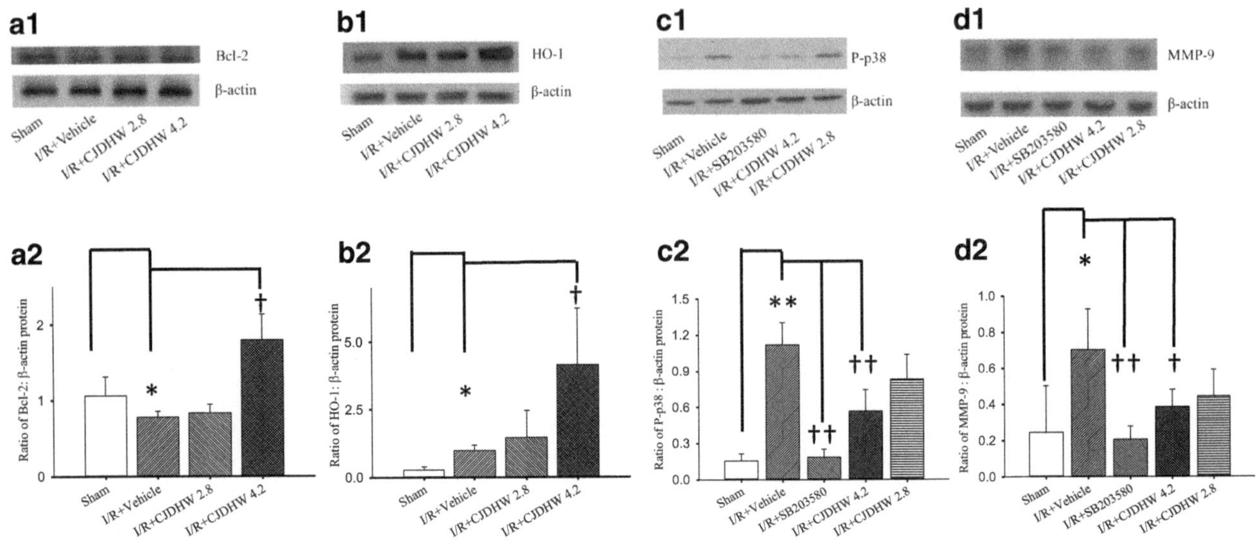

Fig. 7 Western blotting. The antibodies against Bcl-2 (**a1**), HO-1 (**a1**), P-p38 (**c1**), MMP-9 (**d1**) and β-actin are respectively shown as 26, 34.6, 43, 92~96 and 43-kDa bands. Each bar represents the ratio of Bcl-2 (n = 4–9; **a2**), HO-1 (n = 4; **b2**), P-p38 (n = 4-9; **c2**), or MMP-9 (n = 4–5; **d2**) to β-actin. * or †represents significance ($P < 0.05$; Group 1 vs. 2) or significance ($P < 0.05$; Group 2 vs. 4, I/R + CJDHW4.2; Group 2 vs. 5, SB203580), respectively. Additionally, for P-p38, ** or ††/†represents significance ($P < 0.01$; Group 1 vs. 2) or significance ($P < 0.01/P < 0.05$; Group 2 vs. 5/Group 2 vs. 4), respectively. These 5 Groups included Group 1 as well as Groups 2, 3, 4 and 5 [(the retina subjected to ischemia plus reperfusion respectively pretreated with vehicle (I/R + Vehicle), 2.8 g/kg/day of CJDHW (I/R + CJDHW2.8), 4.2 g/kg/day of CJDHW (I/R + CJDHW4.2) and SB203580 (p38 MAPK inhibitor)]. The results are presented as the mean ± SD

Table 7 Western blotting. The ratios of the protein expression levels of Bcl-2, HO-1, P-p38 or MMP-9 relative to that of β-actin

Group	1	2	3	4	5
Bcl-2/β-actin (n = 4-9)	1.06 ± 0.25	0.78 ± 0.08*	0.83 ± 0.11	1.80 ± 0.34†	Not available
HO-1/β-actin (n = 4)	0.27 ± 0.12	0.99 ± 0.20*	1.46 ± 0.99	4.15 ± 2.08†	Not available
P-p38/β-actin (n = 4-9)	0.15 ± 0.06	1.12 ± 0.18**	0.83 ± 0.21	0.57 ± 0.18††	0.18 ± 0.07††
MMP-9/β-actin (n = 4-5)	0.25 ± 0.26	0.70 ± 0.23*	0.44 ± 0.15	0.39 ± 0.10†	0.21 ± 0. 07††

This study included 5 Groups, namely, Group 1 (the sham procedure retina) as well as Groups 2, 3, 4 and 5 [(the retina subjected to ischemia plus reperfusion respectively pretreated with vehicle (I/R + vehicle), 2.8 g/kg/day of CJDHW (I/R + CJDHW2.8), 4.2 g/kg/day of CJDHW (I/R + CJDHW4.2) and SB203580 (p38 MAPK inhibitor)]. * or † represents significance ($P < 0.05$; Group 1 vs. 2) or significance ($P < 0.05$; Group 2 vs. 4; Group 2 vs. 5), respectively. Additionally, for P-p38, ** or †† represents significance ($P < 0.01$; Group 1 vs. 2) or significance ($P < 0.01$; Group 2 vs. 5; Group 2 vs. 4), respectively. The results are mean ± SD (Bcl-2, n = 4–9; HO-1, n = 4; P-p38, n = 4–9; MMP-9, n = 4–5). *CJDHW* Chi-Ju-Di-Huang-Wan

the apoptotic pathway. This possibility is also supported by the observation that pretreating ischemic rats with CJDHW led to a significant increase in the expression of the Bcl-2 protein (Fig. 7; Table 7). To our knowledge, this study is the first reported account of CJDHW as a protective agent against retinal ischemic injury. CJDHW could preserve the electrophysiological functions of the retina, counteracting any reduction in the thickness of the inner retina and avoiding cholinergic neuron death. CJDHW achieves these protective effects by attenuating Müller cell vimentin/GFAP glial activation, decreasing the number of apoptotic cells in the RGC layer as well as by attenuating the downregulation of Thy-1 mRNA expression and reducing RGC death, as detected by fluorogold labeling. HO-1 has been reported to act as an antioxidant [27]. The protective properties of CJDHW towards ischemia-injured retinal cells such as amacrine cells and RGCs may be attributable, at least in part, to the antioxidative effects resulting from the overexpression of HO-1 (Fig. 7; Table 7).

P-p38 and MMP-9 are both upregulated during brain ischemia. Under certain circumstances in astrocytes, MMP-9 is activated via the p38 MAPK pathway. The results of the current study showed a significant increase in the expression of MMP-9 mRNA in the retina following 60 min of ischemia plus 24 h of reperfusion (Fig. 7; Table 7), which was consistent with the results of a recent report [23]. This upregulation also coincided

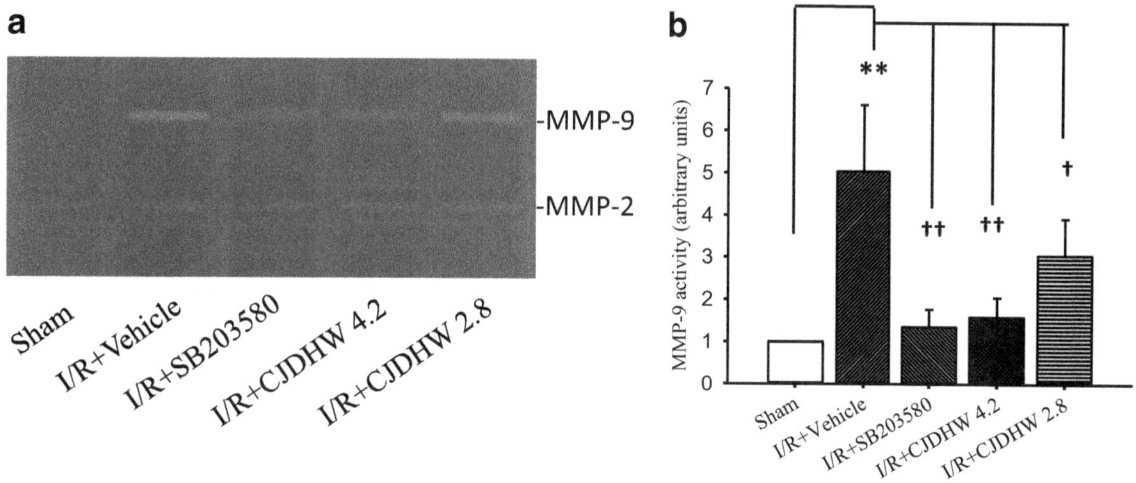

Fig. 8 Gel zymography. An example of a gelatin zymogram (**a**) used for the quantification of matrix metalloproteinase-9 (MMP-9) quantitation protein expression by densitometry. Gelatinolytic bands of 72 and 97 kDa corresponded to MMP-2 and active MMP-9, respectively. *Lane 1*, the sham procedure retina (Group 1); *Lane 2*, the vehicle-pretreated ischemic retina (I/R + Vehicle; Group 2); *Lane 3*, the SB203580 (p38 MAPK inhibitor)-pretreated ischemic retina (I/R + SB203580; Group 5); *Lanes 4* and *5*, the ischemic retina respectively pretreated with 4.2 g/kg/day (I/R + CJDHW4.2; Group 4) and 2.8 g/kg/day of CJDHW (I/R + CJDHW2.8; Group 3). Each bar (**b**) indicates the mean ± SD (B; n = 4–5). **indicates significance ($P < 0.01$; Group 1 vs. 2). ††indicates significance ($P < 0.01$; Group 2 vs. 4; Group 2 vs. 5). †indicates significance ($P < 0.05$; Group 2 vs. 3). In contrast to the results for MMP-9, the expression of MMP-2, when measured at 24 h after ischemia and pretreatment with vehicle (Group 2) or CJDHW4.2 (Group 4)/CJDHW2.8 (Group 3), was found to have a similar protein expression level to that of the control Group (Sham; Group 1)

Table 8 Gel zymography

Group (n = 4–5)	1	2	3	4	5
MMP-9/β-actin	1.00 ± 0.00	5.03 ± 1.57**	3.05 ± 0.88†	1.35 ± 0.41††	1.49 ± 0.47††

The ratios of the protein expression levels of MMP-9 relative to that of β-actin

This study included 5 Groups, namely, Group 1 (the sham procedure retina) as well as Groups 2, 3, 4 and 5 [(the retina subjected to ischemia plus reperfusion respectively pretreated with vehicle (I/R + vehicle), 2.8 g/kg/day of CJDHW (I/R + CJDHW2.8), 4.2 g/kg/day of CJDHW (I/R + CJDHW4.2) and SB203580 (p38 MAPK inhibitor)]

CJDHW Chi-Ju-Di-Huang-Wan

** indicates significance ($P < 0.01$; Group 1 vs. 2)

†† indicates significance ($P < 0.01$; Group 2 vs. 4; Group 2 vs. 5). †indicates significance ($P < 0.05$; Group 2 vs. 3). The results are mean ± SD (n = 4–5)

with a significantly increase in the level of P-p38. Notably, however, these increases in the levels of MMP-9 and P-p38 were significantly attenuated after pretreating the rats with either CJDHW or the p38 MAPK inhibitor, SB203580. CJDHW could downregulate MMP-9 expression by inhibiting the p38 MAPK pathway.

Ischemia might be involved in diabetic retinopathy (DR) [6], neovascular age-related macular degeneration [7] and central/branch retinal vascular occlusion [4]; and anti-VEGF antibodies and various steroids are currently used in clinical practice to treat these conditions [28]. However, these approaches are not completely effective for treating vision-threatening ocular disorders [29]. For example, poor visual outcomes have been reported in some patients treated with anti-VEGF and steroidal agents, even though ocular hemorrhage and macular edema were successfully controlled in these patients. There is therefore an urgent need to develop agents that use novel mechanisms of action against ischemic ocular disorders, such as inhibitors of p38 MAPK and MMP-9. The increased levels of P-p38 and subsequent overexpression of MMP-9 detected during the current study were linked to retinal ischemia and/or wet age-related macular degeneration (wAMD). In such circumstances, based on the current results, CJDHW might provide an alternative way to deal with these defined vision-threatening retinal ischemic disorders.

Hayreh et al. [30, 31] used 38 elderly, atherosclerotic and hypertensive rhesus monkeys (similar to the characteristics of most patients with CRAO) to show that CRAO lasting for approximately 240 min results in massive irreversible retinal damage (i.e., retinal cell death).

Moreover, in human BRAO studies, 46 % (24 of 52) of the eyes tested in the series reported by Mason et al. [32] and 100 % (5 of 5) of eyes tested in the series reported by Hsu et al. [33] were found to present with best corrected visual acuity (BCVA) values of <20/40. Furthermore, Mason et al. [32] indicated that 75 % (18 of 24) of the untreated eyes with a poor presentation of BCVA (<20/40) had a final BCVA of <20/40. Moreover, only 14 % (2 of 14) of eyes with a BCVA of ≤20/100 were improved to a BCVA of ≥20/40. There was a high rate of spontaneous improvement in the vision of BRAO eyes that had an initial poor BCVA, although these data should be treated with caution because these events are generally associated with irreversible retinal damage. The Eurocondor project [34] assessed whether topical brimonidine and somatostatin could be used to prevent or arrest neurodegeneration, and the development and progression of the "early" stages of DR. Pretreatment with CJDHW could become clinically important as a preventive approach for patients with a family history of AMD or diabetes, and/or when there are predisposing factors related to CRAO or BRAO, hypertension, coronary/carotid artery disease, hyperlipidemia or heart valve disorder.

Conclusions

CJDHW inhibited apoptosis, increased antioxidative activity, downregulated MMP-9 and inhibited p38 MAPK.

Abbreviations

wAMD: wet age related macular degeneration; Bcl-2: B-cell lymphoma 2; BCVA: best corrected visual acuity; ChAT: choline acetyltransferase; CJDHW: Chi-Ju-Di-Huang-Wan; CRAO: central retinal artery occlusion; DAPI: 4′,6-diamidino-2-phenylindole; DMSO: dimethyl sulfoxide; DR: diabetic retinopathy; ERG: electroretinogram; GCL: ganglion cell layer; GFAP: glial fibrillary acidic protein; HE: hematoxylin–eosin; HIOP: high intraocular pressure; HO-1: heme oxygenase-1; HRP: horseradish peroxidase; INL: inner nuclear layer; IPL: inner plexiform layer; I/R: ischemia/reperfusion; P-p38: phosphorylated-p38; MAPK: mitogen-activated protein kinases; MMP-9: matrix metallopeptidase-9; PCR: polymerase chain reaction; RGC: retinal ganglion cell; RPE: retinal pigment epithelium; SDS-PAGE: sodium dodecyl sulfate polyacrylamide gel electrophoresis; TBS: tris-buffered saline; TUNEL: terminal deoxynucleotidyl-transferase (TdT)-mediated dUTP nick end-labeling; VEGF: vascular endothelial growth factor.

Authors' contributions

HMC, LH and JMC designed the study. JMC, XQL performed the experiments, and wrote the manuscript. JHL, HTP, XMZ, LH and HMC analyzed the data and revised the manuscript. All authors read and approved the final manuscript.

Author details

[1] Department of Ophthalmology, Affiliated Hospital of Taishan Medical University, Shandong, China. [2] Department of Pharmacology, School of Medicine, Shandong University, Jinan, Shandong, China. [3] Department of Ophthalmology, Cheng Hsin General Hospital, Taipei, Taiwan. [4] Institute of Pharmacology, School of Medicine, National Yang-Ming University, Taipei, Taiwan. [5] Department of Chinese Medicine, School of Chinese Medicine, China Medical University, Taichung, Taiwan.

Acknowledgements

Heartfelt gratitude is conveyed for the financial support from the project [CHGH102-21]. Great thanks is given to Ms. Shih-Hsin Wang and Ms. Huei-Wen Shiu as well as to Professor Ralph Kirby for their skillful techniques in molecular biological assays and his expert correction of the manuscript, respectively. We are also indebted to Professor Gordon J. Johnson, Honorary Professor, London School of Hygiene and Tropical Medicine, UK, for carefully reading and professionally commenting on the final draft of this revised manuscript.

Competing interests

The authors declare that they have no competing interests.

References

1. Chao HM, Chen IL, Liu JH. S-allyl L-cysteine protects the retina against kainate excitotoxicity in the rat. Am J Chin Med. 2014;42(3):693–708.
2. Osborne NN, Casson RJ, Wood JP, Chidlow G, Graham M, Melena J. Retinal ischemia: mechanisms of damage and potential therapeutic strategies. Prog Retin Eye Res. 2004;23:91–147.
3. Peng PH, Chao HM, Juan SH, Chen CF, Liu JH, Ko ML. Pharmacological preconditioning by low dose cobalt protoporphyrin induces heme oxygenase-1 overexpression and alleviates retinal ischemia-reperfusion injury in rats. Cur Eye Res. 2011;36:238–46.
4. Park SJ, Choi NK, Seo KH, Park KH, Woo SJ. Nationwide incidence of clinically diagnosed central retinal artery occlusion in Korea 2008 to 2011. Ophthalmology. 2014;121(10):1933–8.
5. Zhao Y, Fu JL, Li YL, Li P, Lou FL. Epidemiology and clinical characteristics of patients with glaucoma: an analysis of hospital data between 2003 and 2012. Indian J Ophthalmol. 2015;63(11):825–31.
6. Thomas RL, Dunstan FD, Luzio SD, Chowdhury SR, North RV, Hale SL, Gibbins RL, Owens DR. Prevalence of diabetic retinopathy within a national diabetic retinopathy screening service. Br J Ophthalmol. 2015;99(1):64–8.
7. Park SJ, Kwon KE, Choi NK, Park KH, Woo SJ. Prevalence and incidence of exudative age-related macular degeneration in South Korea: a nationwide population-based study. Ophthalmology. 2015;122(10):2063–70.
8. Wurm A, Iandiev I, Uhlmann S, Wiedemann P, Reichenbach A, Bringmann A, Pannicke T. Effects of ischemia-reperfusion on physiological properties of Muller glial cells in the porcine retina. Invest Ophthalmol Vis Sci. 2011;52:3360–7.
9. He S, Masland RH. Retinal direction selectivity after targeted laser ablation of starburst amacrine cells. Nature. 1997;389:378–82.
10. Guo L, Moss SE, Alexander RA, Ali RR, Fitzke FW, Cordeiro MF. Retinal ganglion cell apoptosis in glaucoma is related to intraocular pressure and IOP-induced effects on extracellular matrix. Invest Ophthalmol Vis Sci. 2005;46:175–82.
11. Zhao J, Tan S, Liu F, Zhang Y, Su M, Sun D. Heme oxygenase and ocular disease: a review of the literature. Curr Eye Res. 2012;37:955–60.
12. Frank RN, Amin RH, Puklin JE. Antioxidant enzymes in the macular retinal pigment epithelium of eyes with neovascular age-related macular degeneration. Am J Ophthalmol. 1999;127:694–709.
13. Ralay Ranaivo H, Hodge JN, Choi N, Wainwright MS. Albumin induces upregulation of matrix metalloproteinase-9 in astrocytes via MAPK and reactive oxygen species-dependent pathways. J Neuroinflammation. 2012;9:68.
14. Wang JJ, Huan SK, Hsieh KH, Chou HC, Hsiao G, Jayakumar T, Sheu JR. Inhibitory effect of midazolam on MMP-9, MMP-1 and MMP-13 expression in PMA-stimulated human chondrocytes via recovery of NF-kappaB signaling. Arch Med Sci. 2013;9:332–9.
15. Chang YH, Lin HJ, Li WC. Clinical evaluation of the traditional chinese prescription Chi-Ju-Di-Huang-Wan for dry eye. Phytother Res. 2005;19:349–54.

16. Leung I, Tso M, Li W, Lam T. Absorption and tissue distribution of zeaxanthin and lutein in rhesus monkeys after taking Fructus lycii (Gou Qi Zi) extract. Invest Ophthalmol Vis Sci. 2001;42:466–71.
17. Perucho J, Casarejos MJ, Gomez A, Solano RM, de Yebenes JG, Mena MA. Trehalose protects from aggravation of amyloid pathology induced by isoflurane anesthesia in APP(swe) mutant mice. Curr Alzheimer Res. 2012;9:334–43.
18. Jenkins ES, Combes RD. FRAME's response to an APC questionnaire on emerging biotechnologies and the animals (scientific procedures) Act 1986. Altern Lab Anim. 2000;28(2):333–8.
19. Buchi ER, Suivaizdis I, Fu J. Pressure-induced retinal ischemia in rats: an experimental model for quantitative study. Ophthalmologica. 1991;203(3):138–47.
20. Miller RF, Dowling JE. Intracellular responses of the Muller (glial) cells of mudpuppy retina: their relation to the b-wave of the electroretinogram. J Neurophysiol. 1970;33:323–41.
21. Chao H, Chidlow G, Melena J, Wood J, Osborne N. An investigation into the potential mechanisms underlying the neuroprotective effect of clonidine in the retina. Brain Res. 2000;877:47–57.
22. Schatz A, Arango-Gonzalez B, Fischer D, Enderle H, Bolz S, Röck T, Naycheva L, Grimm C, Messias A, Zrenner E. Transcorneal electrical stimulation shows neuroprotective effects in retinas of light-exposed rats. Invest Ophthalmol Vis Sci. 2012;53:5552–61.
23. Chao HM, Chuang MJ, Liu JH, Liu XQ, Ho LK, Pan WHT, Zhang XM, Liu CM, Tsai SK, Kong CW, Lee SD, Chen MM, Chao FP. Baicalein protects against retinal ischemia by antioxidation, antiapoptosis, downregulation of HIF-1alpha, VEGF, and MMP-9 and upregulation of HO-1. J Ocul Pharmacol Ther. 2013;29:539–49.
24. Liu JH, Wann H, Chen MM, Pan WH, Chen YC, Liu CM, Yeh MY, Tsai SK, Young MS, Chuang HY. Baicalein significantly protects human retinal pigment epithelium cells against H2O2-induced oxidative stress by scavenging reactive oxygen species and downregulating the expression of matrix metalloproteinase-9 and vascular endothelial growth factor. J Ocul Pharmacol Ther. 2010;26:421–9.
25. Marecko I, Cvejic D, Selemetjev S, Paskas S, Tatic S, Paunovic I, Savin S. Enhanced activation of matrix metalloproteinase-9 correlates with the degree of papillary thyroid carcinoma infiltration. Croat Med J. 2014;55:128–37.
26. Dong W, Sun W, Zhang Y, Chen X, He S. Dendritic relationship between starburst amacrine cells and direction-selective ganglion cells in the rabbit retina. J Physiol. 2004;556:11–7.
27. Dulak J, Deshane J, Jozkowicz A, Agarwal A. Heme oxygenase-1 and carbon monoxide in vascular pathobiology: focus on angiogenesis. Circulation. 2008;117:231–41.
28. Opremcak E, Rehmar AJ, Ridenour CD, Borkowski LM, Kelley JK. Restoration of retinal blood flow via translumenal Nd:YAG embolysis/embolectomy (TYL/E) for central and branch retinal artery occlusion. Retina. 2008;28:226–35.
29. Zarbin MA. Current concepts in the pathogenesis of age-related macular degeneration. Arch Ophthalmol. 2004;122:598–614.
30. Hayreh SS, Jonas JB. Optic disk and retinal nerve fiber layer damage after transient central retinal artery occlusion: an experimental study in rhesus monkeys. Am J Ophthalmol. 2000;129:786–95.
31. Hayreh SS, Zimmerman MB, Kimura A, Sanon A. Central retinal artery occlusion. Retinal survival time. Exp Eye Res. 2004;78:723–36.
32. Mason JO III, Shah AA, Vail RS, Nixon PA, Ready EL, Kimble JA. Branch retinal artery occlusion: visual prognosis. Am J Ophthalmol. 2008;146:455–7.
33. Hsu TK, Chen SJ, Lei J, Wu Z, Lin CC, Chen MM, Lin TC, Liu JH, Chao HM. Embolus-induced branch retinal artery occlusion with a presenting best-corrected visual acuity of <6/12 and visual field defect: yag embolectomy safely restores arteriolar perfusion and/or visual function. Retin Cases Brief Rep. 2013;7(3):210–6.
34. Hernandez C, Simo R. Somatostatin replacement: a new strategy for treating diabetic retinopathy. Curr Med Chem. 2013;20(26):3251–7.

Full component analysis of *Tianma-Gouteng-Yin*

Ying-Yu Huang[1,2†], Liang-Feng Liu[1,2†], Rui-Qi Yue[1], Jun Xu[1], Alan Ho[1], Min Li[1,2*] and Quan-Bin Han[1,2*]

Abstract

Background: *Tianma-Gouteng-Yin* (TGY), which is common Chinese medicine formulation consisting of 11 different herbs and being used in China for the treatment of Parkinson's disease, inflammatory conditions and cardiovascular diseases, was selected for full component analysis. The aim of this study was to quantitatively analyze the chemical profiles of ten commercial TGY samples and one sample produced in our laboratory.

Methods: Ultra-high performance liquid chromatography (UHPLC) coupled with quadrupole-tandem time-of-flight mass spectrometry (Q-TOF-MS) was used to analyze the non-saccharide small molecule components of the different TGY samples. The established method was validated in terms of its linearity, sensitivity, precision, accuracy and stability. High performance liquid chromatography coupled with evaporative light scattering detection (HPLC-ELSD) was also used to quantify three major saccharides (fructose, glucose and sucrose).

Results: The relative standard deviations for the precision, repeatability and stability of these compounds were less than 5 %, while the accuracy of the method was 95–105 %. Twenty-eight of the compounds found in TGY were successfully identified, with 20 being quantified. The macromolecules present in these samples were also identified using an ethanol precipitation method, representing 294.68–696.64 mg/g of the total material depending on the batch. Notably, the components identified using this method represented up to 78 % of the total weight of the TGY samples.

Conclusions: The developed UHPLC/Q-TOF-MS and HPLC-ELSD methods successfully identified 28 of the complex compounds found in TGY.

Background

Tianma-Gouteng-Yin (TGY) is commonly used in Chinese medicine for calming liver wind, clearing heat, promoting blood flow and nourishing the liver and kidney [1]. Several clinical studies [2–4, 12] showed that TGY can reduce the motor fluctuations of Parkinson's disease (PD) patients. Pharmacological studies showed that TGY can prevent the apoptosis of dopaminergic neurons [2]. Furthermore, some of the active compounds isolated from the constituent of TGY exhibit neuroprotective, anti-inflammatory and cardiovascular protective effects [5–11]. In particular, the results of our recent studies revealed that some of the active compounds isolated from *Uncaria rhynchophylla* (*Gouteng*) and *Scutellaria baicalensis* (*Huangqin*), which are two of the key herbs used in TGY, promoted the clearance of pathogenic proteins and suppressed the progression of PD [5, 6, 10].

Although the clinical and pharmacological evaluation of TGY and its component herbs have been attracting interest in relevant fields, the quality analysis of TGY remains unsatisfactory. TGY consists of 11 herbs, including *Gastrodia elata* (*Tianma*), *U. rhynchophylla (Gouteng), Cyathula officinalis (Chuan Niu Xi), Gardenia jasminoides (Zhizi), S. baicalensis (Huangqin), Eucommia ulmoides (Du Zhong), Leonurus japonicus (Yimucao), Taxillus chinensis (Sang Ji Sheng), Polygonum multiflorum (Ye Jiao Teng), Poria cocos (Fuling)* and *Haliotis diversicolor (Shi Jue Ming)* [1]. TGY contains a complex mixture of chemical ingredients, including numerous small molecules (e.g., glycosides, quinic acids, terpenes and flavonoids) and a large amount of carbohydrates (e.g.,

*Correspondence: limin@hkbu.edu.hk; simonhan@hkbu.edu.hk
†Ying-Yu Huang and Liang-Feng Liu contributed equally to this work
[1] School of Chinese Medicine, Hong Kong Baptist University, Hong Kong, China
Full list of author information is available at the end of the article

monosaccharides, oligosaccharides and polysaccharides). The only small molecules listed as quality control markers for TGY in the Chinese Pharmacopeia are baicalin and gastrodin [1]. Several methods have been reported for the analysis of a few marker compounds in TGY, including geniposide, rhynchophylline and isorhynchophylline by thin layer chromatography (TLC) and high performance liquid chromatography (HPLC) [13–15]. However, these methods found that the contents of these markers were only 2.05 %, suggesting that a large number of the compounds in TGY were being left undetermined. As a product of decoction, TGY also contains several other constituents such as macromolecules, including a large amount of carbohydrates (e.g., monosaccharides, oligosaccharides and polysaccharides) [16]. However, the analytical methods published to date for the analysis of TGY have missed this critical part. The existing analytical methods for the quality control of TGY are therefore not suitable to deliver consistent quality control.

The aim of this study was to develop a quantitative analytical method for evaluating the chemical profiles of ten commercial TGY samples and one sample produced in our laboratory. Ultra-high performance liquid chromatography (UHPLC) coupled with quadrupole-tandem time-of-flight mass spectrometry (Q-TOF-MS) was used to analyze 17 non-saccharide compounds, and high performance liquid chromatography coupled with an evaporative light scattering detector (HPLC-ELSD) was used to quantitatively determine three major saccharides. The macromolecular contents of these samples (i.e., polysaccharides, proteins and nucleic acids) were also determined by the precipitation of these molecules with ethanol.

Methods

Reagents, chemicals and materials

Acetonitrile (MS grade) was purchased from RCI Lab scan Ltd (Bangkok, Thailand). Analytical grade formic acid was purchased from Sigma-Aldrich (St. Louis, MO, USA). HPLC grade methanol and ethanol were obtained from Merck (Darmstadt, Germany). Deionized water was prepared using a Millipore MilliQ-Plus water purification system (Millipore, Bedford, MA, USA).

Reference standards of L-phenylalanine (**1**), catechin (**2**), genipin-1-gentiobioside (**3**), epicatechin (**4**), geniposide (**5**), leonurine (**6**), 2,3,5,4′-tetrahydroxystilbene-2-*O*-β-D-glucoside (**7**), cyasteron (**8**), corynoxeine (**9**), isorhynchophylline (**10**), isocorynoxeine (**11**), baicalin (**12**), rhynchophylline (**13**), oroxylinA-7-*O*-glucuronide (**14**), bacalein-6-*O*-beta-glucopyranoside (**15**), wogonoside (**16**) and wogonin (**17**) were purchased from Chengdu Preferred Biotechnology Co., Ltd (Chengdu, China). The identities of the reference standards were confirmed by mass spectrometry prior to being used. The purities of the reference standards were determined to be greater than 98 % by UPLC-DAD analysis based on peak area normalization. Reference standards of fructose, glucose and sucrose were purchased from Sigma-Aldrich. The structures of the reference standards are shown in Fig. 1.

Commercial samples (TGY1–10) were purchased from different pharmacies in several different regions of China, including Jilin, Beijing, Nanchang, Shenzhen and Hong Kong. The sample designated TGY11 evaluated in the current study was prepared in our laboratory using herbal materials purchased from the Mr & Mrs Chan Hon Yin Chinese Medicine Specialty Clinic and Good Clinical Practice Centre, Hong Kong Baptist University, China. All of the herbs used in the current study were identified and authenticated by Professor Zhong-Zhen Zhao from the School of Chinese Medicine, Hong Kong Baptist University, China. Voucher specimens were deposited at the School of Chinese Medicine, Hong Kong Baptist University, Hong Kong, China (Collection numbers A110607, 110991, A1202151, 1300942, A121017, 131110, 140102, 140112, 130906, 130603).

Sample solutions preparation

The commercial samples (TGY1–10) were ground into fine powders and passed through a 60–80 mesh filter. A small accurately weighed sample (20 mg) of each powder was then dissolved in distilled water in a 10 mL volumetric flask at room temperature. All of the resulting sample solutions were filtered through a 0.22 μm nylon-membrane filter (Millipore, Barcelona, Spain) prior to being analyzed to determine the 17 non-saccharide small molecules.

The TGY11 material prepared in our laboratory consisted of the following materials: *G. elata* (*Tianma*) (9 g), *U. rhynchophylla* (*Gouteng*) (12 g), *C. officinalis* (*Chuan Niu Xi*) (18 g), *G. jasminoides* (*Zhizi*) (9 g), *S. baicalensis* (*Huangqin*) (9 g), *C. officinalis* (*Chuan Niu Xi*) (9 g), *E. ulmoides* (*Du Zhong*) (9 g), *L. japonicus* (*Yimucao*) (9 g), *T. chinensis* (*Sang Ji Sheng*) (9 g), *P. multiflorum* (*Ye Jiao Teng*) (9 g) and *P. cocos* (*Fuling*) (9 g) [1]. All of the crude materials were powdered and extracted three times by refluxing in boiling water (1:10, w/v) for 1 h. The combined extracts were then filtered and evaporated under reduced pressure, before being freeze-dried to give the TGY11 material as a powder. This powders were then prepared according to the procedure described above for the preparation of the commercial samples.

For the analysis of the saccharides, a small accurately weighed portion (10 mg) of each sample was dissolved in 2 mL of water. Ethanol (8 mL) was then added slowly

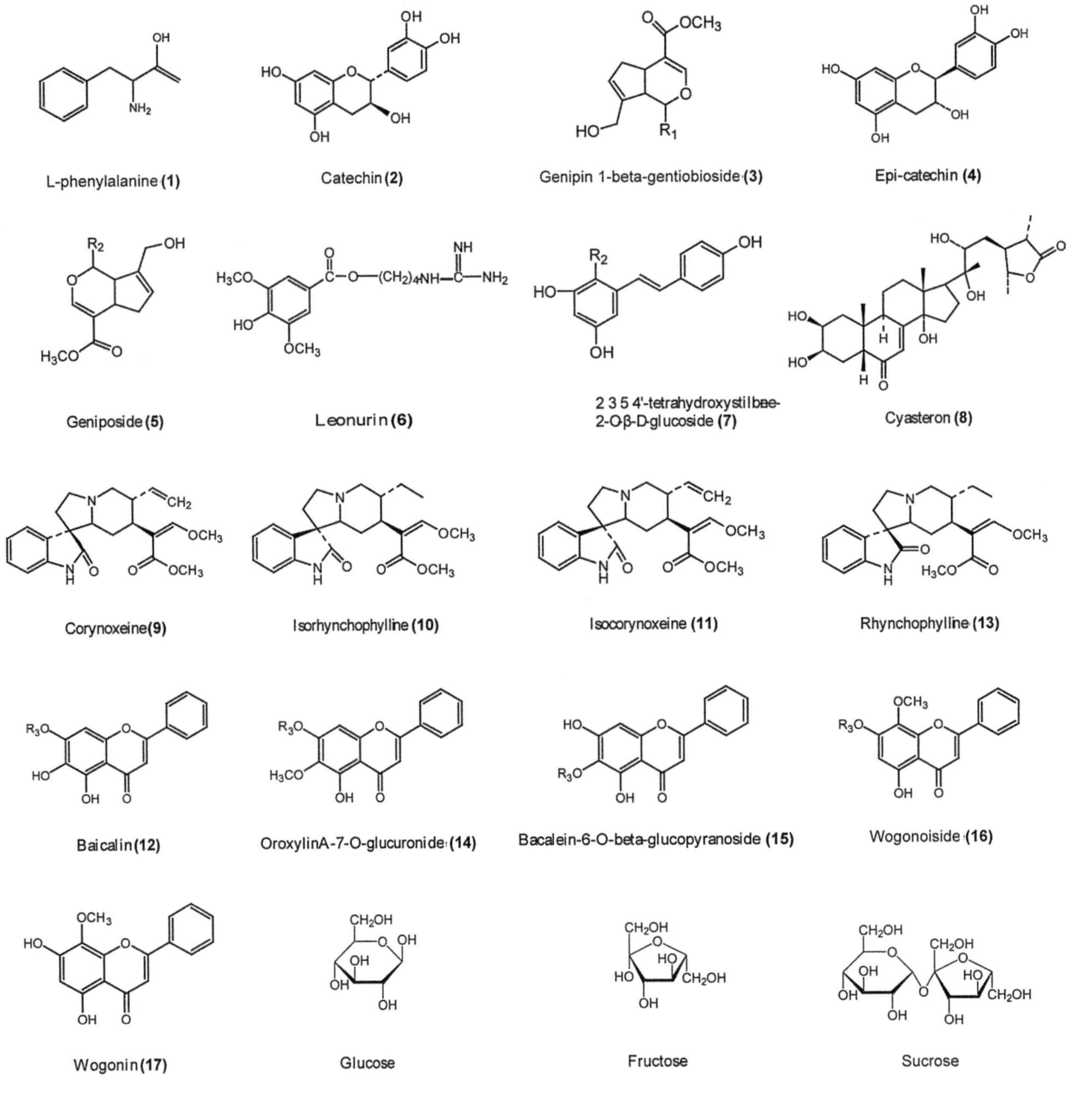

R_1 = 1-6-O-beta-D-Glucose-beta-D-Glucose R_2=Glucose R_3=Glucuronide

Fig. 1 Chemical structures of the positively identified constituents of the TGY decoction

added to each aqueous solution to precipitate any macromolecular components. The resulting mixtures were held for 24 h at room temperature, before being centrifuged on a 5804 Eppendorf multi-purpose centrifuge (Eppendorf Bio Tools, Radnor, PA, USA) at 3250×*g* for 15 min. The supernatant was collected and evaporated to dryness to give a residue, which was dissolved in a 1:1 (v/v) mixture of ACN and water (1 mL) and filtered through a 0.22 nylon-membrane filter (Millipore). The resulting filtrates were subjected to HPLC-ELSD analysis to determine their fructose, glucose and sucrose levels. The precipitate from the centrifugation step was dried and weighed to determine the macromolecular content of each sample [17].

Standard solutions preparation

Reference standards of L-phenylalanine, catechin, genipin-1-gentiobioside, epicatechin, geniposide, leonurine, 2,3,5,4′-tetrahydroxystilbene-2-*O*-β-D-glucoside, cyasteron, corynoxeine, isorhynchophylline, isocorynoxeine, rhynchophylline, baicalin, oroxylinA-7-*O*-glucuronide, wogonoside, baicalein and wogonin were weighed and dissolved in different volumes of methanol containing distilled water to prepare stock solutions. Samples of these stock solutions were then mixed together to prepare a mixed standard solution. The standard saccharide solutions were prepared according to the methods described in our previous publication [18]. Reference markers of fructose, glucose and sucrose were accurately weighed and dissolved in a 1:1 (v/v) mixture of ACN and water. Calibration curves were obtained by the appropriate dilution of these mixed standard solutions.

Analytical methods

Chromatographic analysis was performed on an Agilent 1290 UHPLC system (Agilent Technologies, Santa Clara, CA, USA) equipped with a binary pump, a thermostat-controlled column compartment, an auto sampler and a DAD detector. Separations were conducted over an Acquity UPLC BEH C18 column (2.1 × 100 mm, 1.7 μm, Waters, Milford, CT, USA) at 40 °C with a gradient elution consisting of 0.1 % formic acid in water (mobile phase A) and 0.1 % formic acid in ACN (mobile phase B). The column was eluted with the following gradient program: 0–3 min, 2 % B; 3–9 min, 2–12 % B; 9–24 min, 12–32 % B; 24–29 min, 32–75 % B; 29–29.1 min, 75–100 % B; 29.1–32 min, 100 % B. The flow rate was set at 0.4 mL/min.

An Agilent 6540 Q-TOF mass spectrometer (Agilent Technologies) equipped with a jet stream electrospray ionization (ESI) source was used to acquire the MS and MS/MS data in the positive and negative ionization modes. Data acquisition was controlled using MassHunterB.03 software (Agilent Technologies, Wilmington, USA). The operating parameters were set as follows: nebulizing gas (N_2) flow rate, 8.0 L/min; nebulizing gas temperature, 300 °C; jet stream gas flow, 9 L/min; sheath gas temperature, 350 °C; nebulizer gas pressure, 45 psi; capillary voltages, 3000 V; skimmer voltage, 65 V; Oct RFV, 600 V; fragment voltage, 150 V. Mass spectra were recorded for *m/z* values in the range of 100–1700 with accurate mass measurements for all of the mass ions. The peak areas determined in the extracted ion chromatograms were placed into calibration curves, which were prepared by plotting the peak areas of samples containing different concentrations to calculate the non-saccharide small molecule contents contained in this decoction.

The HPLC-ELSD conditions used for the determination of the saccharides were described in our previous publication [18]. An Agilent 1100 liquid chromatograph system (Agilent Technologies, Palo Alto, CA, USA) equipped with an Alltech 2000 evaporative light-scattering detector (Grace, Deerfield, MA, USA) was used. The chromatographic separations were performed over an Asahipak NH2P-50 4E column (4.6 × 250 mm, Shodex, Tokyo, Japan) at a column temperature of 30 °C. The column was eluted with a mixture of water (mobile phase A) and ACN (mobile phase B) at a flow rate of 0.8 mL/min. The elution conditions were as follows: 0–16 min, 78 % B; 16–20 min, 78–62 % B; 20–30 min, 62–60 % B. The drift tube temperature of the ELSD was set at 120 °C, and the nitrogen flow rate was set at 3.2 L/min. The peak areas in the ELSD chromatograms were collected to calculate the concentrations of the different components. Calibration curves were generated by plotting the logarithmic values of the different peak areas against the logarithmic values of the corresponding concentrations.

Method validation

The optimum method for the quantitative analysis of the samples was validated in terms of its linearity, sensitivity, precision, accuracy and stability. Stock solutions of the mixed standards were diluted to a variety of different concentrations to allow for the construction of calibration curves. At least six concentrations of each reference standard were analyzed in triplicate. The calibration curves were constructed by plotting the peak areas versus the concentrations of the corresponding constituents. The limit of detection (LOD) and limit of quantification (LOQ) values for the optimum conditions were determined at signal-to-noise ratios (S/N) of 3 and 10, respectively. The intra- and inter-day variations were used to evaluate the precision of our newly developed method. Six independently prepared solutions of TGY11 were analyzed within 1 day to evaluate the intra-day variability of the optimum method. To evaluate the inter-day variability of this method, we examined the same sample twice a day over 3 consecutive days. Variations were expressed as relative standard deviations (RSDs) of the data, which were calculated using the following formula: RSD (%) = (standard deviation/mean) × 100 %. A recovery test was performed to evaluate the accuracy of the optimum method by adding three different concentrations of a standard solution (i.e., low, medium and high) to TGY11, which contained known quantities of the target compounds. These samples were then analyzed in parallel using our newly established method. Each experiment was conducted in triplicate at each level. The spike recoveries were calculated using the following equation:

$$Spike\ recovery\ (\%) = (total\ amount\ detected - amount\ original) / amount\ spiked \times 100\,\%$$

The stability of the optimal method was evaluated by analyzing the TGY11 extracts over periods of 0, 2, 4, 8, 12 and 24 h. The RSDs of the peak areas of each compound were used as an indication of the stability.

Results and discussion

Optimization of the chromatographic conditions

The MS experiments were performed on an LC–MS system equipped with an ESI source to optimize the resolution, sensitivity and analytical time of this method. A full MS scan was obtained in the form of a total ion chromatogram (TIC). With regard to MS conditions, all of the samples were simultaneously evaluated in the positive and negative ionization modes. The positive ionization mode provided much more ESI information than the negative ionization mode and was therefore selected for the subsequent experiments. The gradient elution program was also optimized eluting with 0.1 % formic acid in water (mobile phase A) and 0.1 % formic acid in ACN (mobile phase B) under the following conditions: 0–3 min, 2 % B; 3–9 min, 2–12 % B; 9–24 min, 12–32 % B; 24–29 min, 32–75 % B; 29–29.1 min, 75–100 % B; 29.1–32 min, 100 % B. These conditions provided the best separation and peak shapes for all of compounds evaluated in the current study. Formic acid was added to the mobile phase to give a final concentration of 0.1 % to allow for the complete ionization of TGY. Representative chromatograms of the reference standards and TGY samples are shown in Fig. 2.

Identification of chemical compounds

The peaks observed in the chromatograms of the TGY samples were primarily identified based on a comparison of their accurate molecular mass data with those of the reference standards and data from the literature [19–23]. In this way, we were able to identify 28 compounds. Data for the MS/MS fragments of the different peaks were also obtained and these results are summarized in Table 1. Representative TICs of TGY in the positive ionization mode are shown in Fig. 2a. Chromatograms of the mono- and oligosaccharides found in the different TGY samples were obtained by HPLC-ELSD for the analysis of the saccharides, and the results are shown in Fig. 3. Three peaks were identified following this analysis, including fructose, glucose and sucrose by comparing their retention times with those of the reference standards.

A comparison of the retention time and MS/MS fragmentation data for the TGY samples with those of the reference standards led to the successful identification of 17 non-saccharide compounds. Specifically, peaks 1–17 were unambiguously identified as L-phenylalanine, catechin, genipin-1-gentiobioside, epicatechin, geniposide, leonurine, 2,3,5,4′-tetrahydroxystilbene-2-*O*-β-D-glucoside, cyasteron, corynoxeine, isorhynchophylline, isocorynoxeine, rhynchophylline, baicalin, oroxylinA-7-*O*-glucuronide, wogonoside, baicalein and wogonin, respectively. The chemical structures of these compounds are shown in Fig. 1.

Based on a comparison with data from the literature, peaks 18–25 were tentatively attributed to vanillin, pinoresinol diglucoside, chrysin-6-C-ara-8-C-glu, chrysin-6-C-glu-8-C-ara, quercitrin, norwogonin-7-*O*-glucuronide, 5,7,8-trihydroxy-6-methoxyflavone-7-glucuronide and 5,6,7-trihydroxy-8-methoxyflavone-7-glucuronide, respectively.

Peak 18 was determined to be vanillin based on its mass spectrum, which contained a molecular ion peak with an *m/z* value of 153.0546 for $[M+Na]^+$ [24]. The mass spectrum for peak 19 contained a molecular ion peak with an *m/z* value of 705.2367 for $[M+Na]^+$, which corresponded well with pinoresinol diglucoside [20, 25]. The mass spectra of peaks 20 and 21 contained molecular ion peaks with *m/z* values of 549.1646 and 549.1620, respectively, for $[M+H]^+$. These peaks could be attributed to chrysin-6-C-ara-8-C-glu or chrysin-6-C-glu-8-C-ara. Although the MS/MS fragmentation spectra of these peaks contained identical signals with *m/z* values of 489, 459 and 429, the intensities of these ions varied considerably for the different peaks. Data from the literature suggested that chrysin-6-C-ara-8-C-glu would have a shorter retention time than chrysin-6-C-glu-8-C-ara. Based on this information, peak 20 was tentatively attributed to chrysin-6-C-ara-8-C-glu, whereas peak 21 was attributed to chrysin-6-C-glu-8-C-ara [21, 26]. Peak 22 was attributed to quercitrin based on a comparison of its MS and MS/MS fragmentation spectra with those reported in the literature [20]. It is noteworthy that the mass spectrum for quercitrin contained a molecular ion with an *m/z* value of 449.1178 for $[M+H]^+$, whereas the MS/MS fragmentation spectrum contained a peak with an *m/z* value of 303.0486. This new peak was attributed to the formation of a quercetin aglycone fragment following the loss of a fragment with a molecular weight of 176. The ESI analysis of peak 23 in the positive ionization mode gave a molecular ion with an *m/z* value of 447.0922 for $[M+H]^+$, along with a fragment ion with an *m/z* value of 271.0617 for the aglycone cation. Based on these data, peak 23 was tentatively identified as norwogonin-7-*O*-glucuronide [27]. Peaks 24 and 25 were attributed to isomeric compounds and eluted with retention times of 18.9 and 19.8 min, respectively. Furthermore, these peaks gave molecular ions with *m/z* values of 477.1065 and 447.1058, respectively. The MS/MS fragmentation spectra of these

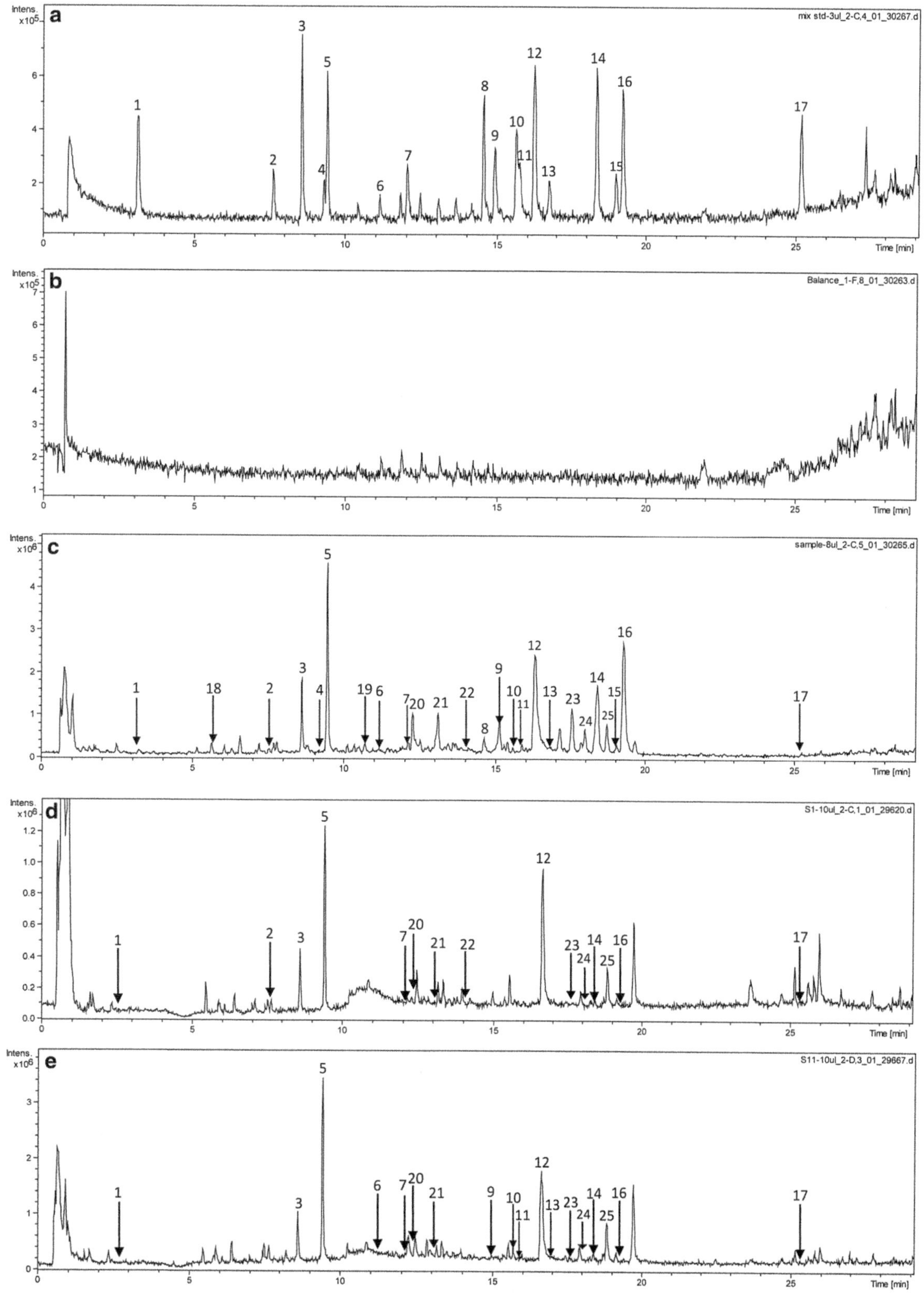

Fig. 2 Typical UPLC-Q-TOF chromatograms. Reference standards (**a**); blank solvent (**b**); self-made sample TGY11 (**c**); Commercial samples TGY1 (**d**) and TGY6 (**e**)

Table 1 Chromatographic and MS data (positive mode) of the constituents identified using our newly developed UPLC-Q-TOF-MS method

	R.T. (min)	Mass		Error (ppm)	Fragment ions (m/z)	Molecular formula	Identification	Herbal origin	Confirmed with reference standard
		Observed	Calculated						
1	2.80	166.0871	166.0863	4.8	120.0792 $[M+H-COOH]^+$	$C_9H_{11}NO_2$	L-Phenylalanine	*H. diversicolor*	Yes
2	7.50	291.0862	291.0863	5.3	139.0396 $[M+H-C_8H_7O_3]^+$, 123.0434 $[M+H-C_8H_7O_4]^+$	$C_{15}H_{14}O_6$	Catechin	*U. rhynchophylla*	Yes
3	8.59	551.2007	551.1970	4.3	573.2007 $[M+Na]^+$, 227.0753 $[M+H-maltose]^+$ 209.0656 $[M+H-maltose-OH]^+$	$C_{23}H_{34}O_{15}$	Genipin 1-beta-gentiobioside	*G. jasminoides*	Yes
4	9.30	291.0866	291.0863	1.0	139.0381 $[M+H-C_8H_7O_3]^+$, 123.0422 $[M+H-C_8H_7O_4]^+$	$C_{15}H_{14}O_6$	Epi-catechin	*U. rhynchophylla*	Yes
5	9.40	389.1452	389.1442	2.6	411.0792 $[M+Na]^+$, 231.0366 $[M+H-glucose-2H]^+$	$C_{17}H_{24}O_{10}$	Geniposide	*G. jasminoides*	Yes
6	11.2	312.1554	312.1554	1.6	181.0498 $[M-C_5H_{13}N_3O]$, 132.1125 $[M+H-C_9H_9N_4O]^+$	$C_{14}H_{22}N_3O_5$	Leonurine	*L. japonicus*	Yes
7	12.3	407.1337	407.1351	3.4	245.0768 $[M+H-glucose]^+$	$C_{20}H_{22}O_9$	2 3 5 4′-tetrahydroxystilbene-2-*O*-β-D-glucoside	*P. multiflorum*	Yes
8	14.9	521.3146	521.3109	5.2	503.2947 $[M+H-H_2O]^+$, 485.2896 $[M+H-2H_2O]^+$	$C_{29}H_{44}O_8$	Cyasteron	*C. officinalis*	Yes
9	15	383.1978	383.1965	3.4	383.1978$[M+H]^+$	$C_{22}H_{26}N_2O_4$	Corynoxeine	*U. rhynchophylla*	Yes
10	15.8	385.2131	385.2122	2.3	241.1337	$C_{22}H_{28}N_2O_4$	Isorhynchophylline	*U. rhynchophylla*	Yes
11	15.9	383.1976	383.1965	2.9	383.1976$[M+H]^+$	$C_{22}H_{26}N_2O_4$	Isocorynoxeine	*U. rhynchophylla*	Yes
12	16.7	447.0944	447.0922	4.9	271.0621 $[M+H-glucuronide]^+$	$C_{21}H_{18}O_{11}$	Baicalin	*S. baicalensis*	Yes
13	16.9	385.2126	385.2122	1.0	353.1854 $[M+H-OCH_3]^+$, 160.0754	$C_{22}H_{28}N_2O_4$	Rhynchophylline	*U. rhynchophylla*	Yes
14	18.9	461.1110	461.1078	5.1	285.0762 $[M+H-glucuronide]^+$, 270.0507 $[M+H-glucuronide-CH_3]^+$	$C_{22}H_{20}O_{11}$	OroxylinA-7-*O*-glucuronide	*S. baicalensis*	Yes
15	19.6	447.0951	447.0922	3.7	271.0601$[M+H-glucuronide]^+$	$C_{21}H_{18}O_{11}$	Bacalein-6-*O*-beta-glucopyranoside	*S. baicalensis*	Yes
16	19.8	461.1105	461.1078	5.9	285.0754 $[M+H-glucuronide]^+$	$C_{22}H_{20}O_{11}$	Wogonoside	*S. baicalensis*	Yes
17	25.6	285.0773	285.0757	5.6	270.0535 $[M+H-CH_3]^+$	$C_{16}H_{12}O_5$	Wogonin	*S. baicalensis*	Yes

Table 1 continued

	R.T. (min)	Mass		Error (ppm)	Fragment ions (m/z)	Molecular formula	Identification	Herbal origin	Confirmed with reference standard
		Observed	Calculated						
18	5.6	153.0546	153.0507	4.9	175.0380 $[M+Na]^+$	$C_8H_8O_3$	Vanillin	*G. elata*	Not yet
19	10.9	683.2537	683.2507	4.4	705.2363 $[M+Na]^+$	$C_{32}H_{42}O_{16}$	Pinoresinol diglucoside	*E. ulmoides*	Not yet
20	12.2	549.1646	549.1616	5.5	531.1493 $[M+H-H_2O]^+$	$C_{26}H_{28}O_{13}$	Chrysin-6-C-ara-8-C-glu	*S. baicalensis*	Not yet
21	13.1	549.1620	549.1616	0.7	531.1482 $[M+H-H_2O]^+$	$C_{26}H_{28}O_{13}$	Chrysin-6-C-glu-8-C-ara	*S. baicalensis*	Not yet
22	14.0	449.1143	449.1178	5.4	303.0486 $[M+H-rhamnose]^+$	$C_{21}H_{20}O_{11}$	Quercitrin	*L. japonicus*	Not yet
23	18.5	447.0946	447.0922	5.4	271.0617 $[M+H-glucuronide]^+$	$C_{21}H_{19}O_{11}$	Norwogonin-7-*O*-glucuronide	*S. baicalensis*	Not yet
24	18.9	477.1065	447.1028	4.9	301.0719 $[M+H-glucuronide]^+$	$C_{22}H_{20}O_{12}$	5,7,8,-Trihydroxy-6-methoxyflavone-7-glucuronide	*S. baicalensis*	Not yet
25	19.8	477.1058	477.1028	3.7	301.0718 $[M+H-glucuronide]^+$	$C_{22}H_{20}O_{12}$	5,6,7,-Trihydroxy-8-methoxyflavone-7-glucuronide	*S. baicalensis*	Not yet

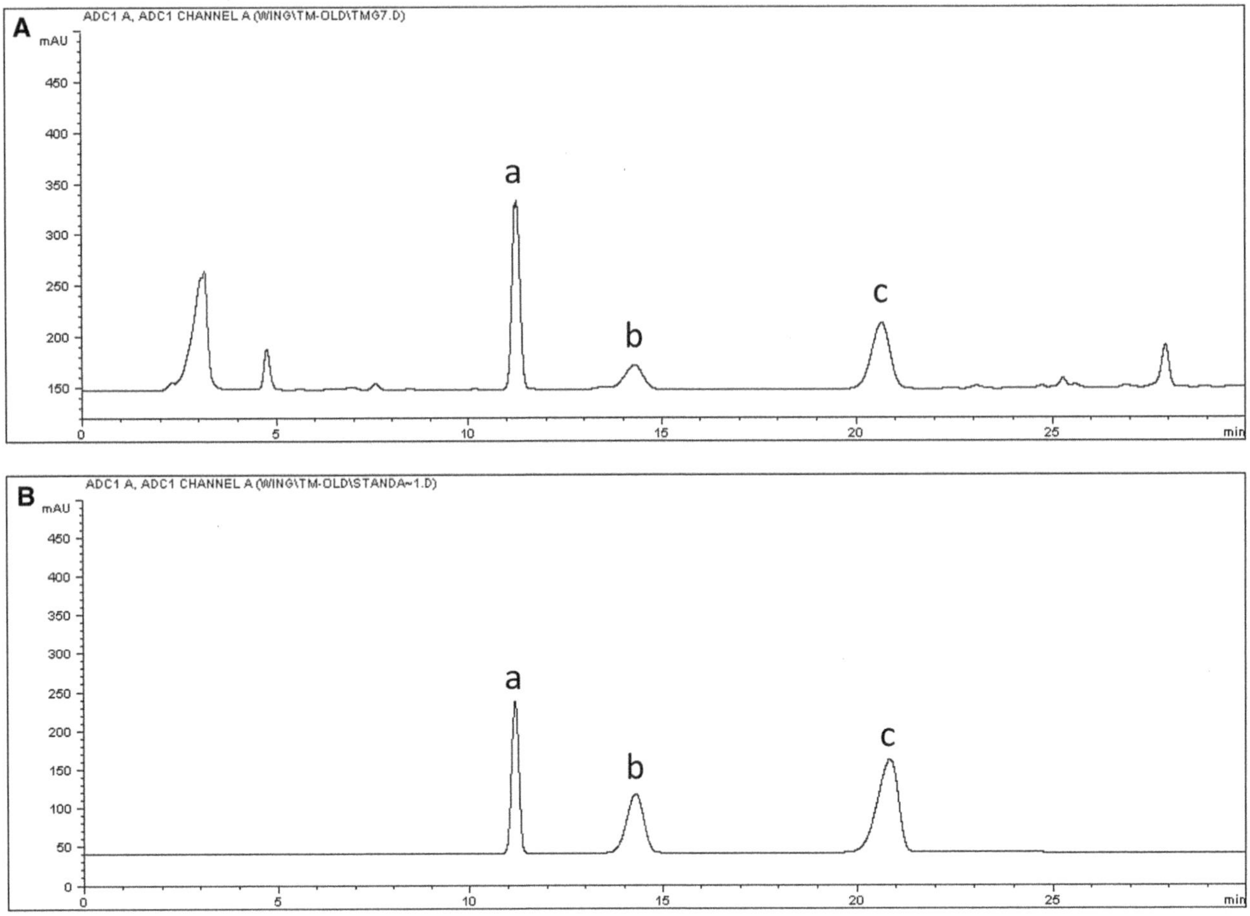

Fig. 3 Typical HPLC-ELSD chromatograms. TGY sample (TGY11) (**A**); reference standards (**B**) (*a*: fructose, *b*: glucose, *c*: sucrose)

peaks both produced an ion with an *m/z* value 301. The loss of a fragment with a molecular weight of 176 in the MS/MS fragmentation spectrum was consistent with the presence of a glucuronide group. Peaks 24 and 25 were therefore tentatively attributed to 5,7,8-trihydroxy-6-methoxyflavone-7-glucuronide and 5,6,7-trihydroxy-8-methoxyflavone-7-glucuronide, respectively, based on their accurate mass and MS/MS fragmentation data [27].

Method validation

Linearity calibration curves were constructed using at least six different concentrations of the reference standards. Each concentration of the reference standards was analyzed in duplicate. The results revealed that there was a good correlation between the concentration and peak area of these compounds, as indicated by the high coefficients of determination ($r^2 > 0.999$). The linear ranges of the 17 different compounds evaluated in this way are summarized in Table 2. The LOD and LOQ values were measured using signal to noise ratios of 3:1 and 10:1, respectively, and the results are also listed in Table 2. A solution of the TGY11 material prepared in our laboratory was analyzed six times within 24 h under the optimized conditions to evaluate the intra-day variation of the method. The same solution was also analyzed on 3 successive days to assess the inter-day variation of the optimized method, as well as its precision and accuracy. The RSDs of the intra- and inter-day variations were 4.06 and 5.54 %, respectively, which indicated that our newly established method had satisfactory precision and repeatability properties. The results of spiking recovery experiments showed that our newly developed method performed well with a mean recovery in the range of 94.37–105.99 with RSDs of less than 4.5 % for the 17 positively identified compounds. The stability of our newly developed method was determined by assessing the RSDs of the peaks of the 17 positively identified compounds within 24 h. The results of this analysis revealed that the RSDs of all 17 compounds were less than 4.6 %. Taken together, these results demonstrated that our newly developed UPLC-Q-TOF method was sufficiently reliable and accurate for the simultaneous quantification

Table 2 Results of methodology validation in terms of linear regression, LOD, LOQ, repeatability, accuracy, and stability

Analyte	Linearity			LOD (ng/mL)	LOQ (ng/mL)	Repeatability (RSD, %, n = 6)		Spike recovery (RSD, %, n = 3)			Stability (RSD, %, n = 6)
	Range (ng/mL)	Equation	r^2			Intra-day	Inter-day	High	Middle	Low	
1	50.60–404.80	Y = 148.2X − 704.4	0.9996	13.67	45.58	3.45	4.81	96.37 (2.08)	96.55 (0.18)	105.99 (2.65)	3.16
2	397.50–3180.00	Y = 33.8X − 721.8	0.9989	104.61	348.68	2.93	4.84	98.86 (2.16)	98.67 (0.65)	94.99 (2.00)	2.46
3	329.10–10530.00	Y = 56.9X + 10454.0	0.9997	43.38	144.60	1.20	3.37	101.88 (2.21)	101.73 (0.65)	94.37 (1.72)	1.81
4	3187.50–25500.00	Y = 7.3X + 2059.8	0.9997	233.80	779.34	2.53	5.54	96.96 (2.22)	104.26 (0.78)	102.12 (5.48)	4.59
5	1659.40–53100.00	Y = 16.9X + 18376.0	0.9989	174.67	582.64	4.06	4.64	102.71 (1.99)	96.39 (0.31)	102.31 (1.94)	2.59
6	59.48–237.93	Y = 1203.4X + 9810.8	0.9992	11.65	38.84	3.78	4.66	101.38 (5.10)	104.00 (0.69)	104.50 (1.23)	3.98
7	126.28–5387.76	Y = 493.9X + 11718.0	0.9999	25.25	84.18	2.58	4.17	97.14 (2.19)	95.46 (1.27)	95.10 (0.37)	2.58
8	116.50–1864.00	Y = 170.7X + 5289.2	0.9996	17.83	59.44	1.05	4.54	96.77 (0.99)	101.81 (0.77)	104.52 (0.51)	1.56
9	13.02–208.33	Y = 378.9X + 1346.2	0.9994	2.77	9.24	1.55	3.66	101.45 (4.45)	97.26 (1.42)	104.54 (2.29)	1.29
10	13.27–106.12	Y = 12974.0X − 33626.0	0.9994	2.14	7.13	1.19	4.71	101.76 (2.68)	103.99 (1.79)	105.29 (1.15)	1.51
11	52.95–211.80	Y = 592.1X + 6742.6	0.9993	9.57	31.05	2.42	3.97	102.07 (1.53)	95.27 (0.78)	105.62 (0.58)	2.37
12	1273.44–81500.00	Y = 44.0X + 62221.0	0.9996	49.97	166.57	2.50	4.59	100.78 (2.65)	98.85 (3.36)	101.55 (3.70)	4.67
13	33.04–198.21	Y = 2767.1X − 52144.0	0.9988	7.62	25.41	3.46	4.43	95.89 (0.71)	99.58 (3.47)	94.63 (0.77)	2.85
14	204.10–13062.50	Y = 132.0X + 17621.0	0.9992	28.98	96.62	1.69	4.89	97.72 (3.65)	98.26 (0.72)	99.54 (3.98)	4.28
15	259.38–4150.00	Y = 47.4X − 1173.4	0.9989	71.38	237.95	2.64	3.89	102.64 (2.18)	99.14 (0.64)	106.11 (1.39)	2.29
16	1767.19–28275.00	Y = 117.5X + 127121.0	0.9989	26.61	88.71	1.89	4.29	97.29 (2.79)	98.27 (0.29)	96.19 (2.40)	1.87
17	118.64–2548.47	Y = 1291.1X − 78900.0	0.9998	27.23	90.76	1.07	1.69	96.64 (1.39)	101.78 (0.77)	94.88 (1.05)	1.73

All *P* values for linear regression were <0.001

Table 3 Contents of 17 constituents in eleven batches of TMGTY samples (mg/g)

Analyte	TGY-01	TGY-02	TGY-03	TGY-04	TGY-05	TGY-06	TGY-07	TGY-08	TGY-09	TGY-10	TGY-11
1[a]	0.03[b] ± 2.57[c]	–[d]	–	–	0.04 ± 2.50	0.08 ± 2.82	–	–	–	–	0.05 ± 3.45
2	0.39 ± 3.42	0.38 ± 2.27	0.40 ± 1.53	0.27 ± 2.72	0.25 ± 0.56	–	–	0.18 ± 1.09	–	–	0.93 ± 2.93
3	1.02 ± 1.95	0.99 ± 2.50	1.42 ± 0.13	1.27 ± 3.00	1.89 ± 2.48	1.65 ± 2.65	2.02 ± 3.16	2.54 ± 4.39	1.84 ± 0.67	2.03 ± 1.71	0.23 ± 1.20
4	–	–	–	–	–	–	–	–	–	–	4.59 ± 2.53
5	2.10 ± 3.11	2.12 ± 0.48	3.18 ± 1.90	2.92 ± 4.33	5.04 ± 4.73	5.98 ± 1.94	8.00 ± 0.63	5.69 ± 1.71	5.74 ± 2.10	6.67 ± 0.63	13.15 ± 4.06
6	–	–	–	–	–	0.05 ± 0.65	0.04 ± 1.68	0.04 ± 1.16	0.02 ± 4.77	0.02 ± 4.16	0.053 ± 3.78
7	0.03 ± 3.40	0.03 ± 0.64	0.27 ± 4.12	0.24 ± 2.86	0.09 ± 1.95	1.79 ± 1.83	1.79 ± 3.25	1.67 ± 1.96	1.72 ± 3.28	1.44 ± 2.65	0.10 ± 2.58
8	–	–	–	–	–	–	–	–	–	–	0.36 ± 1.05
9	–	–	–	–	–	0.06 ± 1.34	0.02 ± 4.10	0.02 ± 4.43	0.01 ± 1.51	0.01 ± 2.96	0.02 ± 1.55
10	–	–	–	–	–	0.03 ± 4.30	0.01 ± 1.51	0.01 ± 5.02	0.01 ± 2.85	0.01 ± 3.09	0.01 ± 1.19
11	–	–	–	–	–	0.14 ± 1.26	0.06 ± 1.13	0.04 ± 1.90	0.03 ± 2.29	0.03 ± 0.67	0.05 ± 2.42
12	1.83 ± 2.28	1.64 ± 2.29	2.08 ± 2.07	1.30 ± 4.48	5.55 ± 1.81	8.33 ± 0.95	8.18 ± 3.38	9.22 ± 1.83	10.94 ± 0.40	12.11 ± 3.41	31.34 ± 2.50
13	–	–	–	–	–	0.08 ± 1.84	0.03 ± 1.70	0.02 ± 1.13	0.03 ± 1.50	0.02 ± 1.38	0.03 ± 3.46
14	0.24 ± 4.02	0.21 ± 1.87	0.25 ± 1.41	0.22 ± 2.63	0.53 ± 0.50	0.85 ± 0.62	0.90 ± 2.66	1.02 ± 1.90	1.21 ± 1.29	1.38 ± 1.75	3.59 ± 1.69
15	–	–	–	–	–	–	–	–	–	–	0.26 ± 2.64
16	0.41 ± 3.08	0.32 ± 3.72	0.52 ± 1.53	0.44 ± 3.37	0.95 ± 1.29	1.33 ± 2.08	1.31 ± 4.36	1.60 ± 4.13	1.74 ± 0.40	2.06 ± 0.56	5.98 ± 1.89
17	0.09 ± 2.50	0.05 ± 2.12	0.06 ± 3.66	–	–	0.17 ± 0.20	0.08 ± 4.89	0.09 ± 3.89	0.11 ± 1.69	0.12 ± 3.12	0.57 ± 1.07
Fructose	38.03 ± 1.45	70.92 ± 0.99	30.26 ± 3.02	41.04 ± 1.03	45.46 ± 1.21	38.08 ± 1.66	80.56 ± 1.86	26.79 ± 1.45	40.15 ± 3.67	38.12 ± 0.71	69.60 ± 2.86
Glucose	45.70 ± 1.07	46.34 ± 0.39	34.31 ± 0.41	37.30 ± 0.50	46.35 ± 3.21	30.64 ± 4.48	52.21 ± 1.59	32.79 ± 4.38	33.07 ± 4.93	27.89 ± 2.10	67.87 ± 4.12
Sucrose	14.50 ± 0.63	14.71 ± 0.04	13.52 ± 1.02	12.92 ± 4.74	16.18 ± 4.79	4.72 ± 1.78	5.85 ± 1.23	5.01 ± 2.13	3.83 ± 4.33	4.10 ± 4.56	4.03 ± 1.02
Mac. molecular	549.36 ± 2.81	643.87 ± 4.33	559.69 ± 3.69	483.25 ± 0.48	655.19 ± 0.94	618.28 ± 0.02	535.61 ± 0.06	696.64 ± 4.11	611.02 ± 2.92	636.59. ± 0.03	294.98 ± 1.11

[a] The compound numbers are the same as in Fig. 1

[b] The data was present as average of triplicate determinations

[c] SD value of two times determination results

[d] Under the limit of quantification (LOQ)

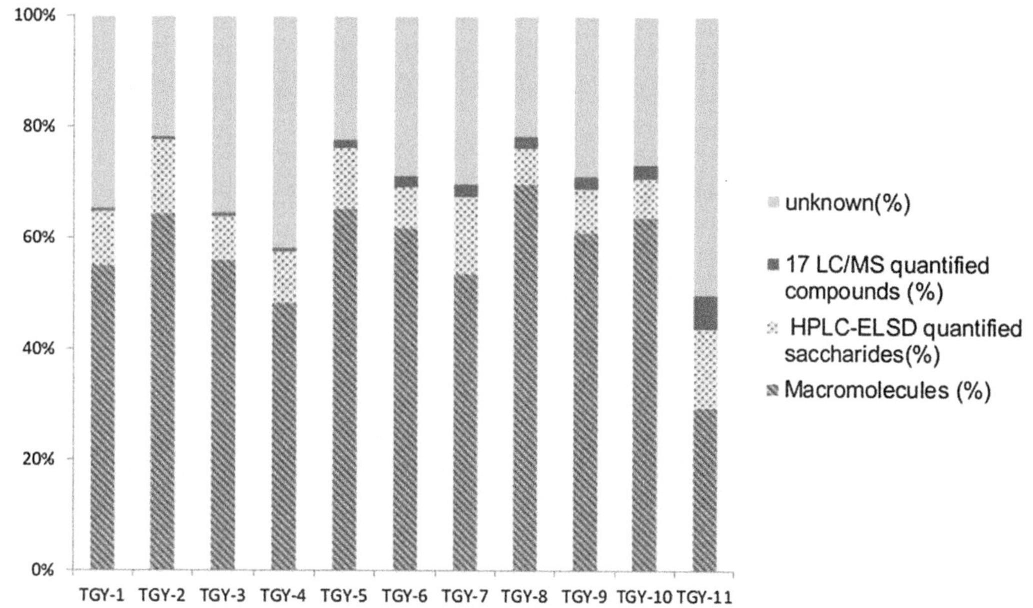

Fig. 4 Content percentages of the chemicals determined in this study

of the 17 positively identified non-saccharide compounds in TGY.

Quantification of compounds in commercial samples

Our newly developed UPLC-Q-TOF and HPLC-ELSD methods were successfully applied to the simultaneous determination of 20 identified compounds in 10 commercial TGY samples (TGY1–10) and one lab-prepared sample (TGY11). The results of these analyses are summarized in Table 3 and Fig. 4. The 17 positively identified non-saccharide compounds accounted for 0.5–6.1 % of the overall weight of the TGY samples, whereas the three mono- and di-saccharides accounted for 7–14.2 %. The biggest contribution to the weight of the TGY samples came from macromolecules, which account for 30–70 % of the total weight. The quantification percentage of the commercial TGY samples reached up to 78.33 %, thereby demonstrating the suitability of our newly developed method for the quality control of TGY samples in terms of accounting for most of the major components.

All 17 of the positively identified non-saccharide compounds were found in the lab-prepared sample (TGY11), with baicalin being the most abundant. The contents of these compounds varied considerably in the samples collected from the different manufacturers. For example, rhynchophylline, isorhynchophylline, corynoxeine and isocorynoxeine are considered to be the four main bioactive constituents of *U. rhynchophylla* [6, 13, 28]. However, the amount of corynoxeine detected in TGY6 was six times greater than that detected in TGY9. Furthermore, none of these four alkaloids were detected in TGY1–5. This result implied that there were inconsistencies in the quality of the TGY decoctions. These variations in the quality could be attributed to various factors, including differences in the origins of the plants, as well as differences in the planting methods, harvest time, geographical climate and processing methods. The fructose, glucose and sucrose contents of the samples also fluctuated considerably between the different samples. Once again, these variations could be attributed in part to differences in the pretreatment processes or manufacturing procedures. It is noteworthy that much larger amounts of sucrose were found in TGY1–5 than any of the other samples. In terms of the macromolecular contents of these samples, the contents of TGY8 and TGY11 were 696.64 and 294.98 mg/g, respectively. This variation may have been introduced as a consequence of the difference in the raw materials, extraction process or processing procedures. Also, the presence of excipients in the sample matrix could have a significant impact on the contents of the sample being investigated.

Compared with other methods reported in the literature [1, 13–15, 29], which have been used to determine the total contents of only a few chemical markers at concentrations as low as 2.05 %, the method described herein was used to quantify almost 60–80 % of the compounds found in TGY, representing a clear majority. The percentage ratios of the components determined in the current study are shown in Fig. 4. These results show that the quantification percentages of the commercial samples could reach up to 78.33 %, whereas that of TGY11 was much lower at 50 %. Notably, more than 40 % of the chemicals present in TGY11 remained unidentified. These chemicals could include amino acids, inorganic salts or some other ingredients. However, it is also possible that the addition of 80 % ethanol was not sufficient to precipitate all of the polysaccharides completely, and that those with lower molecular weights remained in solution [17] and their content could not be determined.

Conclusions

The developed UHPLC/Q-TOF-MS and HPLC-ELSD methods successfully identified 28 of the complex compounds found in TGY, and quantified 20 of them.

Abbreviations

TGY: *Tianma-Gouteng-Yin*; PD: Parkinson disease; UHPLC: ultra high-performance liquid chromatography; Q-TOF-MS: quadrupole-tandem time-of-flight mass spectrometry; HPLC: high performance liquid chromatography; ELSD: evaporative light scattering detection; RSD: relative standard deviation.

Authors' contributions

All authors designed the study. YYH completed the HPLC analysis and LFL prepared the samples tested. LFL, RQY, JX and AH analyzed the data. YYH and LFL wrote the manuscript. ML and QBH revised this paper. All authors read and approved the final manuscript.

Author details

[1] School of Chinese Medicine, Hong Kong Baptist University, Hong Kong, China. [2] Mr. & Mrs. Ko Chi Ming Centre for Parkinson's Disease Research (CPDR), Hong Kong Baptist University, Kowloon Tong, Hong Kong SAR.

Acknowledgements

This study was supported by GRF Grant (HKBU 121009/14), Innovation & Technology Fund (ITS/274/12) and Health and Medical Research Fund (HMRF 12132091) from the Hong Kong Government and research Grants IRMS/12-13/1A, MPCF-004-2012/2013 and FRG2/13-14/094, FRG2/11-2/048, FRG1/12-13/018, FRG2/12-13/006, FRG2/13-14/026, MPCF-001-2014/2015 and RC-start up grant from Hong Kong Baptist University. The authors would like to thank Dr. Siva Sundara Kumar Durairajan, Ms. Leilei Chen, Ms. Yu Zeng, Dr. Juxian Song, Ms. Huaixue Mu, Mr. Zhaoliang Zhou, Ms. Dongdong Hu, Ms. Tianbo Zhang and Mr. Kakit Chua. The authors would also like to thank Dr. Martha Dahlen for her English editing of this manuscript.

Competing interests

The authors declare that they have no competing interests.

References

1. The State Pharmacopoeia Commission of P. R. China. Pharmacopoeia of the People's Republic of China. 1st ed. Beijing: Chemical Industry Press; 2010. pp. 519–520.
2. He JC, Wang WW. Effect of Tianma Gouteng Yin on apoptosis of dopaminergic neurons in Parkinson's disease model rats. Zhong Yi Za Zhi. 2010;51:1024–7.
3. Zhang ZQ, Tan WL, Lu H, Ren D. 62 cases of Parkinson's disease treated by TianMa GouTeng Yin with Madopar. Shan Xi Zhong Yi Za Zhi. 2008;29:666–7.
4. Kum WF, Durairajan SSK, Bian ZX, Man SC, Lam YC, Xie LX. Treatment of idiopathic Parkinson's disease with traditional Chinese herbal medicine: a randomized placebo-controlled pilot clinical study. Evid Based Complt Alt. 2009;2011:1–8.
5. Lu JH, Tan JQ, Durairajan SSK, Liu LF, Zhang ZH, Ma L. Isorhynchophylline, a natural alkaloid, promotes the degradation of alpha-synuclein in neuronal cells via inducing autophagy. Autophagy. 2012;8:98–108.
6. Chen LL, Song JX, Lu JH, Yuan ZW, Liu LF, Durairajan SSK, Li M. Corynoxine, a natural autophagy enhancer, promotes the clearance of alpha-synuclein via Akt/mTOR pathway. J Neuroimmune Pharm. 2014;9:380–7.
7. Wang SW, Wang YJ, Su YJ, Zhou WW, Yang SG, Zhang R. Rutin inhibits β-amyloid aggregation and cytotoxicity, attenuates oxidative stress, and decreases the production of nitric oxide and proinflammatory cytokines. Neurotoxicology. 2012;33:482–90.
8. Tanaka M, Yamazaki M, Chiba K. Neuroprotective action of genipin on tunicamycin-induced cytotoxicity in Neuro2a cells. Biol Pharm Bull. 2009;32:1220–3.
9. Xu X, Lu Y, Bie X. Protective effects of gastrodin on hypoxia-induced toxicity in primary cultures of rat cortical neurons. Planta Med. 2007;73:650–4.
10. Lu JH, Ardah MT, Durairajan SSK, Liu LF, Xie LX, Fong WFD. Baicalein inhibits formation of α-synuclein oligomers within living cells and prevents Aβ peptide fibrillation and oligomerisation. Chem Bio Chem. 2011;12:615–24.
11. Stratil P, Klejdus B, Kubáň V. Determination of phenolic compounds and their antioxidant activity in fruits and cereals. Talanta. 2007;71:1741–51.
12. Ma DL. Clinical observations of 42 cases of Parkinson's disease treated by integration of Chinese and Western Medicine. J Integr Chin West Med Card Cerebr Vasc Dis. 2003;1:2.
13. Xu Y, Tan H, Li T. Determination of rhynchophylline and baicalin in Tianma Gouteng Yin by RP-HPLC. Zhong Guo Yao Xue Za Zhi. 2001;36:414–5.
14. Yu C, Yang LJ, Ma B, Liu SK, Yuan Y, Yuan D. Simultaneous determination of rhynchophylline, isorhynchophylline, corynoxeine, and isocorynoxeine in the traditional Chinese prescriptions by HPLC. Shen Yang Yao Ke Da Xue Xue Bao. 2010;27:897–901.
15. Zhang R, Zhang CL, Fang PF, Xu Y, Wan X, Chen Y. TLC identification of Tianma gouteng granules. Hua Xi Yao Xue Za Zhi. 2001;16:384–6.
16. Lu W, Zhang JM, Hong YL, Feng Y, Chen MW, Wang YT. Phytochemical and pharmacological review of Da Chuanxiong formula: a famous herb pair composed of Chuanxiong Rhizoma and Gastrodiae Rhizoma for headache. Evid-Based Compl Alt. 2013;16:425369.
17. Xu J, Yue RQ, Liu J, Ho HM, Yi T, Chen HB, Han QB. Structural diversity requires individual optimization of ethanol concentration in polysaccharide precipitation. Int J Biol Macromol. 2014;67:205–9.
18. Zhang TB, Yue RQ, Xu J, Ho HM, Ma DL, Leung CH, Chau SL, Zhao ZZ, Chen HB, Han QB. Comprehensive quantitative analysis of Shuang-Huang-Lian oral liquid using UHPLC–Q-TOF-MS and HPLC-ELSD. J Pharm Biomed Anal. 2015;102:1–8.
19. Nurul Islam M, Downey F, Ng CKY. Comprehensive profiling of flavonoids in *Scutellaria incana* L. using LC-Q-TOF-MS. Acta Chromatogr. 2013;25:555–69.
20. Zhang D, Zhang CF, Yang ZL. Identification of chemical compounds on fingerprint of Cortex Eucommiae. Zhong Yi Yao Xue Bao. 2012;40:58–61.
21. Wu W, Yan C, Li L, Liu Z, Liu S. Studies on the flavones using liquid chromatography–electrospray ionization tandem mass spectrometry. J Chromatogr A. 2004;1047:213–20.
22. Xie S, Shi Y, Wang Y, Wu C, Liu W, Feng F, Xie N. Systematic identification and quantification of tetracyclic monoterpenoid oxindole alkaloids in Uncaria rhynchophylla and their fragmentations in Q-TOF-MS spectra. J Pharm Biomed Anal. 2013;81:56–64.
23. Nováková L, Spáčil Z, Seifrtová M, Opletal L, Solich P. Rapid qualitative and quantitative ultra-high performance liquid chromatography method for simultaneous analysis of twenty nine common phenolic compounds of various structures. Talanta. 2010;80:1970–9.
24. Fernandes A, Sousa A, Mateus N, Cabral M, Freitas V. Analysis of phenolic compounds in cork from *Quercus suber* L. by HPLC-DAD/ESI-MS. Food Chem. 2011;125:1398–405.
25. He F, Wang YL, Zheng L, Liu LJ, Wang AM, Li YJ, Huang Y. Identification of compounds in herb of *Eucommia ulmoides* by UPLC-PDA-ESI-MS. Zhong Guo Shi Yan Fang Ji Xue Za Zhi. 2014;20:59–62.
26. Han J, Ye M, Xu M, Sun J, Wang B, Guo DA. Characterization of flavonoids in the traditional Chinese herbal medicine-Huangqin by liquid chromatography coupled with electrospray ionization mass spectrometry. J Chromatogr B. 2007;848:355–62.

27. Liu GZ, Ma JY, Chen YZ, Tian QQ, Shen Y, Wang XS, Chen B. Investigation of flavonoid profile of *Scutellaria bacalensis* Georgi by high performance liquid chromatography with diode array detection and electrospray ion trap mass spectrometry. J Chromatogr A. 2009;1216:4809–14.
28. Xian YF, Lin ZX, Mao QQ, Hu Z, Zhao M, Che CT, Ip SP. Bioassay-guided isolation of neuroprotective compounds from *Uncaria rhynchophylla* against beta-amyloid-induced neurotoxicity. Evid-Based Compl Alt. 2012;2012:1–8.
29. Mao SF, Chao RB. Determination of baicalin in Tianma Gouteng granules by HPLC. Hua Xi Yao Xue Za Zhi. 2003;18:127–9.

10

Loki zupa (Luooukezupa) decoction reduced airway inflammation in an OVA-induced asthma mouse model

Ying Wei[1,2†], Muhammadjan Abduwaki[1,3†], Mihui Li[1,2], Qingli Luo[1,2], Jing Sun[1,2], Yubao Lv[1,2], Mammat Nurahmat[1,3] and Jingcheng Dong[1,2*]

Abstract

Background: *Loki zupa* (*Luooukezupa*) decoction, consisting of the roots of *Hyssopuscuspidatus Boriss* (*Shenxiangcao*) and *Irishalophila Pall* root (*Yuanweigen*), is commonly used in Uygur medicine to treat asthma. However, the mode of action of this material has yet to be elucidated. This study aims to investigate the effects of *Loki zupa* decoction on the airway inflammation of an ovalbumin (OVA)-induced asthma mouse model.

Methods: Mice were divided into normal control (NC), asthma (A), high, medium and low doses of *Loki zupa* decoction (L 14.0, L 7.0, L 3.5), water extract (LW), *n*-butanol extract (LN), ethyl acetate extract (LE) and dexamethasone (DEX) groups. Anti-asthmatic model was induced by OVA sensitization and challenged using BALB/c mice. Airway hyperresponsiveness (AHR) toward methacholine (Mch) was assessed using Buxco equipment. Lung inflammation was measured by hematoxylin and eosin staining and bronchoalveolar lavage fluid (BALF) cell count and classification. Inflammatory cytokines in BALF and serum were analyzed by Bio-Plex assay, and mRNA levels were investigated by qPCR analysis. The roots of *H. Boriss* (250 g) and *I. Pall* (250 g) were decocted, concentrated and diluted to 14.0, 7.0 and 3.5 g crude herb/kg body weight. The LW, LN and LE of the *Loki zupa* decoction were prepared and diluted to a dose equivalent to 7 g of crude herb/kg body weight.

Results: *Loki zupa* decoction and its extracts significantly attenuated the AHR towards Mch (all $P < 0.05$). Treatment with *Loki zupa* decoction and its extracts relieved the infiltration of inflammatory cells in and around the airways, and reduced the total white blood cell (all $P < 0.05$), neutrophil (all $P < 0.05$), monocyte (all $P < 0.05$) and eosinophil (all $P < 0.05$) counts in the BALF. The BALF samples collected from the mice treated with the *Loki zupa* decoction and its extracts had lower levels of IL-1β (all $P < 0.05$), TNF-α (all $P < 0.05$), IL-2 (all $P < 0.05$), IL-4 ($P = 0.047$) and IL-5 (all $P < 0.05$). The serum samples of these mice also had lower IL-1β (all $P < 0.05$), TNF-α (all $P < 0.05$), IL-4 (all $P < 0.05$) and IL-5 (all $P < 0.05$) levels and higher levels of IFN-γ ($P < 0.001$) compared with the OVA-induced asthma mouse model. qPCR analysis revealed that *Loki zupa* decoction and its extracts inhibited mRNA expression of IL-4 (all $P < 0.05$), IL-5 (all $P < 0.05$) and IL-13 (all $P < 0.05$) and promoted mRNA expression of IFN-γ (all $P < 0.05$) in asthmatic mice.

Conclusion: *Loki zupa* decoction reduced AHR, attenuated airway inflammation, promoted Th1 and suppressed Th2 cell functions in an OVA-induced asthma mouse model.

Background

Asthma is one of the most prevalent respiratory diseases in the world, and the prevalence of this disease is increasing on an annual basis [1]. Asthma is characterized by the inflammation of the airways, with the airways also becoming hyperresponsive. Furthermore, the inflammatory cells can infiltrate the airways, resulting in the secretion of related pro-inflammatory mediators [2]. Inhaled corticosteroids are currently the most effective drugs available for the treatment of asthma [3, 4]. However, the use of these drugs is often accompanied by undesirable side effects.

*Correspondence: jcdong2004@126.com
†Ying Wei and Muhammadjan Abduwaki contributed equally to this work
[2] Institute of Integrated Traditional Chinese and Western Medicine, Fudan University, 12 Middle Urumqi Road, Shanghai 200040, China
Full list of author information is available at the end of the article

The Th2-driven inflammation of the eosinophilic airways is responsible for upto 50 % of all cases of asthma, and is generally considered to be the major pathogenetic factor in this disease [4–6]. Asthmatic patients typically have elevated levels of Th2 cytokines in their BALF and bronchial mucosa [7]. It is well known that Th2-activated cells orchestrate pulmonary immune responses and mediate the inflammation of lung tissues, as well as airway hyperresponsiveness [8–10]. Th1-activated cells also inhibit the inflammation of asthmatic airways [11]. It is noteworthy that mice deficient in the Th1-type transcription factor T-bet develop spontaneous AHR and augmented airway eosinophilia [12]. The immunomodulation of the Th1/Th2 imbalance encountered in asthma patients is therefore considered to be a practical strategy for controlling asthma [11].

Loki zupa (*Luooukezupa*) decoction, which consists of a 1:1 mixture (w/w) of the roots of *Hyssopuscuspidatus Boriss* (*Shenxiangcao*) and *Irishalophila Pall* (*Yuanweigen*), is commonly used in Uygur medicine for the treatment of asthma [13, 14]. Although the oral administration of *Loki zupa* decoction alleviates asthmatic symptoms, the exact mode of action of this drug has not been elucidated.

This study aims to investigate the effects of *Loki zupa* decoction on the inflammation of the airways in an ovalbumin (OVA)-induced asthma mouse model.

Methods

Animals

Female BALB/c mice (6 weeks old) were purchased from Shanghai Sippr BK Laboratory Animal Co., Ltd (Shanghai, China) and raised in a pathogen-free rodent facility according to the procedures approved (2013-06-HSYY-DJC-02; Additional file 1) by the Committee on the Ethics of Animal Experiments of Fudan University. The mice were housed in separate stainless steel cages (six mice per cage) in a temperature-controlled environment (20–24 °C) on 12 h light–dark cycles with unrestricted access to food and water. All procedures of this study were in accordance with "Experimental Animal Ordinance" of Fudan University. The animal studies were performed following the ARRIVE guideline (Additional file 2).

Reagents

OVA and Mch were purchased from Sigma-Aldrich (St. Louis, MO, USA).The Bio-Plex kit used in this study was purchased from Bio-Rad (Hercules, CA, USA). The roots of *H. Boriss* and *I. Pall* were provided by the Xinjiang Uygur Medical College Affiliated Hospital, China. Small samples of these herbs were identified [15–17] by experts at the Testing Center of Jiangyin Tianjiang Pharmaceutical Co., Ltd (Jiangyin, China), where samples were also deposited with the following voucher specimen numbers: LZ-2013-01 to 02. Dexamethasone (DEX) was purchased from Chenxin pharmaceutical Co. Ltd (Jining, China) (Fig 1).

Preparation and extraction of a *Loki zupa* decoction

The roots of *H. Boriss* (250 g) and *I. Pall* (250 g) were decocted in water (3.6 L) for 1 h (two times). The decoction was then filtered through a sterile gauze and concentrated to 1000 mL (equivalent to 500 g of crude herb per 1000 mL of decoction) using a concentration heater. The concentrated decoction was subsequently diluted to several different concentrations (i.e., 14.0, 7.0 and 3.5 g of crude herb/kg body of weight) before being used.

For the extraction of the *Loki zupa* decoction, the roots of *H. Boriss* (1250 g) and *I. Pall* (1250 g) were ground into a fine powder using a pestle and mortar. The

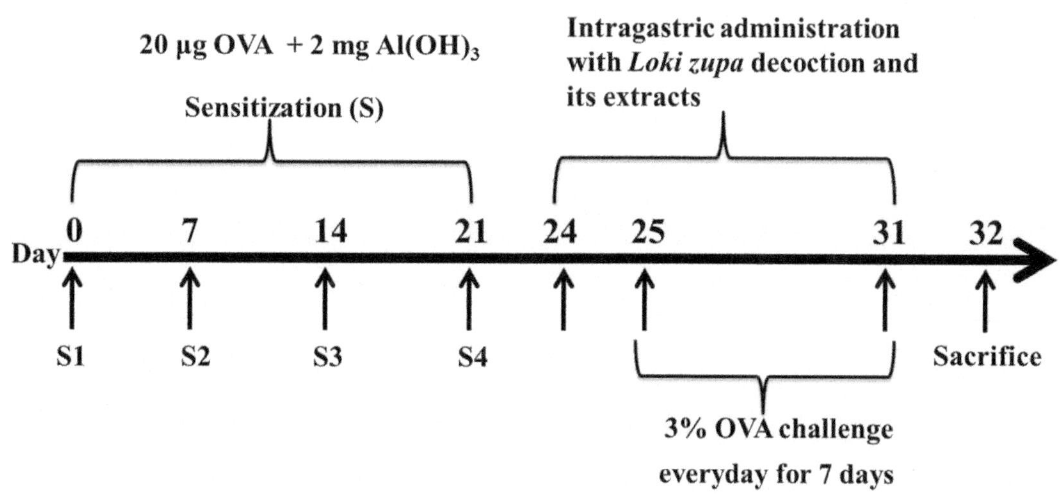

Fig. 1 Experimental protocol for the OVA-induced asthmatic model and treatment processes

resulting powder was degreased with petroleum ether and extracted three times with 70 % ethanol. The combined extracts were then filtered through sterile gauze and concentrated under vacuum on a rotary evaporator (EYELAN-1000, EYELA, Tokyo, Japan). The concentrated solution (predominantly aqueous) was extracted sequentially with petroleum ether, *n*-butanol and ethyl acetate. The water (LW), *n*-butanol (LN) and ethyl acetate (LE) extracts of the *Loki zupa* decoction were diluted to a concentration equivalent to 7 g of crude herb/kg body weight before being used.

Asthmatic model establishment and treatment

Female BALB/c mice (n = 108) were arbitrarily divided into nine groups (n = 12 each group), including normal control (NC), asthma (A), *Loki zupa* decoction (L 14.0, L 7.0, L 3.5), LW, LN, LE and DEX groups. As shown in Fig. 1, mice in group A and the other treatment groups were sensitized with an intraperitoneal injection of 0.2 mL saline containing 20 μg OVA and 2 mg aluminum hydroxide on days 0, 7, 14 and 21. From day 25, the mice in group A and the other treatment groups were challenged for 7 consecutive days with a 3 % (w/v) OVA solution, which was administered using an ultrasonic nebulizer (402AI ultrasonic nebulizer, Yuyue, China). The mice in the NC group were sensitized and challenged with saline. From day 24, the mice in the NC and A groups were intragastrically administrated with saline, whereas the other treatment groups were administrated with 14.0, 7.0 and 3.5 g/kg *Loki zupa* decoctions and its extracts, as well as DEX.

Measurement of AHR to Mch

Twenty-four hours after their last OVA challenge, the mice were anesthetized with pentobarbital sodium (50 mg/kg) to allow for their AHR to be measured using an invasive approach, as described previously, using Buxco resistance and compliance measurements (FinePointe RC System, Buxco, Wilmington, NC, USA) [18]. Increasing doses of Mch (0, 3.125, 6.25 and 12.5 mg/mL) were inhaled by nebulization to allow for the measurement of the AHR of the mice. Changes in airway resistance (R_L) and lung dynamic compliance (Cdyn) were measured and these data were subsequently expressed as a percent change from the baseline value.

Blood and bronchoalveolar lavage fluid (BALF) collection

Blood samples were collected from the mice immediately after the AHR measurements and stored at 4 °C for 2 h before being centrifuged at 5000×*g* for 15 min at 4 °C (5804R, Eppendorf, Leipzig, Germany). The resulting serum was collected, repackaged and stored at −80 °C prior to being analyzed in a Bio-Plex assay (Bio-Plex 200 System, Bio-Rad, Hercules, CA, USA). BALF collection was performed by lavaging the left lung with 0.3 mL aliquots of PBS (two times) through the tracheal cannula (total volume 0.6 mL). The resulting mixture was centrifuged at 1000×*g* for 10 min at 4 °C. The supernatant was collected and stored at −80 °C for further assay. The pellet from the BALF was resuspended in PBS (0.1 mL) for cell count and classification analysis using an automatic hematology analyzer (BC-5300 Vet, Mindray, China).

Pulmonary histopathology analysis

Samples of the lung tissues were collected, fixed in 4 % paraformaldehyde, embedded in paraffin and cut into 5 μm sections for histopathological analysis. Lung sections were stained with hematoxylin and eosin (H&E) to evaluate any inflammatory changes. Ten mice from each group and six arbitrarily selected fields in each mouse were photographed using an optical microscope (ECLIPSE 80i, Nikon, Japan) and the resulting images were analyzed in detail. The severity of any inflammatory cell infiltration in the lung samples was evaluated using a 5 point scoring system: 1, no cells; 2, a few cells; 3, a ring of cells with a depth of one-cell layer; 4, a ring of cells with a depth of 2–4 cells; and 5, a ring of cells with a depth of >4 cells. The degree of airway inflammation in each group was determined by two independent analysts. If their results were different, a third analyst was considered for further analysis of the related data.

Inflammatory mediators assay in BALF and serum

Cytokines present in the BALF and serum, including IL-1β, TNF-α, IFN-γ, IL-2, IL-4 and IL-5 were assayed by Bio-Plex according to the manufacturer's instructions.

Real-time quantitative PCR (qPCR) analysis

qPCR analysis of the cytokine expression levels in the lung samples collected from the mice was performed according to the manufacturer's instructions. The total RNA isolated from the lung tissue in each group was reverse transcripted into the first strand of cDNA using the Trizol reagent and a RevertAid TM First Strand cDNA Synthesis Kit (Fermentas, Vilnius, Republic of Lithuania). The qPCR amplification experiments were subsequently performed according to the manufacturer's instructions using a PCR Amplifier (ViiA7, life technologies, Carlsbad, CA, USA). The final data were normalized to determine the level of GAPDH expression in each group, and the results were presented as fold changes compared with the expression levelsin mice belonging to the NC group. The primers' sequences used for IL-4, IL-5, IL-13, IFN-γ and GAPDH are shown in Table 1.

Table 1 Primer sequences used for qPCR amplification

Gene	Primer sequence
IL-4 (NM_021283.2)	Forward primer: 5′-CAGCAACGAAGAACACCACA-3′ Reverse primer: 5′-AATCCAGGCATCGAAAAGCC-3′
IL-5 (NM_010558.1)	Forward primer: 5′-CAGTGTGAATGAGAGCCAGC-3′ Reverse primer: 5′-TTCTGTTGGCATGGGGTAGT-3′
IL-13 (NM_008355.3)	Forward primer: 5′-TTGAGGAGCTGAGCAACA-3′ Reverse primer: 5′-CCATGCTGCCGTTGCA-3′
IFN-γ (NM_008337.3)	Forward primer: 5′-AGCTCTTCCTCATGGCTGTT-3′ Reverse primer: 5′-TCCTTTTGCCAGTTCCTCCA-3′
GAPDH (NM_008084.2)	Forward primer: 5′-GTGGAGTCTACTGGTGTCTTC-3′ Reverse primer: 5′-CTCAGTGTCCCACCACCCT-3′

Statistical analysis

Data were expressed as the mean ± standard deviation (SD). SPSS 19.0 for Windows (IBM, Chicago, Illinois, USA) was used to analyze the significance of the differences between the different groups, using 10 mice from each group. Statistical analysis of these data was performed by one-way analysis of variance (ANOVA) for multiple comparisons followed by the least significantly different or Games-Howell test for a comparison of the different groups. *P* values less than 0.05 were considered statistically significant.

Results

Loki zupa decoction and its extracts treatment decreased AHR of OVA-induced asthmatic mice

The results of this study showed that the short-term OVA challenge of mice with Mch led to a significant decrease in AHR in the R_L group compared with mice in the NC group ($P = 0.037$, $P = 0.003$, $P = 0.001$; Fig. 2a). Treatment of the mice with *Loki zupa* decoction or its extracts resulted in a significant decrease in the AHR of the R_L group towards Mch compared with the OVA-induced asthmatic mice ($P < 0.05$; Fig. 2a). Furthermore, the treatment of the mice with *Loki zupa* decoction and its extracts led to an obvious increase in their inhibitory effects towards Mch in the R_L group. For example, at a Mch dose of 3.125 mg/mL, LE and DEX demonstrated significant inhibitory activity towards the R_L group ($P = 0.041$, $P = 0.047$; Fig. 2a). Furthermore, all of the *Loki zupa*-and DEX-treated groupsled to a considerable decreasein AHR in the $R_L$groups at a Mch dose of 6.25 mg/mL compared with OVA-induced asthmatic mice ($P = 0.001$, $P < 0.001$, $P < 0.001$, $P < 0.001$, $P < 0.001$, $P < 0.001$, $P < 0.001$). At aMch dose of 12.5 mg/mL, all of the treatment groups resulted in a significant decrease in AHR in the R_L group compared with the asthmatic mice ($P = 0.002$, $P < 0.001$, $P < 0.001$, $P < 0.001$, $P < 0.001$, $P < 0.001$, $P < 0.001$; Fig. 2a). The L 3.5 and LE-treated groups showed the greatest inhibitory effect of all of the groups tested in the current study towards AHR in the R_L group, which were the same as that of DEX at a Mch dose of 12.5 mg/mL ($P = 0.364$, $P = 0.362$; Fig. 2a).

Short-term OVA challenge in the mice also led to a significant reduction in Cdyn towards progressive doses of Mch compared with the mice in the NC group ($P = 0.021$, $P = 0.002$, $P < 0.001$; Fig. 2b). Treatment with *Loki zupa* decoction or its extracts resulted in improved Cdyn compared with the OVA-induced asthmatic mice. Furthermore, DEX treatment led to a dramatic increase in Cdyn compared with the asthmatic mice ($P = 0.035$, $P = 0.004$, $P < 0.001$). Different doses of *Loki zupa* decoction and its extracts resulted in a diverse range of effects on Cdyn to progressive doses of Mch. At a Mch dose of 3.125 mg/mL, all three doses of the *Loki zupa* decoction treatment tested in the current study led to significant increases in Cdyn ($P = 0.031$, $P = 0.027$, $P = 0.032$) compared with the asthmatic mice, representing a similar effect to that of DEX ($P = 0.871$, $P = 0.329$, $P = 0.877$).

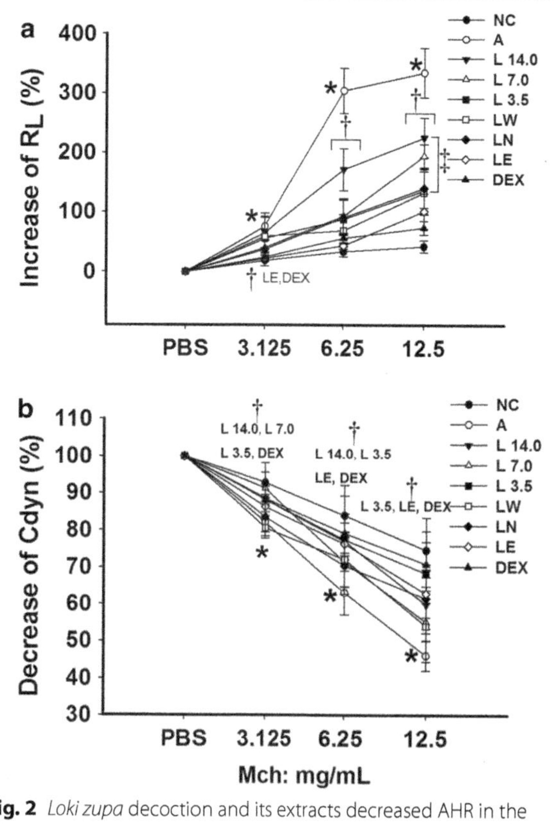

Fig. 2 *Loki zupa* decoction and its extracts decreased AHR in the OVA-induced asthmatic mice compared with the untreated mice. AHR towards progressive doses of Mch was measured by an invasive approach 24 h after the last OVA challenge. Changes in R_L and Cdyn have been expressed as percentage changes from the corresponding baseline values. The abbreviations for NC, A, L, LW, LN, LE, DEX are as follows: *NC* normal control, *A* asthma, *L 14.0, L 7.0, L 3.5 Loki zupa* decoction, *LW* water extract, *LN n*-butanol extract, *LE* ethyl acetate extract, *DEX* dexamethasone. $^{*}P < 0.05$ *vs.* NC group, $^{\dagger}P < 0.05$ *vs.* A group, $^{\ddagger}P < 0.05$ *vs.* DEX group

At a Mch dose of 6.25 mg/mL, the L 14.0 and L 3.5 treatment groups, as well as the LE treatment group, showed significant increases in Cdyn ($P = 0.010$, $P = 0.012$, $P = 0.017$) compared with the asthmatic mice, which were similarto the effect of DEX ($P = 0.630$, $P = 0.633$, $P = 0.513$). At a Mch dose of 12.5 mg/mL, only the L 3.5 and LE treatment groups showed significant increases in Cdyn ($P = 0.003$, $P = 0.007$) compared with asthmatic mice, with DEX treatment resulting in no significant changes ($P = 0.693$, $P = 0.217$).

Treatment with the *Loki zupa* decoction and its extracts attenuated pulmonary inflammation in the OVA-induced asthmatic mice

Short-term OVA challenge led to significant increase in the infiltration of inflammatory cells into the peribronchiolar tissues ($P < 0.001$; Fig. 3). A pronounced increase in the level of mucus secretion and marked thickening of the basement-membrane were also observed in the bronchi of the OVA-induced asthmatic mice compared with the mice in the NC group. A reduction in inflammatory infiltrates was observed in the mice treated with the *Loki zupa* decoction and its extracts, as well as the DEX treatment groups, compared with mice in the A group ($P < 0.001$). The LN and LE treatment groups were more effective in terms of their ability to alleviate inflammation compared with the L 7.0, L 3.5 and LW treatment groups ($P < 0.001$), and no significant differences were observed for the DEX treatment group ($P = 0.062$, $P = 0.223$).

Loki zupa decoction and its extracts treatment inhibited inflammatory cells in BALF of OVA-induced asthmatic mice

The total white blood cell (WBC), neutrophil (Neu), lymphocyte (Lym), monocyte (Mon), eosinophil (Eos) and basocyte (Bas) counts in the BALF samples were analyzed to investigate the effects of the *Loki zupa* decoction and its extracts on the inflammatory cells in the lung tissue. OVA inhalation led to significant increases in the total WBC, Neu, Lym, Mon, Eos and Bas counts in the BALF samples ($P = 0.001$, $P < 0.001$, $P = 0.047$, $P < 0.001$, $P = 0.007$, $P = 0.041$; Fig. 4). Treatment with *Loki zupa* decoction and its extracts, as well as DEX, led to a decrease in the total WBC ($P = 0.013$, $P = 0.044$, $P = 0.009$, $P = 0.029$, $P = 0.001$, $P = 0.014$, $P = 0.004$), Neu ($P = 0.001$, $P = 0.001$, $P = 0.001$, $P = 0.047$, $P < 0.001$, $P = 0.003$, $P = 0.001$), Mon ($P < 0.001$, $P < 0.001$, $P < 0.001$, $P = 0.001$, $P < 0.001$, $P < 0.001$, $P < 0.001$) and Eos ($P = 0.003$, $P = 0.004$, $P = 0.001$, $P = 0.047$, $P < 0.001$, $P = 0.004$, $P = 0.001$) counts in the BALF samples. However, treatment with the *Loki zupa* decoction and DEX did not led to a decrease in the Lym ($P = 0.519$, $P = 0.848$, $P = 0.543$, $P = 0.212$, $P = 0.089$, $P = 0.273$, $P = 0.133$) or Bas ($P = 0.309$, $P = 0.860$, $P = 0.337$, $P = 0.209$, $P = 0.123$, $P = 0.807$, $P = 0.631$) counts in the BALF samples collected from the OVA-induced asthmatic mice.

Loki zupa decoction and its extracts treatment regulated inflammatory cytokines in BALF and serum of OVA-induced asthmatic mice

Marked increases were observed in the IL-1β (Fig. 5a, $P = 0.042$), TNF-α (Fig. 5b,$P = 0.045$), IL-4 (Fig. 5e, $P = 0.038$) and IL-5 (Fig. 5f, $P = 0.002$) levels in the BALF (Fig. 5) and serum (Fig. 6a, $P = 0.045$, Fig. 6b, $P = 0.042$, Fig. 6e, $P = 0.008$, Fig. 6f, $P = 0.047$) (Fig. 6) samples collected from the OVA-induced asthmatic mice, as well as a decrease in their IFN-γ levels (Fig. 5c, $P = 0.039$, Fig. 6c, $P = 0.038$). Treatment with the *Loki zupa* decoction or its extracts led to a reduction in the levels of IL-1β, TNF-α, IL-4 and IL-5 in the BALF and serum samples, as well as an increase in IFN-γ levels (Fig. 5 or Fig. 6).

The LN and LE treatment groups showed reduced levels of IL-1β in their BALF samples ($P = 0.039$, $P = 0.042$; Fig. 5a) compared with the OVA-induced asthma mice. However, DEX was found to be ineffective for lowering the IL-1β levels in BALF ($P = 0.466$; Fig. 5a). The three different doses of *Loki zupa* decoction used in the current study, as well as the LE and DEX treatment groups showed dramatic decreases in the TNF-α levels found in their BALF samples ($P = 0.037$, $P = 0.043$, $P = 0.009$, $P = 0.028$, $P = 0.016$; Fig. 5b) compared with A group. The L 3.5 and DEX treatment groups showed a tendency towards increased IFN-γ levels in their BALF samples, although these results were not statistically different ($P = 0.247$, $P = 0.173$; Fig. 5c). The L 14.0, L 3.5, LN and DEX treatment groups showed reduced IL-2 levels in their BALF sampled ($P = 0.049$, $P = 0.019$, $P = 0.019$, $P = 0.023$; Fig. 5d) compared with A group. The L 14.0 treatment group showed a decrease in the IL-4 levels in its BALF sampled ($P = 0.047$; Fig. 5e) compared with A group. Furthermore, the L 3.5 and LW treatment groups showed reduced levels of IL-5 compared with the OVA-induced asthmatic mice ($P = 0.004$, $P = 0.004$; Fig. 5f). However, treatment with DEX had no effect on the IL-4 and IL-5 levels in the BALF samples of the mice in A group.

The L 14.0, L 7.0, LN and LE treatment groups showed significant decreases in the IL-1β levels observed in the serum samples taken from the OVA-induced asthmatic mice ($P = 0.044$, $P = 0.045$, $P = 0.049$, $P = 0.047$; Fig. 6a) compared with mice in A group. However, DEX treatment did not result in a significant decrease in IL-1β levels in the serum ($P = 0.63$; Fig. 6a). The L 7.0, LN, LE and DEX treatment groups showed significant decreases in the TNF-α levels of the serum samples collected from the asthmatic mice ($P = 0.001$, $P = 0.01$, $P < 0.001$, $P = 0.012$; Fig. 6b) compared with the mice from the untreated

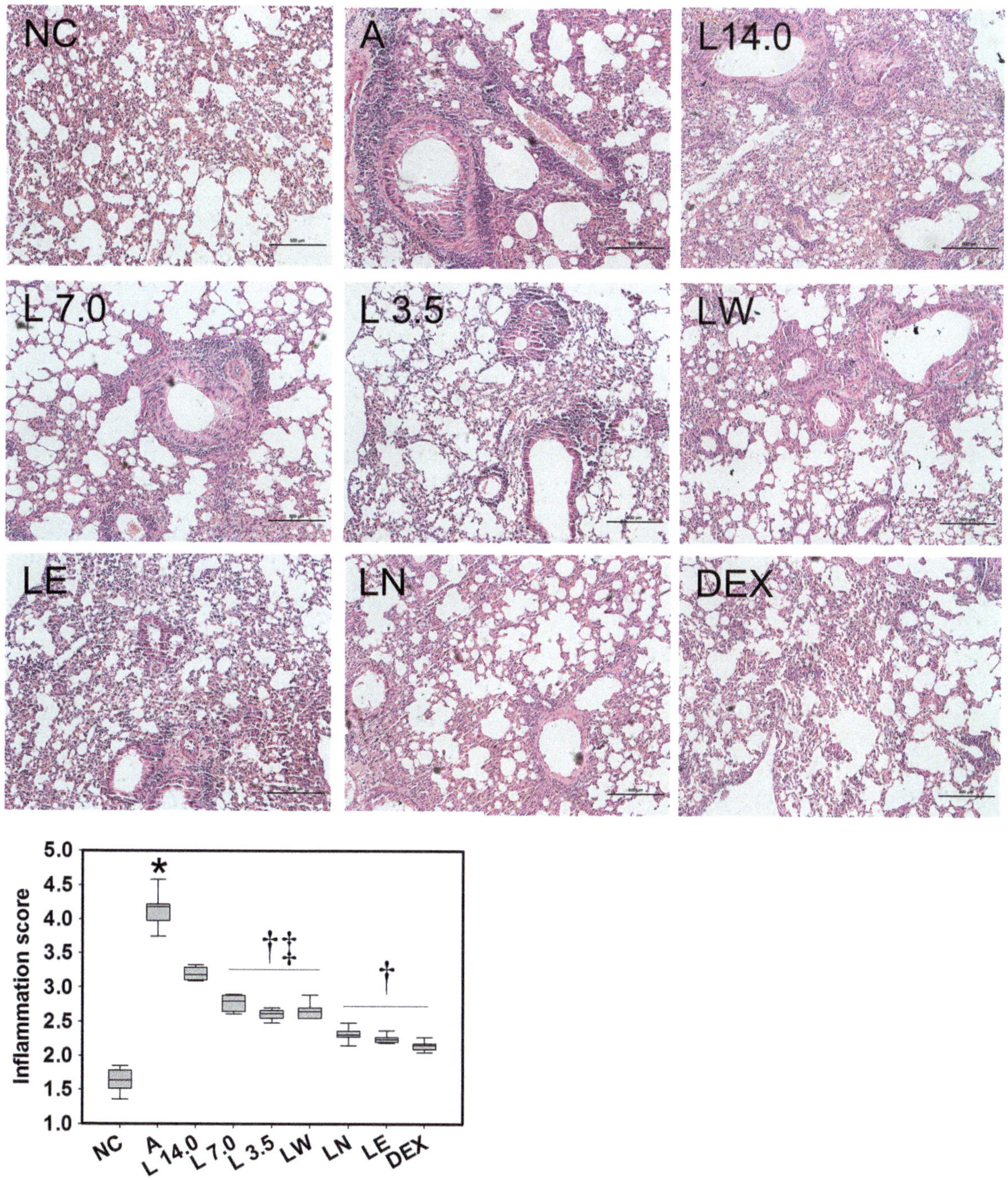

Fig. 3 *Loki zupa* decoction and its extracts attenuated airway inflammation of OVA-induced asthmatic mice. The airway inflammatory changes in each group were assessed by H&E staining of the lung slices and examined at 10× magnification by light microscopy. At least ten mice in each group and six arbitrarily selected fields in each mouse were assessed. Inflammatory scores in each group were assessed. Bar = 500 μm. *$P < 0.05$ *vs.* NC group, †$P < 0.05$ *vs.* A group, ‡$P < 0.05$ *vs.* DEX group

group. The LE and DEX treatment groups showed a significant increase in the IFN-γ levels of the serum samples compared with the OVA-induced asthmatic mice ($P < 0.001$, $P = 0.03$; Fig. 6c). Moreover, LE treatment was found to be more effective than DEX for promoting the levels of IFN-γ in serum ($P = 0.001$). None of the treatment groups tested in the current study had a discernible impact on the levels of IL-2 secretion in the serum (Fig. 6d). However, the LW and DEX treatment groups showed a marked decrease in the IL-4 levels of the serum

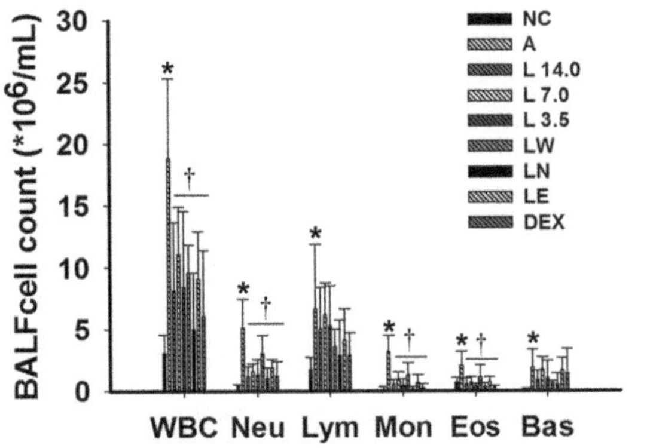

Fig. 4 *Loki zupa* decoction and its extracts inhibited the inflammatory cells in BALF. The total white blood cell (WBC), neutrophil (Neu), lymphocyte (Lym), monocyte (Mon), eosinophil (Eos) and basocyte (Bas) counts in BALF were analyzed and the resulting data expressed as the mean ± SD. * $P < 0.05$ *vs.* NC group, †$P< 0.05$ *vs.* A group

($P = 0.021$, $P = 0.049$; Fig. 6e) compared with A group. Lastly, the serum samples collected from the L 14.0, LW and LE treatment groups showed significant reductions in the secretion of IL-5 ($P = 0.036$, $P = 0.04$, $P = 0.049$; Fig. 6f) compared with the untreated mice. However, DEX exhibited no inhibitory activity towards the IL-5 levels in serum.

Treatment with *Loki zupa* decoction or its extracts regulated mRNA expression of Th2 and Th1 cytokines in OVA-induced asthmatic mice

OVA inhalation led to enhanced levels of IL-4 (Fig. 7b), IL-5 (Fig. 7c) and IL-13 (Fig. 7d) mRNA expression, as well as reduced levels of IFN-γ (Fig. 7a) mRNA expression in the OVA-induced asthmatic mice compared with mice in the NC group ($P < 0.001$, $P = 0.045$, $P = 0.049$, $P = 0.047$; Fig. 7). Treatment with the *Loki zupa* decoction or its extracts led to reduced IL-4 (Fig. 7b) , IL-5 (Fig. 7c) and IL-13 (Fig. 7d) mRNA expression levels in asthmatic mice, as well as improved IFN-γ(Fig 7a) mRNA expression. With the exception of the L 7.0 group, all of the other treatment groups exhibited a significant promotion effect towards the mRNA expression of IFN-γ ($P = 0.039$, $P = 0.04$, $P = 0.048$, $P = 0.035$, $P < 0.001$, $P < 0.001$; Fig. 7a). The L 3.5, LN and LE treatment groups also showed a dramatic decrease in the mRNA expression of IL-4 ($P = 0.021$, $P = 0.023$, $P = 0.017$; Fig. 7b). Furthermore, mice in the L 3.5, LW and LE treatment groups demonstrated a marked reduction in their IL-5 mRNA expression ($P = 0.043$, $P = 0.044$, $P = 0.04$; Fig. 7c). The L 7.0, LN and LE treatment groups led to an obvious decrease in the mRNA expression of IL-13 ($P < 0.001$, $P = 0.037$, $P = 0.046$; Fig. 7d). DEX treatment had no effect on the mRNA expression levels of IL-4, IL-5 and IL-13 in our study ($P = 0.91$, $P = 0.83$, $P = 0.792$).

Discussion

Several characteristic features of acute asthma are observed in the OVA-induced mice asthma model, including an exaggerated airway response to Mch and eosinophil-rich airway inflammation [19]. Short-term OVA inhalation resulted in a marked increase in R_L, as well as a pronounced decrease in Cdyn towards increasing doses of Mch. H&E staining of the lung slices revealed that there was a significant increase in the infiltration of Eos into the airways of the asthmatic mice, as well as the levels of mucus secretion. Treatment with *Loki zupa* decoction led to a dramatic decrease in the elevated AHR towards progressive Mch doses in asthmatic mice. Furthermore, the L 3.5 and LE treatment groups showed a reduction in R_L, which was almost identical to that of DEX, highlighting the potential value of these materials for the treatment of asthma. Treatment withthe *Loki zupa* decoction resulted in a decrease in the number of WBC, Neu, Eos and Mon cell counts in the lungs of the asthmatic mice. There was a direct correlation between Eos counts and asthma symptom scores [20]. According to the results of several previous studies [21, 22], treatments aimed at reducing airway eosinophilia numbers are effective for controlling asthma symptoms. Treatment with the *Loki zupa* decoction also had a direct impact on Eos numbers in the airways, highlighting its efficacy for controlling asthma.

In our study, *Loki zupa* decoction exerted prominent inhibitory effects towards the levels of IL-1β and TNF-α. Elevated Th2 cell levels and cytokine functions are characteristic features of allergic asthma, which have been implicated in eosinophilic inflammation as well as AHR [5, 23, 24]. The administration of L 14.0 and LW resulted in a dramatic reduction in IL-4 levels in the BALF and serum samples collected from the asthmatic mice. IL-4 is essential for the development of AHR in murine models [25, 26], indicating that the decrease observed in AHR following the treatment of the mice with *Loki zupa* decoction could be attributed to a reduction in IL-4 levels. IL-5 is involved in Eos maturation, differentiation, recruitment, and survival [6]. L 3.5 and LW, as well as L 14.0 and LE inhibited the OVA-induced increase in IL-5 levels in the BALF and serum samples collected from the mice. However, DEX had no effect on the levels of IL-4 and IL-5 in the BALF samples or the IL-5 levels in the serum samples. Th2 blockade is effective for suppressing the features of allergic disease in mice [27]. Anti-IL-5 antibody has therefore been reported to reduce the risk of exacerbation in patients with severe eosinophilic asthma [28]. Approximately 50 % of asthmatic patients have a Th2-driven phenotype [29]. The treatment of the mice with *Loki zupa* decoction inhibited the expression of the Th2 cytokines, indicating that its related anti-asthmatic effect

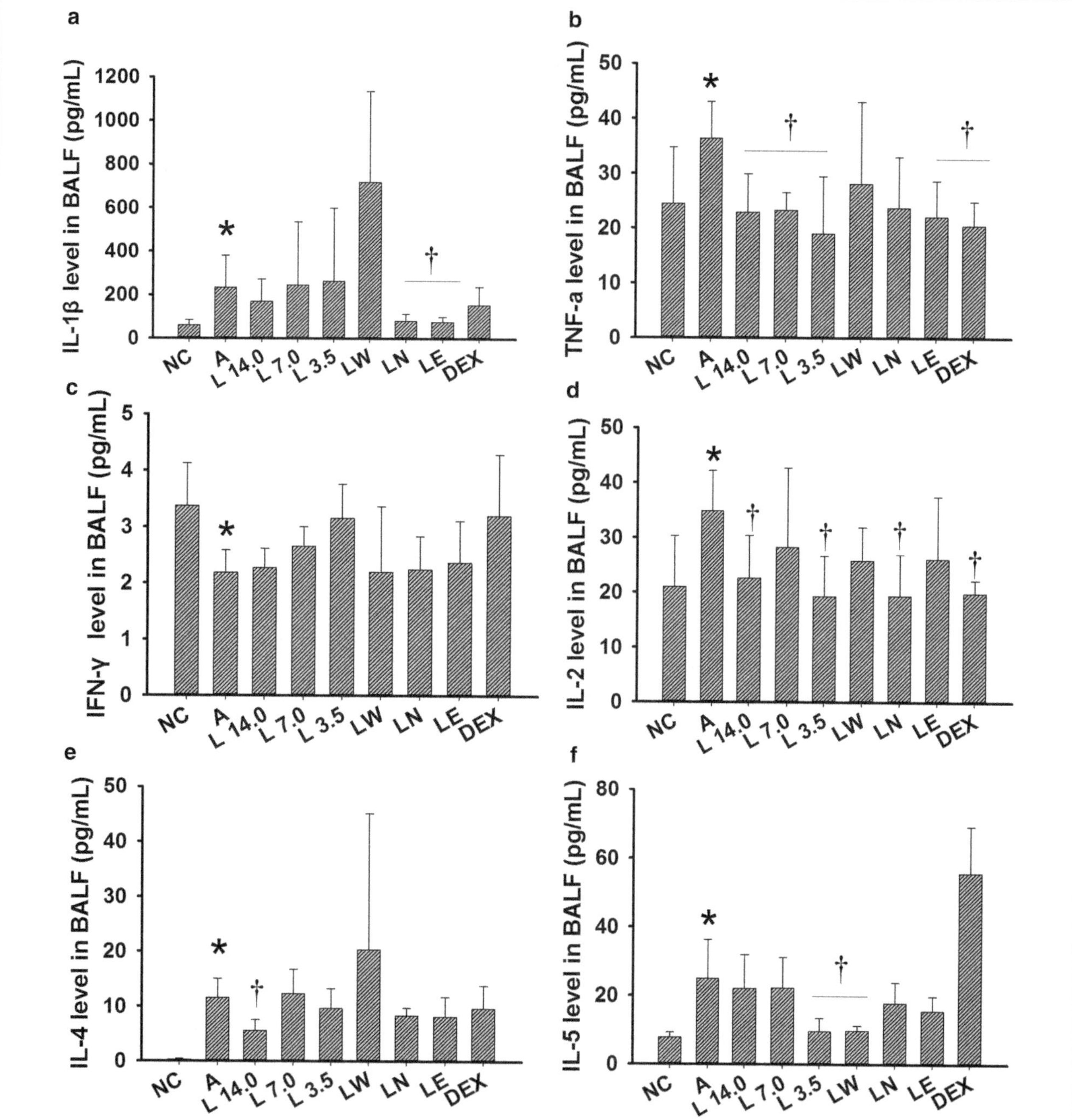

Fig. 5 *Loki zupa* decoction and its extracts regulated the secretion of several inflammatory cytokines in BALF. The IL-1β, TNF-α, IFN-γ, IL-2, IL-4 and IL-5 levels in BALF were measured by Bio-Plex and the resulting data expressed as mean ± SD. **a** IL-1β level in BALF, **b** TNF-α level in BALF, **c** IFN-γ level in BALF, **d** IL-2 level in BALF, **e** IL-4 level in BALF, **f** IL-5 level in BALF. *$P < 0.05$ *vs.* NC group, $^{\dagger}P < 0.05$ *vs.* A group

could be attributed to its ability to inhibit the activity of the Th2 cells. Treatment with *Loki zupa* decoction or its extracts also led to a significant down-regulatory effect on the gene amplification levels of IL-4, IL-5 and IL-13. However, DEX treatment had no discernible impact on the levels of these cytokines. IL-13 is a key Th2 cytokine that might be involved in the development of asthma [30, 31]. Transgenic mice over-expressing IL-13 in their lung develop some of the features of airway inflammation typically observed in asthma [32]. Treatment with L 7.0, LN and LE led to a remarkable decrease in the mRNA amplification of IL-13, indicating that the anti-inflammatory

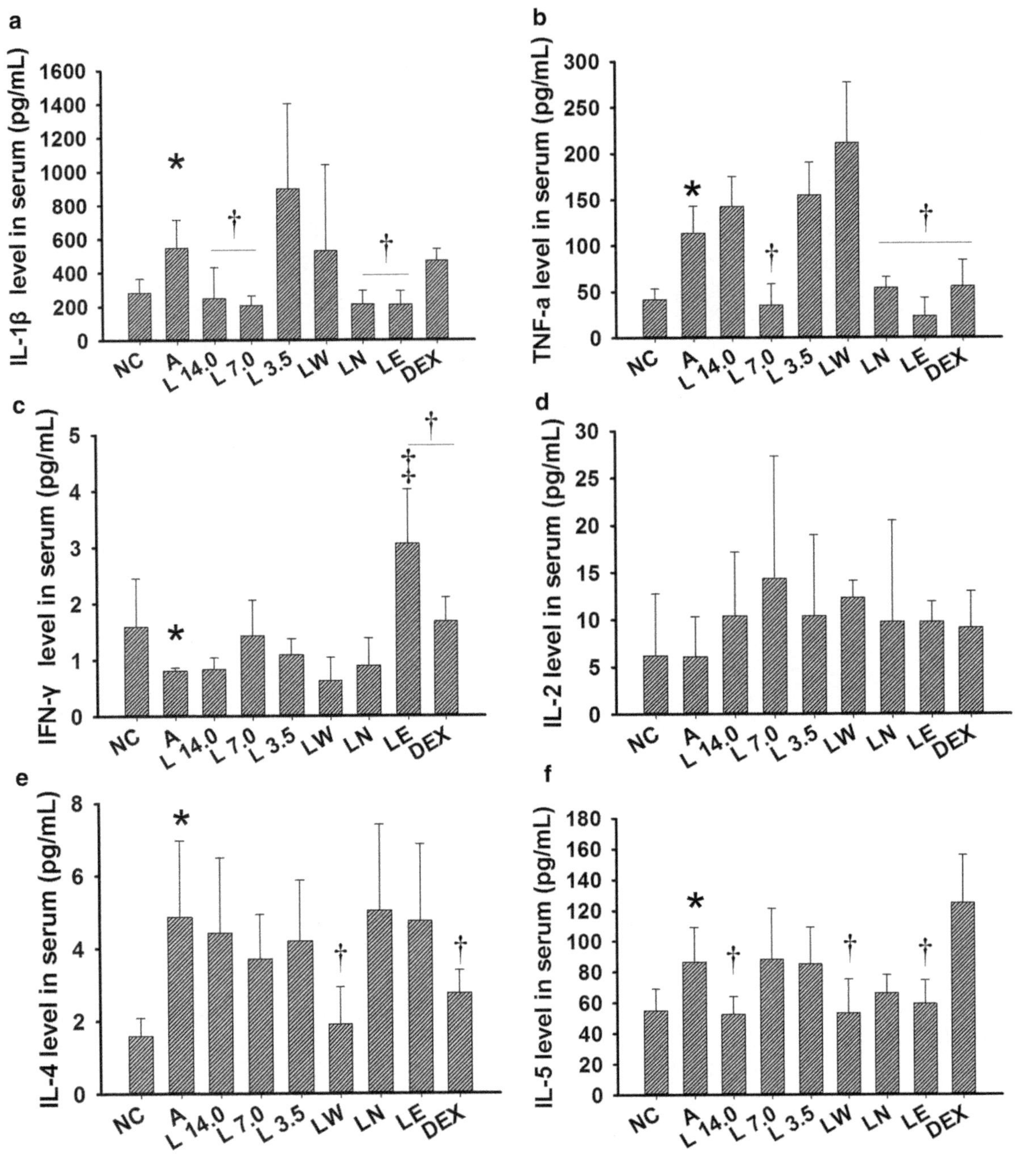

Fig. 6 *Loki zupa* decoction and its extracts regulated the secretion of several inflammatory cytokines in serum. The IL-1β, TNF-α, IFN-γ, IL-2, IL-4 and IL-5 levels in serum were measured by Bio-Plex and the resulting data expressed as mean ± SD. **a** IL-1β level in serum, **b** TNF-α level in serum, **c** IFN-γ level in serum, **d** IL-2 level in serum, **e** IL-4 level in serum, **f** IL-5 level in serum. *$P < 0.05$ *vs.* NC group,†$P < 0.05$ *vs.* A group, ‡$P < 0.05$ *vs.* DEX group

effects of these materials could be related to their ability to inhibit the expression of this cytokine.

Th1 cells have been reported to exhibit inhibitory effects towards the inflammation of asthmatic airways by inhibiting Th2 cytokine responses [33]. Furthermore, there are generally lower levels ofthe Th1 cytokine IFN-γ in asthma [34, 35]. The treatment of the mice with *Loki zupa* decoction or its extracts and DEX effectively promoted the expression of IFN-γ at the gene and protein levels. This result therefore indicated that the anti-inflammatory activity of *Loki zupa* decoction towards asthma could be attributed to its ability to promote the activity of Th1 cells, as well as its antagonistic potential towards the function of Th2 cells. IFN-γ

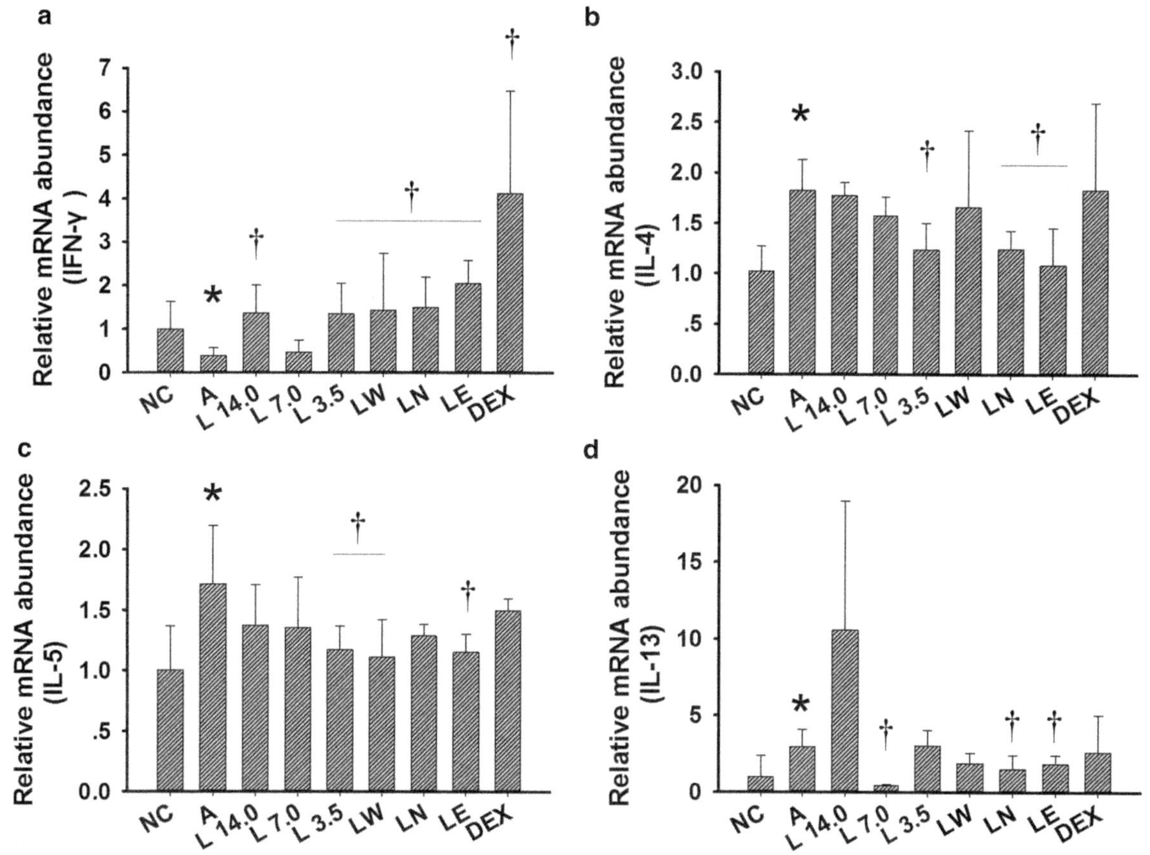

Fig. 7 *Loki zupa* decoction and its extracts inhibited and promoted the Th2 and Th1 cytokine mRNA expression levels of asthmatic mice, respectively. The mRNA expression levels of IL-4, IL-5, IL-13 and IFN-γ in the lung tissues were measured by qPCR and the data expressed as the mean ± SD. **a** mRNA expression level of IFN-γ, **b** mRNA expression level of IL-4, **c** mRNA expression level of IL-5, **d** mRNA expression level of IL-13. *$P < 0.05$ *vs.* NC group, $^{\dagger}P < 0.05$ *vs.* A group

has been shown to inhibit antigen-induced AHR in mice [36], indicating that elevated levels of IFN-γ might be involved in the responses observed in the *Loki zupa* decoction-treated groups.

Except for the decrease observed in the serum level of IL-4, DEX promoted the expression of the Th1 cytokine IFN-γ in the serum and lung tissue samples, but did not lead to a decrease in the expression levels of IL-4 and IL-5 in BALF. In contrast, *Loki zupa* decoction exhibited inhibitory activity towards the expression of IL-4 and IL-5 in the BALF and serum samples, as well as the lung tissues. However, *Loki zupa* decoction also exhibited a significant promotion effect towards IFN-γ, indicating that the anti-inflammatory effect of the *Loki zupa* decoction treatment could be attributed to the promotion and suppression of the Th1 and Th2 cytokine expression levels, respectively. This promotion of the Th1 cell function could therefore be responsible for the effect of DEX on asthma.

The JAK-STAT pathway promotes the differentiation of naive T cells into Th2 cells, as well as inducing the secretion of Th2 cytokines [37–39]. STAT4 has been implicated in IL-12-dependent Th1 cellular responses, and mice lacking STAT4 have been reported to show severe deficiencies in mounting a Th1 response [40]. Furthermore, IL-4-induced STAT6 activation has been reported to contribute to the differentiation of Th2 cells [41]. The JAK-STAT pathway could therefore be involved in regulating the Th1/Th2 imbalance observed in asthma patients following their treatment with *Loki zupa* decoction.

Conclusion

The treatment of mice with *Loki zupa* decoction and its extracts resulted in a decrease in AHR and attenuated airway inflammation in an OVA-induced asthma mouse model by promoting and suppressing the cellular functions of Th1 and Th2, respectively.

Abbreviations

OVA: ovalbumin; AHR: airway hyperresponsiveness; Mch: methacholine; NC: normal control; A: asthma; *Loki zupa* decoction 14.0 g/kg: L 14.0; *Loki zupa* decoction 7.0 g/kg: L 7.0; *Loki zupa* decoction 3.5 g/kg: L 3.5; H&E: hematoxylin and eosin; BALF: bronchoalveolar lavage fluid; LW: water extract; LE: ethyl acetate extract; LN: *n*-butanol extract; DEX: dexamethasone; R_L: airway resistance; Cdyn: lung dynamic compliance; WBC: white blood cell; Neu: neutrophil; Mon: monocyte; Eos: eosinophil; Lym: lymphocyte; Bas: basocyte.

Authors' contributions

YW, MA, JS and JCD conceived and designed the study, and wrote the manuscript. YW and MHL performed the animal model-making of asthma, the qPCR and Bio-Plex assay, QLL performed the AHR detection, MN prepared the Loki zupa decoction and extracts and performed the intragastric administration to mice, YBL performed pulmonary histopathology analysis. YW, MA, MHL, QLL, YBL, MN and JCD analyzed the data and revised the manuscript. All the authors read and approved the final manuscript, and agree to be accountable for all aspects of the work.

Author details

[1] Department of Integrative Medicine, Huashan Hospital, Fudan University, 12 Middle Urumqi Road, Shanghai 200040, China. [2] Institute of Integrated Traditional Chinese and Western Medicine, Fudan University, 12 Middle Urumqi Road, Shanghai 200040, China. [3] Xinjiang Uygur Medical College, 370 West Beijing Road, Hotan, Xinjiang 848000, China.

Acknowledgements

This work was supported by the National Natural Science Program of China (81173390, 81403476 and 81573758) and Development Project of Shanghai Peak Disciplines-Integrated Chinese and Western Medicine.

Competing interests

The authors declare that they have no competing interests.

References

1. van Schayck OC. Global strategies for reducing the burden from asthma. Prim Care Respir J. 2013;22(2):239–43.
2. Saglani S, Lloyd CM. Novel concepts in airway inflammation and remodelling in asthma. Eur Respir J. 2015;46(6):1796–804.
3. Tourangeau LM, Kavanaugh A, Wasserman SI. The role of monoclonal antibodies in the treatment of severe asthma. Ther Adv Respir Dis. 2011;5(3):183–94.
4. Caramori G, Ito K, Adcock IM. Targeting Th2 cells in asthmatic airways. Curr Drug Targets Inflamm Allergy. 2004;3(3):243–55.
5. Lloyd CM, Saglani S. T cells in asthma: influences of genetics, environment, and T-cell plasticity. J Allergy Clin Immunol. 2013;131(5):1267–74.
6. Shalaby KH, Martin JG. Overview of asthma; the place of the T cell. Curr Opin Pharmacol. 2010;10(3):218–25.
7. Barrett NA, Austen KF. Innate cells and T helper 2 cell immunity in airway inflammation. Immunity. 2009;31(3):425–37.
8. Diamant Z, Tufvesson E, Bjermer L. Which biomarkers are effective for identifying Th2-driven inflammation in asthma. Curr Allergy Asthma Rep. 2013;13(5):477–86.
9. Fajt ML, Gelhaus SL, Freeman B, Uvalle CE, Trudeau JB, Holguin F, Wenzel SE. Prostaglandin D(2) pathway upregulation: relation to asthma severity, control, and TH2 inflammation. J Allergy Clin Immunol. 2013;131(6):1504–12.
10. Lin WH, Wu CR, Lee HZ, Kuo YH, Wen HS, Lin TY, Lee CY, Huang SY, Lin CY. Induced apoptosis of Th2 lymphocytes and inhibition of airway hyperresponsiveness and inflammation by combined lactic acid bacteria treatment. Int Immunopharmacol. 2013;15(4):703–11.
11. Nagai H. Recent research and developmental strategy of anti-asthma drugs. Pharmacol Ther. 2012;133(1):70–8.
12. Finotto S, Neurath MF, Glickman JN, Qin S, Lehr HA, Green FH, Ackerman K, Haley K, Galle PR, Szabo SJ. Development of spontaneous airway changes consistent with human asthma in mice lacking T-bet. Science. 2002;295(5553):336–8.
13. Ekim M, Rozi N, Yusup A. Effect of Uighur medicine *Hyssopus officinalis* L ethyl aectate on inflammatory response in asthma rats. Ke ji dao bao. 2011;29(30):52–6.
14. Hou M, Zhu M, Ma XM, Ding JB, Ma J, Ma XP, Wang XX, Wang YN. Effect of Uighur Medicine *Hyssopus officinalis* L. on serum IL-17 level and balance of Th1/Th2 of asthma rats. *Zhongguo xian dai yi xue* 2010,03(02):365-368.
15. Zdolsek HA, Janefjord CK, Falth-Magnusson K, Jenmalm MC. Reduced IL-2-induced IL-12 responsiveness in atopic children. Pediatr Allergy Immunol. 2003;14(5):351–7.
16. Xu F, Zhao J, He J, Chen Y, Tan W. Pharmacognostic identification of Uygur medicine *Hyssopus cuspidatus* and its adulterant *Nepeta bracteata*. Zhongguo yao fang. 2012;23(35):3321–3.
17. Yang XJ, Yang WJ. Quality Standard of Xinjiang Uygur medicine *Iris halophila*. Zhongguo yao fang. 2011;22(31):2924–7.
18. Jin H, Luo Q, Zheng Y, Nurahmat M, Wu J, Li B, Lv Y, Wang G, Duan X, Dong J. CD4 + CD25 + Foxp3 + T cells contribute to the antiasthmatic effects of Astragalus membranaceus extract in a rat model of asthma. Int Immunopharmacol. 2013;15(1):42–9.
19. Reddy AT, Lakshmi SP, Reddy RC. Murine model of allergen induced asthma. J Vis Exp JoVE. 2012;63:e3771.
20. Nair P. What is an "eosinophilic phenotype" of asthma? J Allergy Clin Immunol. 2013;132(1):81–3.
21. Steinke JW, Negri J, Liu L, Payne SC, Borish L. Aspirin activation of eosinophils and mast cells: implications in the pathogenesis of aspirin-exacerbated respiratory disease. J Immunol. 2014;193(1):41–7.
22. Fulkerson PC, Rothenberg ME. Targeting eosinophils in allergy, inflammation and beyond. Nat Rev Drug Discov. 2013;12(2):117–29.
23. Hams E, Fallon PG. Innate type 2 cells and asthma. Curr Opin Pharmacol. 2012;12(4):503–9.
24. Corrigan C. Mechanisms of asthma. Medicine. 2012;40(5):223–7.
25. Perkins C, Yanase N, Smulian G, Gildea L, Orekov T, Potter C, Brombacher F, Aronow B, Wills-Karp M, Finkelman FD. Selective stimulation of IL-4 receptor on smooth muscle induces airway hyperresponsiveness in mice. J Exp Med. 2011;208(4):853–67.
26. Tanaka H, Nagai H, Maeda Y. Effect of anti-IL-4 and anti-IL-5 antibodies on allergic airway hyperresponsiveness in mice. Life Sci. 1998;62(13):169–74.
27. Finkelman FD, Hogan SP, Hershey GK, Rothenberg ME, Wills-Karp M. Importance of cytokines in murine allergic airway disease and human asthma. J Immunol. 2010;184(4):1663–74.
28. Pavord ID, Korn S, Howarth P, Bleecker ER, Buhl R, Keene ON, Ortega H, Chanez P. Mepolizumab for severe eosinophilic asthma (DREAM): a multicentre, double-blind, placebo-controlled trial. Lancet. 2012;380(9842):651–9.
29. Apte K, Salvi S. Vitamin D reduces eosinophilic airway inflammation in nonatopic asthma: are we sure? J Allergy Clin Immunol. 2015;136(2):516–7.
30. Ingram JL, Kraft M. IL-13 in asthma and allergic disease: asthma phenotypes and targeted therapies. J Allergy Clin Immunol. 2012;130(4):829–42.
31. Elias JA, Lee CG. IL-13 in asthma. The successful integration of lessons from mice and humans. Am J Respir Crit Care Med. 2011;183(8):957–8.
32. Qaseem AS, Sonar S, Mahajan L, Madan T, Sorensen GL, Shamji MH, Kishore U. Linking surfactant protein SP-D and IL-13: implications in asthma and allergy. Mol Immunol. 2013;54(1):98–107.
33. Kips JC, Brusselle GJ, Joos GF, Peleman RA, Tavernier JH, Devos RR, Pauwels RA. Interleukin-12 inhibits antigen-induced airway hyperresponsiveness in mice. Mol Immunol. 1996;153(2):535–9.
34. Brooks GD, Buchta KA, Swenson CA, Gern JE, Busse WW. Rhinovirus-induced interferon-gamma and airway responsiveness in asthma. Mol Immunol. 2003;168(9):1091–4.
35. Akpinarli A, Guc D, Kalayci O, Yigitbas E, Ozon A. Increased interleukin-4 and decreased interferon gamma production in children with asthma: function of atopy or asthma? J Asthma. 2002;39(2):159–65.
36. Yoshida M, Leigh R, Matsumoto K, Wattie J, Ellis R, O'Byrne PM, Inman MD. Effect of interferon-gamma on allergic airway responses in interferon-gamma-deficient mice. Am J Respir Crit Care Med. 2002;166(4):451–6.
37. Espinosa K, Bosse Y, Stankova J, Rola-Pleszczynski M. CysLT1 receptor upregulation by TGF-beta and IL-13 is associated with bronchial smooth muscle cell proliferation in response to LTD4. J Allergy Clin Immunol. 2003;111(5):1032–40.

38. Matsuse H, Kong X, Hu J, Wolf SF, Lockey RF, Mohapatra SS. Intranasal IL-12 produces discreet pulmonary and systemic effects on allergic inflammation and airway reactivity. Int Immunopharmacol. 2003;3(4):457–68.
39. Ashino S, Takeda K, Li H, Taylor V, Joetham A, Pine PR, Gelfand EW. Janus kinase 1/3 signaling pathways are key initiators of TH2 differentiation and lung allergic responses. J Allergy Clin Immunol. 2014;133(4):1162–74.
40. Shirai T, Suzuki K, Inui N, Suda T, Chida K, Nakamura H. Th1/Th2 profile in peripheral blood in atopic cough and atopic asthma. Clin Exp Allergy. 2003;33(1):84–9.
41. Gao Z, Kang Y, Xu Y, Shang Y, Gai J, He Q. Inhibition of allergic responsiveness in a murine asthma model via IFN-gamma transgene expression. Chin Med J. 2002;115(10):1470–4.

11

Analyzing the Chinese landscape in anti-diabetic drug research: leading knowledge production institutions and thematic communities

Junling Deng[1†], Kaweng Sitou[1†], Yongping Zhang[2], Ru Yan[1] and Yuanjia Hu[1*]

Abstract

Background: The discovery of anti-diabetic drugs is an active Chinese medicine research area. This study aims to map out anti-diabetic drug research in China using a network-based systemic approach based on co-authorship of academic publications. We focused on identifying leading knowledge production institutions, analyzing interactions among them, detecting communities with high internal associations, and exploring future research directions.

Methods: Target articles published in 2009–2013 under the topic "diabetes" and subject category "pharmacology & pharmacy," with "China," "Taiwan," "Hong Kong," or "Macao" (or "Macau") in the authors' address field were retrieved from the science citation index expanded database and their bibliographic information (e.g., article title, authors, keywords, and authors' affiliation addresses) analyzed. A social network approach was used to construct an institutional collaboration network based on co-publications. Gephi software was used to visualize the network and relationships among institutes were analyzed using centrality measurements. Thematic analysis based on article keywords and R_{sc} value was applied to reveal the research hotspots and directions of network communities.

Results: The top 50 institutions were identified; these included Shanghai Jiao Tong University, National Taiwan University, Peking University, and China Pharmaceutical University. Institutes from Taiwan tended to cooperate with institutes outside Taiwan, but those from mainland China showed low interest in external collaboration. Fourteen thematic communities were detected with the Louvain algorithm and further labeled by their high-frequency and characteristic keywords, such as *Chinese medicines*, *diabetic complications*, *oxidative stress*, *pharmacokinetics*, and *insulin resistance*. The keyword *Chinese medicines* comprised a range of Chinese medicine-related topics, including *berberine*, *flavonoids*, *Astragalus polysaccharide*, *emodin*, and *ginsenoside*. These keywords suggest potential fields for further anti-diabetic drug research. The correlation of −0.641 ($P = 0.013$) between degree centrality and the R_{sc} value of non-core keywords indicates that communities concentrating on rare research fields are usually isolated by others and have a lower chance of collaboration.

Conclusion: With a better understanding of the Chinese landscape in anti-diabetic drug research, researchers and scholars looking for experts and institutions in a specific research area can rapidly spot their target community, then select the most appropriate potential collaborator and suggest preferential research directions for future studies.

Keywords: Greater China, Anti-diabetes drug, Chinese medicines, Research collaboration networks, Network analysis

*Correspondence: yuanjiahu@umac.mo
†Junling Deng and Kaweng Sitou contributed equally to this work
[1] State Key Laboratory of Quality Research in Chinese Medicine, Institute of Chinese Medical Sciences, University of Macau, Macao, China
Full list of author information is available at the end of the article

Background

Diabetes mellitus (DM) is a chronic disease that is defined as a long period of having a high blood glucose level [1], which results in excessive thirst, frequent urination, and hunger. DM complications include ketoacidosis and nonketotic hyperosmolar [2, 3]. According to the latest statistics of the International Diabetes Federation, the global prevalence of diabetes among adults aged between 20 and 79 years reached 8.3 % in 2013 [4]. A total of 382 million people worldwide are affected by the disease; of these, 80 % live in either mid- or low-income countries [4]. The number of people living with the disease worldwide is predicted to rise to 592 million by 2035 [4]. The prevalence of DM in China escalated from 0.9 % in 1980 to 11.6 % in 2010 [5, 6]. In 2013, diabetes caused 5.1 millions deaths, accounting for 8.39 % of global mortality [4]. The financial cost of diabetes in the U.S. exceeded $548 billion in 2013, accounting for 11 % of global expenditure on health care [4]. The rapidly growing prevalence of diabetes has placed an enormous burden on both social and economic development [4].

The discovery of anti-diabetic drugs has become an active research area in Chinese medicine [7]. Many institutes located in different regions of Greater China are currently engaged in the research and development (R&D) of anti-diabetic drugs. They cooperate on diabetes research projects and work concurrently on self-developed products. Some of these products, such as *Xiaoke wan* (消渴丸), *Yuquan pill* (玉泉片), and *Ginseng–milkvetch declining sugar granule* (參芪降糖顆粒) are among the most popular and well-known anti-diabetic drugs in China. Several studies have investigated the R&D of anti-diabetic drugs in China using bibliometrics to examine the distribution of publication years and journals, document types, keywords, citation counts, and journal impact factors [8, 9]. However, the network-based systematic method has not been applied to evaluate China's pharmaceutical research in relation to diabetes, creating a gap in the understanding of the R&D landscape.

This study aims to map the R&D landscape of anti-diabetic drugs in Greater China (which includes mainland China, Taiwan, Hong Kong, and Macao) using a network-based systematic review. By analyzing co-authorship in the diabetic literature to include Chinese researchers published in international journals during the period 2009–2013, the active institutes in this field were identified, the relationship between research units was explored, communities with high internal associations were detected, and the interests of a research community were characterized.

Methods

Data

This systematic review was based on the web of science's science citation index expanded (SCIE) database, a multidisciplinary index of more than 8500 peer-reviewed international journals [10]. Retrieved articles were those published during the period 2009–2013 under the topic "diabetes" and subject category "pharmacology & pharmacy," with "China," "Taiwan," "Hong Kong," or "Macao" (or "Macau") in the authors' address field.

Bibliographic information such as article title, authors, keywords, and authors' affiliation addresses was extracted for analysis. Records of authors affiliated with non-Chinese institutes were eliminated. We standardized and combined authors and their affiliated organizations. The data retrieval process is illustrated in Fig. 1.

Network visualization and analysis

The network was visualized using the Gephi software package (Version 0.8.2; The Gephi Consortium, Paris, France) and the relationships were analyzed to extract the associations between organizations. Each node in the network represents a research unit, and an edge between two nodes indicates the strength of co-authoring between these two units. Nodes were positioned using the Fruchterman–Reingold algorithm [11] in Gephi. The algorithm belongs to a class of algorithms known as force-directed algorithms; these are used to calculate

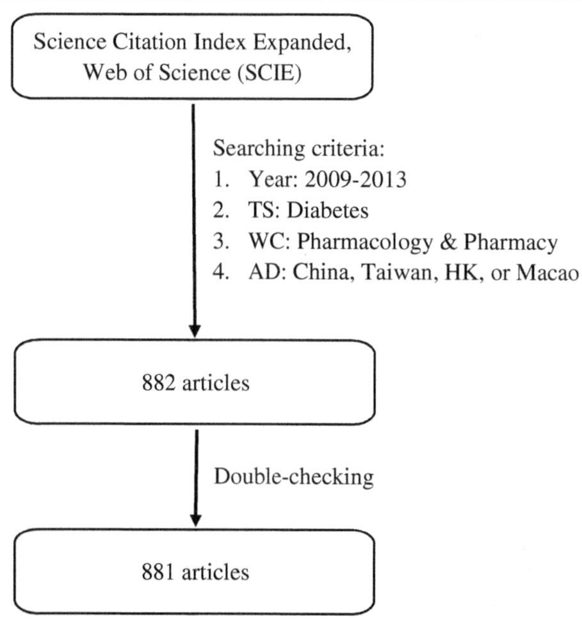

Fig. 1 Flowchart of the inclusion and exclusion criteria. Combined search strategy: "AD = (China or Taiwan or Hong Kong or Macau or Macao or Hongkong) and WC = (Pharmacology & Pharmacy) and TS = (Diabetes) and Indexes = SCIE and Timespan = 2009–2013". *AD* address, *TS* topic, *HK* Hong Kong, *WC* Web of Science Category which aims to narrow search result to some specific fields of study. Institutional information was obtained from the addresses provided by authors in the target articles, and was later standardized. Records of authors belonging to a non-Chinese institute were removed

layouts of simple undirected graphs. This method uses a physical analogy to determine the placement of network nodes by minimizing the energy of the system. Nodes behave like atomic particles; they exert repulsive and attractive forces on one another. Repulsive forces exist between all pairs of nodes (like charged particles repelling each other); edges between adjacent nodes cause attraction (like spring force). The position of all nodes continues to adjust until the system reaches its equilibrium state. Thus, the more connected organizations have higher attractive forces and are positioned at the center; in contrast, weaker nodes with less or no connections to others are found on the periphery of the map.

In this study, we applied four centrality metrics to identify the key institutes: degree centrality, weighted degree centrality, betweenness centrality, and closeness centrality.

Degree centrality measures centrality. This shows the number of ties associated with a node in an undirected graph and is reflected in node size. In our research, the degree centrality of an institute represents its number of collaborating organizations. Nodes with a high degree of centrality are usually found in the dense area of the network because they are working with many different research units.

Each node's weighted degree was used to measure an institution's actual performance in productivity and how active the organization was in the system. Weighted degree centrality corresponds to the sum of weighted edges connected to a vertex. In the present study, it signified an organization's total number of co-publications.

Betweenness and closeness centrality describe the importance and role of a node in the system. Betweenness centrality measures how often a node appears on the shortest path between two nodes. In a collaboration network, some nodes do not interact directly; instead, they depend on an intermediary for communication. An intermediary with high betweenness functions as a "gatekeeper" to control the flow of interactions in the network. However, a high-betweenness node need not necessarily be one with a high degree centrality [12]. The closeness centrality of a vertex is the total geodesic distance between a vertex and all other vertices; it can be defined as how close an organization is to all others. A lower closeness value indicates that it is a more central node; that is, a node that can access or disseminate new information quicker than others [13, 14].

The above analysis focused mainly on absolute strength between nodes, but the relative strength between them was also considered. The Jaccard index is a statistic that shows how similar two sample sets are by calculating the ratio of intersection of the sets by the union of the sample sets [15]. Jaccard index values range from 0 to 1; a value closer to 1 indicates a higher mutual dependence between the two units. This value is defined as

$$J_{ij} = \frac{N_{ij}}{\sum_{j=1}^{n} N_{ij} + \sum_{i=1}^{n} N_{ij} - N_{ij}} \quad (i,j = 1,\ldots,n;\ i \neq j)$$

where N_{ij} and J_{ij} stand for number of co-publications and relative strength of co-publication between institutions i and j, respectively. Referring to Scherngell and Hu's use of this index [16], we used it to measure each institution's level of mutual dependence on its collaborating pair for co-publication. We separately collected the top 50 institutional pairs measured by absolute (edge weight) and relative (Jaccard index) values. We selected the overlapping pairs between two rankings to determine the top institutional pairs in the Chinese anti-diabetic drug research network; this indicated those strongly connected institutional pairs that rely heavily on each other for publication.

Community detection and thematic analysis

In the undirected network, some tightly interconnected nodes formed relatively stable community subnetworks. To quantify the notion of community, we used modularity, a measure that assigns a numeric value assessing how well a partition of the network nodes matches the informal notion of community. We used the Louvain algorithm, an efficient and widely used Gephi method to detect high-modularity communities, to determine the relevant communities in the network [17].

To characterize the themes of each identified community, the occurrence of each article keyword in the community was calculated and its relevance to that particular community was measured by its R_{sc} value, which is defined as $R_{sc} = f_{sc}/f_s$ [18]. This value is the ratio of occurrence of keyword S in community C's articles to its occurrence in the article set as a whole. A high R_{sc} value indicates that a keyword's occurrence in a specific community is relatively higher than in the whole system and is more significant to that community. Moreover, for each community, we categorized all non-core keywords as "Others" and calculated its R_{sc} value. The term "non-core keywords" describes keywords that appeared in the article set less than five times in total. Considering the linear and normally distributed characteristics of the data at the interval or ratio level, we then performed a Pearson's correlation test (SPSS Statistics software, Version 20; IBM Corp., Armonk, NY, USA) between the R_{sc} value of "Others" and the degree centrality of that community to identify the relationship between research topics and collaboration opportunities of communities in the network.

Results

General description of data sample

Using the retrieval criteria mentioned in the Methods section, a total of 882 articles were retrieved. Excluding one correction article, we obtained 881 articles after the exclusion process. A majority of the sampled items were research articles (86.85 %); the rest comprised review articles (9.75 %), meeting abstracts (3.29 %), and proceedings papers (1.02 %). Most of these publications were funded by government or non-profit organizations. The top three funding sources were the National Natural Science Foundation of China (25.26 %), the National Basic Research Program (also called "973 Program") (2.15 %), and the Fundamental Research Funds for the Central Universities (1.81 %). In this article set, the number of publications rose from 128 to 241 over the 5-year period of 2009–2013, representing a growth rate of 88.28 % or an annual rate of increase of 17.14 %. Increasing attention has been paid to anti-diabetic drug research in China and the discovery of new therapeutics for the disease has become increasingly important and urgent.

After standardizing and combining authors and their affiliated organizations, 430 research units were identified. Universities and their affiliated hospitals accounted for the largest proportion (48.84 %), followed by hospitals and clinics (24.88 %). There were fewer research centers and enterprises, accounting for only 16.98 and 9.30 %, respectively. Of all research units, 79.53 % were located in mainland China while 17.44 % were from Taiwan; the rest were from Hong Kong (2.56 %) and Macao (0.47 %).

Institutional collaboration network

Figure 2 illustrates the current collaborative relationship between Chinese institutes involved in the anti-diabetic drug research. There are 430 nodes on the map and 7673 undirected weighted edges, indicating that these 430 institutes have cooperated 7673 times. Node size depends on degree centrality and edge thickness between two nodes is determined by the number of co-publications between them [19]; more frequently collaborating institutional pairs are connected by a thicker edge.

In this figure, research units from mainland China and Taiwan are represented in cyan and yellow, respectively, and magenta represents those from both Hong Kong and Macao. Only the names of the more active nodes are shown here.

The structure of this network can be broadly divided into two parts. The left part is dominated by institutions from mainland China and those from Hong Kong and Macao, and the right part comprises mainly Taiwanese organizations. Although there were few connections between these two parts, each part contained abundant internal connections. The research units in Taiwan tended to collaborate with organizations from the same region, but less with those from mainland China, Hong Kong, or Macao.

Leading knowledge producers

Table 1 shows the top 50 institutes in weighted degree, indicating the total number of an institute's co-publications. In addition, the influence of a particular institute on others' collaborative behavior was explored using betweenness and closeness centrality.

The majority of mainland Chinese organizations on the list are outstanding academic institutes; these include the universities of project 985 and 211 and some of the country's best-known hospitals and research centers. Most of these are located in Shanghai (18.42 %) and Beijing (15.79 %).

The weighted degree comprises two parts: internal and external degrees. The internal degree represents the number of articles authored by scholars within the same research unit. The external degree reflects the number of co-publications by authors from different institutes. As characterized by their high weighted degrees, Shanghai Jiao Tong University, National Yang Ming University, China Pharmaceutical University, Chang Gung Medical Foundation, Taipei Veterans General Hospital, and Peking Union Medical College are the key institutes in Greater China's anti-diabetic drug research. Organizations that tend to collaborate externally rather than internally had a higher level of external collaboration (LEC). The average LEC value of Taiwanese institutes listed here was 66.99 %, indicating that they tended to cooperate more externally than internally. Conversely, mainland China's LEC was much lower than that of Taiwan, at only 32.98 %, indicating a rather closed collaboration network. As an example, Shanghai Jiao Tong University ranked first in weighted degree but its LEC was only 17 %. In contrast, Peking University had the highest betweenness centrality in the whole system, acting as a gatekeeper of knowledge flow. Other organizations that showed strong betweenness performance include Fudan University, National Taiwan University, Shandong University, Sun Yat-Sen University, and the University of Hong Kong; all of these acted as information intermediaries located in different regions across Greater China.

Many high-betweenness organizations were also the ones with low closeness centrality, emphasizing their important position as knowledge brokers who could access and share new information more quickly than others (Table 1). Some organizations occupied the highest positions for co-publication numbers, betweenness, and closeness, demonstrating their extraordinary contributions to knowledge creation and dissemination. These institutions were Shanghai Jiao Tong University,

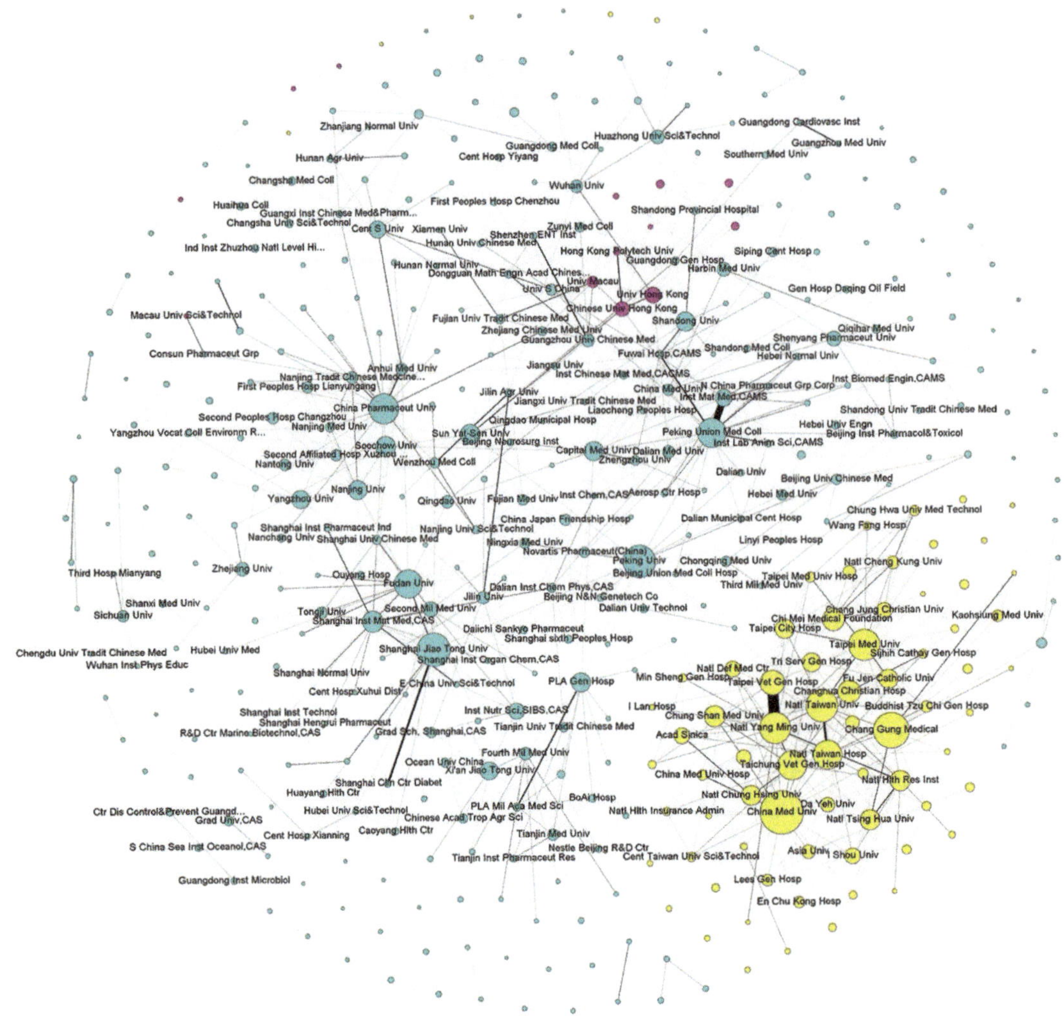

Fig. 2 Institutional collaboration network of anti-diabetic drug research in China. This network is visualized and analyzed by using software Gephi, it comprises 430 *nodes* and 7673 *undirected weighted edges*. A *node* represents a research institution and node size depends on degree centrality while *edge* thickness between two nodes is determined by the number of co-publications between them. Research institutions from mainland China and Taiwan are represented in *cyan* and *yellow* respectively, and *magenta* represents those from both Hong Kong and Macao. Only the names of the more active nodes are shown here

China Pharmaceutical University, Peking Union Medical College Hospital, Fudan University, Peking University, National Taiwan University, University of Hong Kong, and Sun Yat-Sen University.

Top institutional pairs

Institutional pairs that concurrently ranked in the top 50 in terms of edge weight and Jaccard index were chosen to identify the most frequently collaborating pairs with highest mutual dependence. Table 2 shows the 12 pairs meeting these criteria. Closed collaborators that depend heavily on each other included National Yang Ming University and Taipei Veterans General Hospital in Taiwan, and Peking Union Medicine College and the Institute of Materia Medica of the Chinese Academy of Medical Science in Beijing. The data suggested that some pairs showing strong, solid collaborations (83.33 %) were geographically adjacent.

Thematic communities

The basic elements of an institutional collaboration network are the nodes and subgroups of the network, with various subgroups combining to form a complex institution network. As shown in Fig. 3, closely collaborating organizations were clustered into various community subnetworks. The 14 major subnetworks in this system were labeled in descending order of number of institutes. For example, community 1 was the largest community,

Table 1 Top 50 institutions ranked by weighted degree

Rank	Organizations	WD (LEC, %)	BC	CC
1	Shanghai Jiao Tong Univ	1756 (17.0)	8300	3.029
2	Natl Yang Ming Univ (TW)	1539 (63.7)	1222	3.841
3	China Pharmaceut Univ	1311 (22.8)	7233	3.441
4	Chang Gung Medical (TW)	1257 (14.6)	4579	3.809
5	Taipei Vet Gen Hosp (TW)	1112 (72.6)	623	3.859
6	Peking Union Med Coll	1101 (70.6)	6402	3.271
7	Fudan Univ	783 (27.7)	10,980	2.962
8	Inst Mat Med, CAS	750 (76.1)	500	3.894
9	Cent S Univ	725 (15.3)	3654	4.347
10	Chinese Univ Hong Kong (HK)	707 (20.9)	1251	3.718
11	Shanghai Inst Mat Med, CAS	690 (38.6)	3153	3.506
12	Jilin Univ	632 (21.5)	1662	4.365
13	Harbin Med Univ	597 (8.4)	242	3.994
14	Huazhong Univ Sci & Technol	566 (13.3)	1650	4.638
15	Peking Univ	556 (20.7)	21,524	2.729
16	Natl Taiwan Univ (TW)	502 (72.7)	9998	3.212
17	Fourth Mil Med Univ	482 (15.8)	1788	3.72
18	Wenzhou Med Coll	450 (26.2)	1456	3.703
19	Zhejiang Univ	397 (13.9)	1555	3.785
20	Natl Hlth Res Inst (TW)	395 (52.2)	568	3.988
21	Second Mil Med Univ	373 (27.6)	1475	3.588
22	Sichuan Univ	363 (11.8)	2018	5.829
23	Shanghai Clin Ctr Diabet	348 (38.8)	0	4.021
24	PLA Gen Hosp	324 (47.8)	4045	3.500
25	Natl Taiwan Hosp (TW)	309 (79.3)	642	3.888
26	Capital Med Univ	298 (35.2)	4486	3.194
27	Taipei Med Univ (TW)	281 (81.9)	1245	3.93
28	Univ S China	280 (25.4)	2700	4.079
29	Guangzhou Med Univ	278 (25.9)	0	6.147
30	Fuwai Hosp, CAMS	277 (50.9)	325	4.126
31	Third Mil Med Univ	267 (7.1)	339	4.374
32	Nanjing Tradit Chinese Medcine Univ	261 (39.5)	1282	4.076
33	China Med Univ (TW)	254 (78.3)	2810	3.932
34	Taichung Vet Gen Hosp (TW)	237 (88.6)	569	3.971
35	Anhui Med Univ	229 (52.0)	3161	3.641
36	Shenyang Pharmaceut Univ	208 (29.3)	2938	3.938
37	Hebei Med Univ	206 (13.6)	228	3.568
38	Guangzhou Univ Chinese Med	204 (71.6)	1468	3.694
39	Univ Hong Kong (HK)	198 (41.9)	3317	3.471
40	Nanjing Univ	196 (39.3)	1459	3.547
41	Wuhan Univ	188 (22.3)	2114	4.171
42	Nanjing Med Univ	188 (35.1)	113	4.197
43	Weifang Med Univ	187 (13.9)	0	1.000
44	Shanghai Univ Chinese Med	186 (33.3)	128	3.744
45	Shandong Univ	185 (61.6)	4118	3.815
46	Xuzhou Med Coll	184 (32.6)	339	4.429
47	Beijing Inst Technol	174 (29.9)	2	1.000
48	Sun Yat Sen Univ	166 (51.8)	4493	3.300
49	Jilin Agr Univ	162 (69.1)	815	4.371
50	Natl Chung Hsing Univ (TW)	159 (66.0)	364	3.926

Institutions based in Hong Kong and Taiwan are labelled HK and TW respectively, while others are from the mainland of China

WD weighted degree, *LEC* level of external collaborations, *BC* betweenness centrality, *CC* closeness centrality

with 71 organizations, whereas community 14 was the smallest, with only three organizations. Community size increases with number of articles, and edge thickness between any two nodes corresponds to the frequency of co-publications involving authors from those two communities. Table 3 contains additional information about the 14 communities.

The internal structure mining of communities revealed geographic features. For community 2, only one out of the 64 institutes was outside Taiwan, indicating that this community was dominated by Taiwanese organizations that seldom communicate with mainland China, Hong Kong, or Macao. Community 3 was composed mainly of outstanding institutes from Shanghai, such as Shanghai Jiao Tong University, Fudan University, Shanghai Institute of Materia Medical of Chinese Academy of Sciences, and The Second Military Medical University. In contrast, all six research units in community 11 were found in Northwest China, including five from Shaanxi Province and one from the Xinjiang Uygur Autonomous Region.

The research interests of communities were identified by calculating the R_{sc} value of article keywords. For each community, keywords were arranged in descending order of frequency; those accounting for the top 50 % of cumulative frequency were shown and those in bold and in italic were the ones with top 10 R_{sc} values and more related to Chinese medicines respectively. As an example, community 2 focuses not only on *Chinese medicines*, *diabetic complications*, and *hyperglycemia*, but also on *cohort study* and *structural biology*.

All keywords appearing in the system were standardized for statistical analysis. Those occurring more than five times were classified as core keywords and the rest were classified as non-core keywords. The top core keywords were *Chinese medicines*, *diabetic complications*, *oxidative stress*, *hyperglycemia*, *insulin resistance*, *mice model*, *inflammatory*, *pharmacokinetics*, and *GLP-1*. The most frequent *Chinese medicines* keywords included *berberine*, *flavonoids*, *Astragalus polysaccharide*, *emodin*, *ginsenoside*, *quercetin*, *curcumin*, *Ganoderma lucidum*, and *resveratrol*. Table 4 shows the most frequently used keywords in Chinese medicine anti-diabetes research; these are categorized into "Herbs" and "Compounds." More than three research articles focused on "Herbs" and more than five articles focused on "Compounds."

Table 2 Top institutional pairs in Chinese diabetes drug research network

No.	Institutional pairs (region)		Co-publication frequency	Jaccard index (J_{ij}; 0-1)
1	Natl Yang Ming Univ (Taiwan)	Taipei Vet Gen Hosp (Taiwan)	709	0.365
2	Peking Union Med Coll (Beijing)	Inst Mat Med, CAMS (Beijing)	446	0.317
3	Natl Taiwan Hosp (Taiwan)	Natl Taiwan Univ (Taiwan)	135	0.200
4	PLA Military Academy of Medical Sciences (Beijing)	PLA Gen Hosp (Beijing)	81	0.209
5	Guangzhou Univ Chinese Med (Guangdong)	Shenzhen ENT Inst (Guangdong)	72	0.290
6	Guangdong Cardiovasc Inst (Guangdong)	Guangzhou Med Univ (Guangdong)	64	0.204
7	Nanjing Mil Command, Nanjing Gen Hosp (Jiangsu)	Xuzhou Med College (Jiangsu)	50	0.249
8	Macau Univ Sci & Technol (Macao)	Consun Pharmaceut Grp (Guangdong)	32	0.457
9	Univ Macau (Macao)	Fujian Univ Tradit Chinese Med (Fujian)	32	0.182
10	Beijing BIT&GY Pharmaceut R&D (Beijing)	Beijing Inst Technol (Beijing)	32	0.174
11	Xiamen Univ (Fujian)	Fujian Univ Tradit Chinese Med (Fujian)	27	0.197
12	State Adm Tradit Chinese Med (Beijing)	Hunan Agr Univ (Hunan)	25	0.379

Institution's regional location is the provincial-level administrative divisions of China

The Pearson's test of correlations between degree centrality and the R_{sc} value of non-core keywords across communities produced a negative correlation coefficient of -0.641 ($P = 0.013$), indicating that when a community focuses on a research topic that is of common interest to all communities, it can easily build up its collaboration network. However, communities that concentrate on rare research fields are usually isolated by others and have a lower chance of collaboration. For more details regarding the collaboration network and thematic communities, please refer to the Additional files 1, 2, 3, 4.

Discussion

In the present study, the sample data included 881 scientific articles published by 430 Chinese institutes over the 5-year period of 2009–2013. This study identified the most productive institutes and leading academic communities in anti-diabetic drug development.

The average LEC of mainland China's organizations was only half that of Taiwan, indicating that institutes in China were less dependent on external collaboration. This might be explained by a number of factors: (1) the organization had sufficient resources to meet the needs of research projects; (2) there might be no adequate communication platform for knowledge sharing; and (3) geographic distance resulted in a negative impact on information flow between institutes. In contrast, although Taiwan exhibited a high LEC, it was rather disconnected from organizations in mainland China, Hong Kong, and Macao.

The network visualized data in this article may help researchers and scholars to navigate in this active research area and to find potential collaborators specializing in a particular research area. For instance, a researcher affiliated with Jilin University (a member of community 8) who specializes in the research of *ginsenoside*, is planning to explore the therapeutic effect of a combination of *ginsenoside* and *medicinal mushrooms* on diabetic complications. In Fig. 3, community 2 was the only group to focus on *medicinal mushrooms* research; therefore, the researcher could probably identify potential collaborators from this community. Knowledge of the list of institutes that belong to community 2, and with the help of the co-authorship network, the researcher could select the most appropriate expert for research collaboration based on centrality measurements. In this case, the researcher might approach China Medical University in Taiwan, as it ranked at the top in the three aspects of centrality measurements among institutes studying *medicinal mushrooms*. This kind of research collaboration does not simply represent the building of a new partnership between two researchers or institutions, but also fosters knowledge exchange across various diabetes research communities in China and further stimulates innovation and productivity.

In addition, each community studied here is labeled with a list of keywords, covering a diverse range of topics that included *herbology, chemical component, molecular biology, clinical medicine, pharmacokinetics, therapeutic drugs*, and *animal experimental models*. *Chinese medicines, diabetic complications, oxidative stress, hyperglycemia*, and *insulin resistance* were common topics that could be found on the keyword list across different communities, indicating their significance in the field. Only minimal adverse effects were reported for Chinese medicines used in treating type 2 DM, indicating certain advantages in the prevention of diabetes and delay of its complications [7]. Studying the role of oxidative stress in the pathogenesis of diabetes provides a theoretical basis for the prevention and treatment of the disease [20], as oxidative stress could be

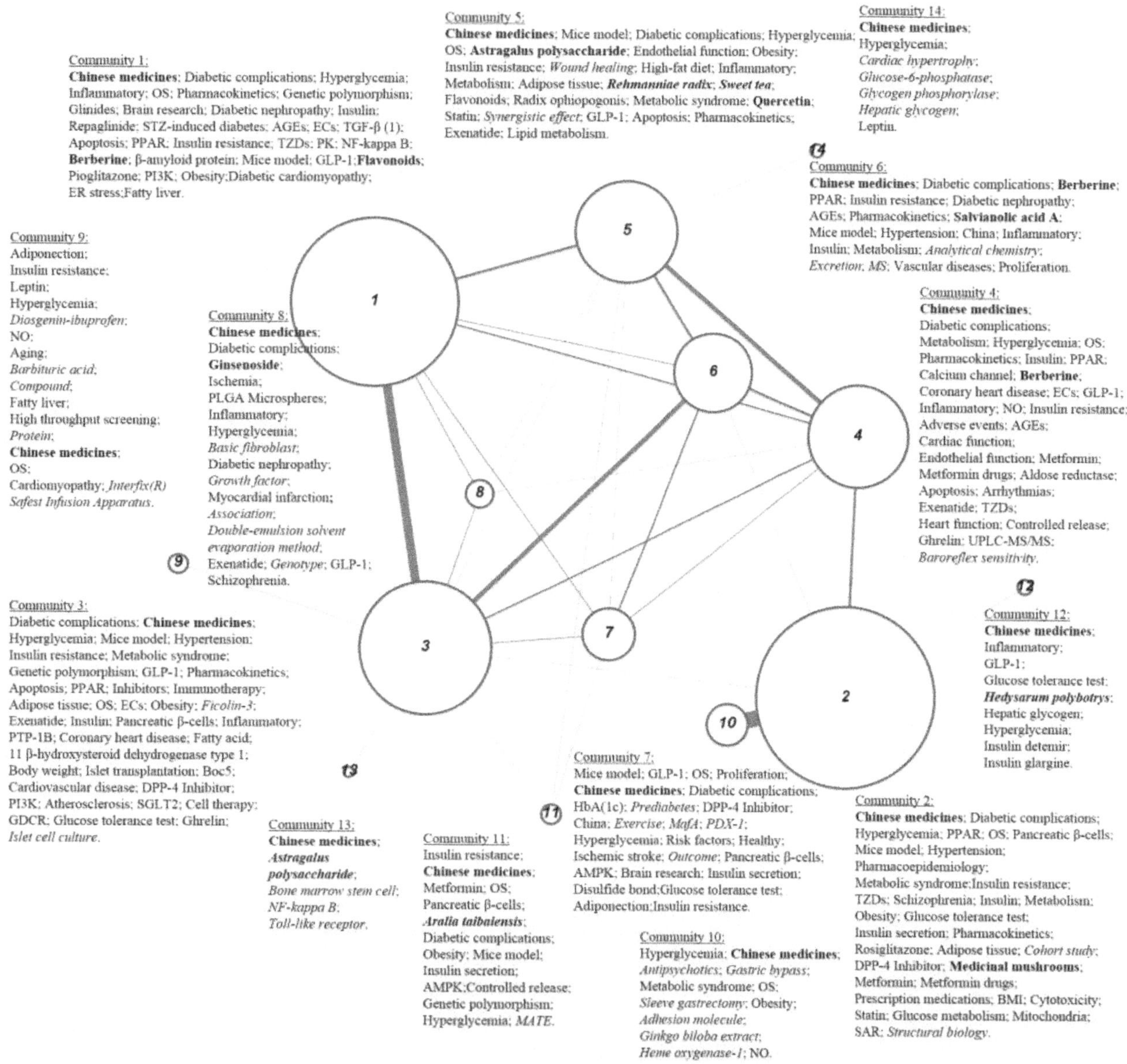

Fig. 3 Thematic community network of diabetes drug research in greater China. This figure consists of 14 communities which are shown as *nodes* and labelled by their high frequency keywords in which *italic words* are research topics more relevant to a given community than to the others and those letters in *bold* are more related to Chinese medicines. Community size increases with number of articles, and *edge* thickness between any two nodes corresponds to the frequency of co-publications involving authors from those two communities. These subnetworks are labelled in descending order of number of institutes

a major cause of the development of type 2 DM [21]. Furthermore, *Chinese medicines* in combination with insulin exhibited better clinical effect in the treatment of gestational diabetes [22]. Similarly, *berberine* exhibited beneficial anti-inflammation effects, indicating that it could be a potential therapeutic drug in type 1 DM treatment [23].

Each of the 14 communities in the studied system has its own area of expertise, which is usually a non-mainstream topic. Community 2, a subnetwork primarily composed of Taiwanese organizations, focuses on *cohort study* and *structural biology* while Community 3 is a Shanghai-based group that specializes in *ficolin-3* and *islet cell culture*. Community 5 focuses on *wound healing, radix Rehmanniae, sweet tea*, and *synergistic effect*; most of its constituent organizations are from Guangdong Province, Hong Kong, and Macao. Finally, the Beijing-dominated

Table 3 Detailed information of 14 communities

Community codes	Number of institutes	Number of articles	Frequency of co-publications
1	71	275	1159
2	64	285	769
3	44	197	881
4	34	152	618
5	33	151	564
6	30	117	413
7	21	77	252
8	11	41	215
9	8	28	122
10	7	52	234
11	6	29	137
12	6	12	34
13	3	5	22
14	3	9	65

Community size increases with number of articles, and the subnetworks are labelled in descending order of number of institutes. The edge thickness between any two nodes reflects the frequency of co-publications involving authors from those two communities

Table 4 Frequent keywords relevant to Chinese medicines

Herbs (frequency ≥ 3)		Compounds (frequency ≥ 5)	
Items (Chinese)	**Frequency**	**Items (Chinese)**	**Frequency**
Coptidis Rhizoma (黃連)	27	*Berberine* (黃連素)	27
Medicinal mushrooms (藥用蘑菇)	8	*Flavonoids* (黃酮類化合物)	25
Ginseng (人參)	7	*Astragalus polysaccharide* (黃芪多醣)	12
Ganoderma lucidum (靈芝)	5	*Polysaccharide* (多聚糖)	10
Potentilla discolor bunge (翻白草)	4	*Emodin* (大黃素)	8
Radix ophiopogonis (麥冬)	4	*Ginsenoside* (人參皂苷)	7
Salvia miltiorrhiza (丹參)	4	*Quercetin* (槲皮素)	7
Buckwheat (蕎麥)	3	*Curcumin* (薑黃素)	6
Cinnamon (肉桂)	3	*Salvianolic acid A* (丹酚酸A)	6
Folium Eriobotryae (枇杷葉)	3	*Triterpenes* (三萜類化合物)	6
Paeonia lactiflora (芍藥)	3	*Resveratrol* (白藜蘆醇)	5
Selaginella tamariscina (卷柏)	3		
Swertia (獐牙菜)	3		

Community 6 concentrates on *analytical chemistry*, *excretion*, and *mass spectrometry*.

The collaboration opportunities available to a community are strongly affected by the level of interest in its research topics. Communities dedicated to less-studied research areas usually have more difficulty in identifying suitable collaborators. This community thematic analysis provides a reference for researchers and institutes looking for potential collaborators based on research direction.

Researchers would find it easier to create research partnerships if the key researchers' information was also directly available. However, this study explored the research landscape of Chinese anti-diabetic drugs only at an institutional level. It is more difficult to study research at a personal level because of data sensitivity and privacy protection, although we did have available personal publication data to identify the most prolific or influential authors in specific research areas, units, or communities in the system. Those researchers interested in author-related information can consult the list of articles for each thematic community in Additional file 4. For instance, a researcher searching for information related to *berberine* can search for the keyword *berberine* in Additional file 3, which provides the "Article No." that contains this keyword. As each article carries a unique article number, this code can directly identify the article title, authors of the paper, authors' affiliations and geographic region, and the thematic community to which the article belongs.

Because of the need for a homogeneous sample composed of cutting-edge research articles and regional biases, we chose to use just the SCIE data source and to not include Chinese literature indexed in CNKI and other Chinese databases. In using co-authorship academic publication data, this study mainly focuses on basic research and is limited to academic collaborations. A similar exercise for applied and competitive research would be an important addition to the current study and could, for instance, focus on collaboration in patenting and R&D projects. In addition, the arbitrary selection of keywords and the lack of keywords in a small proportion of sample articles may have caused potential bias in the thematic analysis. Future studies could construct a more complex and more influential collaboration network by expanding sample size or time span, or by widening the scope from domestic to international organizations. A dynamic network analysis could also be introduced to investigate how the network evolves over time.

Conclusion

By characterizing communities and noting their research themes, the results of this study could provide guidance to researchers seeking potential collaborators and could suggest a precise research direction for future studies.

Abbreviations
CAMS: Chinese Academy of Medical Science; CAS: Chinese Academy of Sciences; DM: diabetes mellitus; GDM: gestational diabetes mellitus; GLP-1: glucagon-like peptide-1; IDF: International Diabetes Federation; IMM: Institute of Materia Medica; LEC: level of external collaboration; MS: mass spectrum; NO: nitric oxide; OS: oxidative stress; R&D: Research and development; SCIE: science citation index expanded; T1DM: type 1 diabetes mellitus; T2DM: type 2 diabetes mellitus.

Authors' contributions
JLD, KS and YJH conceived and designed the study. JLD collected the data. JLD, KS, YPZ and RY performed the data analysis. JLD, KS and YJH wrote the manuscript. All authors read and approved the final manuscript.

Author details
[1] State Key Laboratory of Quality Research in Chinese Medicine, Institute of Chinese Medical Sciences, University of Macau, Macao, China. [2] Guiyang College of Traditional Chinese Medicine, Guiyang, Guizhou, China.

Acknowledgements
We thank Ms. Han You for her assistance in the preliminary data processing, and the University of Macau for financial support for this research by the project MYRG2015-00172-ICMS-QRCM.

Competing interests
The authors declare that they have no competing interests.

References
1. World Health Organization. Diabetes Action Online: About Diabetes. http://www.who.int/diabetes/action_online/basics/en. Accessed 18 Nov 2014.
2. World Health Organization. Media Centre Fact Sheet: Diabetes Fact Sheet N 312. http://www.who.int/mediacentre/factsheets/fs312/en. Accessed 19 Nov 2014.
3. Kitabchi AE, Umpierrez GE, Miles JM, Fisher JN. Hyperglycemic crises in adult patients with diabetes. Diabetes Care. 2009. doi:10.2337/dc09-9032.
4. International Diabetes Federation: Sixth Edition of the IDF Diabetes Atlas. Brussels; 2014.
5. National Diabetes Prevention and Control Cooperative Group. A mass survey of diabetes mellitus in a population of 300,000 in 14 provinces and municipalities in China. Zhonghua Nei Ke Za Zhi. 1981;20:83–678.
6. Xu Y, Wang LM, He J, Bi YF, Li M, Wang TG, Wang LH, Jiang Y, Dai M, Lu JL, Xu M, Li YC, Hu N, Li JH, Mi SQ, Chen CSA, Li GW, Mu YM, Zhao JJ, Kong LZ, Chen JL, Lai SH, Wang WQ, Zhao WH, Ning G. Prevalence and control of diabetes in Chinese adults. JAMA. 2013;310:59–948.
7. Li WL, Zheng HC, Bukuru J, De Kimpe N. Natural medicines used in the traditional Chinese medical system for therapy of diabetes mellitus. J Ethnopharmacol. 2004;92:1–21.
8. Wang SB, Meng QG. Bibliometric analysis on treatment of type 2 diabetes mellitus by traditional Chinese medicine. Chin Arch Trad Chin Med. 2014;32:273–6.
9. Hu H, Zhao WL. Analysis of diabetes papers indexed by SCI. Med Inf. 2008;21:53–7.
10. Thomson Reuters. Science Citation Index Expanded. http://thomsonreuters.com/science-citation-index-expanded. Accessed 18 Nov 2014.
11. Fruchterman Thomas MJ, Reingold EM. Graph drawing by force-directed placement. Softw-Pract Exp. 1991;21:1158–62.
12. Lin JR. Social network analysis: theory, method and application. 1st ed. Beijing: Beijing Normal University Press; 2009.
13. Newman M. Who is the best connected scientist? A study of scientific coauthorship networks: complex networks. Berlin: Springer; 2004.
14. Newman M. The structure of scientific collaboration networks. Proc Natl Acad Sci USA. 2004;101:5200–5.
15. Leydesdorff L. On the normalization and visualization of author co-citation data: Salton's Cosine versus the Jaccard index. J Assoc Inf Sci Technol. 2008;59:77–85.
16. Scherngell T, Hu YJ. Collaborative knowledge production in china: regional evidence from a gravity model approach. Reg Stud. 2011;45:755–72.
17. Blondel VD, Guillaume JL, Lambiotte R, Lefebvre E. Fast unfolding of communities in large networks. J Stat Mech. 2008. doi:10.1088/1742-5468/2008/10/P10008.
18. Barber MJ, Fischer MM, Scherngell T. The Community Structure of Research and Development Cooperation in Europe: evidence from a social network perspective. Geogr Anal. 2011;43:415–32.
19. Freeman LC. Centrality in social networks conceptual clarification. Soc Networks. 1979;1:215–39.
20. Ren CJ, Yao Z, Cui WZ, Mu ZM. Progress in the role of oxidative stress in the pathogenesis of type 2 diabetes. Acta Physiologica Sinica. 2013;65:664–73.
21. Fardoun RZ. The use of vitamin E in type 2 diabetes mellitus. Clin Exp Hypertens. 2007;29:135–48.
22. Zhang L, Wang LP, Zhang GF, Zhang XL. Traditional Chinese medicine combined with insulin in the treatment of gestational diabetes clinical comparative study. J Med Theor Pract. 2014;27:3250–1.
23. Cui GL, Qin X, Zhang YB, Gong ZW, Ge BX, Zang YQ. Berberine differentially modulates the activities of ERK, p38 MAPK, and JNK to Suppress Th17 and Th1 T Cell differentiation in type 1 diabetic mice. J Biol Chem. 2009;284:28421–2.

12

Ameliorating effect of *Erxian* decoction combined with Fructus *Schisandrae chinensis* (*Wu Wei Zi*) on menopausal sweating and serum hormone profiles in a rat model

Shi Wei Wang[1], Fei Hua Wu[2], Yan Bo Zhang[1], Liang Zhang[1], Jing Su[1], Hei Kei Wong[1], Ai Hua Liu[1,3], Ho Pan Cheung[1], Tzi Bun Ng[4], Yao Tong[1] and Stephen Cho Wing Sze[1*]

Abstract

Background: Modified *Erxian decoction* (MEXD), i.e., *Erxian* decoction (EXD) with Fructus *Schisandrae chinensis* (*Wu Wei Zi*) added, has been used to alleviate menopausal symptoms. This study aimed to investigate the effects of MEXD on menopausal sweating and serum hormone levels in a rat model of menopause after oral administration of MEXD.

Methods: Quality control of MEXD was conducted by employing a reversed-phase high performance liquid chromatography column. The three treatment groups received oral administration of MEXD in 0.5% sodium carboxylmethyl cellulose (CMC-Na) at three different doses (5.5, 11, and 22 g/kg body weight) once-daily for 6 consecutive weeks, with 10 animals per group. *Huangqijing* oral liquor (5 mL/kg) prepared from the roots of *Huang qi* (*Astragalus membranaceus*) with an antiperspirant effect was used as a positive control. The negative control group received the same volume of vehicle (0.5% CMC-Na). Ten 3-month-old Sprague–Dawley rats were used as a young group for comparison with the treatment groups (12–14 months old rats). Blood was collected from all animals after 3–6 weeks of treatment. At the end of the treatment, the uterine weight, ovarian weight, and body weight were recorded. Serum malondialdehyde contents and superoxide dismutase activities were determined by thiobarbituric acid colorimetric assays and chemoluminescence assays, respectively. Serum levels of estradiol, follicle-stimulating hormone, and luteinizing hormone were measured by radioimmunoassays. Rat foot pad assays were used to determine the antiperspirant activity of MEXD and histological examinations were conducted on plantar sweat glands.

Results: Treatment with MEXD (11 g/kg) significantly inhibited sweat excretion in the menopause model rats after treatment for 3 ($P = 0.0026$) and 6 ($P < 0.0001$) weeks. The decoction markedly decreased the number of secretory cells in plantar sweat glands. In addition, MEXD (11 g/kg) significantly increased the serum estradiol levels ($P < 0.001$) and superoxide dismutase activities ($P = 0.0405$). Furthermore, MEXD (11 g/kg) markedly decreased the serum levels of follicle-stimulating hormone ($P = 0.001$), luteinizing hormone ($P = 0.0213$), and malondialdehyde ($P = 0.01$).

Conclusion: Modified *Erxian decoction* significantly inhibited sweat excretion, regulated serum levels of pituitary gonadotropins and estradiol, and exhibited antioxidative effects in a rat model of menopause.

*Correspondence: stephens@hku.hk
[1] School of Chinese Medicine, LKS Faculty of Medicine, The University of Hong Kong, 10 Sassoon Road, Pokfulam, Hong Kong SAR
Full list of author information is available at the end of the article

Background

Menopausal syndrome refers to symptoms that appear during the menopausal transition, including hot flashes, sweating, dysphoria, and insomnia. Sweating is the main menopausal vasomotor symptom, and can significantly affect the quality of life in middle-aged females [1]. More than 80% of middle-aged women suffer from vasomotor symptoms, including hot flashes and night sweats, during menopause [2, 3]. One of the underlying mechanisms involves decreased secretion of sex hormones [4] through deterioration of ovarian functions in an age-related free radical-predominant environment [5], which in turn elevates the production of the gonadotropins luteinizing hormone (LH) and follicle-stimulating hormone (FSH) [6]. This hormonal dysregulation eventually results in autonomic dysfunction, thereby disturbing the coordination of the neuroendocrine system. Hormone replacement therapy (HRT) has been adopted as the conventional treatment for menopausal syndrome to compensate for the reduction in ovarian estrogen production. However, concerns about increased risks of some chronic diseases, such as breast cancer, heart attack, and stroke, with HRT have stimulated interest in the development of safer alternative therapies [7].

Herbal medicines with estrogenic activity or enriched with phytoestrogens have frequently been employed as complementary therapies to relieve menopausal symptoms [8–15]. However, only a few studies have investigated the treatment of menopausal vasomotor symptoms using herbal medicines.

In Chinese medicine, menopausal syndrome is attributed to insufficiency of *kidney essence*, and deficiency of *kidney yin* and *yang*. At the age of about 49 years, the *kidney qi* gradually becomes insufficient, the function of *ChongRen* declines, and *Tian gui* (an important reproduction essence) begins to dry up, thereby causing the loss of reproductive capacity. Clinically, menopausal women often suffer from menstrual disorders, hot flashes, and night sweats. *Erxian* decoction (EXD) has been used in the treatment of menopausal syndrome, and consists of six Chinese medicinal herbs, namely rhizoma *Curculigo orchioides* (*Xian mao*), herba *Epimedium brevicornum* (*Yin yang huo*), radix *Morinda officinalis* (*Ba ji tian*), radix *Angelica sinensis* (*Dang gui*), cortex *Phellodendron chinense* (*Huang bo*), and rhizome *Anemarrhena asphodeloides* (*Zhi mu*) [11, 16]. In EXD, constituent herbs *C. orchioides*, *E. brevicornum*, and *M. officinalis* can warm the *kidney yang*, and was used to restore the *kidney yin*. *A. asphodeloides* goes into the central part of the body, where it removes the heat of the stomach and nourishes the *stomach Yin*. *P. chinense* goes into the lower part of the body, nourishes the *kidney yin*, and brings *pathogenic fire* back to the *kidneys*. *A. sinensis*, a medicine that nourishes *blood*, can also restore *qi*, and was used to restore both *blood* and *qi*. The night sweats during menopause arise through the deficiency of *kidney yin* and *yang*. However, a clinical study reported that EXD alone did not exert marked effects on perspiration [17]. The fruit of *Schisandrae chinensis* (*Wu wei zi*), with the pharmacologic effect of arresting discharge to decrease sweating, is commonly used to treat insomnia and as an antiperspirant clinically [17, 18]. A clinical study showed that modified EXD (MEXD) consisting of EXD with other added herbs, including the fruit of *S. chinensis*, can relieve menopausal sweating [18, 19]. However, related basic research data have not yet been reported.

This study aimed to investigate the effects of MEXD on menopausal sweating and serum hormone profiles in menopausal rats after oral administration of MEXD. We hypothesized that MEXD would alleviate the sweating symptom in menopausal females via increased expression of antioxidative enzymes and estradiol (E2), and decreased production of serum gonadotropins, LH, FSH, and malondialdehyde (MDA). As the study model, we used 12–14-month-old aged menopausal Sprague-Dawley (SD) rats with irregular estrous cycles, as well as elevated serum FSH levels and decreased serum E2 levels, in accordance with our previous publication [11]. The effects of MEXD on sweat excretion, uterine and ovarian weights, serum levels of E2, FSH, LH, and MDA, and activity of serum superoxide dismutase (SOD) were determined. The effects of MEXD on the morphology of plantar sweat glands were also examined. Functional assays of sweating after MEXD treatment were performed to validate its therapeutic efficacy.

Methods

Herbal materials and MEXD extract

The seven medicinal plants of MEXD, namely *C. orchioides*, *E. brevicornum*, *M. officinalis*, *A. sinensis*, *P. chinense*, *A. asphodeloides* and *S. Chinensis* (voucher no. CME140706-03, CME150906-11, CME050406-02, CME090706-12, CME100606-09, CME180806-01 and JWE030806-05 respectively) were collected from various sources and their identities were confirmed by Dr. Yanbo Zhang, School of Chinese Medicine, the University of Hong Kong based on their morphological appearances. One kilogram of each of the six component herbs of EXD, and 1 kg of *S. Chinensis* fruit (composition ratio = 12:12:10:10:9:9:12) was decocted separately with distilled water in a ratio of 10:1 (v/w) at 100 °C for one hour, and the extraction was repeated twice. The procedures followed those of our previous publication [20, 21].

Quality control and high performance liquid chromatography (HPLC)

For evaluation of the quality consistency of MEXD extracts, nine chemical standards were utilized as markers, namely berberine, ferulic acid, icariin, jatrorrhizine, palmatine, schizandrol, schizandrol B, schizandrin A and schizandrin B. All these standard chemicals were purchased from Beijing Century Biotechnology Co., Ltd (Beijing, China). These nine selected chemical standards and three batches of MEXD extracts were accurately weighed out and extracted with 10 mL of methanol in a water bath at 60 °C for 15 min, followed by ultrasonication for 30 min. After centrifugation at 1500×*g* for 15 min, the supernatant was filtered with a 0.45 μm Millex® Syringe filter unit, and then injected in a volume of 10 μL into a HPLC. Reproducibility and linearity were estimated by repetitive injections. The external standard method, employing a series of mixed standard solutions ranging in concentration from 4.0625 to 145 μg/mL, was utilized. The column used was a reversed-phase column (XBridge® C_{18}, 5 μm, 250 mm × 4.6 mm i.e., Waters, Ireland). The mobile phase consisted of acetonitrile (A) and 0.05% sodium dodecyl sulfate (SDS) in 0.1% acetic acid (B) using a gradient program of 95–70% (B) in 0–30 min, 70–70% (B) in 30–35 min, 70–50% (B) in 35–45 min, 50–45% (B) in 50–70 min, 45–35% (B) in 70–90 min, and 35–30% (B) in 90–100 min. The flow rate was 1.0 mL/min. The UV spectra from 200 to 400 nm were acquired with the photodiode array detector and chromatogram at 254 nm was extracted. Peak integration was analyzed by the software of Empower Pro, Waters®.

Experimental animals and drug treatment

Sixty-five female SD rats aged 12–14 months (weight: 290–370 g) and 10 SD rats aged 3 months (weight: 160–190 g) were obtained from the Animal Center of Nanjing Qinglongshan. The animals were housed in an air-conditioned room at an ambient temperature of 24 °C and a relative humidity of 50–65% under automatic 12- /12-h light/dark cycles. All efforts were made to minimize suffering of the animals and to reduce the number of animals used. Animal experiment has been conducted in China Pharmaceutical University since 2007, which was in accordance with the regulations for animal care and use in Department of Health, the Government of the Hong Kong Special Administrative Region (Reference no. 07-298 and 09-92) (Additional files 1, 2). The animal studies were performed following the ARRIVE guideline (Additional file 3).

Using vaginal smear tests, 50 of the 65 rats with both irregular estrous cycles and lowered serum E2 levels were classified as menopausal rats, and selected as the experimental animals. These rats were arbitrarily divided into a negative control group and four treatment groups, with 10 rats per group. The four treatment groups received oral administration of MEXD in 0.5% sodium carboxylmethyl cellulose (CMC-Na) at three different doses (5.5, 11, and 22 g/kg body weight) or *Huangqijing* oral liquor at 5 mL/kg (Z32020370; Yangtze River Pharmaceutical Co. Ltd.), prepared from the roots of *Astragalus membranaceus* with an antiperspirant effect, as a positive control once-daily for 6 consecutive weeks. The drug ratios in MEXD (12:12:10:10:9:9:12), namely rhizoma *Curculigo orchioides* (*Xian mao*) 12 g, herba *Epimedium brevicornum* (*Yin yang huo*) 12 g, radix *Morinda officinalis* (*Ba ji tian*) 10 g, radix *Angelica sinensis* (*Dang gui*) 10 g, cortex *Phellodendron chinense* (*Huang bo*) 9 g, rhizome *Anemarrhena asphodeloides* (*Zhi mu*) 9 g, and Fructus *Schisandrae chinensis (Wu Wei Zi*) 12 g are commonly used clinically [20]. The dosage of 11 g/kg/day applied to rats corresponded to an equivalent dosage in humans [22], and thus three dosages of MEXD (5.5, 11, and 22 g/kg) were selected for this study. The negative control group received the same volume of vehicle (0.5% CMC-Na). The 10 SD rats aged 3 months were used as a young group for comparison with the aged rats.

Rat foot pad assay for antiperspirant activity

Sweat secretion in the rats was detected by rat foot pad assays after MEXD treatment for 3–6 weeks. The method was originally developed by Helman et al. [23] and has been used in previous studies [23–25]. Briefly, the foot pads of all rats were cleaned with 70% ethanol to remove debris, and then swabbed with iodine solution (2% w/v in 95% ethanol). After evaporation of the ethanol at room temperature, the foot pads were coated with castor oil containing 50% starch for 15 min. As the sweating parts of the foot pads showed coloration by starch–iodine reactions, the colored points on the foot pads (i.e., number of sweat glands) were enumerated under a microscope and the degree of perspiration was measured.

Measurement of serum antioxidant biochemical parameters and hormones

At 24 h after the last gavage, blood samples were collected from the femoral artery of the rats to determine the serum levels of MDA, SOD activity, E2, FSH, and LH. The collected blood was centrifuged at 1000×*g* for 10 min and the serum supernatant was stored at −20 °C until analysis. The serum MDA concentrations and SOD activities were determined by thiobarbituric acid colorimetric assays and chemoluminescence assays (Nanjing Jiancheng Bioengineering Institute, Nanjing, China), respectively. The serum levels of E2, FSH, and LH were measured by radioimmunoassays using an E2 assay kit (Cat. No. B05PZA), FSH assay kit (Cat. No. B03PZB), and LH assay kit (Cat. No. B04PZB) from Beijing North Institute of Biological Technology (China), respectively.

Measurement of organ indices

All rats were killed by cervical dislocation after blood collection. The uteri and ovaries were excised and weighed immediately on an electronic balance. The organ indices were calculated by dividing the organ weights by the body weight.

Histological examination

The epidermis of the foot pads was dissected into pieces, fixed in 10% formalin, and processed for paraffin sectioning. Tissue sections were stained with hematoxylin and eosin and examined under an optical microscope [26].

Statistical analysis

All data were expressed as the mean ± standard deviation. Differences among groups were evaluated for statistical significance by one-way ANOVA followed by a Tukey multiple-comparisons test using GraphPad Prism 6.0 (GraphPad Software, USA). Values of $P < 0.05$ were considered statistically significant.

Results

HPLC for quality analysis

The UV spectra of all eluted peaks from 200 to 400 nm in chromatograms of MEXD were measured by photodiode array detection, and the majority of the detectable peaks in the HPLC chromatograms were found at 254 nm. The chromatograms were thus extracted at the detection wavelength of 254 nm. A chromatographic fingerprint indicating the elution peaks of nine standard compounds and other common peaks is shown in Fig. 1. Three batches of MEXD preparations were examined by HPLC using the optimum running conditions. The inter assay relative standard deviation (RSD) values were less than 5% for all of the standard compounds. The results are shown in Table 1.

Antioxidant activity of MEXD in menopausal rats

The serum SOD activities were significantly lower (Fig. 2) and the serum MDA levels were significantly higher (Fig. 3) in the control group compared with the young

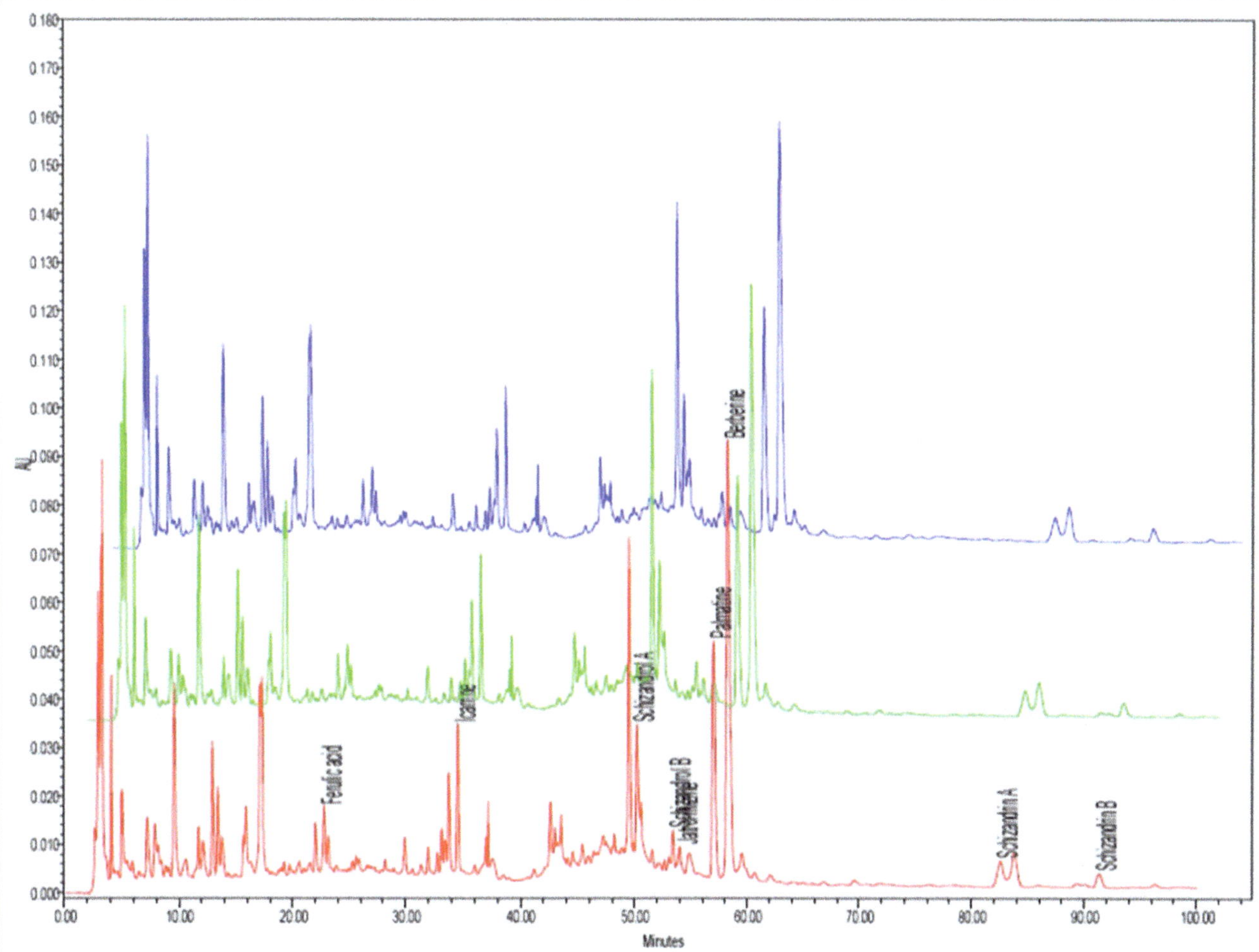

Fig. 1 Overlaid HPLC chromatographic fingerprint of three batches of MEXD extract monitored at 254 nm. Nine standard compounds and their respective retention times are shown

Table 1 Contents of nine compound standards in MEXD

Standards (μg/mg)	Batch 1	Batch 2	Batch 3	Mean	Standard deviation	Relative standard deviation (%)
Berberine	0.961	0.945	0.924	0.943	0.019	1.983
Ferulic acid	0.200	0.189	0.191	0.193	0.006	3.137
Icariine	0.414	0.411	0.408	0.411	0.003	0.783
Jatrorrhizine	0.054	0.054	0.053	0.054	0.000	0.078
Palmatine	0.611	0.598	0.586	0.598	0.013	2.106
Schizandrol A	0.341	0.334	0.354	0.343	0.010	2.990
Schizandrol B	0.114	0.109	0.118	0.113	0.004	3.891
Schizandrin A	0.107	0.107	0.107	0.107	0.000	0.217
Schizandrin B	0.136	0.134	0.133	0.134	0.002	1.469

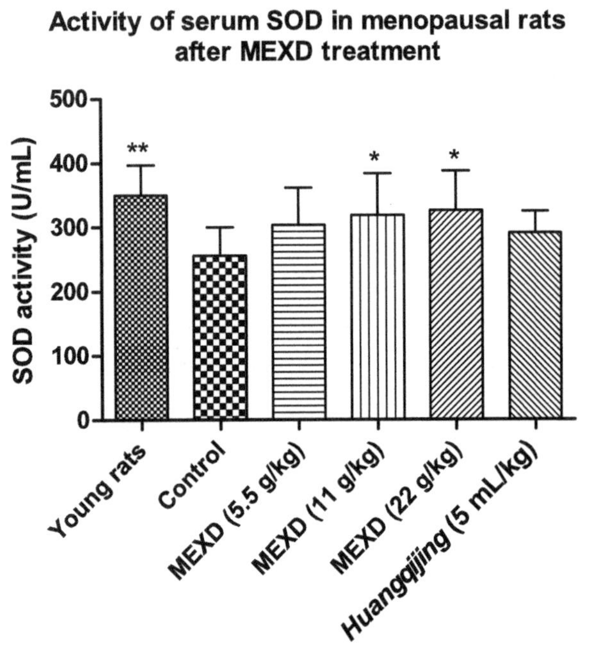

Fig. 2 Serum levels of SOD in menopausal rats after MEXD treatment (n = 10, mean ± standard deviation). One-way ANOVA followed by multiple comparisons. $^{*}P < 0.05$, $^{**}P \leq 0.01$ compared with control. Young rats vs. control: $P = 0.0026$, MEXD (22 g/kg) vs. control: $P = 0.0474$

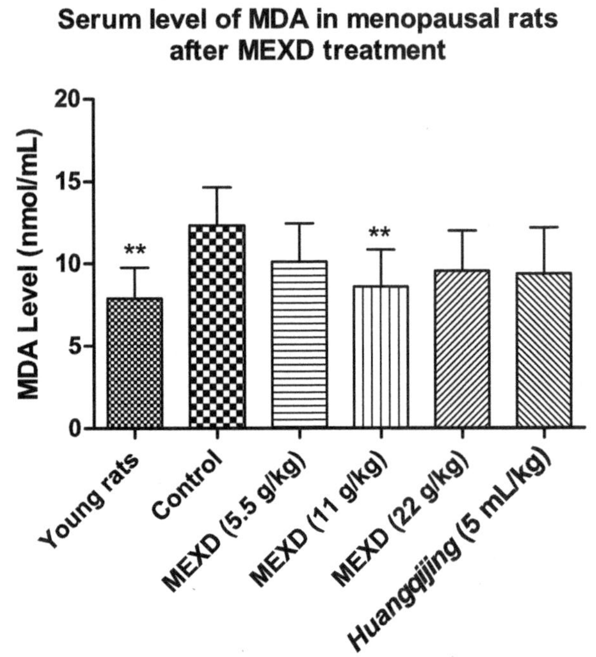

Fig. 3 Serum levels of MDA in menopausal rats after MEXD treatment (n = 10, mean ± standard deviation). One-way ANOVA followed by multiple comparisons $^{*}P < 0.05$, $^{**}P \leq 0.01$ compared with control. Young rats vs. control: $P = 0.0013$, MEXD (11 g/kg) vs. control: $P = 0.01$

rats. Treatment with MEXD at all dosages and *Huangqijing* was able to significantly reverse these changes.

Regulatory effects of MEXD on serum gonadotropic and gonadal hormones in menopausal rats

Significantly reduced serum E2 levels (Fig. 4) accompanied by increased serum levels of FSH (Fig. 5) and LH (Fig. 6) were found in the menopausal rats in the control group compared with the young rats. After treatment with MEXD at 11 g/kg, the serum E2 levels increased significantly. Meanwhile, treatment with MEXD at 5.5 and 11 g/kg decreased the serum LH and FSH levels compared with the control group.

Effects of MEXD on organ indices of the ovaries and uteri

Compared with the young rats, the organ indices of the ovaries of the menopausal rats in the control group were significantly decreased. However, the organ indices of the ovaries and uteri in all four treatment groups (MEXD and *Huangqijing*) did not differ significantly compared with those in the control group (Table 2). These findings

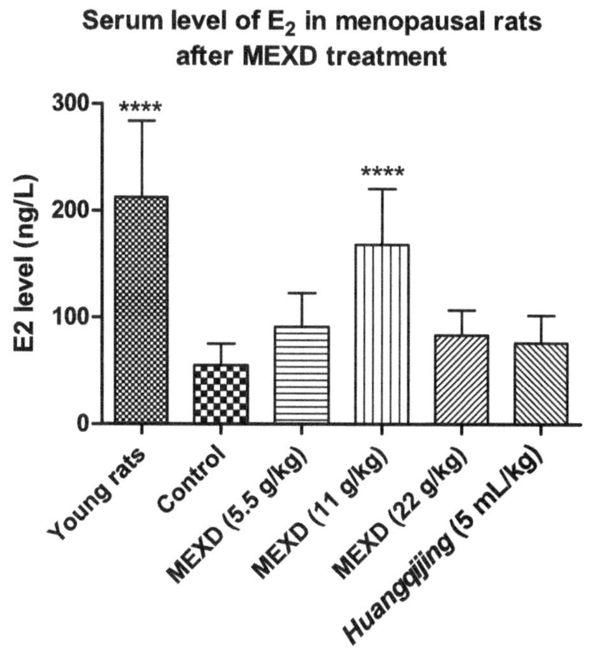

Fig. 4 Serum levels of E2 in menopausal rats after MEXD treatment (n = 10, mean ± standard deviation). One-way ANOVA followed by multiple ***$P < 0.001$ compared with control. Young rats vs. control: $P < 0.0001$, MEXD (11 g/kg) vs. control: $P < 0.0001$

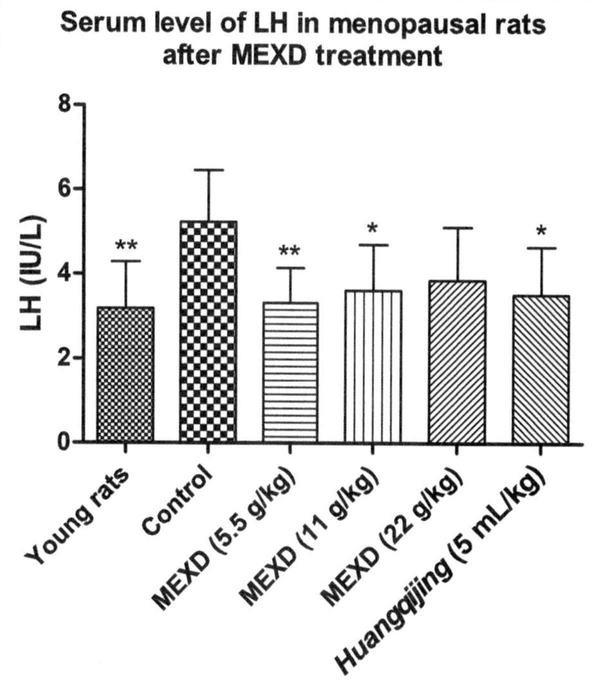

Fig. 6 Serum levels of LH in menopausal rats after MEXD treatment (n = 10, mean ± standard deviation). One-way ANOVA followed by multiple **$P \leq 0.01$ and *$P < 0.05$ compared with control. Young rats vs. control: $P = 0.0017$, MEXD (5.5 g/kg) vs. control: $P = 0.004$, MEXD (11 g/kg) vs. control: $P = 0.0213$, *Huangqijing* vs. control: $P = 0.0131$

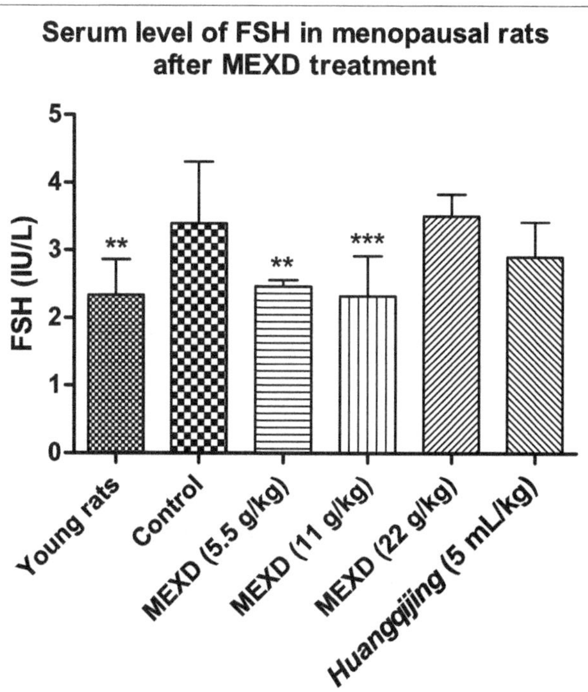

Fig. 5 Serum levels of FSH in menopausal rats after MEXD treatment (n = 10, mean ± standard deviation).One-way ANOVA followed by multiple comparisons. **$P \leq 0.01$, ***$P < 0.001$ compared with control. Young rats vs. control: $P = 0.001$, MEXD (5.5 g/kg) vs. control: $P = 0.005$, MEXD (11 g/kg) vs. control: $P = 0.0008$

indicated that MEXD treatment exerted no observable adverse effects on the ovaries and uteri.

Antiperspirant activity of MEXD on the foot pads of menopausal rats

Sweat secretion of rat foot pads was determined by the iodine–starch reaction in all groups and the results are shown in Fig. 7. The number of active sweat glands in the menopausal rats in the control group was significantly higher than that in the young rats ($P = 0.0012$). At the

Table 2 Organ indices of ovaries and uteruses in menopausal rats after MEXD treatment (n = 10, mean ± standard deviation)

Group	Organ index	
	Uterus ($\times 10^{-3}$)	Ovary ($\times 10^{-4}$)
Young	2.33 ± 0.81	3.38 ± 0.33**
Control	2.34 ± 0.58	2.30 ± 0.51
MEXD (5.5 g/kg)	1.80 ± 0.35	2.37 ± 0.67
MEXD (11 g/kg)	1.88 ± 0.32	2.21 ± 0.25
MEXD (22 g/kg)	2.23 ± 0.63	2.54 ± 0.84
Huangqijing (5 mL/kg)	2.00 ± 0.38	2.27 ± 0.47

** $P < 0.001$ (one way ANOVA, n = 10) compared with control

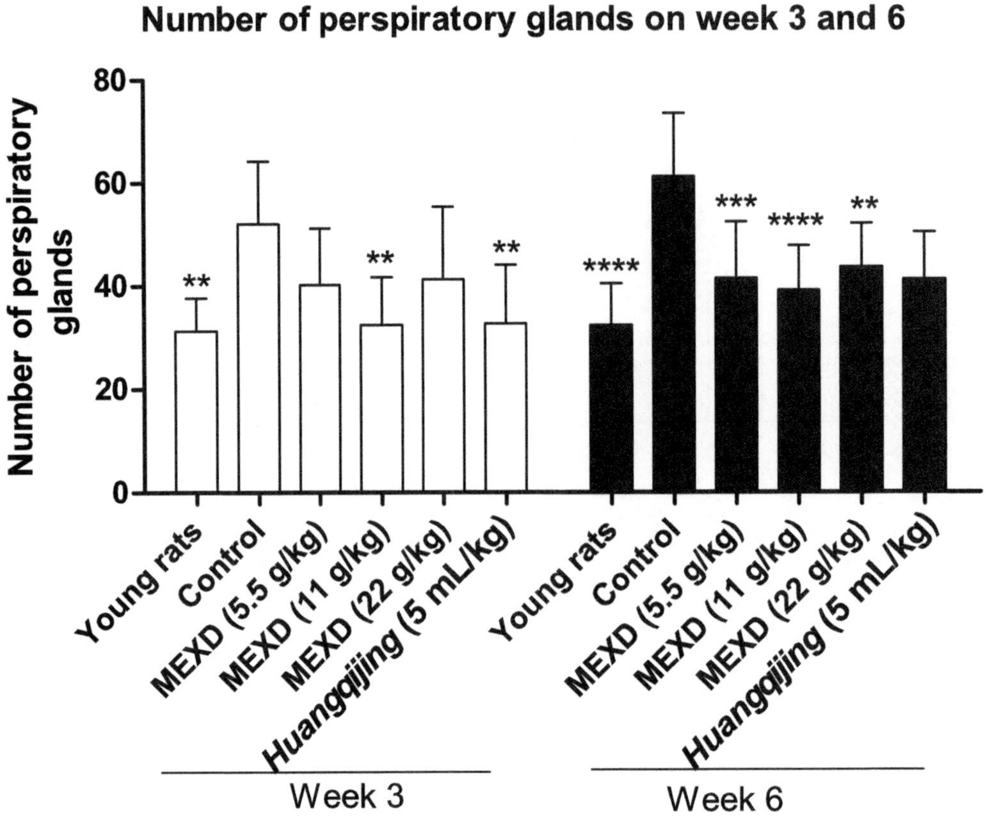

Fig. 7 Antiperspirant effect of MEXD on rats foot pads ($n = 10$, mean ± standard deviation) one-way ANOVA followed by multiple. $^{*}P < 0.05$, $^{**}P \leq 0.01$ and $^{***}P < 0.001$ compared with control. *Week 3* young rats vs. control: $P = 0.0012$, MEXD (11 g/kg) vs. control: $P = 0.0026$, *Huangqijing* vs. control: $P = 0.0032$. *Week 6* young rats vs. control: $P < 0.0001$, MEXD (5.5 g/kg) vs. control: $P = 0.0005$, MEXD (11 g/kg) vs. control: $P < 0.0001$, MEXD (5.5 g/kg) vs. control: $P = 0.0034$

dosage of 11 g/kg, MEXD significantly decreased the number of sweat glands in the menopausal rats after 3 weeks of treatment. All dosages of MEXD were able to inhibit sweat secretion, especially the dose of 11 g/kg, which significantly decreased the number of sweat glands ($P < 0.001$) in the menopausal rats after 6 weeks of treatment.

In the plantar sweat glands of the young rats, the secretory portions lay in clusters among the fat cells of the hypodermis. Irregular connective tissue of the dermis and numerous blood vessels were in the vicinity of the secretory portions (Fig. 8a). In the plantar sweat glands of the menopausal rats in the control group, the number of secretory cells had increased (Fig. 8b). Both the number of secretory cells and the number of vacuoles in the cells were significantly lower in the plantar sweat glands of the menopausal rats after treatment with all dosages of MEXD and *Huangqijing* (Fig. 8c–f).

Discussion

In this study, the anti-menopausal sweating effects of MEXD were evaluated using a 12–14-month-old aged menopausal SD rat model with both irregular estrous cycles and lowered serum E2 levels. All animal models have some limitations, and in this case, the age and physiology of the rats cannot completely mimic human female menopause. The duration of the estrous cycle in SD rats is 3–4 days [27], and the lifespan of the rats is only 2.5–3.5 years [28], while the human menstrual cycle occurs at approximately monthly intervals. During menopause, the ovarian function declines, but the ovaries still synthesize some steroid hormones such as androstenedione, testosterone, and E2 [29]. Thus, the use of ovariectomized female SD rats as an animal model of menopause cannot mimic the physiological states of menopause and ovarian aging in humans. A previous study demonstrated that SD rats have a fertility duration of 3–9 months, indicating that rats aged 12 months and older would correspond to the perimenopause phase in humans [28]. Our unpublished data showed that 12-month-old SD rats undergoing natural aging demonstrated markedly reduced circulating E2 levels compared with 3-month-old rats, indicating that these rats may mimic the human female entering the menopause transition phase. Therefore, our animal model employing 12–14-month-old female SD

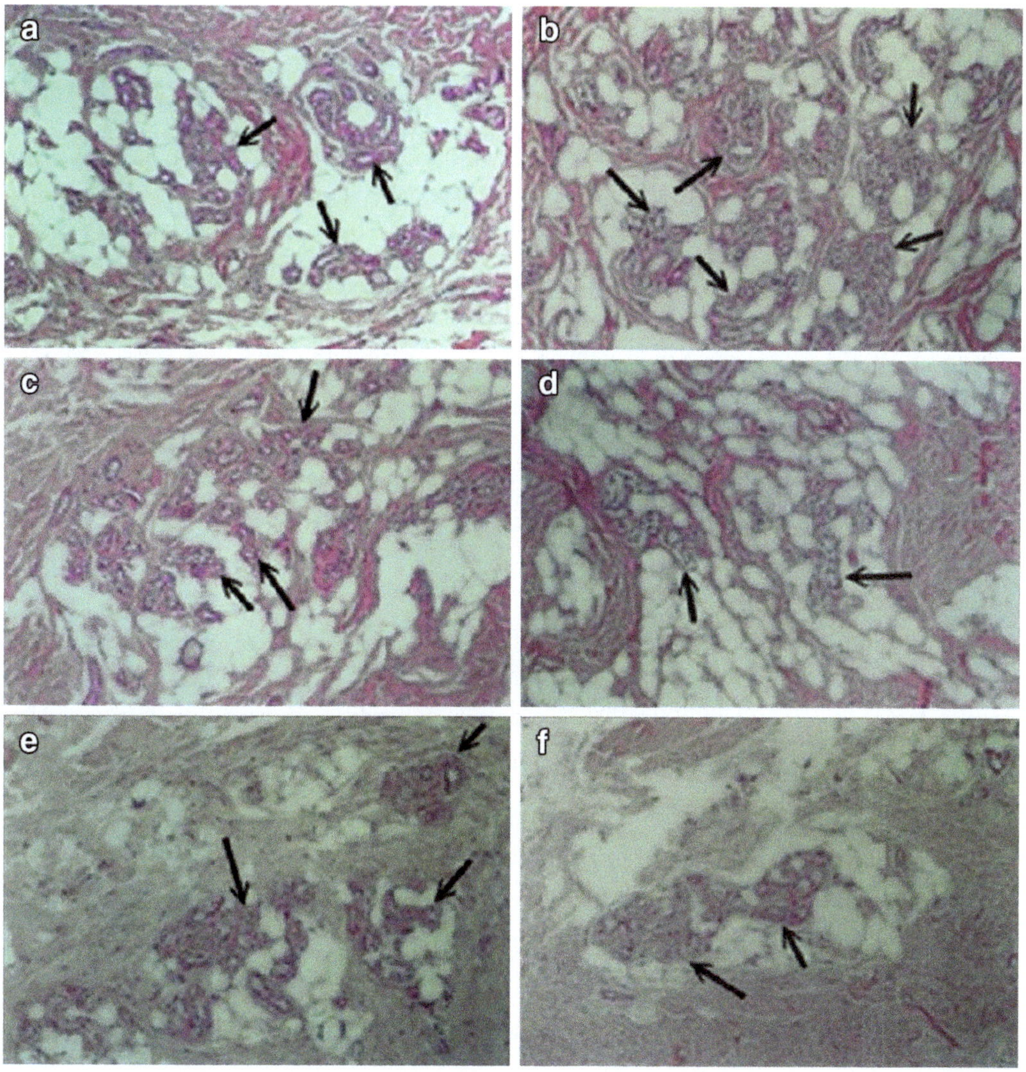

Fig. 8 Secretory portions of rat plantar sweat glands in foot pads (indicated by *solid black arrows*). **a** Young rats; **b** control; **c–e** MEXD (5.5, 11 and 22 g/kg) treated menopausal rats; **f** *Huangqijing* (5 mL/kg) treated menopausal rats. (H&E stain × 100)

rats undergoing natural aging is reasonable. In this study, the estrous phase was determined by vaginal smears, and rats with irregular estrous cycles were regarded as menopausal rats.

To exclude variations in bioactivity caused by inconsistency of herbal extract preparations, HPLC was used to evaluate the quality consistency of the MEXD extract prior to the animal experiments. Nine standard compounds, namely berberine, ferulic acid, icariin, jatrorrhizine, palmatine, schizandrol A, schizandrol B, schizandrin A, and schizandrin B, were selected as markers for evaluating the quality of MEXD (Fig. 1).

Five of these standard chemicals (jatorrhizine, berberine, palmatine, ferulic acid, and icariin) are well-known compounds in EXD according to the Pharmacopoeia of the People's Republic of China [30] and our previous publication [11]. All of these chemicals possess antioxidant activities. Moreover, three of them (ferulic acid, icariin, and berberine) exhibit estrogenic activity. Therefore, these constituents used for quality control are important for the biological activity of the extract. Meanwhile, the markers for *S. chinensis* were not only the major components, but also possessed related pharmaceutical activities [31], including estrogenic and antioxidant activities. Besides, polysaccharides, free amino acids, lignans including schizandrol A, schizandrol B, schizandrin A, and schizandrin B were the major components in *S. chinensis*, and have been commonly used for quality control of *S. chinensis* [32–34]. Based on modern pharmacological studies, schizandrol A and schizandrin B possess antioxidant properties [35]. Schisantherin A manifests estrogenic effects [36]. The interassay RSD values were less than 5% for all nine standard compounds, indicating good quality of the MEXD extract and consistency between different batches of the MEXD extract (Table 1).

Aging is associated with higher levels of oxidative biomolecules reacting with free radicals [36–38]. Menopause or ovariectomy (estrogen deficiency) can induce hot flashes and oxidative stress [38]. In addition, reactive oxygen species attack the heme group of aromatase to inhibit E2 biosynthesis [39]. Previous studies demonstrated that pulsatile release of FSH and LH is related to the mechanism underlying the initiation of hot flashes [40, 41]. Commonly, HRT effectively decreases oxidative stress and relieves hot flashes [42], indicating that estrogen deficiency may increase oxidative stress and hot flashes physiologically. Besides, other studies indicated that increased oxidative stress and MDA levels and decreased antioxidant enzyme SOD levels accompany hot flashes in menopausal women, and these symptoms were reversed after receiving HRT or undertaking yoga exercise [43–45]. The increased production of oxygen free radicals concomitant with aging accelerates the depletion of SOD and hinders SOD synthesis, leading to decreased SOD activity. In this study, the serum SOD activities of menopausal rats in the control group were significantly lower compared with those in the young rats (Fig. 2). The increased MDA contents indicated that lipid peroxidation became more active in menopausal rats, and the antioxidant abilities were declining. Our results revealed that MEXD at the dose of 11 g/kg effectively reduced serum MDA levels and promoted SOD activities (Figs. 2, 3). These findings demonstrate that MEXD treatment can improve the antioxidant ability in aged female rats and potentially slow down the aging process.

The antioxidant activity of MEXD indicates its role in preventing reproductive aging. Along with reproductive aging, the activities of antioxidant enzymes and steroidogenic enzymes including aromatase become lower, suggesting the association between an age-related environment predominated by free radicals and a decrease in estrogen production through the effect on aromatase (Cyp19) activity in the human ovary [5]. It is known that E2 synthesis is mainly mediated by aromatase in ovarian granulosa cells [46]. Our previous publication [11] demonstrated that one of the possible mechanisms underlying the EXD-mediated relief of menopausal syndrome involves increases in endocrine function and serum E2 levels through activation of ovarian aromatase. Moreover, recent findings suggest that the depletion of estrogen in the postmenopausal period can cause oxidative stress in addition to the known symptoms [47], given that E2 itself possesses antioxidative properties. Oxidative stress stimulates hydroperoxide-dependent hydroxylation of E2 to catecholestrogen metabolites, which in turn can undergo reactive oxygen species-producing redox cycling, thus setting up a self-generating toxic cascade offsetting the antioxidant effects generated by the parent E2 [48]. In this study, treatment of menopausal female rats with MEXD promoted the serum activities of the antioxidative enzyme SOD (Fig. 2), thus possibly preventing the damaging effect of free radicals on the aging ovaries.

Apart from the oxidative stress theory of reproductive aging, it is known that as the number of immature follicles declines with age, the negative feedback control of E2 on FSH secretion is relaxed, and therefore the basal circulating level of FSH increases. FSH orchestrates the termination of folliculogenesis in ovaries, and high levels of FSH promote inappropriate maturation of the granulosa cells of the residual prenatal follicles. This asynchronous maturation of the germinal and somatic components results in follicular atresia, leading to a decrease in E2 production [49]. Among the MEXD-treated groups, MEXD at the dosage of 11 g/kg restored the serum E2 levels (Fig. 4) and significantly reversed the increased FSH (Fig. 5) and LH (Fig. 6) levels compared with the control group. These results demonstrated that MEXD can improve the estrogen-deficient state in aged female rats and prevent reproductive aging. Moreover, the weights of the ovaries and uteri as well as their organ indices did not change after MEXD treatment, indicating that MEXD does not exert any observable adverse effects on the rat ovaries and uteri.

The regulatory effects of MEXD on menopausal hormone profiles provide insights into interventions for vasomotor symptoms during menopause. According to the Dynamic Hypothesis, the most widely-accepted current theory [4, 50], hot flashes and sweating result from the dynamic reduction or sudden deprivation of sex hormones rather than their absolute plasma concentrations. Application of MEXD may reverse the estrogen decline during menopause, and thus prevent hot flashes and sweating. To elucidate the effects of MEXD on menopausal sweating, *Huangqijing* oral liquor, an oral preparation composed of *Radix Astragali* extract, with the functions of replenishing *Qi*, nourishing *blood*, and reinforcing *vital Qi* to stop sweating according to Traditional Chinese Medicine theory [51], was selected as the positive control. Our results revealed that sweating in the soles of menopausal rats in the control group increased significantly, while MEXD at the dosage of 11 g/kg significantly reduced such sweating after both 3–6 weeks of treatment (Fig. 7). The results of the histological study also demonstrated an increase in the number of sweat glands in the soles of the menopausal rats (Fig. 8b). On the contrary, the MEXD-treated groups at all dosages (5.5, 11 and 22 g/kg) exhibited conspicuous decreases in the number of secretory cells (Fig. 8c–e). Therefore, the potential efficacy of MEXD against menopausal perspiration involves increases in endocrine function and serum E2 levels through the antioxidant activity pathways.

In Chinese medicine, through insufficiency of *yin*, *yang* cannot be preserved and the asthenia *yang* cannot guard *yin*, and thus *yin* is excreted in the form of sweat. Therefore, clinically, for restoring the *kidney yin* and *yang*, clinicians usually add *S. chinensis*. In Chinese medicine, the flavor of *S. chinensis* is sour, which can restrain *body essence* and nourish *yin*. *A. sinensis* together with *S. chinensis* can restore both *liver blood* and *kidney essence*, which is in accord with the theory of Chinese medicine that the liver and kidney share the same source. Taken together, the whole formula can nourish *kidney yin* by warming the *kidney yang*, and nourish *yin* to preserve asthenia *yang*, and when yin and *yang* reach a balance, menopausal sweating will cease. Chinese medicine mentions that *Tian gui* may refer to steroid hormones, including E2, which play a vital role in the reproductive system and the process of female menopause. In Chinese medicine, kidney-nourishing herb medicines can restore *Tian gui*, which mimics HRT in supplementing E2. This study also indicated that MEXD was able to promote E2 biosynthesis (Fig. 4). Oral HRT was reported to be highly effective in alleviating hot flushes and night sweats [52]. The results of the present study using a menopausal rat model not only provide evidence to support the traditional Chinese medicine theory, but also shed new light on the effects of drugs in alleviating menopausal sweating and menopausal vasomotor symptoms. Interestingly, our study showed that the pharmacological activities of a Chinese medicine formula are different from those a pure chemical drug, as they did not show a dose-dependent response. This finding also indicates that the complexity of Chinese medicines may be attributed to the interactions among multiple compounds within herbal medicines, and that their interactions in the body should be mediated in the manner of a network of intermolecular interactions. Further studies should investigate the unique pharmacological activities of this herbal formula.

In essence, sweating falls within the scope of automatic temperature regulation. Previous studies suggested that hot flashes, consisting of sweating and peripheral vasodilation, are triggered by small elevations in the core body temperature (CBT) acting within a reduced thermoneutral zone in symptomatic postmenopausal women [53]. The narrowing of the zone may be caused by elevated central noradrenergic activation and is probably precipitated by changes in estrogen [54]. Estrogen withdrawal increases the sensitivity of thermoregulatory neural pathways and modifies the activation of heat loss mechanisms. It was also reported that postmenopausal women with symptomatic hot flashes have a significantly lower rectal temperature for the sweating threshold, and their sweating rate is elevated, compared with their premenopausal counterparts [53]. In other words, sweating or hot flashes can reflect thermoregulatory dysfunction in menopausal females. If the effects of MEXD can be identified by dynamic CBT monitoring, we speculate that the alleviation of menopausal sweating by MEXD may be induced by restoration of the narrowed thermoneutral zone. Further studies on the mechanism through which MEXD ameliorates menopausal perspiration are in progress.

Conclusion

Modified *Erxian decoction* significantly inhibited sweat excretion, regulated sex hormones, and exhibited antioxidative effects in menopausal model rats.

Abbreviations

EXD: *Erxian* decoction; MEXD: modified *Erxian* decoction; HRT: hormone replacement therapy; LH: luteinizing hormone; FSH: follicle-stimulating hormone; SD: Sprague–Dawley; E2: estradiol; MDA: malondialdehyde; SOD: superoxide dismutase; CMC-Na: sodium carboxylmethyl cellulose; TBA: thiobarbituric acid; R.S.D.: inter-assay relative standard deviation.

Authors' contributions

SCWS, YBZ and FHW conceived and designed the study. YBZ extracted herbal medicine. WHK and SWW conducted quality control analysis. FHW treated animal and conduct hormone assay and rat foot pad assay. FHW and AHL measured serum antioxidant biochemical parameters. SWW interpreted the data. SWW, ZL, HPC and AHL wrote the manuscript. SCWS, JS, TBN and YT revised the manuscript critically for important intellectual content. All authors read and approved the final manuscript.

Author details

[1] School of Chinese Medicine, LKS Faculty of Medicine, The University of Hong Kong, 10 Sassoon Road, Pokfulam, Hong Kong SAR. [2] Department of Pharmacology, China Pharmaceutical University, Nanjing, China. [3] Department of Physiology, School of Basic Medicine, Shanghai University of Traditional Chinese Medicine, Shanghai, China. [4] School of Biomedical Sciences, Faculty of Medicine, The Chinese University of Hong Kong, Shatin, N.T., Hong Kong SAR.

Acknowledgements

This study was supported by the Industrial Support Fund (No: 200707160012) and research fund (No: 10208016) from the University of Hong Kong. This study was partially supported by the Seed Funding Programme for Basic

Research (project Number 201211159146 and 201411159213), the University of Hong Kong.

Competing interests

The authors declare that they have no competing interests.

References

1. Avis NE, Crawford SL, Greendale G, Bromberger JT, Everson-Rose SA, Gold EB, Hess R, Joffe H, Kravitz HM, Tepper PG, et al. Duration of menopausal vasomotor symptoms over the menopause transition. JAMA Intern Med. 2015;175:531–9.
2. Gold EB, Colvin A, Avis N, Bromberger J, Greendale GA, Powell L, Sternfeld B, Matthews K. Longitudinal analysis of the association between vasomotor symptoms and race/ethnicity across the menopausal transition: study of women's health across the nation. Am J Public Health. 2006;96:1226–35.
3. Richard-Davis G, Manson JE. Vasomotor symptom duration in midlife women-research overturns dogma. Jama Intern Med. 2015;175:540–1.
4. Kouriefs C, Georgiou M, Ravi R. Hot flushes and prostate cancer: pathogenesis and treatment. BJU Int. 2002;89:379–83.
5. Okatani Y, Morioka N, Wakatsuki A, Nakano Y, Sagara Y. Role of the free radical-scavenger system in aromatase activity of the human ovary. Horm Res. 1993;39(Suppl 1):22–7.
6. Meldrum DR, Defazio JD, Erlik Y, Lu JK, Wolfsen AF, Carlson HE, Hershman JM, Judd HL. Pituitary hormones during the menopausal hot flash. Obstet Gynecol. 1984;64:752–6.
7. Cheema D, Coomarasamy A, El-Toukhy T. Non-hormonal therapy of post-menopausal vasomotor symptoms: a structured evidence-based review. Arch Gynecol Obstet. 2007;276:463–9.
8. Huntley A. Drug-herb interactions with herbal medicines for menopause. J Br Menopause Soc. 2004;10:162–5.
9. Kashani L, Bathaei F, Ojaghi M, Bathaei M, Akondzadeh S. A systematic review of herbal medicinal products for the treatment of menopausal symptoms. J Med Plants Res. 2004;3:1–13.
10. Zhang C, Wang S, Zhang Y, Chen J, Liang X. In vitro estrogenic activities of Chinese medicinal plants traditionally used for the management of menopausal symptoms. J Ethnopharmacol. 2005;98:295–300.
11. Sze SCW, Tong Y, Zhang YB, Zhang ZJ, Lau AS, Wong HK, Tsang KW, Ng TB. A novel mechanism: Erxian Decoction, a Chinese medicine formula, for relieving menopausal syndrome. J Ethnopharmacol. 2009;123:27–33.
12. Newton KM, Grady D. Soy isoflavones for prevention of menopausal bone loss and vasomotor symptoms: comment on "Soy isoflavones in the prevention of menopausal bone loss and menopausal symptoms". Jama Intern Med. 2011;171:1369–70.
13. Sze SCW, Wong WK, Tong Y, Zhang YB, Cheung HP. Novel bioactive protein isolated from Chinese yam. Alexandria: USPTO; 2011.
14. Wong KL, Lai PYM, Li KW, Lee KF, Ng TB, Cheung HP, Zhang YB, Lao L, Wong RNS, Shaw PC, Wong JH, Zhang ZJ, Lam JK, Ye WC, Sze SCW. A novel, stable, estradiol-stimulating, osteogenic yam protein with potential for the treatment of menopausal syndrome. Sci Rep. 2015;5:10179.
15. Wang SW, Tong Y, Ng TB, Lao L, Lam JK, Zhang KY, Zhang ZJ, Sze SCW. Network pharmacological identification of active compounds and potential actions of Erxian decoction in alleviating menopause-related symptoms. Chin Med. 2015;10:19.
16. Sze SCW, Ip CW, Ng TB, Zhang KY, Zhang Z-J, Cheung HP, Cheng CLY, Tong Y. Compatibility of multiple herbal components in Erxian decoction, a Chinese medicinal formula, for treating osteoporosis. Eur J Intergr Med. 2012;4:e187–96.
17. Guo LQ, Zang P, Huang L, Xu GH. Research progress on pharmacological action of Fructus Schisandrae Chinensis. Acta Chin Med Pharmacol. 2006;34:51–3.
18. Su YM, Zhang Z. The treatment of the peri-menopausal syndrome by EXD added-other herbs on 56 cases. Hebei J Tradit Chin Med. 2006;28:290.
19. Am Z. Treatment menopausal symptom by modified Er-xian decoction in 106 women. Yunan J Tradit Chin Med. 2008;29:36.
20. Wang X, Song P, Zhang Q, Wang ZQ. Experience on application of convergence method to treat the menopause hyperhidrosis. World Chin Med. 2013;8:1.
21. Wang CH, Li F, Xing L, Zhang ZH. Er-xian decoction treating menopausal symptoms in 50 women. Shanxi J Tradit Chin Med. 1997;18:253.
22. Huang JH, Huang HX, Chen ZY, Zheng C, Jui Y. Dose conversion among different animals and healthy volunteers in pharmacological study. Chin J Clin Pharmacol Ther. 2004;9:3.
23. Helman MD, Re TA, Lukacsko AB. Antiperspirant activity of H1-histamine blockers as determined by a modified rat foot pad assay. Pharm Res. 1989;6:883–6.
24. Marcy R, Quermonne M. Inhibition of palmar skin conductance in mice by antiperspirants. J Soc Cosmet Chem. 1976;27:333.
25. Habecker BA, Symes AJ, Stahl N, Francis NJ, Economides A, Fink J, Yancopoulos GD, Landis SC. A sweat gland-derived differentiation activity acts through known cytokine signaling pathways. J Biol Chem. 1997;272:30421–8.
26. Myers M, Britt KL, Wreford NG, Ebling FJ, Kerr JB. Methods for quantifying follicular numbers within the mouse ovary. Reproduction. 2004;127:569–80.
27. Butcher R, Collins W, Fugo N. Plasma concentration of LH, FSH, prolactin, progesterone and estradiol-17β throughout the 4-day estrous cycle of the rat. Endocrinology. 1974;94:1704–8.
28. Sengupta P. The laboratory rat: relating its age with human's. Int J Prev Med. 2013;4:624–30.
29. Shifren JL, Schiff I. The aging ovary. J Women's Health Gend Based Med. 2000;9:3–7.
30. Zaban A, Ban XS. Pharmacopoeia of the People's Republic of China. People's Medical Publishing House. 2005; 66, 229, 289, 255, 214, 148.
31. Ye C. Formulation design and development of transdermal delivery system-nanoemulsion of Schizandrol A. Singapore: Thesis NUS; 2013.
32. Guangxin F. Study on the quality control method and the extraction of the antioxidant activity of the extract of Fructus. Changchun: The University of Jilin; 2012.
33. Caili Z, Xueli H. Research progress of Fructus *Schisandrae Chinensis*. J Baoding Teach Coll. 2004;10:36–9.
34. Yang Qing QX, Li H, Jin D, Lyu G, Wang J, Wang B, Li NA. Schisandra chemical composition and pharmacological action research. Jilin J Tradi Chin Med. 2015;35:3.
35. Chiu PY, Leung HY, Poon MK, Ko KM. Chronic schisandrin B treatment improves mitochondrial antioxidant status and tissue heat shock protein production in various tissues of young adult and middle-aged rats. Biogerontology. 2006;7:199–210.
36. Liu HW, Yu XZ, Padula D, Pescitelli G, Lin ZW, Wang F, Ding K, Lei M, Gao JM. Lignans from *Schisandra* sphenathera Rehd. et Wils. and semisynthetic schisantherin A analogues: absolute configuration, and their estrogenic and anti-proliferative activity. Eur J Med Chem. 2013;59:265–73.
37. Oliveira BF, Nogueira-Machado JA, Chaves MM. The role of oxidative stress in the aging process. Sci World J. 2010;10:1121–8.
38. Mendoza CCC, Zamarripa CAJ. Menopause induces oxidative stress. Oxidative Stress and Chronic Degenerative Diseases - A Role for Antioxidants. InTech. 2013. doi:10.5772/52082. Available from: http://www.intechopen.com/books/oxidative-stress-and-chronic-degenerative-diseases-a-role-forantioxidants/menopause-induces-oxidative-stress.
39. Fujii J, Iuchi Y, Okada F. Fundamental roles of reactive oxygen species and protective mechanisms in the female reproductive system. Reprod Biol Endocr. 2005;3:43.
40. Tataryn IV, Meldrum DR, Lu K, Fruraar AM, Judd HL. LH, FSH and skin temperature during the menopausal hot flas. J Clin Endocr Metab. 1979;49:152–4.
41. Randolph JF Jr, Sowers M, Bondarenko I, Gold EB, Greendale GA, Bromberger JT, Brockwell SE, Matthews KA. The relationship of longitudinal change in reproductive hormones and vasomotor symptoms during the menopausal transition. J Clin Endocrinol Metab. 2005;90:6106–12.
42. Leal M, Díaz J, Serrano E, Abellán J, Carbonell LF. Hormone replacement therapy for oxidative stress in postmenopausal women with hot flushes. Am J Obstet Gynecol. 2000;95:804–9.
43. Yasui T, Uemura H, Takikawa M, Irahara M. Hormone replacement therapy in postmenopausal women. Int J Med Invest. 2003;50:136–45.

44. Unfer TC, Conterato GM, da Silva JC, Duarte MM, Emanuelli T. Influence of hormone replacement therapy on blood antioxidant enzymes in menopausal women. Clin Chim Acta. 2006;369:73–7.
45. Ross A, Thomas S. The health benefits of yoga and exercise: a review of comparison studies. J Altern Complement Med. 2010;16:3–12.
46. Simpson ER, Mahendroo MS, Means GD, Kilgore MW, Hinshelwood MM, Graham-Lorence S, Amarneh B, Ito Y, Fisher CR, Michael MD, et al. Aromatase cytochrome P450, the enzyme responsible for estrogen biosynthesis. Endocr Rev. 1994;15:342–55.
47. Sanchez-Rodriguez M, Zacarias-Flores M, Arronte-Rosales A, Correa-Muñoz E, Mendoza-Nunez VM. Menopause as risk factor for oxidative stress. Menopause. 2012;19:361–7.
48. Nilsen J. Estradiol and neurodegenerative oxidative stress. Front Neuroendocrinol. 2008;29:463–75.
49. Alviggi C, Humaidan P, Howles CM, Tredway D, Hillier SG. Biological versus chronological ovarian age: implications for assisted reproductive technology. Reprod Biol Endocrinol. 2009;7:101.
50. Shanafelt TD, Barton DL, Adjei AA, Loprinzi CL. Pathophysiology and treatment of hot flashes. Mayo Clin Proc. 2002;77:1207–18.
51. Ziming ZM. Effect of XueHanjing oral fluid on mice hidropoiesis inhibition function. Sichuan J Physiol Sci. 2004;26:104–6.
52. MacLennan A, Lester S, Moore V. Oral estrogen replacement therapy versus placebo for hot flushes: a systematic review. Climacteric. 2001;4:58–74.
53. Freedman RR. Pathophysiology and treatment of menopausal hot flashes. Semin Reprod Med. 2005;23:117–25.
54. Sturdee DW. The menopausal hot flush–anything new? Maturitas. 2008;60:42–9.

13

Antidiabetic and antioxidant effects of catalpol extracted from *Rehmannia glutinosa* (Di Huang) on rat diabetes induced by streptozotocin and high-fat, high-sugar feed

Huifeng Zhu[1,2], Yuan Wang[1,2], Zhiqiang Liu[3], Jinghuan Wang[1,2], Dong Wan[4*], Shan Feng[1,2], Xian Yang[1,2] and Tao Wang[1,2]

Abstract

Background: Diabetes, associated with hyperlipidemia and oxidative stress, would lead to an increased production of reactive oxygen species. *Rehmannia glutinosa* (Di Huang) is widely used to nourish *yin*, invigorate the *kidney* (*shen*), and treat *xiao ke* (a diabetes-like syndrome in Chinese medicine). This study aims to investigate the antidiabetic and antioxidant effects of catalpol from *R. glutinosa* on rat diabetes induced by streptozotocin (STZ) and high-fat, high-sugar feed.

Methods: Rats (eight rats in each group at least) were induced diabetes by an initial high-fat high-sugar feed for 3 weeks, followed by an intraperitoneal injection of STZ (30 mg/kg) for 3 days, and rats were fasted overnight before treatments. Catalpol at a dose of 0, 5, 10, 20 or 50 mg/kg was administrated through bolus intravenous injection to the experimental rats to find the most effective anti-hyperglycemic dose of catalpol to further study body weight loss, water intake, and food intake. The most effective catalpol dose was given to the diabetic model rats with hyperlipidemia, and the levels of blood sugar, plasma total cholesterol (TC), triglyceride (TG), and high-density lipoprotein cholesterol (HDL-C) were measured after catalpol administration once a day for 2 weeks. An oral glucose challenge test (OGCT) was performed after above experiments in which the most effective dose of catalpol has been determined. Levels of glutathione peroxidase (GSH-PX), catalase (CAT), superoxide dismutase (SOD), and malondialdehyde (MDA) were measured by corresponding reagent kits and morphological changes of the pancreas were observed with histopathological examination using H&E stain.

Results: Catalpol at a dose of 50 mg/kg ameliorated body weight loss and increased water and food intake. Catalpol also attenuated the increase of plasma TC ($P = 0.0067$) and TG ($P = 0.0084$) and increased HDL-C ($P = 0.0336$). The OGCT revealed that catalpol reduced the increase of plasma glucose. The activities of antioxidative enzymes (SOD, $P = 0.0037$; GSH-PX, $P = 0.0066$; CAT, $P = 0.005$) were enhanced and MDA was reduced ($P = 0.003$). Furthermore, catalpol reduced the morphological impairment of the pancreas.

Conclusion: Catalpol protected against STZ-induced diabetes with high-fat and high-sugar feed with ameliorated structural impairment of the pancreas and restored balance between oxidative enzymes and antioxidative enzymes.

*Correspondence: wandongcqykdx@126.com
[4] Department of Emergency, The First Affiliated Hospital of Chongqing Medical University, POB 400016, Chongqing, China
Full list of author information is available at the end of the article

Background

Diabetes mellitus is a heterogeneous metabolic disorder characterized by chronic hyperglycemia. It is associated with long-term complications and results in various bodily dysfunctions [1]. Diabetes often leads to the vascular complications of coronary artery disease and cerebrovascular disease and can cause renal failure, blindness, limb amputation, neurological complications, and premature death. With rapid therapeutic advancements, novel treatments with fewer side effects have become more feasible for long-term management of this disorder [2].

Rehmannia glutinosa (Di Huang) is a widely used herb in Chinese medicine (CM) that belongs to the Scrophulariaceae family. It has a high medicinal value and is taken to nourish *yin* and invigorate the *kidney* in CM [3]. *R. glutinosa* is often used to treat *xiao ke* [4], both *xiao ke* and diabetes patients experience the "3Ps": polyuria (frequent urination), polydipsia (increased thirst), and polyphagia (increased hunger). CM theory attributes *yin* deficiency to diabetes [4] and *R. glutinosa* is often clinically used to ameliorate patients' symptoms.

Catalpol, an iridoid glucoside of *R. glutinosa*, has many biological effects, including anticytotoxic and anti-inflammatory properties. Catalpol protected mesencephalic neurons from 1-methyl-4-phenylpyridinium [MPP(+)]-induced oxidative stress [5]. It also protected against hydrogen peroxide-induced apoptosis by preventing cytochrome c release and inactivating the caspase cascade, [6] against hydrogen peroxide-induced oxidative damage [7], and against ischemia-induced damage in astrocytes. Moreover, in an animal model, catalpol treatment ameliorated cognitive deficits and attenuated oxidative damage in brains of aging mice induced by d-galactose, increased the activities of SOD and GSH-PX, and reduced MDA levels in the liver and spleen [8].

Recent works have demonstrated catalpol's anti-hyperglycemic effect in streptozotocin (STZ)-induced [2] and alloxan-induced rat diabetes [9, 10]. Catalpol could increase glucose use to lower plasma glucose in diabetic rats lacking insulin [2] through increasing beta-endorphin secretion from the adrenal gland in STZ-diabetic rats [11]. Moreover, oral supplementation of catalpol ameliorates diabetic encephalopathy by attenuating oxidative stress and increasing nerve growth factor concentration [1]. It ameliorated diabetic nephropathy [12] in rats by reducing the expression of pro-inflammatory mediators, such as monocyte chemotactic protein-1, tumor necrosis factor-alpha, inducible nitric oxide synthase, and receptors for advanced glycation endproducts (AGE). Catalpol suppressed AGE-induced phosphorylation of mitogen activated protein kinases, degradation of IkappaBalpha, and the nuclear localization of nuclear factor-kappaB [13]. Most studies of the effects of catalpol on diabetes mellitus have used normal diets in experimental models of chemical diabetes. However, type 2 diabetes mellitus is usually accompanied by glycolipid metabolism disorders and the effect of catalpol on type 2 diabetes mellitus with hyperlipid syndrome after a high-fat diet is still unknown.

This study aims to investigate the antidiabetic and antioxidant effects of catalpol from *R. glutinosa* on rat diabetes induced by STZ and high-fat, high-sugar feed. STZ and alloxan have been used to induce a diabetes mellitus model and damage the pancreas. Oxidative stress produced by STZ and alloxan is involved in diabetes mellitus and catalpol seems to have good anti-oxidative stress properties. In the present study, STZ-induced diabetes mellitus with a high-sugar and high-fat diet was used to imitate human type 2 diabetes mellitus. We investigated the effects of catalpol on glucose and fat metabolism in STZ-induced diabetic rats and measured oxidative enzyme and antioxidative enzyme plasma levels to explore the possible mechanisms of catalpol on type 2 diabetes mellitus.

Methods

Materials

STZ was obtained from Sigma-Aldrich Inc. (Sigma, S0130, USA). Analytical grade catalpol (product >99 % purity) was purchased from Liubobainiao Biotechnology Co., Ltd (Shijiazhuang, China). Blood glucose Span Diagnostic kit and Jinque test strips was obtained from Shanghai MicroSence Inc. (Shanghai, China). Blood lipid commercially available kits, CAT, GSH-PX, SOD and MDA commercially available kits were from Nanjing Jiancheng Bioengineering Institute (China).

Experimental animals and feeds

One hundred twenty male Wistar rats (200–250 g) were procured from the Experimental Animal Center, Chongqing Medical University, China. The rats were arbitrarily divided into four groups: normal group ($n = 8$), high-sugar and high-fat feed (high-fat, $n = 8$) group, STZ-diabetic animals with high-sugar and high-fat feed (STZ-fat, $n = 12$), and STZ-diabetic animals with high-sugar and high-fat feed treated with catalpol (STZ-fat-cat, $n = 12$).

Rats were kept in an air-conditioned room maintained at a constant temperature (24–26 °C) and humidity (50–60 %) under a 12-h light/dark cycle (07:00 on and 19:00 off). Standard rat feed and water were provided ad libitum. The rats were allowed to acclimatize to the laboratory environment for 7 days before the start of the experiment. All experimental procedures were conducted in conformity with institutional guidelines for the care and use of laboratory animals in China (Permit:

SCXK 2002A040), and the international guidelines on the ethical use of animals (NIH publications No. 80–23, revised 1996).

The high-sugar, high-fat diet was comprised of normal diet 54 kg, sucrose 16.5 kg, lard 8.31 kg, egg yolk 4.14 kg, and salt 83.4 g, with a total combined weight of 83.784 kg [14, 15]. The normal diet was purchased from Beijing China Fukang Biotechnology Co., Ltd (Beijing, China). The main components of the normal diet were crude protein $\geq$18 %, crude fat $\geq$4 %, crude fiber $\geq$5 %, crude ash $\leq$8 %, moisture $\leq$10 %, lysine $\geq$0.82 %, calcium 1–1.8 %, phosphorus 0.6–1.2 %, and salt 0.2–0.8 %.

Induction of diabetes in rats

Diabetes was induced by an initial high-sugar and high-fat feed for 3 weeks, followed by an intraperitoneal injection of STZ (30 mg/kg) for 3 days. STZ was dissolved in a freshly prepared 0.01 M citrate buffer (pH 4.5). The normal control group was injected with buffer alone. Rats with blood glucose $\geq$16.7 mmol/L for 3 weeks were considered as diabetic [16] and the death rates for modeling of STZ-fat were 22–28 %.

Experimental design and catalpol treatment of rats

At the first stage, catalpol was injected into the rat tail vein at a dose of 0, 5, 10, 20, or 50 mg/kg. Blood was collected after catalpol treatment for 14 days to assess the blood glucose-lowering effect of catalpol.

At the second stage, the most effective dose of catalpol was selected for further study. The plasma lipid level was detected in the normal, high-sugar and high fat feed, STZ-fat, and STZ-fat-cat groups at 14 days after treatment with catalpol. The plasma in each group was collected and then antioxidative enzymes such as GSH-PX, SOD, CAT, and the MDA oxidative products were detected with corresponding kits. Oral glucose challenge tests (OGCT) were then performed on experimental rats using a Roche blood glucose monitor (Roche Diagnostics, Rotkreuz, Switzerland.) with Jinque test strips. During the experiment, body weight, food intake, and water intake were recorded every 2 days. Finally, a splenic portion of pancreatic tissue was removed immediately after sacrifice to observe morphological changes of the pancreas.

Determination of plasma glucose

Blood samples were collected from the inner canthus using a capillary tube under chloral hydrate anesthesia at each time point. Concentration of blood glucose was determined by a glucose meter (Roche Diagnostics, Rotkreuz, Switzerland) with Jinque test strips (Span Biotech Ltd, India).

Plasma collection and biochemical determination

Blood samples were collected from the inner canthus using a capillary tube under chloral hydrate anesthesia after catalpol treatment for 14 days. The samples were centrifuged at 2810×*g* for 10 min at 4 °C within 1 h after collection, and then supernatants were collected. The concentration of plasma total cholesterol (TC), triglyceride (TG), and high-density lipoprotein cholesterol (HDL-C); the activities of SOD, GSH-PX, CAT and the concentration of MDA were determined by a series of commercially available kits including SOD, GSH-PX, CAT, and MDA kits (Nanjing Jiancheng Bioengineering Institute, China) according to the manufacturers' instructions.

Oral glucose challenge test

An OGCT was performed according to a method previously described with minor modifications [17–19]. Briefly, catalpol at the most effective dose, or the same volume of vehicle, was injected intravenously into rats for 14 days. Then a glucose dose of 2.5 g/kg was intragastrically administrated to the rats. Blood samples were collected sequentially from the tail vein before (0 h) and 0.5, 1, 2, 3, 5, 7, and 9 h post challenge. Plasma glucose changes at the indicated time were determined with a glucose meter (Accu-Chek, Switzerland) and Jinque test strips.

Histological evaluation of pancreas with hematoxylin and eosin (H&E) staining

A splenic portion of pancreatic tissue was removed immediately after sacrifice and rinsed with ice-cold saline. The tissue samples were fixed in 4 % buffered neutral paraformaldehyde solution overnight, embedded in paraffin, and deparaffinized using standard procedures [20, 21]. Thin Sections (5 μm) were dewaxed, dehydrated in a graded series of ethanol, and rehydrated, then stained with H&E for light microscopic examination (Leica, Germany). All histological analyses were performed in arbitrarily selected fields in sections by two investigators blinded to the identity of the treatment groups.

Statistical analysis

All data were analyzed by the SPSS statistical software (version 13.0, SPSS, Chicago, IL, USA), with $P < 0.05$ values were considered as statistically significant. Results were expressed as mean ± standard deviation (SD). Comparisons between the groups were assessed by paired-samples *t* test, and *P* value correction for multiple group comparison by LSD-*t* test. Dose-dependent manner of catalpol's hyperglycemic action was visually determined from a dose–response curve.

Results

Dose-dependent anti-hyperglycemic action of catalpol

Catalpol at higher doses lowered plasma glucose concentrations more effectively in STZ-fat-diabetic rats. A dose-dependent increase of anti-hyperglycemic activity was observed in STZ-fat-diabetic rats upon intravenous injection of catalpol at the dose range 10–50 mg/kg for 2 weeks (Fig. 1). There was no additional effect of catalpol with an increase in dosage beyond 50 mg/kg. The minimal and maximal plasma glucose-lowering activities of catalpol in STZ-fat-diabetic rats were 21.7 ± 1.3 % at 10 mg/kg and 65.8 ± 3.07 % at 50 mg/kg.

Effects of catalpol on body weight

As shown in Fig. 2, after adaptation feed for 1 week, and then high-fat and high-sugar feed for 3 weeks, the initial body weight and the body weight increase in each group were similar. After administration of STZ, the body weight of the STZ-fat-diabetic rats continued to reduce. At the end of the study, the diabetic rats in all groups had lost body weight even when compared with their weight after high-fat and high-sugar feeding for 3 weeks ($P = 0.047$). However, the final body weight in the catalpol group was significantly greater than the body weight in the STZ-fat-diabetic rats ($P = 0.009$) and was close to the starting weight.

Effects of catalpol on feed consumption

After adaptation feed for 1 week, and high-fat and high-sugar feed for 3 weeks, food intake starting in the high-fat and high-sugar feed period increased quickly in the first 2 weeks, then began to decrease, and increased obviously when STZ was given to induce diabetes in the STZ-fat-diabetic group (Fig. 3). When catalpol was given for 4 days, the food intake obviously reduced compared with that of STZ-fat-diabetic rats administered with same volume of vehicle ($P = 0.045$), and continued to reduce for 14 days after catalpol treatment ($P = 0.020$–0.045).

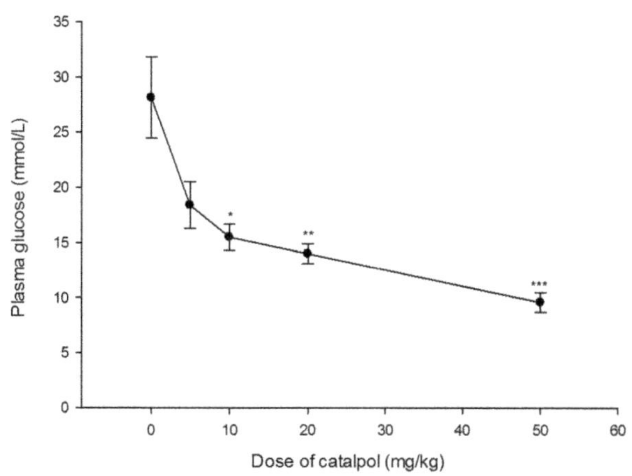

Fig. 1 Anti-hyperglycemic action of catalpol for 2 weeks in STZ-diabetic rats with high-sugar and high-fat diet. Values (mean ± SD) were obtained from eight animals through intravenous injection (iv) of catalpol at the indicated dose. $^*P = 0.02$, $^{**}P = 0.005$ and $^{***}P < 0.001$ as compared with no treatment values (0 mg/kg)

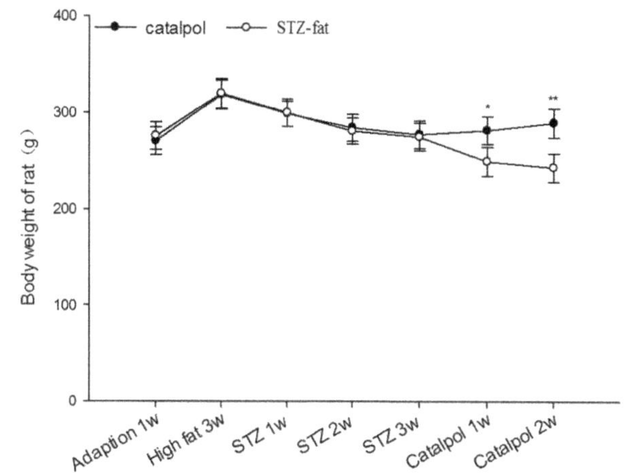

Fig. 2 Effects of catalpol on body weight gains of rats. After given high-sugar high-fat food for 3 weeks, and STZ induced STZ-fat-diabetic rats successfully for 3 weeks, a solution of catalpol at 50 mg/kg or the same volume of vehicle was injected intravenously into rats. Changes of body weight at the indicated time point were compared between the catalpol-treated group (*solid circles*) and the vehicle-treated group (*open circles*). Values (mean ± SD) of each group were obtained from eight animals. $^*P = 0.047$ and $^{**}P = 0.009$ as compared with vehicle-treated group at the same time

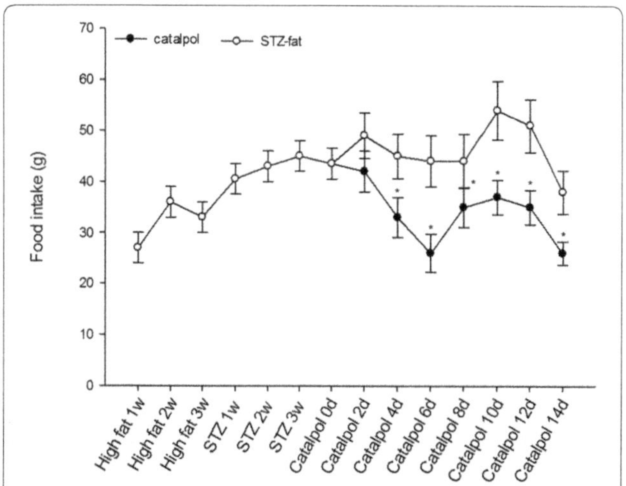

Fig. 3 Effect of catalpol on food consumption of rats. After given high-fat high-sugar food for 3 weeks, and STZ induced STZ-fat-diabetic rats successfully for 3 weeks, a solution of catalpol at 50 mg/kg or the same volume of vehicle was injected intravenously into rats. Changes of food intake at the indicated time point were compared between the catalpol-treated group (*solid circles*) and the vehicle-treated group (*open circles*). Values (mean ± SD) of each group were obtained from eight animals. $^*P < 0.05$ as compared with vehicle-treated group at the same time

Effects of catalpol on water intake

As shown in Fig. 4, after adaptation feed for 1 week, and then high-fat and high-sugar feed for 3 weeks, water intake increased quickly starting in the high-fat and high-sugar feed period, and continued to increase for 3 weeks after STZ-fat-diabetes was successfully induced. After catalpol treatment for 6, 8, and 10 days, the water intake obviously reduced compared with water intake in the STZ-fat-diabetic rats administered with the same volume of vehicle ($P = 0.05$, 0.034, 0.048, respectively). At 12 and 14 days, water intake reduced significantly compared with the control rats ($P = 0.0087$, 0.0089, respectively).

Anti-hyperglycemic action of catalpol in rat diabetes induced by STZ with high-sugar and high-fat feed

No group differences in plasma sugar were found before STZ administration (Fig. 5). Plasma sugar reached 16.7 mmol/L for 1 week after STZ was given, and plasma sugar in each group became gradually elevated. However, plasma sugar decreased significantly after catalpol (50 mg/kg) treatment for 2 weeks, compared with that of the STZ-fat-diabetic rats ($P = 0.0031$), and plasma sugar recovered to the level before STZ administration.

Anti-hyperlipid action of catalpol

As shown in Fig. 6, TC and TG were obviously elevated in rats given the high-fat and high-sugar diet for 3 weeks compared with the normal group ($P = 0.036$, 0.04, respectively) and HDL-C decreased significantly ($P = 0.045$). After STZ administration, TC and TG increased remarkably ($P = 0.0067$, 0.0058, respectively) compared with those of the high-fat group and the HDL-C in the high-fat group was reduced compared with that of the normal group ($P = 0.044$). STZ-fat-diabetic rats treated with catalpol (50 mg/kg) showed

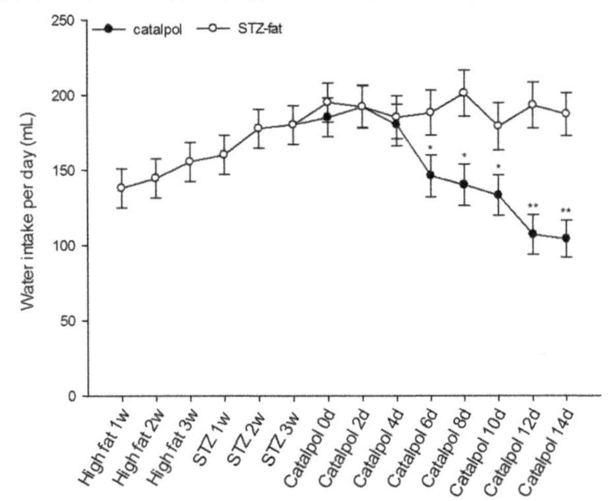

Fig. 4 Effect of catalpol on water intake of rats. After given high-fat high-sugar food for 3 weeks, and treatment by STZ for 3 days induced STZ-fat-diabetic rats successfully for 3 weeks. A solution of catalpol at 50 mg/kg or the same volume of vehicle was injected intravenously into rats. Changes of water intake at the indicated time point were compared between the catalpol-treated group (*solid circles*) and the vehicle-treated group (*open circles*). Values (mean ± SD) of each group were obtained from eight animals. $^*P < 0.05$ and $^{**}P < 0.01$ as compared with vehicle-treated group at the same time

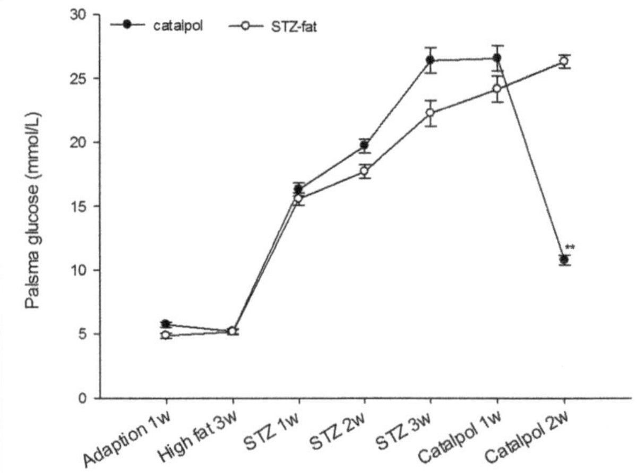

Fig. 5 Anti-hyperglycemic action of catalpol for 2 weeks in STZ-diabetic rats with high-sugar and high-fat feed. Values (mean ± SD) were obtained from eight animals through intravenous injection (iv) of catalpol at 50 mg/kg dose. $^*P = 0.0031$ as compared with non-treated group (*saline*)

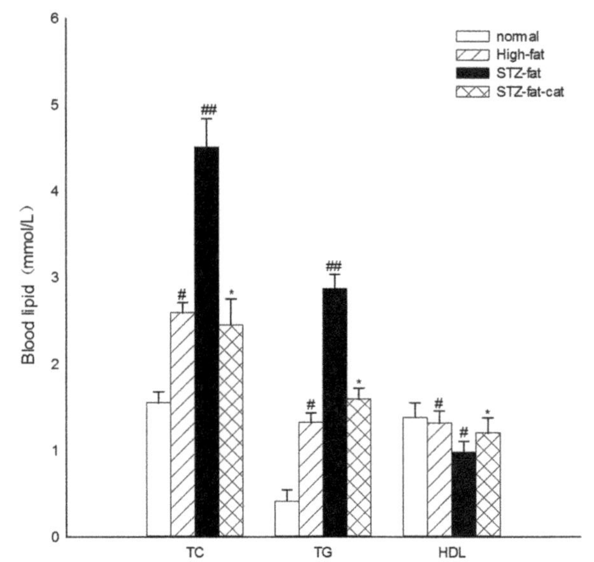

Fig. 6 Anti-hyperlipid action of catalpol for 2 weeks in STZ-diabetic rats with high-sugar and high-fat feed. Values (mean ± SD) were obtained from eight animals through intravenous injection (iv) of catalpol at 50 mg/kg dose. $^{\#}P < 0.05$ vs. normal; $^{\#\#}P < 0.01$ vs. high fat group and $^*P < 0.05$ vs. STZ-fat group

significantly attenuated TC ($P = 0.0067$) and TG ($P = 0.0084$) compared with the high-fat group. The level of HDL-C obviously increased ($P = 0.0336$), although TC, TG, and HDL-C levels did not all return to normal.

Effects of catalpol on the oral glucose challenge test in STZ-fat-diabetic rats

An OGCT was then carried out to determine the glucose clearance. The plasma glucose concentration was elevated in both vehicle- and catalpol-treated rats 30 min after oral glucose administration (Fig. 7). However, there were no statistically significant differences in plasma glucose concentration between the catalpol group and the vehicle group within 3 h after treatment. The increased plasma glucose induced by the oral glucose was significantly lower in the rats at 3 h in the catalpol group compared with the vehicle-treated rats ($P = 0.046$), and this pattern continued for 5 h ($P = 0.0076$), 7 h ($P < 0.001$), and 9 h ($P < 0.001$), finally returning to normal. It means that significantly higher plasma glucose concentrations were detected in the vehicle-treated group at 3, 5, 7, and 9 h time points as compared to that in the catalpol group. This suggested that catalpol could enhance glucose use in vivo.

Effects of catalpol on oxidative stress in STZ-treated diabetic rats

The activities of antioxidative enzymes and the MDA plasma concentrations were shown in Fig. 8. There were

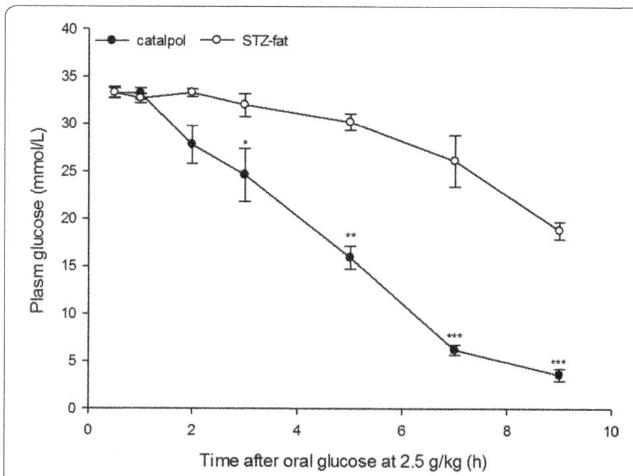

Fig. 7 Effect of catalpol on plasma glucose levels in STZ-fat diabetic rats in an oral glucose challenge test. A solution of catalpol at 50 mg/kg or the same volume of vehicle was intragastrically administrated into rats. Then, a glucose dose of 2.5 g/kg was intragastric administration into each rat. Changes of plasma glucose at the indicated time were compared between the catalpol-treated group (*solid circles*) and the vehicle-treated group (*open circles*). Values (mean ± SD) of each group were obtained from eight animals. **P* < 0.05, ***P* < 0.01, and ****P* < 0.001 as compared with vehicle-treated group at the same time

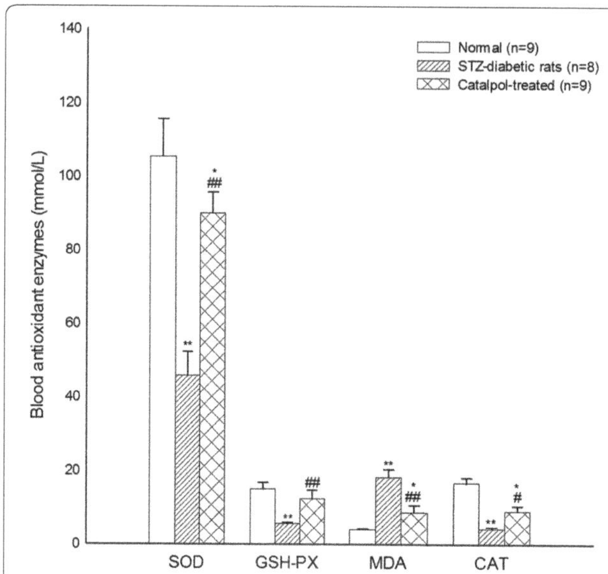

Fig. 8 Effect of catalpol on the activities of antioxidant enzymes and the concentration of MDA in the plasma. **P* < 0.05, ***P* < 0.01 vs. normal group, #*P* < 0.05, ##*P* < 0.01 vs. STZ-treated group

no significant differences in oxidative stress between the high-fat and the normal group, although a rising trend in MDA and a decreasing trend in GSH-PX, SOD, and CAT activity were found in the high-fat group. The activities of GSH-PX, SOD, and CAT ($P = 0.008, 0.002, 0.007$, respectively) in STZ-treated diabetic rats were significantly lower than in the normal control rats and high-fat rats, while the concentration of MDA ($P = 0.006$)in STZ-treated diabetic rats was significantly greater than in the normal control rats. Catalpol significantly improved the activities of antioxidative enzymes and decreased MDA concentration.

Effect of catalpol on morphological changes of the pancreas

Only minimal pancreatic histological changes were observed in the high-fat group, compared with normal pancreatic tissue (Fig. 9a). Minimal inflammatory cells were infiltrated into the intralobular area and around the pancreatic ducts (Fig. 9b). However, in the STZ-fat-diabetic group, the pancreatic ducts were hypertense and markedly dilated, there was much infiltration of inflammatory cells in the intralobular and periductal areas, the exocrine glands of the pancreas were atrophic, and the fibrotic areas were markedly distributed around the pancreatic ducts in the interlobular and intralobular areas (Fig. 9c). In contrast, distribution of fibrosis and inflammatory cells was markedly attenuated in the STZ-fat-cat group and there was no pancreatic ductal hypertension and dilation (Fig. 9d).

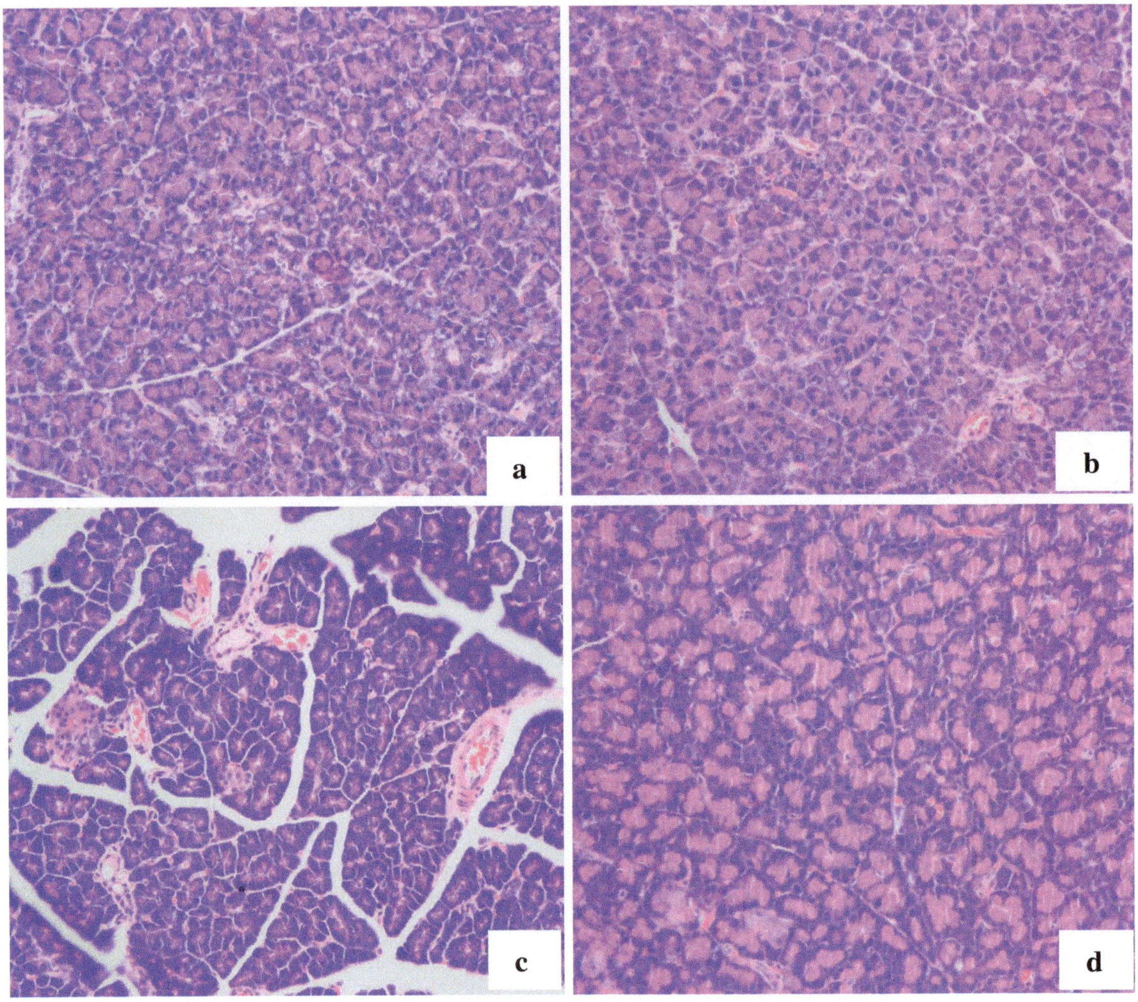

Fig. 9 Representative light microscopic appearances of the pancreas stained with H&E (200x) (**a**–**d**). **a** Normal histological changes were observed in the normal group on day 14. **b** Only minimal histological changes were observed in the control (high-fat and high-sugar) group on day 14. **c** The pancreatic ductal hypertension STZ-fat-diabetic rats group, infiltration of inflammatory cells were found in the interlobular and periductal areas on day 14. The pancreas was atrophic, and fibrosis and inflammatory cells were markedly distributed in the interlobular and interlobular areas. **d** In contrast, distributions of inflammatory cells and fibrosis were slightly noted Leukocyte infiltration in the catalpol group on day 14. The *arrows* represent inflammatory cells infiltration

Discussion

In this study, STZ-induced type 2 diabetes with a high-fat and high sugar diet was used to study the antidiabetic and antioxidant effects of catalpol. STZ is synthesized by *Streptomycetes achromogenes* and is used to induce both insulin-dependent and non-insulin-dependent diabetes mellitus based on the STZ dose [22, 23]. The most frequently used single intravenous dose to induce insulin-dependent diabetes mellitus in adult rats is between 40 and 60 mg/kg by body weight [24]. STZ is also efficacious after intraperitoneal administration of a similar or higher dose, but a single dose below 40 mg/kg body weight may be ineffective [25]. STZ can also be given in multiple low doses. In this paper, rat diabetes was induced by a small dose of STZ (30 mg/kg) for 3 days after the rats were given high-fat and high-sugar feed for 3 weeks; this modeled more closely human type 2 diabetes because it accompanied the lipid abnormality. Before STZ administration, rats were given a high-sugar and high-fat diet for 3 weeks to induce fat and lipid abnormities, and their fasting blood sugar was near normal (less than 7 mmol/L). The plasma sugar and lipids were high after STZ administration for 2 weeks. STZ-diabetic body weight obviously decreased and was accompanied by increased thirst, frequent urination, and increased hunger. These changes indicated diabetes was successfully induced.

We found that catalpol had positive effects on type 2 diabetes. A dose-dependent anti-hyperglycemic action was observed for intravenous injection of catalpol at the dose range 10–50 mg/kg for 2 weeks. An increase in dosage beyond 50 mg/kg produced no additional effects. We chose a catalpol dose of 50 mg/kg for further study. The data showed that diabetic rats consumed more food and water and lost body weight. Interestingly, 50 mg/kg catalpol treatment for 2 weeks significantly ameliorated body weight loss and attenuated water intake and food consumption. Although we did collect urine or measure urine volume in each group, STZ-fat-diabetes rats became increasingly thinner, and the padding was often wet, which meant diuresis was markedly obvious in STZ-fat-diabetic rats; however, catalpol obviously ameliorated these changes.

As a glucose load test, the OGCT was used to test glucose clearance, which reflects pancreatic β cell function. Catalpol treatment 3 h after oral glucose administration obviously reduced plasma glucose and levels returned to normal in 6 h. The OGCT results showed that catalpol treatment improved diabetic rats' ability to adjust blood sugar, perhaps through improved islet β cell function. Histological evaluation of the pancreas showed clearly (Fig. 9c) that the pancreatic tissue was atrophic with the presence of fibrosis. There was infiltration of inflammatory cells and these were markedly distributed in the interlobular and intralobular areas, but there was minimal distribution of inflammatory cells and fibrosis in the catalpol group. These results indicate that catalpol might facilitate glucose uptake, which is in accordance with previous findings [2].

Diabetes can cause glucose-lipid metabolism disturbance. Many diabetes patients show long-term abnormal lipid metabolism. In this study, the animal model induced by STZ with high-sugar and high-fat feed was close to human diabetes type 2. The rat model indicated that high-sugar and high-fat food with STZ produced type 2 diabetes accompanied by lipid metabolism disturbances with increases in TC and TG and decreases in HDL-C. Catalpol lowered plasma TC and TG and increased HDL-C (Fig. 5) when the blood sugar was lowered (Fig. 6). Catalpol not only ameliorated abnormal glucose tolerance, but also relieved the glucose-lipid metabolism disturbance.

Oxidative stress plays an important role in diabetes mellitus induced by STZ. STZ enters β cells via a glucose transporter and causes alkylation of DNA. DNA damage induces the activation of poly adenosine diphosphate-ribosylation, a process that is more important for the diabetogenicity of STZ than DNA damage itself [26]. Poly adenosine diphosphate-ribosylation leads to the depletion of cellular nicotinamide adenine dinucleotide and adenosine triphosphate. Enhanced adenosine triphosphate dephosphorylation after STZ treatment supplies a substrate for xanthenes oxidase resulting in the formation of superoxide radicals, hydrogen peroxide and hydroxyl radicals. Furthermore, STZ liberates toxic amounts of nitric oxide that inhibit aconitase activity and contribute to DNA damage. STZ can cause β cell necrosis [22, 23, 26]. In addition to a plasma lipid and sugar increase in STZ-fat-diabetic rats, the present findings show that endogenous antioxidants, such as SOD, GSH-PX, and CAT, were decreased and MDA levels were increased, which indicates that oxidative stress was strengthened in STZ-fat-diabetic rats. However, catalpol at 50 mg/kg for 2 weeks significantly reversed the lowered antioxidant levels and the increase of oxidative stress induced by STZ with sugar-lipid abnormities. SOD, GSH-PX, and CAT in plasma increased and MDA levels reduced to recover the balance of endogenous oxidants and antioxidants. The main active ingredients of catalpol, which is an iridoid glucoside, are isolated from the roots of *R. glutinosa* and used for treatment of diabetes and its complications. Furthermore, catalpol is a strong antioxidant [5, 27, 28] used to treat aging, stroke, and demyelination disease. The main effects of catalpol are on endogenous oxidant damage [1, 6, 7, 28] and inflammatory reactions [29, 30]. The antioxidant effects of catalpol found here are in accord with previous findings [1, 6, 7, 28]. However, catalpol possessed a stronger anti-inflammatory action and reduced inflammatory cytokines in senescent mice [29, 30], inhibited lipopolysaccharide plus interferon-gamma-induced inflammatory responses in astrocyte primary cultures [29, 30], and suppressed advanced glycation end-products-induced inflammatory responses through the inhibition of reactive oxygen species [13]. Based on the anti-hyperglycemic effect of catalpol and anti-hyperlipid abnormal coupling with markedly reduced oxidative stress in plasma, morphological pancreatic changes were examined by a light microscope (Fig. 9) after treatment with catalpol. Pancreatic damage induced by STZ was manifested as inflammation: infiltration of inflammatory cells was noted in the hypertension and markedly dilated intralobular and periductal areas. The atrophic, fibrotic, and inflammatory cells were markedly distributed in the interlobular and intralobular areas (Fig. 9c). After treatment with catalpol for 14 days, injury was ameliorated and blood glucose was decreased, and lipid levels also decreased as catalpol attenuated oxidative stress in STZ-fat-diabetic rats. In addition, inflammatory cells and fibrosis were minimal (Fig. 9d) and the pancreatic morphological changes were similar to those of the high-fat, high-sugar group (Fig. 9b). This suggests that catalpol might improve insulin levels in plasma through mitigation of pancreas inflammation induced by STZ and preserve pancreas islet structure and function.

We observed protective effects of catalpol on STZ-fat-diabetic rats. To date, only two studies have investigated the effect of catalpol on STZ-induced diabetes; these have focused on catalpol's actions on preventing diabetic encephalopathy [1] and lowering plasma glucose through increasing muscle glucose use [2]. To our knowledge, this is the first study to investigate the effect of catalpol on diabetes induced by STZ with a high-sugar and high-fat diet. Catalpol reduced the damage to the pancreas in STZ-fat-diabetic rats. Catalpol's protective effects are mainly related to decreased oxidative stress and the attenuation of the "3P" symptoms in a severely diabetic animal model. Further mechanisms of action, such as those involving insulin or glycated hemoglobin levels, should be investigated further.

Conclusion

Catalpol protected against STZ-induced diabetes with high-fat and high-sugar feed with ameliorated structural impairment of the pancreas and restored balance between oxidative enzymes and antioxidative enzymes.

Abbreviations

STZ: streptozotocin; ALX: alloxan; CM: Chinese medicine; 3P: polyuria (frequent urination), increasingly thirsty (polydipsia) and hungry (polyphagia); TC: plasma total cholesterol; TG: triglyceride; HDL-C: high-density lipoprotein-cholesterol; H&E: hematoxylin and eosin; OGCT: oral glucose challenge test; GSH-PX: glutathione peroxidase; MDA: malondialdehyde; SOD: superoxide dismutase; CAT: catalase; LPS: lipopolysaccharides.

Authors' contributions

HFZ and DW designed the study. YW detected plasma glucose, observed body weight, food and water intake. ZQL performed determination and XY and TW performed histological evaluation of pancreas. ZHF, SF and ZQL analyzed the data. HFZ and JHW wrote the manuscript. All authors read and approved the final manuscript.

Author details

[1] College of Pharmaceutical Sciences and Traditional Chinese Medicine, Southwest University, Chongqing 400715, China. [2] Chongqing Engineering Research Center for Pharmacological Evaluation, POB 400715, Chongqing, China. [3] Department of Pharmacy, The First People's Hospital of Neijiang, Neijiang 641000, China. [4] Department of Emergency, The First Affiliated Hospital of Chongqing Medical University, POB 400016, Chongqing, China.

Acknowledgements

This work was supported by the National Natural Science Foundation of China (81073084), Natural Science Foundation Project of CQ CSTC (2010BB5127, cstc2014jcyjA10083), Fundamental Research Funds for the Central Universities (XDJK2012B010, XDJK2009C081, XDJK2015C155) and The Start-up Foundation of Southwest University (SWU114055). The authors Gratefully acknowledge to XiaoYan Zhao and Hua Zuo, Ph.D for her review and helpful comments regarding to this paper.

Competing interests

The authors declare that they have no competing interests.

References

1. Wang CF, Li DQ, Xue HY, Hu B. Oral supplementation of catalpol ameliorates diabetic encephalopathy in rats. Brain Res. 2010;1307:158–65.
2. Huang WJ, Niu HS, Lin MH, Cheng JT, Hsu FL. Antihyperglycemic effect of catalpol in streptozotocin-induced diabetic rats. J Nat Prod. 2010;73:1170–2.
3. Zhang RX, Li MX, Jia ZP. *Rehmannia glutinosa*: review of botany, chemistry and pharmacology. J Ethnopharmacol. 2008;117:199–214.
4. Xin S. The overviews of traditional chinese medicine treatment on pre-diabetes and the data mining and research of professor wei zixiao's experiences. Acad Chin Med Sci. 2015. p. 2 **(Doctoral dissertation)**.
5. Tian YY, Jiang B, Annn LJ, Bao YM. Neuroprotective effect of catalpol against MPP(+)-induced oxidative stress in mesencephalic neurons. Eur J Pharmacol. 2007;568:142–8.
6. Jiang B, Liu JH, Bao YM, An LJ. Catalpol inhibits apoptosis in hydrogen peroxide-induced PC12 cells by preventing cytochrome c release and inactivating of caspase cascade. Toxicon. 2004;43:53–9.
7. Zhang Z, Liu Y, Xue B, Wei L. Protective effects of catalpol against H_2O_2-induced oxidative damage in astrocytes. Zhongguo Zhong Yao Za Zhi. 2009;34:1955–8.
8. Zhang X, Zhang A, Jiang B, Bao Y, Wang J, An L. Further pharmacological evidence of the neuroprotective effect of catalpol from *Rehmannia glutinosa*. Phytomedicine. 2008;15:484–90.
9. Su-rong ZH, Yan-wei L, Jin-long CH, Hai-feng D, Zu-z W. Experimental study on the hypoglycemic activity of catalpol from *Rehmannia glutinosa* Libosch. (alloxan-induced diabetic rats). Lishizhen Medicine Materia Medica Research. 2009;20:171–2.
10. Morelli A, Chavalmane AK, Filippi S, Fibbi B, Silvestrini E, Sarchielli E, Zhang X, Vignozzi L, Vannelli G, Forti G, Maggi M, et al. Atorvastatin ameliorates sildenafil-induced penile erections in experimental diabetes by inhibiting diabetes-induced RhoA/Rho-kinase signaling hyperactivation. J Sex Med. 2009;6:91–106.
11. Shieh JP, Cheng KC, Chung HH, Kerh YF, Yeh CH, Cheng JT. Plasma glucose lowering mechanisms of catalpol, an active principle from roots of *Rehmannia glutinosa*, in streptozotocin-induced diabetic rats. J Agric Food Chem. 2011;59:3747–53.
12. Dong Z, Chen CX. Effect of catalpol on diabetic nephropathy in rats. Phytomedicine. 2013;20:1023–9.
13. Choi HJ, Jang HJ, Chung TW, Jeong SIL, Cha J, Choi JY, Han CW, Jang YS, Joo M, Jeong HS, Ha KT. Catalpol suppresses advanced glycation end-products-induced inflammatory responses through inhibition of reactive oxygen species in human monocytic THP-1 cells. Fitoterapia. 2013;86:19–28.
14. Mu SN, Gao SN, Wan ea FS. Rat model of type 2 diabetes induced by streptozotocin and high-carbonhydrate-fat diet. Chin J Comp Med. 2008;18:19–22.
15. Shen YJ, Peng L, Liaoea ZL. Preparation and experience of rat model of type 2 diabetes induced by streptozotocin. J Guangxi Med Univ. 2011;28:821–3.
16. Wang Cheng-Fang, Lib Dan-Qing, Xue Hong-Yu, Hud Bo. Oral supplementation of catalpol ameliorates diabetic encephalopathy in rats. Brain Res. 2010;1307:158–65.
17. Bailbe D, Philippe E, Gorbunov E, Tarasov S, Epstein O, Portha B. The novel oral drug Subetta exerts an antidiabetic effect in the diabetic Goto-Kakizaki rat: comparison with rosiglitazone. J Diabetes Res. 2013;2013:763125.
18. Sosenko JM, Skyler JS, Herold KC, Palmer JP. The metabolic progression to type 1 diabetes as indicated by serial oral glucose tolerance testing in the diabetes prevention trial-type 1. Diabetes. 2012;61:1331–7.
19. Feigh M, Andreassen KV, Neutzsky-Wulff AV, Hansen C, Bay-Jensen AC, Henriksen JE, Beck-Nielsen H, ChristiansenC Henriksen K, Karsdal MA, et al. Oral salmon calcitonin attenuates hyperglycaemia and preserves pancreatic beta-cell area and function in Zucker diabetic fatty rats. Br J Pharmacol. 2012;167:151–63.
20. Wei L, Yamamoto M, Harada M, Otsuki M. Treatment with pravastatin attenuates progression of chronic pancreatitis in rat. Lab Invest. 2013;91:872–84.
21. Jin L, Xue HY, Jin LJ, Li SY, Xu YP. Antioxidant and pancreas-protective effect of aucubin on rats with streptozotocin-induced diabetes. Eur J Pharmacol. 2008;582:162–7.
22. Szkudelski T. The mechanism of alloxan and streptozotocin action in B cells of the rat pancreas. Physiol Res. 2001;50:537–46.

23. Lenzen S. The mechanisms of alloxan- and streptozotocin-induced diabetes. Diabetologia. 2008;51:216–26.
24. Ganda OP, Rossini AA, Like AA. Studies on streptozotocin diabetes. Diabetes. 1976;25:595–603.
25. Katsumata K, Katsumata K Jr, Katsumata Y. Protective effect of diltiazem hydrochloride on the occurrence of alloxan- or streptozotocin-induced diabetes in rats. Horm Metab Res. 1992;24:508–10.
26. Mabley JG, Suarez-Pinzon WL, Hasko G, Salzman AL, Rabinovitch A, Kun E, SzabÓ C. Inhibition of poly (ADP-ribose) synthetase by gene disruption or inhibition with 5-iodo-6-amino-1,2-benzopyrone protects mice from multiple-low-dose-streptozotocin-induced diabetes. Br J Pharmacol. 2001;133:909–19.
27. Bi J, Jiang B, Hao S, Zhang A, Dong Y, Jiang T, An L. Catalpol attenuates nitric oxide increase via ERK signaling pathways induced by rotenone in mesencephalic neurons. Neurochem Int. 2009;54:264–70.
28. Bi J, Jiang B, Liu JH, Lei C, Zhang XL, An LJ. Protective effects of catalpol against H2O2-induced oxidative stress in astrocytes primary cultures. Neurosci Lett. 2008;442:224–7.
29. Zhang X, Jin C, Li Y, Guan S, Han F, Zhang S. Catalpol improves cholinergic function and reduces inflammatory cytokines in the senescent mice induced by d-galactose. Food Chem Toxicol. 2013;58C:50–5.
30. Bi J, Jiang B, Zorn A, Zhao RG, Liu P, An LJ. Catalpol inhibits LPS plus IFN-gamma-induced inflammatory response in astrocytes primary cultures. Toxicol In Vitro. 2012;27:543–50.

14

Integrated chemometric fingerprints of antioxidant activities and HPLC–DAD–CL for assessing the quality of the processed roots of *Polygonum multiflorum* Thunb. (*Heshouwu*)

Hai Fang Chen[1,2], You Hua Chen[1], Chun Hua Liu[1], Lu Wang[1], Xi Chen[1], Bo Yang Yu[3*] and Jin Qi[3*]

Abstract

Background: The processed roots of *Polygonum multiflorum* Thunb. (*Heshouwu*; processed HSW) are commonly used in anti-aging medicine. Few reports have combined chemical profiles with bioactivity to evaluate the quality of the processed HSW. This study aims to integrate chemometric fingerprints of antioxidant activities and high-performance liquid chromatography–diode array detection–chemiluminescence (HPLC–DAD–CL) to assess the quality of processed HSW.

Methods: An online HPLC–DAD–CL based on the three reactive oxygen species (ROS), superoxide anion, hydrogen peroxide, and peroxynitriteanion, was developed to screen the potential anti-aging constituents for a comprehensive quality evaluation of processed HSW. Additionally, antioxidant-activity-integrated fingerprints were constructed and hierarchical cluster analysis and principal component analysis were used to evaluate the variations among 14 batches of processed HSW samples purchased from drug stores in different habitats.

Results: Fourteen batches of processed HSW samples were highly similar and classified into two clusters using hierarchical cluster analysis. Twelve active compounds exhibited antioxidant activity on the ROS with different degrees of sensitivity that constituted specific fingerprints. Among them, protocatechuic acid, catechin, *trans*-2,3,5,4′-tetrahydroxy-stilbene-2-O-β-D-glucoside, 2,3,5, 4′-tetrahydroxy-stilbene-2-O-β-D-(2″-galloyl)-glucoside, torachrysone-8-O-glucoside, and emodin-8-O-β-D-glucoside exerted relatively large influences on the differences between processed HSW samples.

Conclusion: Our study established the antioxidative activity-integrated fingerprint for processed HSW and achieved a screening of the potential anti-aging constituents using the online HPLC–DAD–CL method with H_2O_2, $O_2^{\bullet-}$, and $ONOO^-$ scavenging experiments.

Background

The roots of *Polygonum multiflorum* Thunb. (*Heshouwu*; HSW) (Fig. 1) are often used in either raw or processed form to treat different diseases in Chinese medicine (CM). Raw HSW loosens the bowel and relieves constipation; HSW's anti-aging property is mainly attributed to the processed form [1]. HSW also exhibits neuroprotective [2] and hairgrowth promoting activity [3, 4]. The characteristic constituent of HSW is 2,3,5,4′-tetrahydroxystilbene-2-O-β-D-glucoside, which is a potential natural inhibitor of advanced glycation end products [5] and exhibited anti-atherosclerosis [6] and anti-osteoporosis effects [7].

HSW contains numerous phenols, anthraquinones, and stilbene glycosides [8, 9]. Most studies have used various methods to focus on qualitative or quantitative analysis of HSW constituents, including

*Correspondence: boyangyu59@163.com; yaoyuelingxing@163.com
[3] Department of Complex Prescription of Traditional Chinese Medicine, State Key Laboratory of Natural Medicines, China Pharmaceutical University, 639 Longmian Road, Nanjing 211198, China
Full list of author information is available at the end of the article

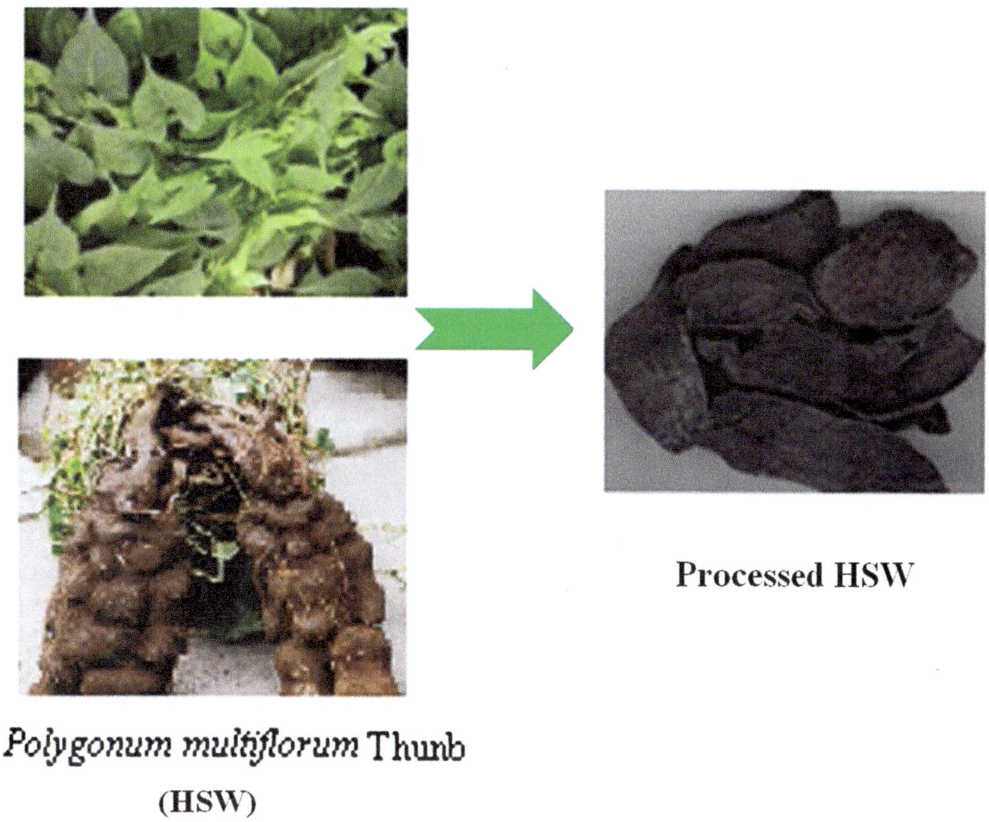

Fig. 1 Photos of *Polygonum multiflorum* Thunb.

high-performance liquid chromatography (HPLC) [10, 11], HPLC–electrospray ionization mass spectrometry (HPLC–ESI–MS) [12], and UHPLC (ultra-HPLC) with linear iontrap–Orbitrap tandem mass spectrometry (UHPLC–LTQ–Orbitrap MS) [13]. However, none of these studies have comprehensively evaluated the quality of HSW by combining chemical components with bioactivity. In addition, research has focused on studies of raw HSW rather than processed HSW. Different processing procedures used by manufacturers could lead to differences in the quality of processed HSW [14]. Therefore, it is necessary to analyze chemical and bioactivity information to comprehensively control the quality of processed HSW.

The fingerprint technique is the predominant tool to evaluate the quality of CM. However, the chromatographic fingerprint only contains the chemical message and is insufficient to demonstrate the overall quality of material [15, 16]. Therefore, activity-integrated fingerprints have been increasingly used to evaluate the quality of CM. High-performance liquid chromatography–diode array detection–chemiluminescence (HPLC–DAD–CL) is a sensitive method and often used in studies of activity-integrated fingerprints. Some studies have used a series of free radicals, such as hydrogen peroxide (H_2O_2), 2,2′-Azinobis-(3-ethylbenzothiazoline-6-sulfonic acid), superoxide anion ($O_2^{\bullet -}$), and 2, 2-diphenyl-1-picrylhydrazyl, to screen bioactive constituents and evaluate the antioxidant activity of CM [15–17]. However, the bioactive constituents obtained using these methods by means of their scavenging activity on one free radical could be insufficient because of their different scavenging capacity on different free radicals. Therefore, it is necessary to develop a multi-free radical scavenging system to obtain chemical and bioactive information to evaluate the quality of CM.

Aging is a complex physiological process and the oxidative stress theory of aging has gained considerable support [18].Numerous studies indicate that reactive oxygen species (ROS), such as $O_2^{\bullet -}$, H_2O_2, and peroxynitriteanion ($ONOO^-$), are involved in the aging process and cause oxidative damage [19–22]. Antioxidative activity may be one index of the anti-aging effect. The anti-aging effect of HSW has been studied in pharmacological experiments [4, 23], but the search for anti-aging constituents is time-consuming, particularly because the content of constituents from different habitats varies markedly. Therefore, the selection of characteristic chemical markers using the

HPLC–DAD–CL method may be a faster way of comprehensively evaluating the quality of HSW.

This study aims to investigate the antioxidant profile of processed HSW by HPLC–DAD–CL combined with chemometrics to rapidly screen potential anti-aging constituents of processed HSW by scavenging three reactive species ($O_2^{\bullet -}$, H_2O_2, and $ONOO^-$).

Methods

Materials and reagents

HPLC grade acetonitrile was obtained from Tedia (Tedia Company Inc., USA). Luminol (Fluka Chemie Buchs, Switzerland), hydrogen peroxide solution (30 % H_2O_2 in water), sodium nitrite ($NaNO_2$), sodium carbonate (Na_2CO_3), sodium bicarbonate ($NaHCO_3$), and hydrochloric acid (HCl) were all purchased from Nanjing Chemical Regent Corporation (Jiangsu, China). Pyrogallol was obtained from Zunyi Second Chemical Corporation (Guizhou, China). Ethylenediaminetetraacetic acid was supplied by Shanghai Chemical Reagent Corporation (Shanghai, China). Sodium hydroxide (NaOH) and manganese dioxide (MnO_2) were purchased from Xilong Chemical Corporation (Guangzhou, China). The reagents used were all of analytical grade. The purified water used was prepared by a Millipore water purification system (Millipore, Bedford, MA, USA).

Preparation of samples

Fourteen batches of processed HSW samples were purchased from different drug stores. The habitats of samples were as follows: Guangdong (20110901, S1), Shanxi (20110702, S2), Hebei (20080526, S3), Guizhou (20080323, S4), Yunnan (20090327, S5), Anhui (20061228, S6), Guangdong (20090705, S7), Hubei (20110523, S8), Sichuan (20110419, S9), Sichuan (20091216, S10), Henan (20120615, S11), Guangxi (20120530, S12), Guizhou (20121129, S13), and Hunan (20120803, S14). All samples were authenticated by Professor Bo-Yang Yu based on their morphological features according to the Chinese Pharmacopoeia [24]. Their voucher specimens were deposited at the Department of Complex Prescription of CM, China Pharmaceutical University, Nanjing, China. Processed HSW samples were ground in a grinder producing a 60-mesh particle size powder. Each sample (1.0 g) was accurately weighed and extracted twice with 50 mL methanol for 30 min in an ultrasonic bath. Then, the extract was vacuum filtered each time. Extraction solutions were mixed together after cooling and evaporated under vacuum at 40 °C. The residue was diluted with methanol (10 mL). The sample solution was further filtered through a 0.22-μm membrane filter prior to injection into the HPLC–CL system.

Preparation of CL solutions

Carbonate buffers (pH 10.0 and 11.0; 0.1 M) were prepared by mixing appropriate volumes of 0.1 M Na_2CO_3 and 0.1 M $NaHCO_3$ solution. A 1.8×10^{-2} M stock solution of luminol was prepared in a 0.1 M Na_2CO_3 solution and stored in a refrigerator for at least 3 days before dilution. A 1.0×10^{-2} M stock solution of pyrogallol was prepared in a 0.1 mM HCl solution and then stored in a dark bottle at 4 °C. Reagent solutions for the determination of H_2O_2, and $O_2^{\bullet -}$ scavenging activity were prepared according to previous work conducted by our research group [15]. Peroxynitrite was prepared according to a previous method [25] and we used an online peroxynitrite scavenging detection method developed by our group [26]. Reagent solutions for the determination of peroxynitrite scavenging activity were as follows: a 9×10^{-6} M luminol solution (Solution I) was prepared with 0.1 M carbonate buffer solution (pH 9, $NaHCO_3$: Na_2CO_3 = 9:1) and a 4.97×10^{-4} M peroxynitrite solution (Solution II) was prepared with a 0.1 M NaOH solution on an ice bath.

HPLC–DAD–CL analysis condition

The HPLC system used was a Shimadzu LC-2010C HT system consisting of a quaternary pump, an autosampler (Shimadzu Corporation, Japan), a thermostated column compartment (Shimadzu Corporation, Japan), and a DAD (SPD-M20A, Shimadzu Corporation, Japan). HPLC separation was achieved with a Venusil MP C_{18} column (250 × 4.6 mm, 5 μm, Agela Technologies, China) with a flow rate of 1.0 mL/min. The column temperature was set at 30 °C. The mobile phase was composed of A (acetonitrile) and B (0.1 % aqueous phosphoric acid, v/v). The gradient elution program was as follows: 0–6 min, isocratic gradient 6 %A; 6–10 min, linear gradient 6 %–10 %A; 10–30 min, linear gradient 10 %–20 %A; 30–70 min, linear gradient 20 %–50 %A; 70–75 min, linear gradient 50 %–60 %A; 75–85 min, isocratic gradient 60 %A.

A BPCL ultraweak bioluminescence system (Academia Sinica Biophysics Institute, Beijing, China) was used to monitor the CL emission. The CL detector was equipped with a flat glass coil (80 μL) as detection cell and a photomultiplier operated at −800 V. The HPLC–DAD–CL detection system was interconnected with PEEK tubes (Mianyang Prochema Commercial Corporation, China). CL reagents, luminal solutions, H_2O_2, pyrogallol, and peroxynitrite were transported by peristaltic pumps at the same flow rate of 1.1 mL/min each. CL reagents were mixed with sample solution eluted from the HPLC detector then passed through the CL detector; the CL emission was detected by the BPCL system (Fig. 2). Resveratrol is a strong, natural antioxidant, therefore, the overall antioxidant activities for processed HSW were evaluated using resveratrol as a positive control (a similar method has

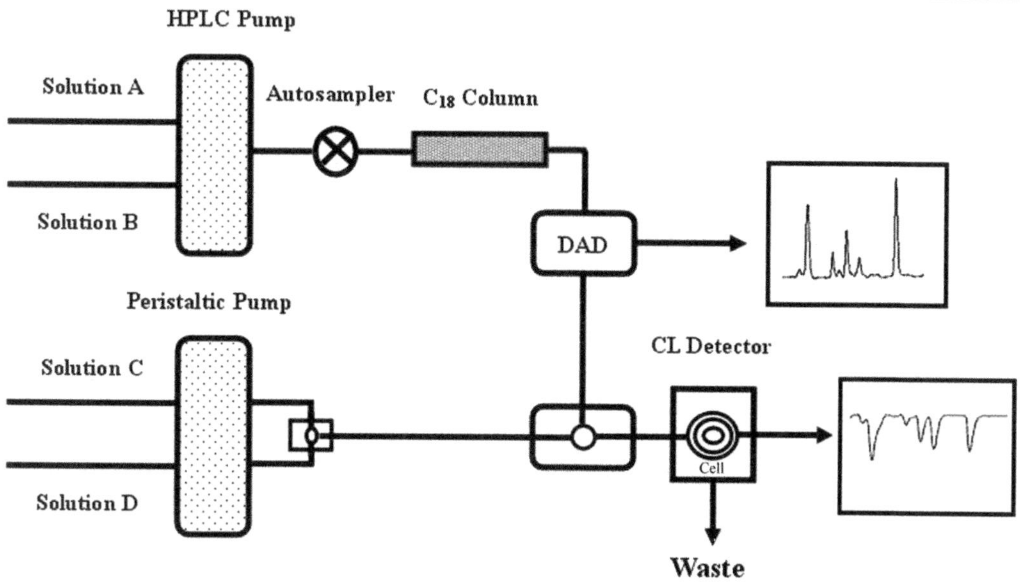

Fig. 2 Detection apparatus for HPLC–DAD–CL

been reported in the literature [15]). The activity of the antioxidant constituents in processed HSW was proportional to the intensity of negative peak and evaluated with the scavenging rate (%), as shown in the following Eq. (1):

$$\text{Scavenging rate (\%)} = \frac{CL_0 - CL_1}{CL_0} \times 100, \quad (1)$$

where CL_0 is the baseline intensity of CL (without sample) and CL_1 is the inhibited CL intensity of every compound in the extracts.

HPLC–ESI–MS analysis condition

An Agilent 1100LC/MSD Trap XCT ESI (Agilent Technologies, MA, USA) was used to obtain information about the structure of the constituents in processed HSW. The mobile phase for HPLC–MS was the same as described for the HPLC analysis conditions but the composition of the B pump substituted 0.1 % aqueous phosphoric acid for 0.1 % aqueous formic acid. The ESI–MS spectra were acquired in negative ionization mode. Capillary voltage was 3300 V. Drying gas temperature was set at 350 °C with a flow rate of 9.0 L/min and nebulizing pressure was set at 275.8 kPa. Data were processed using the 6300 Series HPLC/MSD Trap and Data Analysis 3.4 (Agilent Technologies, MA, USA).

Data analysis of chromatographic profiles and ROS scavenging activity of processed HSW samples

The characteristic constituent in processed HSW samples was selected as the reference peak to calculate relative retention time (RRT) and relative peak area (RPA). The relative standard deviations (RSDs) of RRT and RPA for each common peak were calculated to estimate precision, repeatability, and stability. The method precision was evaluated using intraday and interday variation tests. The intraday variation test was evaluated using five replicate injections of the same sample and the interday variation test was evaluated over 3 days with five replicate injections each day. Method repeatability was analyzed for the six replicate samples. The stability of the sample solution was evaluated at different time points in one day (0, 2, 4, 8, 12, and 24 h).

We used a similarity evaluation system for chromatographic fingerprints of CM (Version 2004 A) to evaluate the similarity of the samples. Six samples from different places were prepared. The similarities between the chromatograms of the samples from different origins were examined by comparing the samples with the reference fingerprint that was generated by the median value of all the chromatograms.

Statistical analysis

Hierarchical cluster analysis (HCA) was performed by SPSS statistics software (SPSS for Windows 11.5, SPSS Inc., Chicago, USA) was used to sort the samples into different groups. The distance between the samples was used to assess the similarities among processed HSW samples. Samples with high similarity were clustered into homogenous groups. Principal components analysis (PCA) is an effective method to determine the main factors in large amounts of data by feature extraction and dimensionality reduction. PCA analysis of the fingerprint data of processed HSW was performed using SIMCA-P 12.0 software (Umetrics AB, Umea, Sweden).

Table 1 Characterization of chemical constituents of the processed HSW samples

Peaks	*TR* (min)	Formula	MS (m/z)	MS^n (m/z)	Identification	λ_{max} (nm)
1	8.20	$C_7H_6O_5$	168.8[M-H]$^-$	124.8 [M-H-CO_2]$^-$,	Gallic acid	270
2	13.262	Unknown	323.1 [M-H]$^-$	–	Unknown	285
3	14.134	$C_7H_6O_4$	152.8 [M-H]$^-$	108.8 [M-H-CO_2]$^-$	Protocatechuic acid	260, 293
4	18.582	Unknown	185.8 [M-H]$^-$	141.8 [M-H-CO_2]$^-$	Unknown	218, 279
5	21.664	$C_{15}H_{14}O_6$	289.0 [M-H]$^-$	244.8 [M-H-CO_2]$^-$	Catechin	278
6	26.645	$C_{15}H_{14}O_6$	289.0 [M-H]$^-$	244.9 [M-H-CO_2]$^-$	Epicatechin	219, 282
7	29.50	$C_{26}H_{32}O_{14}$	567.1 [M-H]$^-$	613.2 [M-H + HCOO]$^-$, 405, 242.9	2, 3, 5, 4′-tetrahydroxystilbene-2-O-(6″-O-α-D-glucopyranosyl)-β-*D*-glucopyranosyl)	320
8	30.28	$C_{20}H_{22}O_9$	405.1 [M-H]$^-$,	441 [M-H + Cl]$^-$, 242.8[M-H-glu]$^-$	*Cis*-2, 3, 5, 4′-tetrahydroxy-stilbene-2-O-β-D-glucoside	283
9	37.17	$C_{20}H_{22}O_9$	405.1 [M-H]$^-$,	441 [M-H + Cl]$^-$, 242.8[M-H-glu]$^-$	*Trans*-2, 3, 5, 4′-tetrahydroxy-stilbene-2-O-β-D-glucoside	213, 322
10	38.112	$C_{22}H_{18}O_{10}$	441.1 [M-H]$^-$	288.9, 330.9	Unknown	273
11	38.538	$C_{27}H_{26}O_{13}$	557.2 [M-H]$^-$	312.9	2, 3, 5, 4′-tetrahydroxy-stilbene-2-O-β-D-(2″- galloyl)-glucoside	214, 293
12	49.58	$C_{20}H_{24}O_9$	407.1 [M-H]$^-$	244.9 [M-H-glu]$^-$	torachrysone-8-O-glucoside	324
13	50.74	$C_{21}H_{20}O_{10}$	431.1 [M-H]$^-$	268.9 [M-H-glu]$^-$	Emodin-8-O-β-D-glucoside	222, 282,422
14	55.64	$C_{22}H_{22}O_{10}$	283 [M-H-glu]$^-$	444.9 [M-H]$^-$, 239.9 [M-CH_3-CO]$^-$, 240.9	Physcion-8-O-β-D-glucoside	222, 271,422
15	69.80	Unknown	283	239.8	Unknown	224, 285,434
16	79.79	$C_{15}H_{10}O_5$	268.9 [M-H]$^-$	224.8 [M-H-CO_2]$^-$	Emodin	287, 439
17	9.0	Unknown	–	–	–	
18	33.09	Unknown	–	–	–	

- Not detected by HPLC–ESI–MS

Data were expressed as the mean ± standard deviation (SD). The statistical significance of differences between means was established by One-way ANOVA with Turkey post hoc tests. Significant differences and highly significant differences were classed as values of $P < 0.05$ and values of $P < 0.01$, $P < 0.001$, respectively.

Results and discussion

HPLC fingerprint method

Trans-2,3,5,4′-tetrahydroxy-stilbene-2-O-β-D-glucoside (peak 9) was selected as the reference peak. The RSDs of RRT and RPA for the precision of each common peak ranged from 0.51 to 2.33 % (n = 6) in the intraday variation test, respectively, and ranged from 0.83 to 3.97 % (n = 5) in the interday variation test, respectively. The RSDs for the repeatability of RRT and RPA of each common peak ranged from 0.9 to 4.1 % (n = 5), respectively. The RSDs of the stability test were below 2.8 % (n = 6) (Additional file1).

Identification of the main constituents in processed HSW by HPLC–ESI–MS

The structures of compounds in processed HSW were identified by comparing retention time and MS data with previous findings [13, 27–30]. The structures of these constituents were further confirmed using available reference standards, including gallic acid, protocatechuic acid, catechin, epicatechin, *trans*-2,3,5,4′-tetrahydroxy-stilbene-2-O-β-D-glucoside, emodin, physcion-8-O-β-D-glucoside, and emodin-8-O-β-D-glucoside (Additional file 2). The MS data are shown in Table 1.

Antioxidant activity of processed HSW samples

The standard potency equation of Ln(*y*) and the scavengingrate (%) (*x*) for resveratrol scavenging $O_2^{\bullet -}$, H_2O_2, and $ONOO^-$ in different concentrations were obtained. The equations for resveratrol scavenging the H_2O_2, $O_2^{\bullet -}$, and $ONOO^-$ were, respectively, as follows: $Ln(y) = 1E - 05x^3 - 0.0015x^2 + 0.1083x - 6.775(R^2 = 0.9997, P < 0.001)$, $Ln(y) = 2E - 05x^3 - 0.0032x^2 + 0.2001x - 6.0478$ ($R^2 = 0.9992$, $P < 0.05$), $Ln(y) = 1E - 05x^3 - 0.0022x^2 + 0.1373x - 6.3504(R^2 = 0.9973, P < 0.001)$. If resveratrol (1 μg) was a potency unit, the relative total activities should be the sums of peak potency. The relative total activities of peaks in 14 batches of processed HSW were calculated according to Eq. (1). The results are shown in Tables 2, 3 and 4. Compared with S1 and S4 samples,the antioxidative activities of S10 and S11 in scavengin ROS were relatively low ($P < 0.001$) and the antioxidative activities of samples S2 and S12 exhibited insignificant differences ($P = 1$). The S2 and S12 samples had strong antioxidative activities, particularly in scavenging

Table 2 The H_2O_2 scavenging rate of the constituents from fourteen batches of the processed HSW samples (n = 6)

No.	Peak 1	Peak17	Peak 3	Peak 5	Peak 8	Peak 18	Peak 9	Peak 11	Peak 12	Total activity (μg)
S1	18.25 ± 0.15	19.19 ± 0.93	32.28 ± 1.76	9.501 ± 0.32	8.89 ± 0.83	22.20 ± 0.17	96.83 ± 3.45	7.12 ± 0.16	16.16 ± 0.23	0.32
S2	22.58 ± 0.23	21.73 ± 1.05	13.30 ± 0.32	59.71 ± 0.67	25.71 ± 0.99	43.73 ± 0.35	94.21 ± 2.36	30.36 ± 0.91	59.29 ± 1.89	0.33
S3	19.78 ± 0.11	9.95 ± 0.51	18.47 ± 0.65	4.88 ± 0.77	17.65 ± 0.71	41.33 ± 0.27	93.09 ± 2.30	9.64 ± 0.66	46.23 ± 2.33	$0.25^{\#\#}$
S4	24.43 ± 0.09	28.72 ± 0.35	29.82 ± 0.89	64.59 ± 2.88	20.44 ± 0.63	31.33 ± 0.38	96.54 ± 4.50	33.40 ± 1.78	7.64 ± 0.59	0.36
S5	17.06 ± 0.05	18.01 ± 0.73	17.77 ± 1.01	11.63 ± 1.20	29.58 ± 0.58	31.17 ± 0.64	94.43 ± 1.19	7.02 ± 0.32	3.15 ± 0.09	$0.26^{\#}$
S6	6.87 ± 0.50	18.93 ± 0.45	12.80 ± 0.25	33.03 ± 1.76	33.27 ± 0.12	33.16 ± 0.47	93.34 ± 0.57	10.20 ± 0.38	25.21 ± 1.75	$0.26^{\#\#\#}$
S7	13.19 ± 0.17	12.04 ± 0.80	11.62 ± 0.17	32.90 ± 1.28	20.72 ± 0.11	21.10 ± 0.32	88.53 ± 1.35	5.69 ± 0.15	1.68 ± 0.18	$0.17^{***,\#\#\#}$
S8	13.60 ± 0.34	22.21 ± 0.66	28.42 ± 0.03	10.72 ± 0.53	30.20 ± 0.27	21.84 ± 0.26	91.29 ± 4.11	4.14 ± 0.32	1.45 ± 0.12	$0.21^{*,\#\#\#}$
S9	18.11 ± 0.57	16.73 ± 0.21	40.53 ± 1.59	50.95 ± 1.27	18.05 ± 0.78	32.71 ± 0.23	93.90 ± 1.61	4.58 ± 0.29	8.31 ± 0.12	0.28
S10	2.74 ± 0.12	14.39 ± 0.15	23.33 ± 0.77	6.13 ± 0.35	7.11 ± 0.21	13.74 ± 0.15	84.91 ± 3.74	1.35 ± 0.08	2.98 ± 0.06	$0.13^{***,\#\#\#}$
S11	10.16 ± 0.18	15.77 ± 0.33	22.35 ± 0.96	3.17 ± 0.12	4.36 ± 0.13	13.86 ± 0.13	77.04 ± 1.23	1.71 ± 0.04	0.39 ± 0.03	$0.09^{***,\#\#\#}$
S12	11.39 ± 0.35	9.34 ± 0.09	6.25 ± 1.23	69.94 ± 3.70	8.28 ± 0.17	38.08 ± 0.59	92.59 ± 2.55	26.50 ± 1.70	63.87 ± 0.73	0.3
S13	–	11.57 ± 0.67	7.30 ± 0.37	46.27 ± 0.98	10.18 ± 0.27	7.88 ± 0.76	83.23 ± 2.37	8.25 ± 0.63	11.74 ± 1.91	$0.13^{***,\#\#\#}$
S14	8.48 ± 0.05	13.51 ± 0.92	37.67 ± 0.95	41.70 ± 1.32	8.18 ± 0.35	16.23 ± 0.84	90.63 ± 5.10	22.13 ± 0.51	5.99 ± 0.57	$0.21^{\#\#\#}$

– Not detected; compared with S1 group, * $P < 0.05$, ** $P < 0.01$,*** $P < 0.01$; compared with S4 group, # $P < 0.05$, ## $P < 0.01$, ### $P < 0.001$

Table 3 The $O_2^{\bullet-}$ scavenging rate of the constituents from fourteen batches of the processed HSW samples (n = 6)

No.	Peak 1	Peak 17	Peak 3	Peak 5	Peak 8	Peak 18	Peak 9	Peak 11	Peak 12	Total activity (μg)
S1	30.48 ± 0.67	28.38 ± 0.15	3.69 ± 0.38	3.77 ± 0.17	5.40 ± 0.06	5.91 ± 0.28	93.88 ± 3.69	5.40 ± 0.13	10.54 ± 0.17	3.17
S2	38.70 ± 1.37	24.42 ± 0.23	–	28.43 ± 0.38	11.82 ± 0.41	13.60 ± 0.72	93.26 ± 4.52	20.84 ± 0.48	43.97 ± 0.72	3.28
S3	23.54 ± 1.57	10.79 ± 0.12	–	27.24 ± 0.23	6.50 ± 0.36	17.81 ± 0.95	87.54 ± 3.21	9.56 ± 0.58	31.16 ± 0.85	$1.74^{\#\#\#}$
S4	39.22 ± 2.36	27.74 ± 0.25	–	37.33 ± 0.95	9.76 ± 0.48	13.66 ± 0.77	96.17 ± 1.48	24.59 ± 0.88	5.94 ± 0.18	4.47
S5	40.91 ± 3.51	24.66 ± 0.49	–	3.06 ± 0.17	13.31 ± 1.07	10.96 ± 0.49	90.88 ± 3.29	4.59 ± 0.34	3.21 ± 0.24	$2.32^{\#}$
S6	23.96 ± 0.74	14.47 ± 0.65	–	15.73 ± 0.67	14.69 ± 0.52	10.30 ± 0.93	89.06 ± 1.78	7.90 ± 0.16	16.63 ± 0.36	$1.87^{\#\#\#}$
S7	30.29 ± 0.26	15.85 ± 0.37	–	13.20 ± 0.42	7.42 ± 0.21	3.96 ± 0.65	87.65 ± 2.35	3.02 ± 0.26	2.46 ± 0.72	$1.62^{*,\#\#\#}$
S8	36.49 ± 0.48	28.09 ± 0.44	4.89 ± 0.40	5.06 ± 0.59	14.57 ± 0.67	7.75 ± 0.49	88.17 ± 2.19	3.31 ± 0.16	1.21 ± 0.53	$1.8^{\#\#\#}$
S9	51.40 ± 1.77	21.26 ± 0.68	5.71 ± 0.31	28.79 ± 0.57	8.11 ± 0.09	13.80 ± 0.13	90.57 ± 3.21	5.01 ± 0.37	5.88 ± 0.39	$2.39^{\#}$
S10	14.34 ± 0.84	15.15 ± 0.22	–	1.97 ± 0.19	2.27 ± 0.56	3.86 ± 0.76	71.00 ± 1.39	–	4.89 ± 0.65	$0.51^{***,\#\#\#}$
S11	28.02 ± 0.73	22.06 ± 0.78	–	1.30 ± 0.17	–	4.432 ± 0.31	70.58 ± 1.21	1.96 ± 0.26	–	$0.58^{***,\#\#\#}$
S12	28.99 ± 0.45	11.29 ± 0.67	–	45.61 ± 0.93	1.92 ± 0.29	15.73 ± 0.55	94.36 ± 1.72	13.82 ± 0.95	46.18 ± 0.91	3.67
S13	17.43 ± 0.55	19.43 ± 0.35	–	27.96 ± 1.27	3.28 ± 0.37	4.00 ± 0.56	83.99 ± 1.80	4.21 ± 0.56	9.28 ± 0.16	$1.21^{**,\#\#\#}$
S14	39.18 ± 0.94	18.63 ± 0.42	–	24.04 ± 1.82	–	6.71 ± 0.21	87.96 ± 2.70	5.99 ± 0.27	4.71 ± 0.22	$1.76^{\#\#\#}$

– Not detected; compared with S1 group, * $P < 0.05$,** $P < 0.01$,*** $P < 0.01$; compared with S4 group, # $P < 0.05$, ## $P < 0.01$, ### $P < 0.001$

$O_2^{\bullet-}$ and H_2O_2. The qualities and antioxidative effects of S7 in scavenging $O_2^{\bullet-}$, H_2O_2 and $ONOO^-$ were significantly different from S1, although the two samples were from Guangdong province (in scavenging $O_2^{\bullet-}$: $P = 0.037$; in scavenging H_2O_2 and scavenging $ONOO^-$: $P < 0.001$). The same was true for samples S4 and S13. Compared with S4, the antioxidative effects of S13 were obviously weak in scavenging $O_2^{\bullet-}$, H_2O_2 and $ONOO^-$ ($P < 0.001$). The detailed comparison data was shown in Additional file 3. Different processing technology may have caused the variation of chemical compositions and differences in bioactivity. This indicates the importance of the standardization of processing technology.

In the reactive species scavenging test, stilbene glucosides, including *cis*-2,3,5,4′-tetrahydroxy-stilbene-2-O-β-D-glucoside (peak 8), *trans*-2,3,5,4′-tetrahydroxy-stilbene-2-O-β-D-glucoside (peak 9), and 2,3,5,4′-tetrahydroxy-stilbene-2-O-β-D-(2″-galloyl)-glucoside (peak 11), were sensitive in scavenging three reactive species, and *trans*-2,3,5,4′-tetrahydroxy-stilbene-2-O-β-D-glucoside exhibited significant antioxidant activity because of its high content in processed HSW. Gallic acid (peak 1),

Table 4 $ONOO^-$ **scavenging rate of constituents from 14 batches of processed HSW samples (n = 6)**

NO.	Peak17	Peak 3	Peak 5	Peak 6	Peak 8	Peak 9	Peak 11	Peak 12	Peak 13	Peak 16	Total activity (μg)
S1	49.93 ± 0.64	69.52 ± 1.24	35.73 ± 1.80	5.01 ± 0.34	43.21 ± 1.33	94.37 ± 3.45	10.40 ± 0.19	3.97 ± 0.17	6.91 ± 0.44	49.05 ± 0.93	0.14***, ###
S2	51.72 ± 1.22	38.09 ± 0.45	90.57 ± 3.76	25.24 ± 0.56	68.83 ± 1.31	91.49 ± 1.37	28.39 ± 0.64	19.48 ± 0.04	21.67 ± 0.88	16.35 ± 0.35	0.15***, ##
S3	29.07 ± 0.65	65.71 ± 0.62	92.42 ± 0.79	60.95 ± 1.33	64.41 ± 2.19	95.39 ± 1.46	12.95 ± 0.45	3.57 ± 0.20	17.26 ± 0.12	6.75 ± 0.20	0.12***, ###
S4	59.74 ± 2.56	67.28 ± 2.61	93.61 ± 2.99	44.33 ± 0.51	67.33 ± 0.64	95.67 ± 4.10	28.38 ± 0.46	3.85 ± 0.10	8.83 ± 0.16	47.59 ± 0.13	0.15***, ###
S5	46.56 ± 3.78	50.42 ± 1.33	45.81 ± 0.79	8.83 ± 0.24	72.21 ± 3.10	97.15 ± 2.08	13.15 ± 0.88	3.84 ± 0.04	7.55 ± 0.30	19.82 ± 0.25	0.13***, ###
S6	42.32 ± 2.19	41.31 ± 1.28	80.45 ± 1.35	20.22 ± 0.11	77.98 ± 1.12	90.65 ± 3.48	15.57 ± 0.33	–	6.80 ± 0.06	18.21 ± 0.08	0.12***, ###
S7	18.97 ± 0.52	26.39 ± 0.77	55.57 ± 0.23	20.50 ± 0.38	39.47 ± 0.93	87.05 ± 2.13		–	–	27.03 ± 0.42	0.12***, ###
S8	22.70 ± 0.72	36.84 ± 0.09	16.73 ± 0.19	5.74 ± 0.10	42.08 ± 0.67	80.86 ± 2.79	3.37 ± 0.11	–	–	21.87 ± 0.61	0.1***, ####
S9	12.97 ± 0.79	32.39 ± 1.88	43.80 ± 1.04	22.23 ± 0.27	20.58 ± 0.88	86.27 ± 1.41	–	–	–	14.92 ± 0.31	0.1***, ###
S10	–	15.44 ± 0.66	–	–	7.04 ± 0.22	64.77 ± 0.39	–	–	–	21.13 ± 0.81	0.04***, ###
S11	8.09 ± 0.19	34.02 ± 0.21	–	–	4.94 ± 0.79	70.21 ± 1.03	–	–	–	27.52 ± 0.13	0.06***, ###
S12	15.23 ± 0.35	16.94 ± 0.16	84.77 ± 0.62	19.66 ± 0.33	19.46 ± 0.44	90.12 ± 1.08	20.67 ± 0.61	14.35 ± 0.37	18.39 ± 0.07	8.11 ± 0.76	0.10***, ###
S13	37.66 ± 1.67	36.12 ± 0.62	88.86 ± 1.34	32.31 ± 1.75	33.76 ± 0.36	93.50 ± 0.49	13.14 ± 0.66	–	–	13.55 ± 0.46	0.12***###
S14	33.40 ± 1.27	80.75 ± 2.36	83.45 ± 2.35	46.39 ± 0.26	39.91 ± 0.66	92.08 ± 0.48	8.21 ± 0.90	–	12.14 ± 0.10	28.29 ± 0.95	0.13**, ###

–Not detected; compared with S1 group, * $P < 0.05$, ** $P < 0.01$, *** $P < 0.01$; compared with S4 group, # $P < 0.05$, ## $P < 0.01$, ### $P < 0.001$

protocatechuic acid (peak 3), catechin (peak 5), and torachrysone-8-O-glucoside (peak 12) exhibited scavenging activity on H_2O_2, $O_2^{\bullet-}$, or $ONOO^-$ (Fig. 3a–d). Compared with other components, epicatechin (peak 6), emodin-8-O-β-D-glucoside (peak 13), and emodin (peak 16) demonstrated higher selectivity in scavenging $ONOO^-$ than on other two reactive species, especially emodin. These constituents had different scavenging capacities on different ROS and could affect different aspects of the aging process, such as directly scavenging free radicals, decreasing the oxidation of nucleic acid and nitration of protein tyrosine residues, and inhibiting apoptosis. In addition, peak 4 had no antioxidant activity, and peaks 17 and 18 showed certain antioxidant activity in the ROS scavenging test despite their weak ultraviolet absorption or unavailable MS messages. The relationship between constituents of processed HSW and the corresponding free radicals are summarized in Fig. 4.

Gallic acid, protocatechuic acid, epicatechin, catechin, *trans(cis)*-2,3,5,4′-tetrahydroxy-stilbene-2-O-β-D-glucoside, torachrysone-8-O-glucoside, emodin-8-O-β-D-glucoside, and emodinall exhibit pharmacological effects on the age-related pathological process [31–35]. In particular, *trans(cis)*-2,3,5,4′-tetrahydroxy-stilbene-2-O-β-D-glucoside, torachrysone-8-O-glucoside, and emodin-8-O-β-D-glucoside all significantly promote hair growth [4]. These constituents were selected as chemical markers for the quality control of processed

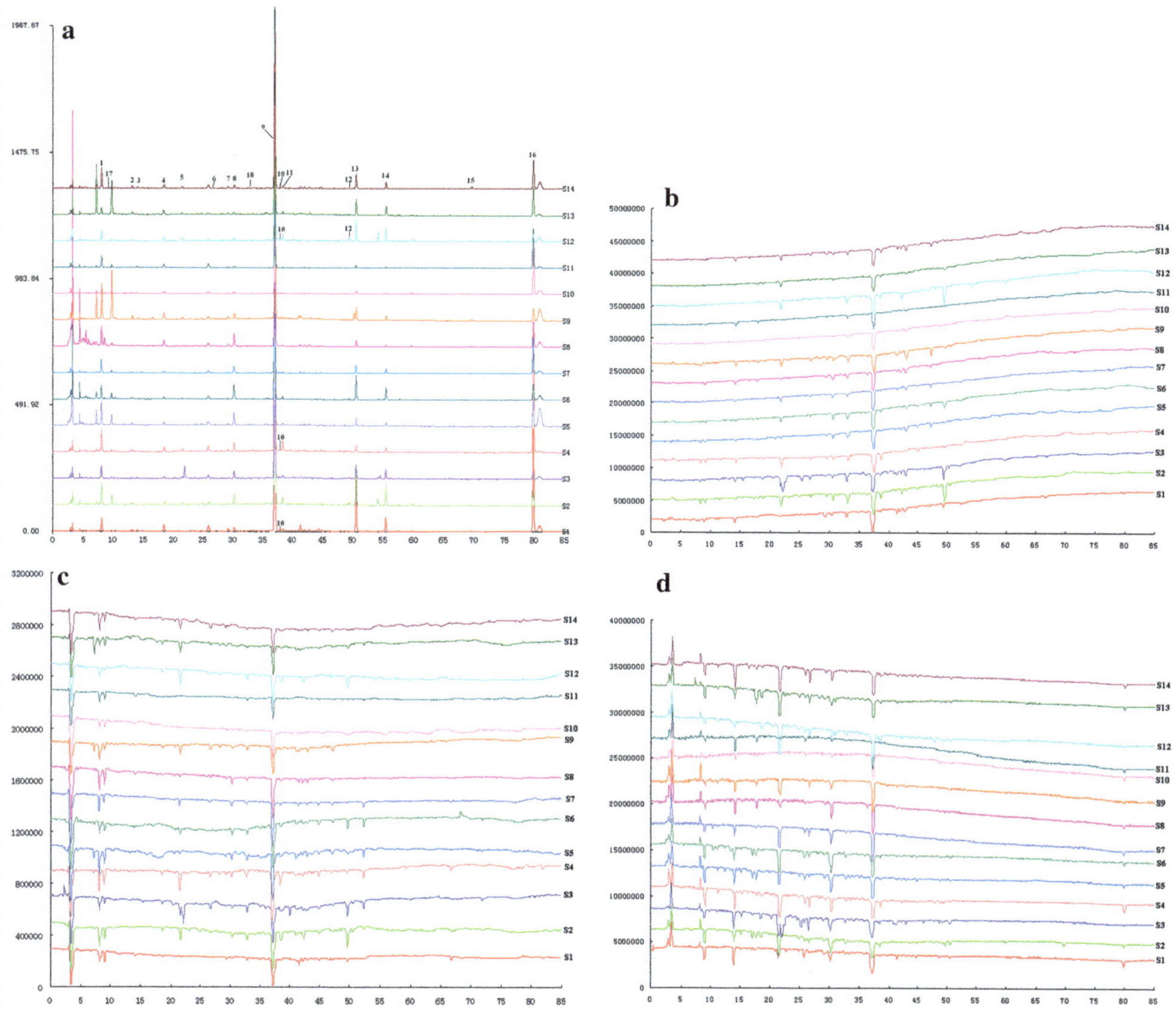

Fig. 3 The HPLC fingerprints (**a**) of processed HSW samples from different habitats, H_2O_2 scavenging profiles (**b**) of processed HSW samples, $O_2^{\bullet-}$ scavenging profiles (**c**) of processed HSW samples and $ONOO^-$ scavenging profiles (**d**) of processed HSW samples (refer to Table 1 for peak numbering)

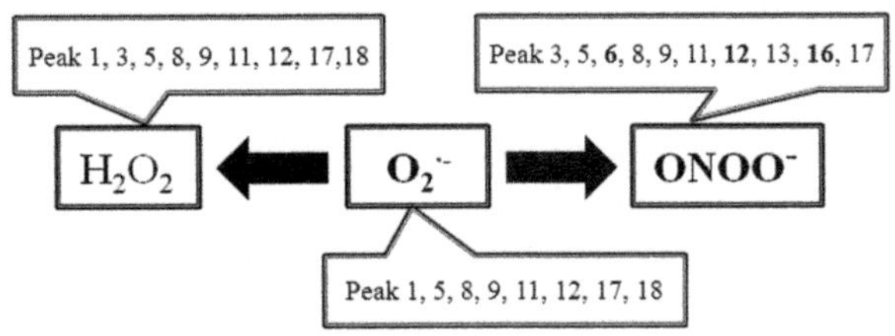

Fig. 4 The antioxidants in processed HSW samples and the corresponding ROS antioxidative effect

HSW in this study. Among the constituents, *cis*-2,3,5,4′-tetrahydroxy-stilbene-2-O-β-D-glucoside, torachrysone-8-O-glucoside, and 2,3,5,4′-tetrahydroxy-stilbene-2-O-β-D-(2″-galloyl)-glucoside were screened and proposed as chemical markers for the quality control of processed HSW. To the best of our knowledge, this is a novel research finding.

HPLC fingerprints and similarities of samples from different origins

Similarities of samples

The relationship among samples was ascertained by comparing the similarity of the samples chromatographic fingerprint series. The relationship between sets of chromatographic fingerprints was analyzed by comparing the similarity between the objects and the reference fingerprints. The similarity values of 14 batches of samples (S01–S14) were 0.989, 0.990, 0.990, 0.989, 0.982, 0.995, 0.995, 0.986, 0.970, 0.870, 0.905, 0.989, 0.945, and 0.996 ($n = 6$), respectively. Overall, the processed HSW samples were very similar. Compared with other samples, the similarity indexes of samples S10 and S11 were relatively lower. The different habitats and processing technology could have caused variation in the content or chemical compositions of processed HSW [14, 36].

Results of HCA

Peak 1, peak 3, peak 5, peak 6, peak 8, peak 9, peak 11, peak 12, peak 13, and peak 16 were the antioxidants in all processed HSW samples. Peak 17 and peak 18 were not examined for weak chemical messages. HCA analysis, was performed by the SPSS statistics software. The samples of processed HSW could be classified into two clusters despite high similarity: samples S10, S11, S5, S9, S6, S8, S14, S7, S13, and S3 were in Cluster 1; samples S2, S12, S1, and S4 were in Cluster 2. The HCA results were similar to the HPLC similarity index results (Fig. 5). The data indicated that these selected constituents were the chemical markers for the quality control of processed HSW.

Results of PCA

The PCA analysis produced a classification of samples similar to that produced by the HCA results (Fig. 6a). S1, S3, S5, S6, S7, S8, S9, S10, S11, S13, and S14 were

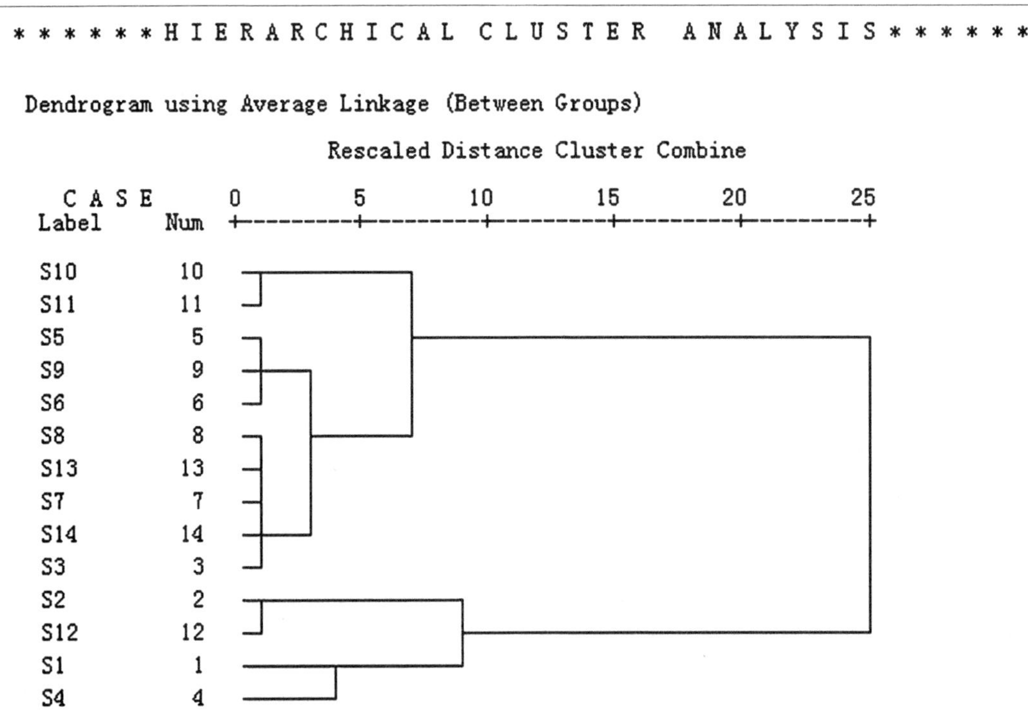

Fig. 5 Hierarchical clustering analysis of processed HSW samples

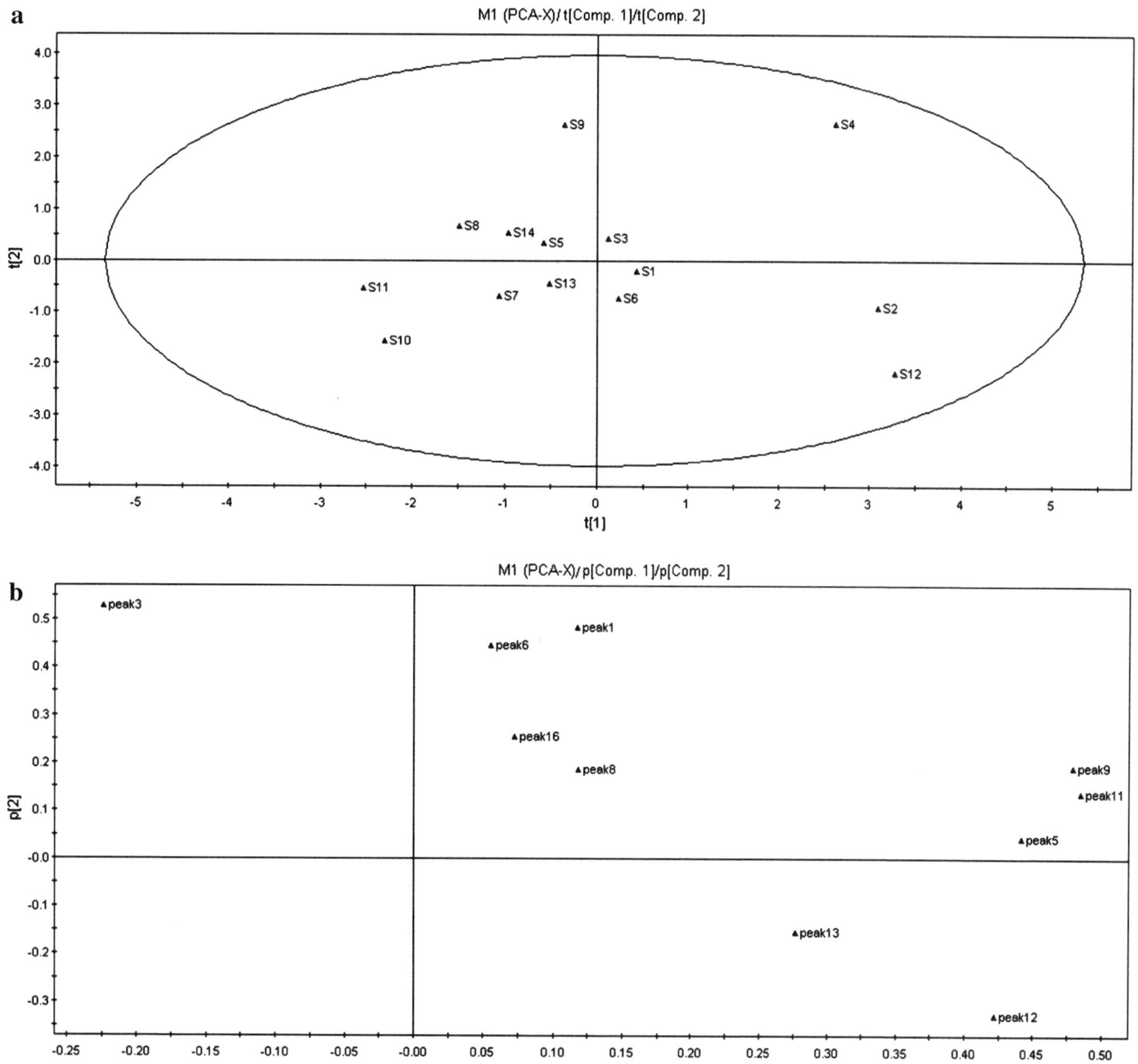

Fig. 6 PCA Scores plot (**a**) for HPLC chromatogram data of processed HSW samples. Loadings plot (**b**) for HPLC chromatogram data of processed HSW samples

classified into group 1; S2, S4, and S12 were classified into group 2. The results of the PCA loading plot indicated that protocatechuic acid, catechin, *trans*-2,3,5,4′-tetrahydroxy-stilbene-2-O-β-D-glucoside, 2,3,5,4′-tetrahydroxy-stilbene-2-O-β-D-(2″-galloyl)-glucoside, torachrysone-8-O-glucoside, and emodin-8-O-β-D-glucoside had relatively large influences on the difference between processed HSW samples (Fig. 6b). In addition to the common chemical markers used in the quality control of processed HSW, orachrysone-8-O-glucoside and 2,3,5,4′-tetrahydroxy-stilbene-2-O-β-D-(2″-galloyl)-glucoside appeared to be chemical markers for the quality control of processed HSW.

Conclusion

Our study established the antioxidative activity-integrated fingerprint for processed HSW and achieved the potential anti-aging constituents using the online HPLC–DAD–CL method with H_2O_2, $O_2^{\bullet-}$, and $ONOO^-$scavenging experiments.

Abbreviations

HSW: roots of *Polygonum multiflorum* Thunb.; HPLC–DAD–CL: high-performance liquid chromatography with diode array detector coupled with chemiluminescence detection; CM: Chinese medicine; UHPLC-LTQ-Orbitrap MS: UHPLC with linear ion trap-Orbitrap tandem mass spectrometry; RSDs: the relative standard deviations; HCA: hierarchical cluster analysis.

Authors' contributions

HFC, YHC, JQ and BYY designed the study. HFC conducted the experiments. HFC,CHL, LW and XC wrote the manuscript. All authors read and approved the final manuscript.

Author details

[1] Jiangsu Key Laboratory of TCM Evaluation and Translational Research, China Pharmaceutical University, 639 Longmian Road, Nanjing 210009, China. [2] Key Laboratory of Modern Preparation of TCM of Ministry of Education, Jiangxi University of Traditional Chinese Medicine, Nanchang 330004, China. [3] Department of Complex Prescription of Traditional Chinese Medicine, State Key Laboratory of Natural Medicines, China Pharmaceutical University, 639 Longmian Road, Nanjing 211198, China.

Acknowledgements

This study was financially supported by National Natural Science Foundation of China (No. 81274004), 2011' Program for Excellent Scientific and Technological Innovation Team of Jiangsu Higher Education and the Priority Academic Program Development of Jiangsu Higher Education Institutions.

Competing interests

The authors declare that they have no competing interests.

References

1. Li SZ. Compendium of materia medica. Beijing: China Medical Science Press; 2011. p. 673–5.
2. Um MY, Choi WH, Aan JY, Kim SR, Ha TY. Protective effect of *Polygonum multiflorum* Thunb. on amyloid β-peptide 25-35 induced cognitive deficits in mice. J Ethnopharmacol. 2006;104:144–8.
3. Park HJ, Zhang NN, Park DK. Topical application of *Polygonum multiflorum* extract induces hair growth of resting hair follicles through upregulating Shh and β-catenin expression in C57BL/6 mice. J Ethnopharmacol. 2011;135:369–75.
4. Sun YN, Cui L, Li W, Yan XT, Yang SY, Kang JI I, Kang HK, Kim YH. Promotion effect of constituents from the root of *Polygonum multiflorum* on hair growth. Bioorg Med Chem Lett. 2013;23:4801–5.
5. Lv LS, Shao X, Wang LY, Huang DR, Ho CT, Sang SM. Stilbene glucoside from *Polygonum Multiflorum* Thunb.: a novel natural inhibitor of advanced glycation end product formation by trapping of methylglyoxal. J Agr Food Chem. 2010;58:2239–45.
6. Yao WJ, Fan WJ, Huang C, Zhong H, Chen XF, Zhang W. Proteomic analysis for anti-atherosclerotic effect of tetrahydroxy stilbene glucoside in rats. Biomed Pharmacother. 2013;67:140–5.
7. Zhang JK, Yang L, Meng GL, Fan J, Chen JZ, He QZ, Chen S, Fan JZ, Luo ZJ, Liu J. Protective effect of tetrahydroxystilbene glucoside against hydrogen peroxide-induced dysfunction and oxidative stress in osteoblastic MC3T3-E1 cells. Eur J Pharmacol. 2012;689:31–7.
8. Yao S, Li Y, Kong LY. Preparative isolation and purification of chemical constituents from the root of *Polygonum multiflorum* by high-speed counter-current chromatography. J Chromatogr A. 2006;1115:64–71.
9. Chen LL, Huang XJ, Li MM, Ou GM, Zhao BX, Chen MF, Zhang QW, Wang Y, Ye WC. Polygonflavanol A, a novel flavonostilbene glycoside from the roots of *Polygonum Multiflorum*. Phytochem Lett. 2012;5:756–60.
10. Han DQ, Zhao J, Xu J, Peng HS, Chen XJ, Li SP. Quality evaluation of *Polygonum Multiflorum*in China based on HPLC analysis of hydrophilic bioactive compounds and chemometrics. J Pharm Biomed Anal. 2013;72:223–30.
11. He DX, Chen B, Tian QQ, Yao SZ. Simultaneous determination of five anthraquinones in medicinal plants and pharmaceutical preparations by HPLC with fluorescence detection. J Pharm Biomed Anal. 2009;49:1123–7.
12. Zhu ZW, Li J, Gao XM, Amponsem E, Kang LY, Hu LM, Zhang BL, Chang YX. Simultaneous determination of stilbenes, phenolic acids, flavonoids and anthraquinones in Radix *Polygonimultiflori* by LC–MS/MS. J Pharm Biomed Anal. 2012;62:162–6.
13. Qiu XH, Zhang J, Huang ZH, Zhu DY, Xu W. Profiling of phenolic constituents in *Polygonum multiflorum* Thunb.by combination of ultra-high-pressure liquid chromatography with linear ion trap-Orbitrap mass spectrometry. J Chromatogr A. 2013;1292:121–31.
14. Liang ZT, Chen HB, Yu ZL, Zhao ZZ. Comparison of raw and processed radix *Polygoni multiflori* (Heshouwu) by high performance liquid chromatography and mass spectrometry. Chin Med-UK. 2010;5:29–37.
15. Ding XP, Qi J, Chang YX, Mu LL, Zhu DN, Yu BY. Quality control of flavonoids in Ginkgo biloba leaves by high-performance liquid chromatography with diode array detection and on-line radical scavenging activity detection. J Chromatogr A. 2009;1216:2204–10.
16. He WH, Liu X, Xu HG, Gong Y, Yuan F, Gao YX. On-line HPLC-ABTS screening and HPLC-DAD-MS/MS identification of free radical scavengers in Gardenia (Gardenia jasminoides Ellis) fruit extracts. Food Chem. 2010;123:521–8.
17. Zhang YT, Li Q, Xing H, Lu XF, Zhao LS, Qu KK, Bi KS. Evaluation of antioxidant activity of ten compounds in different tea samples by means of an on-line HPLC–DPPH assay. Food Res Int. 2013;53:847–56.
18. Sohal RS, Svensson I, Brunk UT. Hydrogen peroxide production by liver mitochondria in different species. Mech Ageing Dev. 1990;53:209–15.
19. Bergamini E, Cavallini G, Donati A, Gori Z. The role of macroautophagy in the ageing process, anti-ageing intervention and age-associated diseases. Int J Biochem Cell Biol. 2004;36:2392–404.
20. Moreira PI, Nunomura A, Nakamura M, Takeda A, Shenk JC, Aliev G, Smith MA, Perry G. Nucleic acid oxidation in Alzheimer disease. Free Radic Bio Med. 2008;44:1493–505.
21. Page MM, Robb EL, Salway KD, Stuart JA. Mitochondrial redox metabolism: aging, longevity and dietary effects. Mech Ageing Dev. 2010;131:242–52.
22. Poulsen HE, Specht E, Broedbaek K, Henriksen T, Ellervik C, Mandrup-Poulsen T, Tonnesen M, Nielsen PE, Andersen HU, Weimann A. RNA modifications by oxidation: a novel disease mechanism? Free Radic Bio Med. 2012;52:1353–61.
23. Zhou XX, Yang Q, Xie YH, Sun JY, Qiu PC, Cao W, Wang SW. Protective effect of tetrahydroxystilbene glucoside against D-galactose induced aging process in mice. Phytochem Lett. 2013;6:372–8.
24. Pharmacopoeia of the People's Republic of China, Part I. The Pharmacopoeia Commission of PRC. Beijing: China Medical Science Press; 2010. p. 164–165.
25. Beckman JS, Chen J, Ischiropoulos H, Crow JP. Oxidative chemistry of peroxynitrite. New York: E-Publishing Inc.; 1994. p. 229–40.
26. Qi J, Chen YH, Wang Y, Chen X, Wang L, Hu YJ, Yu BY. Screening of peroxynitrite scavengers in Flos Lonicerae by using two new methods, an HPLC-DAD-CL technique and a peroxynitrite spiking test followed by HPLC-DAD analysis. Phytochem Anal. 2015; in press.
27. Ye M, Han J, Chen HB, Zheng JH, Guo D. Analysis of phenolic compounds in Rhubarbs using liquid chromatography coupled with electrospray ionization mass spectrometry. J Am Soc. 2007;18:82–91.
28. Chen WS, Liu WY, Yang GJ, Zhang WD, Chu ZY, Chen HS, Qiao CZ. Structural elucidation of a new tetrahydroxystilbene of Radix *Polygoni multiflori* preparata and study on its cardiovascular activity. Acta Pharm Sin. 2000;35:906–8.

29. Kim HK, Choi YH, Choi JS, Choi SU, Kim YS, Lee KR, Kim YK, Ryu SY. A new stilbene glucoside gallate from the roots of *Polygonum multiflorum*. Arch Pharm Res. 2008;31:1225–9.
30. Ashihara H, Deng WW, Mullen W, Crozier A. Distribution and biosynthesis of flavan-3-ols in *Camellia sinensis* seedlings and expression of genes encoding biosynthetic enzymes. Phytochemistry. 2010;71:559–66.
31. Wang WG, He YR, Lin P, Li YF, Sun RF, Gu W, Yu J. Zhao RH. In vitro effects of active components of *Polygonum Multiflorum* Radix on enzymes involved in the lipid metabolism. J Ethnopharmacol. 2014;153:763–70.
32. Haute GV, Eduardo C, Squizania E, Mesquita FC, Pedrazza L, Martha BA, Melo DA, Cassel E, Czepielewski RS, Bitencourt S, Goettert MI, Oliveira JR. Gallic acid reduces the effect of LPS on apoptosis and inhibits the formation of neutrophil extracellular traps. Toxicol In Vitro. 2015;30:309–17.
33. Song Y, Cui T, Xie N, Zhang XY, Qian ZB, Liu JY. Protocatechuic acid improves cognitive deficits and attenuates amyloid deposits, inflammatory response in aged AβPP/PS1 double transgenic mice. Int Immunopharmacol. 2014;20:276–81.
34. Prince PSM. (−) Epicatechin attenuates mitochondrial damage by enhancing mitochondrial multi-marker enzymes, adenosine triphosphate and lowering calcium in isoproterenol induced myocardial infarcted rats. Food Chem Toxicol. 2013;53:409–16.
35. Ma J, Zheng L, Deng T, Li CL, He YS, Li HJ, Ping Li. Stilbeneglucoside inhibits the glucuronidation of emodin in rats through the down-regulation of UDP-glucuronosyltransferases 1A8: application to a drug–drug interaction study in Radix *Polygoni Multiflori*. J Ethnopharmacol. 2013;147:335–40.
36. Zheng W, Zhang M, Zhang CF, Wang ZT. Study on quality evaluation for 36 Samples of Radix *Polygonui Multiflori* by HPLC-fingerprints. Chin Pharm J. 2006;41:257–60.

15

In silico profiling for secondary metabolites from *Lepidium meyenii* (maca) by the pharmacophore and ligand-shape-based joint approach

Fan Yi[1,2], Xiao-lei Tan[1,2], Xin Yan[3] and Hai-bo Liu[1,2*]

Abstract

Background: *Lepidium meyenii* Walpers (maca) is an herb known as a traditional nutritional supplement and widely used in Peru, North America, and Europe to enhance human fertility and treat osteoporosis. The secondary metabolites of maca, namely, maca alkaloids, macaenes, and macamides, are bioactive compounds, but their targets are undefined.

Methods: The pharmacophore-based PharmaDB targets database screening joint the ligand shape similarity-based WEGA validation approach is proposed to predict the targets of these unique constituents and was performed using Discovery Studio 4.5 and PharmaDB. A compounds–targets–diseases network was established using Cytoscape 3.2. These suitable targets and their genes were calculated and analyzed using ingenuity pathway analysis and GeneMANIA.

Results: Certain targets were identified in osteoporosis (8 targets), prostate cancer (9 targets), and kidney diseases (11 targets). This was the first study to identify the targets of these bioactive compounds in maca for cardiovascular diseases (29 targets). The compound with the most targets (46) was an amide alkaloid (MA-24).

Conclusion: In silico target fishing identified maca's traditional effects on treatment and prevention of osteoporosis, prostate cancer, and kidney diseases, and its potential function of treating cardiovascular diseases, as the most important of this herb's possible activities.

Background

Lepidium meyenii Walpers (maca) belongs to the brassica (mustard) family and the *Lepidium* genus, which grows robustly only at altitudes over 4000 m [1]. Maca has three major phenotypes, yellow, red and black, based on its hypocotyl and stem coloration [2]. The underground part of the maca is consumed as a food and as a folk medicine to enhance fertility and sexual behaviors and has multiple bioactivities [3]. Currently, maca is used in nutrition and health care products sold from Peru to North America and Europe [4, 5]. Maca contains abundant valuable nutritional ingredients [6], such as maca alkaloids, macaenes, glucosinolates, sterols, and polyphenols, and other secondary metabolites. The maca alkaloids, especially macamides and macaenes, are the main functional constituents of maca [7, 8]. To date, 31 maca alkaloids and four macaenes have been isolated from *L. meyenii.* Their structures are shown below (Table 1). All of the macamides, which are found only in maca, are *N*-benzylamides. Wu [9] synthesized 11 of the reported macamides as well as a series of structurally related amides that resemble macamides (Table 2). These synthesized compounds were collected in this study and used in our experiments.

*Correspondence: fantasyee8991@163.com
[1] Institute of Medicinal Plant Development, Chinese Academy of Medical Sciences, Peking Union Medical College, 151 Malianwa N, Haidian District, Beijing 100193, China
Full list of author information is available at the end of the article

Table 1 Structures of alkaloids and macaenes isolated from *L. meyenii*

No.	Type	Structure	Reference
MA-1	Amide alkaloid	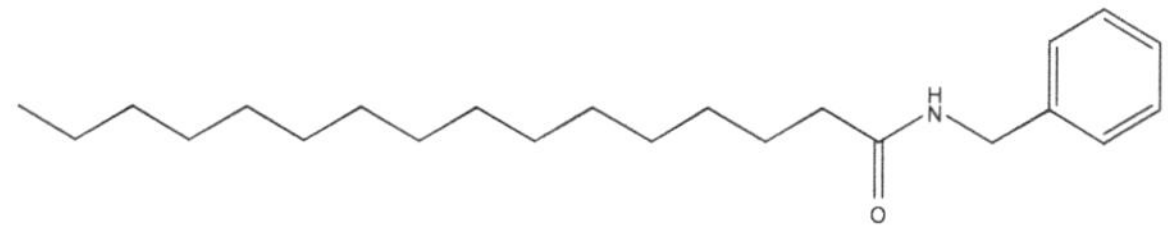	[26]
MA-2	Amide alkaloid	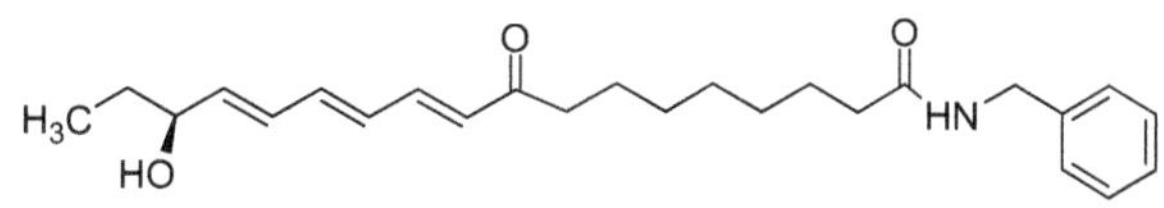	[25]
MA-3	Amide alkaloid	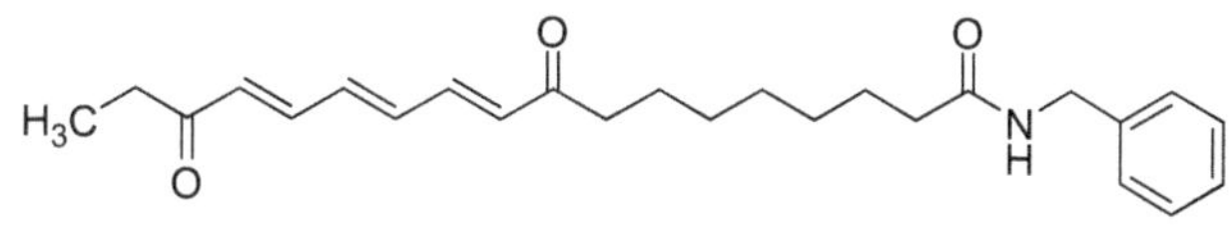	[25]
MA-5	Amide alkaloid	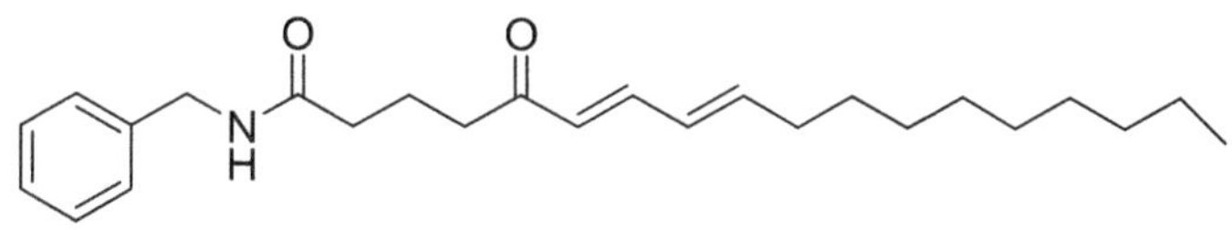	[26]
MA-6	Amide alkaloid	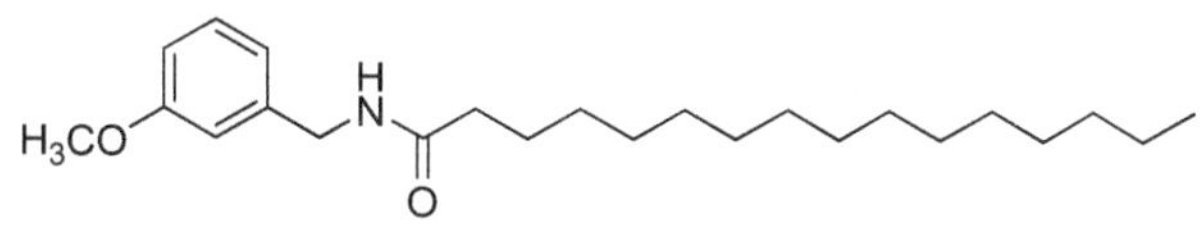	[27]
MA-7	Amide alkaloid	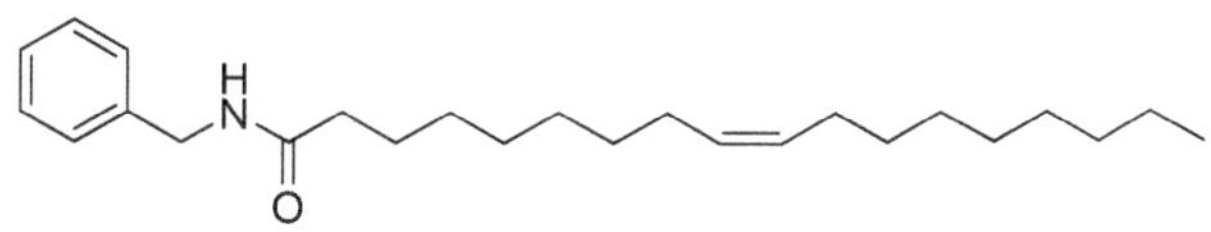	[27]
MA-8	Amide alkaloid	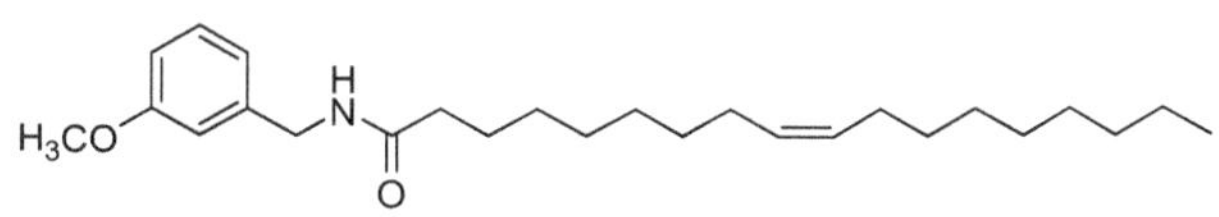	[27]
MA-9	Amide alkaloid	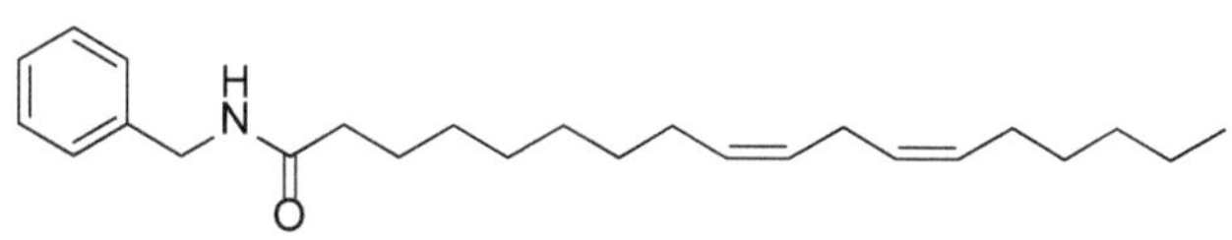	[27]
MA-10	Amide alkaloid	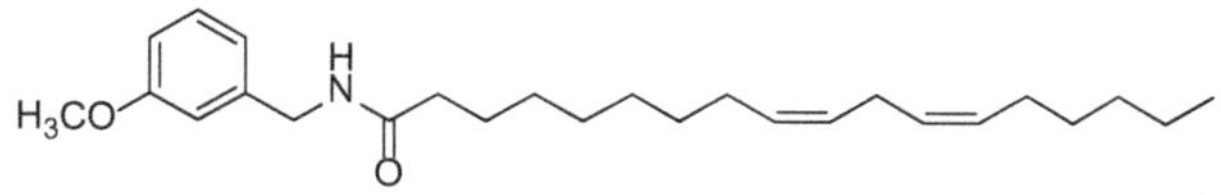	[27]
MA-11	Amide alkaloid	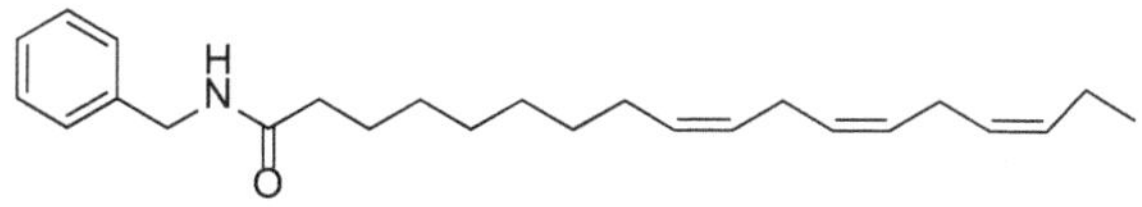	[27]
MA-12	Amide alkaloid	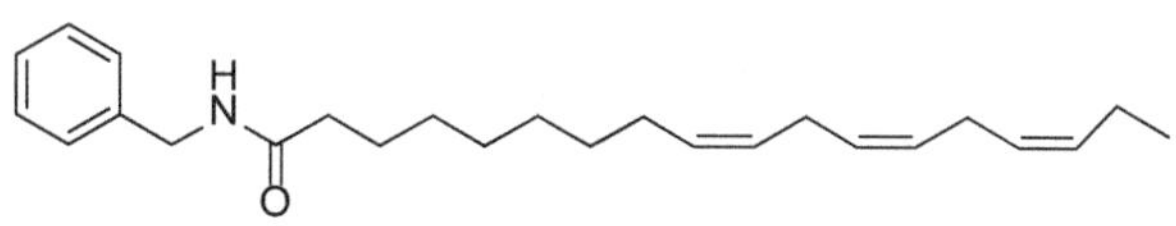	[27]
MA-13	Amide alkaloid	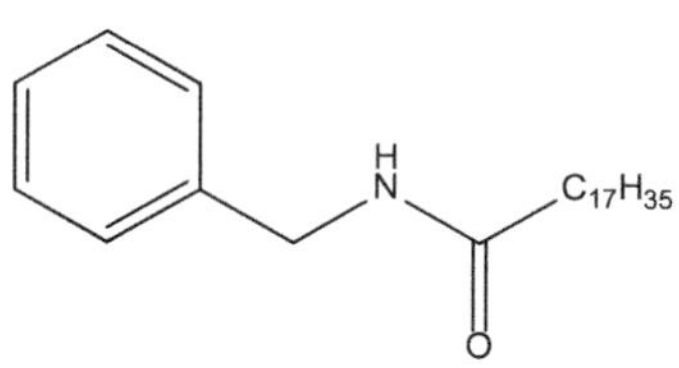	[27]

Table 1 continued

No.	Type	Structure	Reference
MA-14	Amide alkaloid	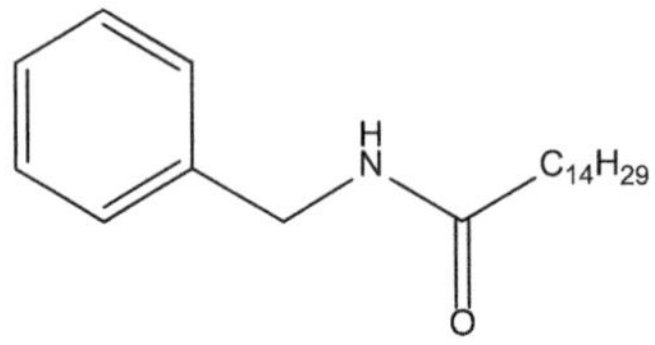	[27]
MA-15	Amide alkaloid	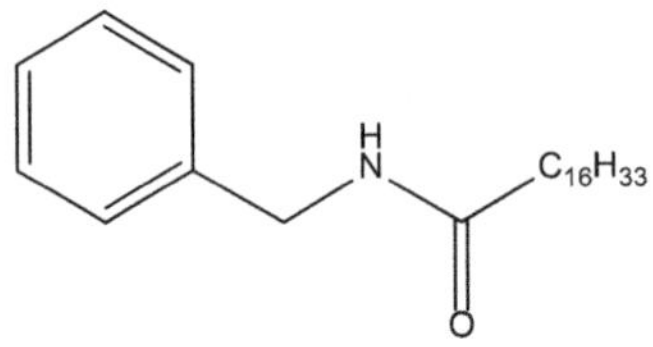	[27]
MA-19	Amide alkaloid	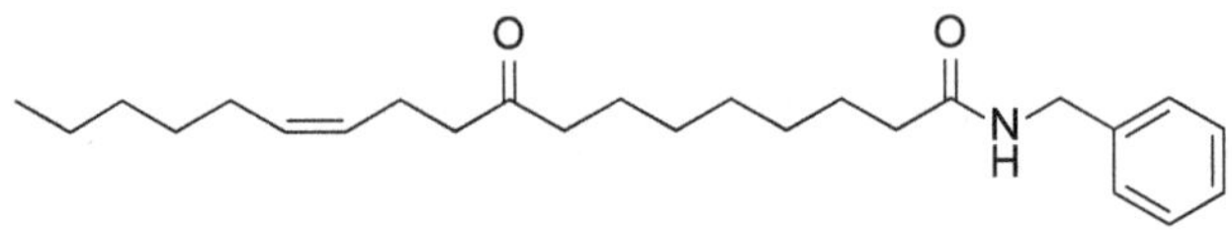	[26]
MA-20	Amide alkaloid	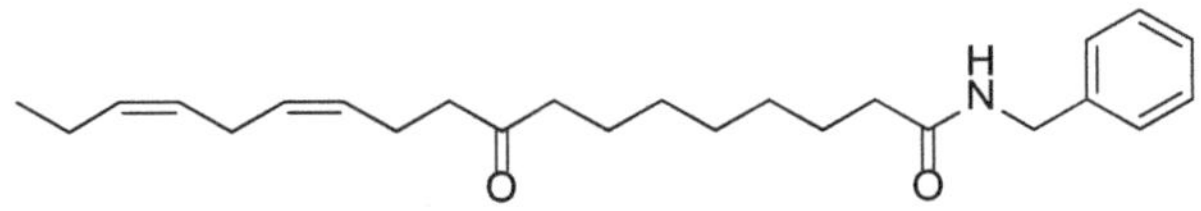	[26]
MA-21	Amide alkaloid	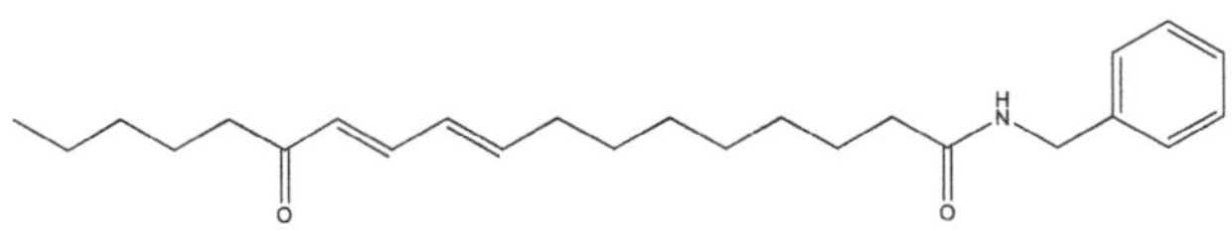	[26]
MA-22	Amide alkaloid	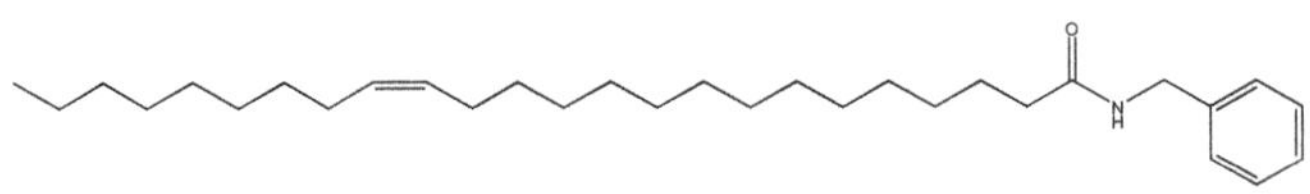	[26]
MA-23	Amide alkaloid	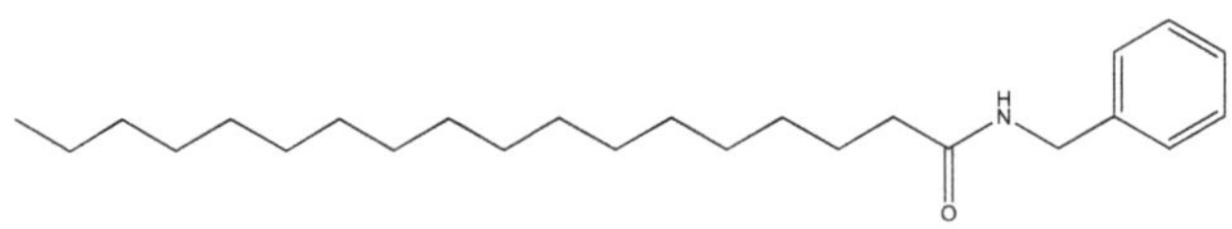	[27]
MA-27	Amide alkaloid	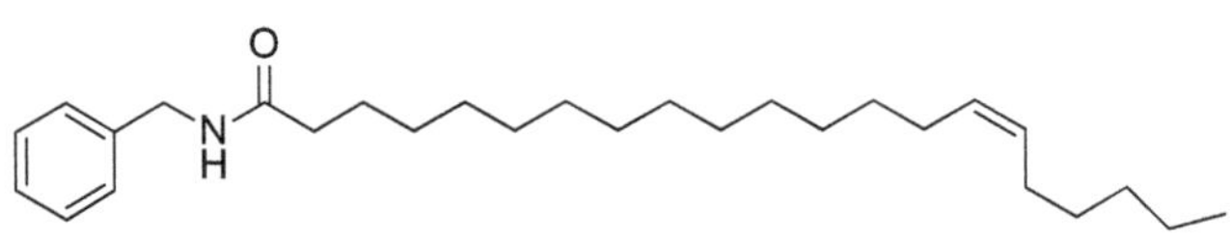	[26]
MA-28	Amide alkaloid	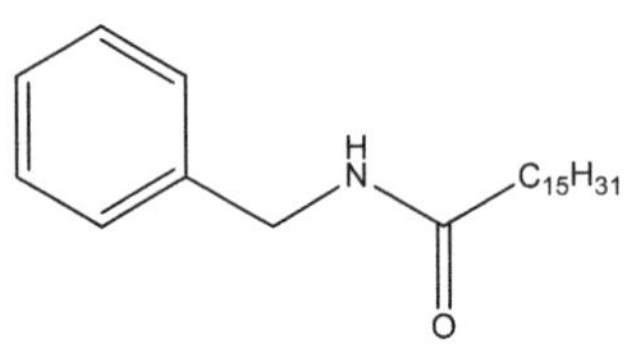	[27]
MA-24	Amide alkaloid	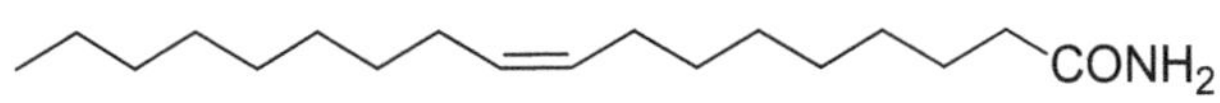	[9]
MA-25	Amide alkaloid	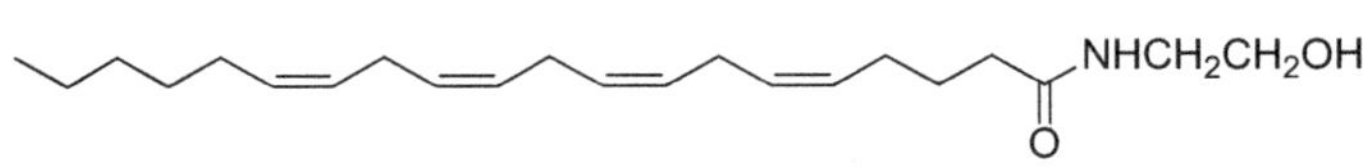	[9]
MA-26	Amide alkaloid	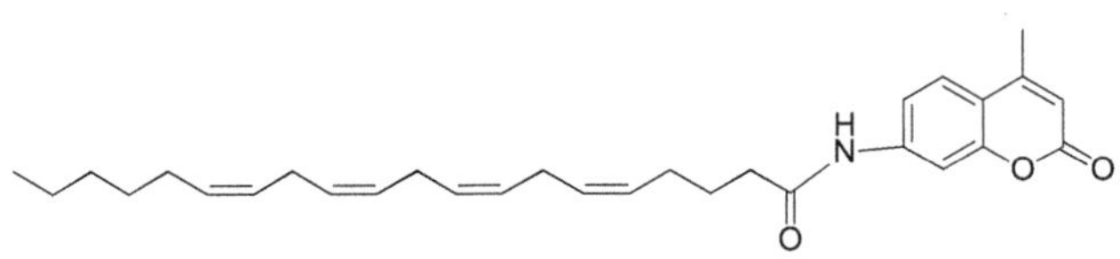	[9]

Table 1 continued

No.	Type	Structure	Reference
MA-4	Pyridine derivatives	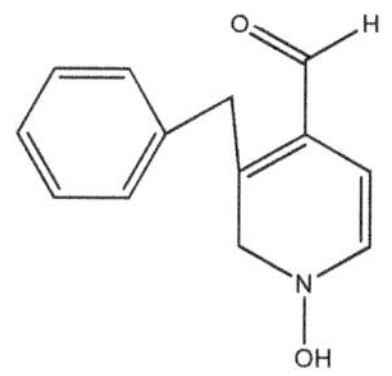	[26]
MA-29	Pyridine derivatives	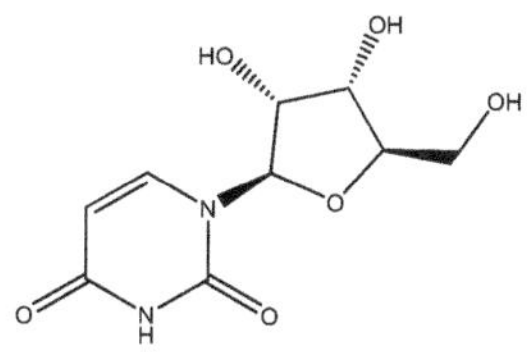	[28]
MA-31	Pyridine derivatives	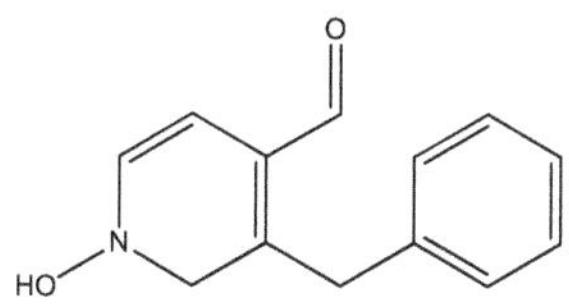	[28]
MA-16	Imidazole alkaloid	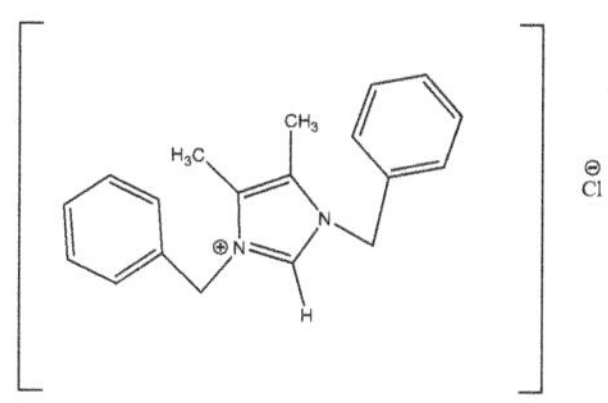	[25]
MA-17	Imidazole alkaloid	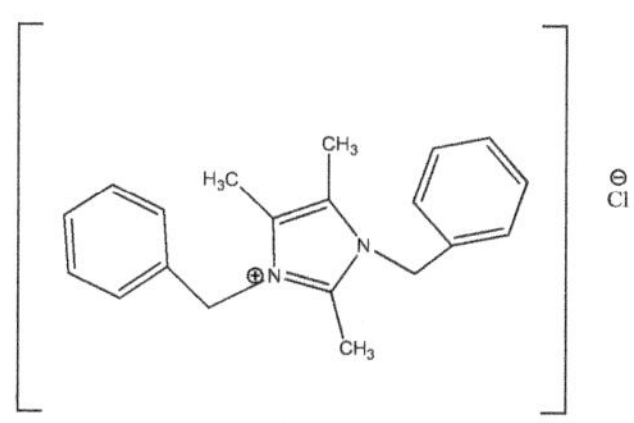	[6]
MA-18	β-carboline alkaloids	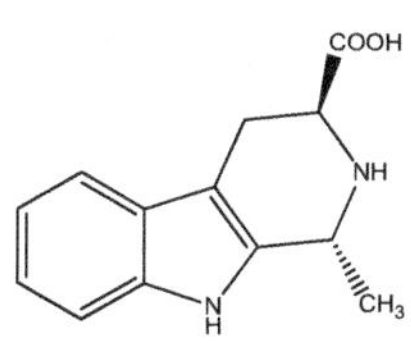	[29]
MA-30	Indole alkaloid	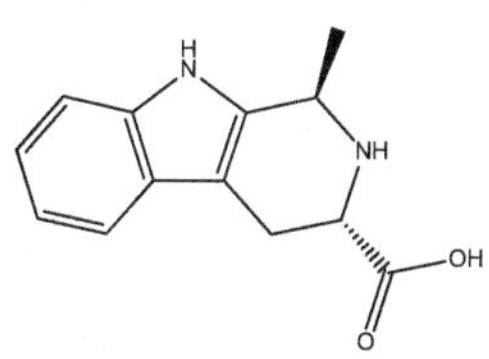	[29]
MA-32	Macaene	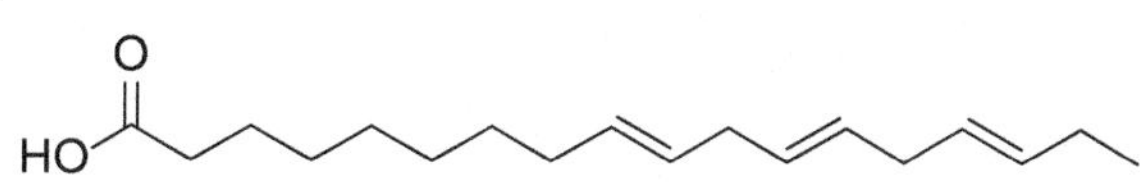	[30]
MA-33	Macaene	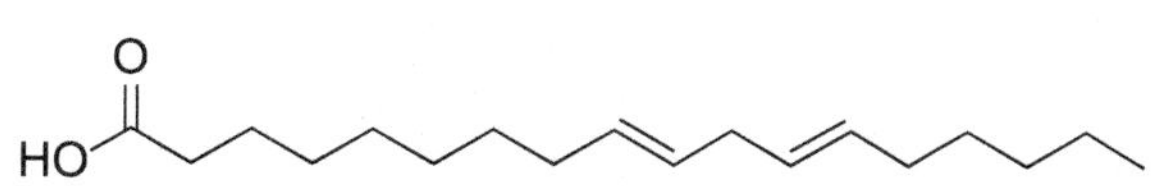	

Table 1 continued

No.	Type	Structure	Reference
MA-34	Macaene	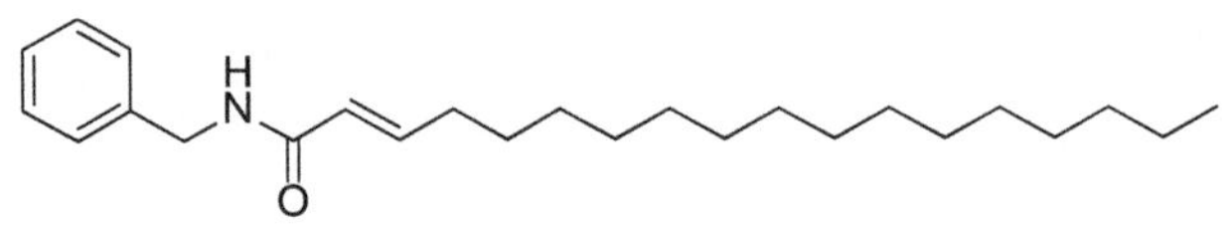	
MA-35	Macaene	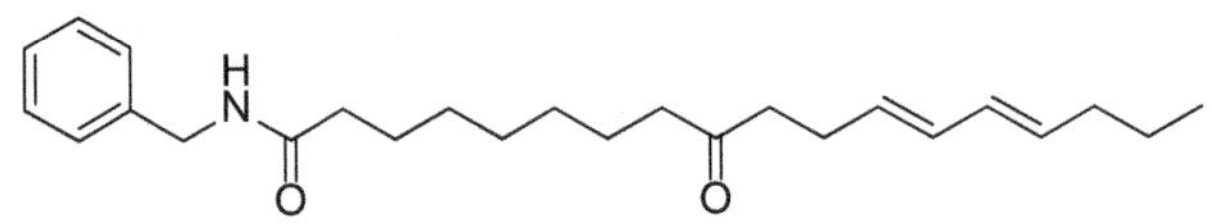	

The biological and pharmacological effects of maca have been investigated in experimental animals such as rats [10], mice [11], fish [12], and bulls [13]. Maca can enhance sexual behavior and increase sperm count [14], improve prostate function related to testosterone enanthate (TE) levels [15], and improve the quality of embryos [16, 17]. Maca also has beneficial effects on learning and memory in scopolamine-induced memory impairment mice [18]. Moreover, maca aqueous extract scavenges free radicals and protects cells against oxidative stress [5].

Several in vitro/in vivo animal experimental studies have shown that secondary metabolites extracted from maca have bioactivities that help treat osteoporosis and enhance prostate function and sexual function [19–21]. However, most in vitro and in vivo experiments have not specified the molecular target of these secondary metabolites and the mechanisms of the functions of the compounds obtained from maca are unclear. The pharmacophore model is reliable for parallel screening to predict and mimic the binding situation of compounds and targets [22, 23]. This study aimed to investigate the network involved in the mechanisms of action of secondary metabolites of maca. We used the pharmacophore-based method in combination with a novel ligand shape similarity strategy and used the weighted Gaussian algorithm (WEGA).

Methods

Collection of chemical constituents

The natural constituents of maca were collected from the literature [9, 24–30] using the search terms "*lepidium* or maca" combined with "constitutes, compounds, chemical or metabolites." Traditionally used maca contains a dominant pattern of secondary metabolites, particularly alkaloids and macaenes [31]. The secondary metabolite constituents from maca were evaluated to precisely predict the active compounds. A total of 47 alkaloids extracted from maca and synthetic amides were categorized into classes.

Conformer generation

All chemical structures were prepared in SD format, converted from a 2D cdx file format to 3D models, using Open Babel GUI [32] version 2.3.2 (OpenBableGUI; Chris Morley, USA). Molecular energy was minimized using the Energy Minimization module of Discovery Studio version 4.5 (DS 4.5; Accelrys Inc., San Diego, CA, USA) under the chemistry at Harvard Macromolecular Mechanics (CHARMM) force field. This survey led to the construction of the 3D multi-conformational maca compounds molecular structure database (i.e., maca-DB), which was generated by a Monte Carlo-based conformational analysis (FAST mode). These compounds are rigid; the number of conformers for each compound is much less than 255. The maca-DB contains a total of 47 constituents and 9976 conformations.

Pharmacophore model collection

In silico profiling of the maca-DB was performed using the generated 3D chemical feature-based pharmacophore models. The pharmacophore models were used to represent the binding mode of particular compounds to specific drug targets [33]. Each pharmacophore model contained several convictive chemical features that determine the chemical functionalities of a certain ligand: H-bond donors or acceptors, hydrophobic groups, aromatic nuclei, and positive or negative ionizable moieties [34]. Unlike common docking methods, pharmacophore-based virtual screening outlines the specific compounds and their multiple pharmacologic targets and determines novel actions of these compounds.

PharmaDB

PharmaDB is the only pharmacophore database implemented in DS 4.5. A total of 68,000 pharmacophores were derived from 8000 protein–ligand complexes in the sc-PDB dataset. sc-PDB is designed to identify binding sites suitable for the docking of a drug-like ligand, and 9276 three-dimensional structures of binding sites were identified using the Protein Data Bank (PDB) [35].

Table 2 Structures of the synthetic amides resembling macamides

No.	Type of compounds	Structure
MA-36	Amide alkaloid	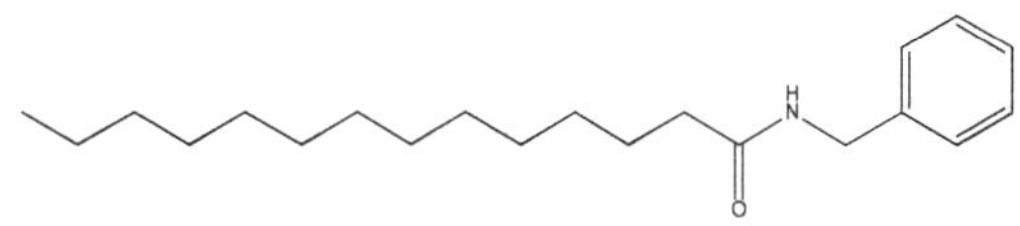
MA-37	Amide alkaloid	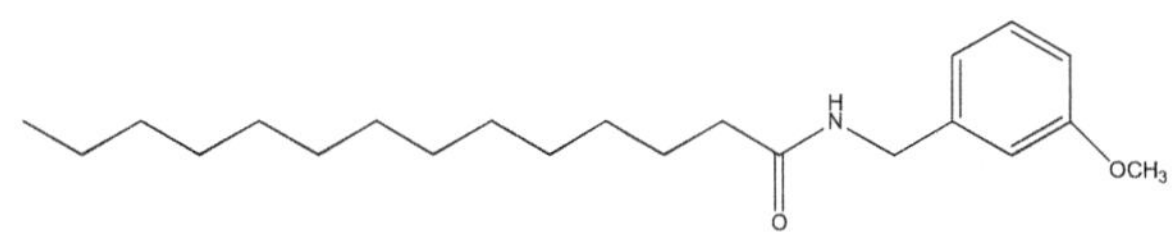
MA-38	Amide alkaloid	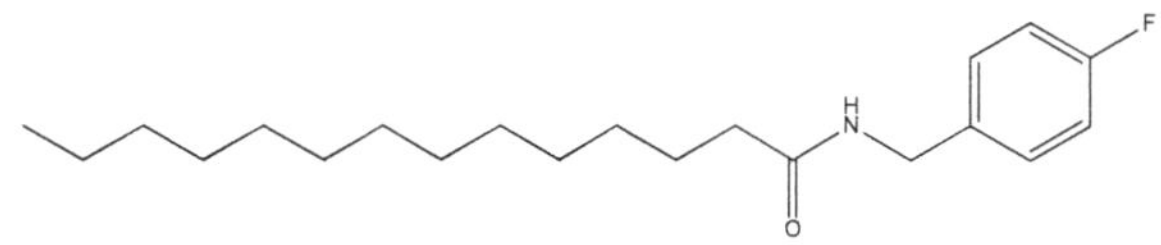
MA-39	Amide alkaloid	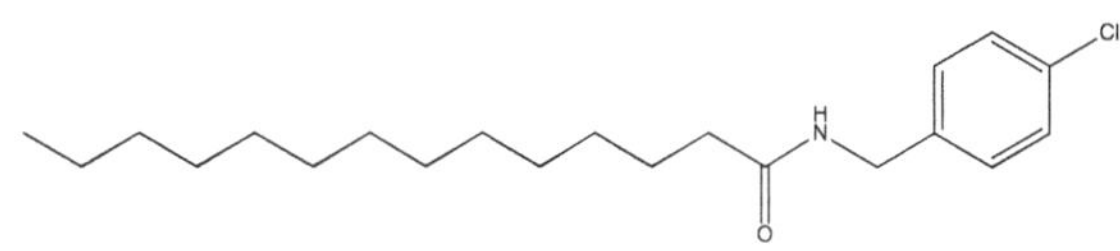
MA-40	Amide alkaloid	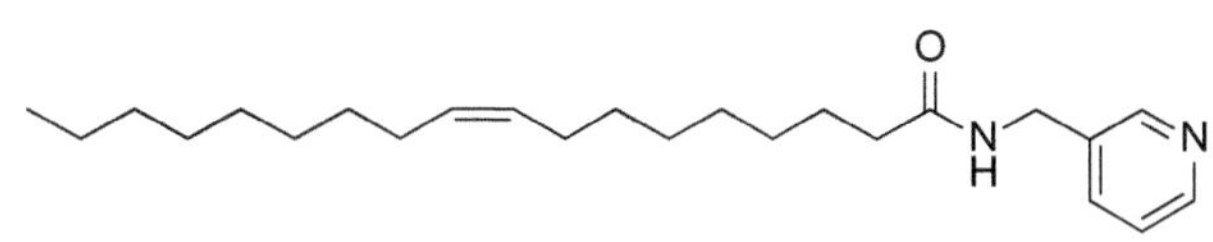
MA-41	Amide alkaloid	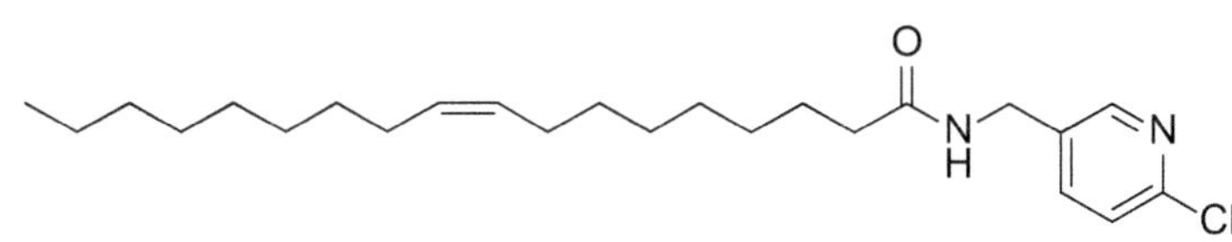
MA-42	Amide alkaloid	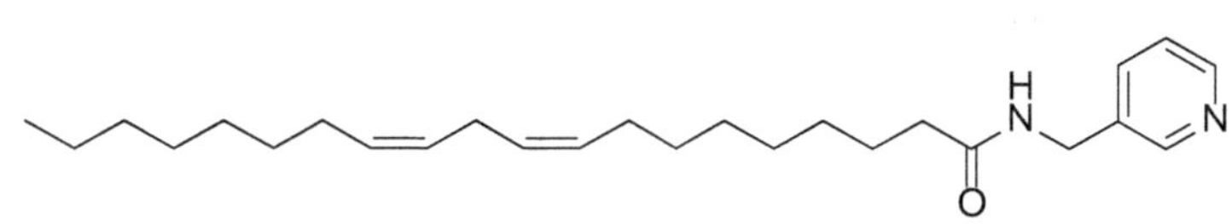
MA-43	Amide alkaloid	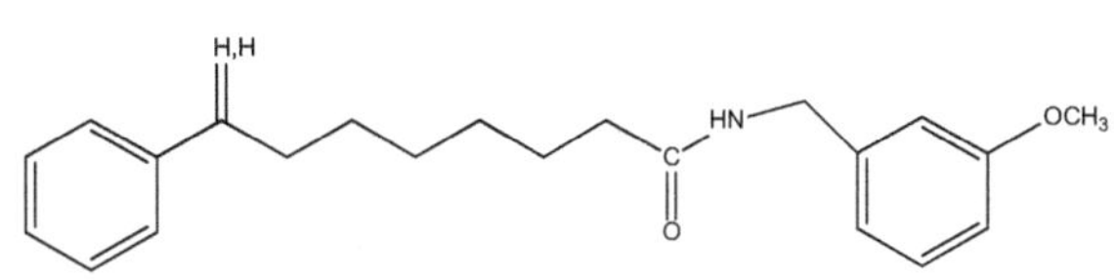
MA-44	Amide alkaloid	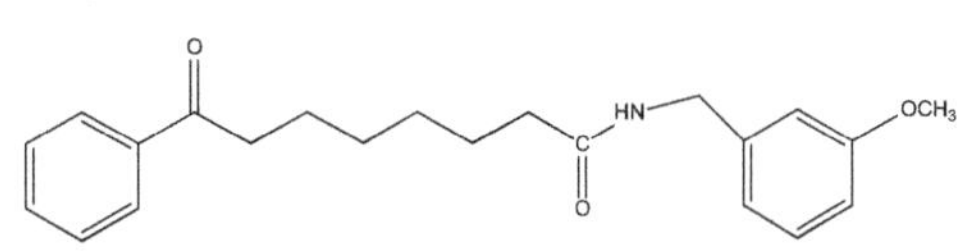
MA-45	Amide alkaloid	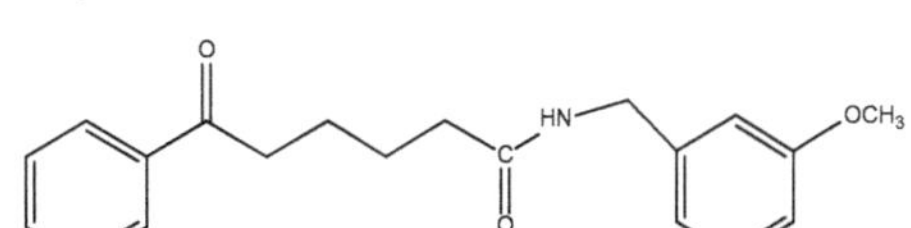
MA-46	Amide alkaloid	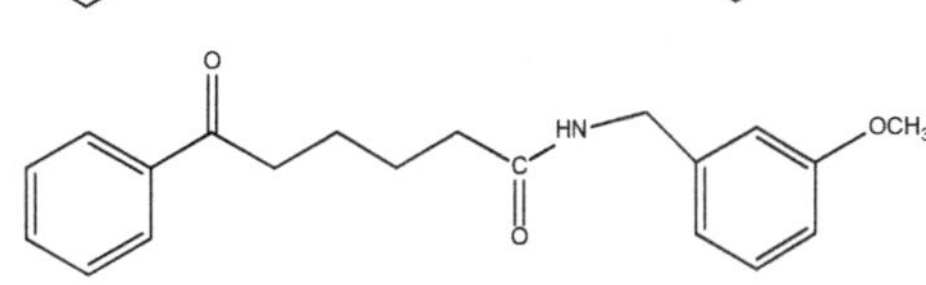
MA-47	Amide alkaloid	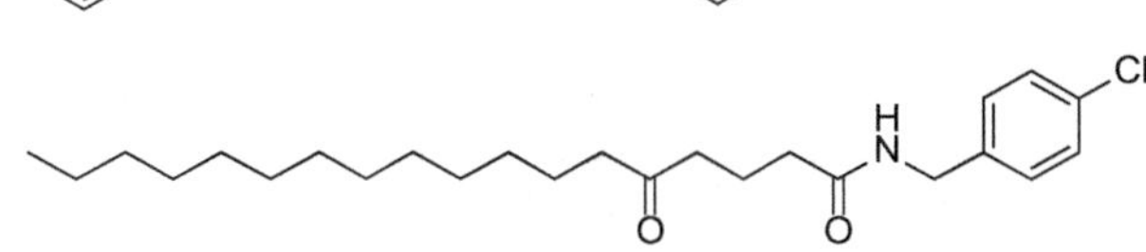

Parameters

In this study, PharmaDB was used for profiling. All pharmacophore models with the shape of the binding pocket were selected for virtual screening using the default settings of the Ligand Profiler module of DS 4.5. In principle, each alkaloid that mapped to a chemical feature of the respective pharmacophore model was counted as one hit. The screening was conducted using the default settings and with a minimal inter-feature distance of 0.5 Å.

Binding mode refinement

All the poses of the ligands mapped to the pharmacophore were preserved. A series of target–ligand pairs were selected for further examination. The selection was based on compatibility with previously reported pharmacological activities and the traditional use of maca. Further refinement was carried in Molecular Operating Environment (MOE; Chemical Computing Group Inc., Canada) to identify the protein–ligand binding modes. Energy minimization was performed by conjugated gradient minimization with the Merck Molecular Force Field 94× (MMFF94×) until a root-mean-square deviation of 0.1 kcal mol^{-1} $Å^{-1}$ was reached.

WEGA validation

The WEGA is an accurate shape-based virtual screening method [36]. In this research, we validated the reliability of the binding model by calculating the binding efficiencies of the compounds and the original ligands of the hit targets using the shape similarity calculations function of WEGA.

The sc-PDB also provides separate MOL2 files for the ligand, its binding site, and the corresponding protein chain(s). Ions and cofactors at the vicinity of the ligand are included in the protein. This helps to evaluate the influence of ligand binding on binding site diversity for docking. MOL2 files of the hit-target protein ligands were selected to create the target-ligands database (tl-DB). WEGA validation was performed by comparing the contents of the maca-DB to those of the tl-DB.

Network construction

The Table 3 showing interactions between all mapped compounds and hit targets shows the ligand profiling results. For each target, the protein name, gene name, and pathway information were collected from the PDB, Kyoto Encyclopedia of Genes and Genomes (KEGG) [37], and Cell Signaling Technology (CST) [38]. The target–target interactions were mapped using GeneMANIA [39]; all targets were analyzed using Ingenuity Pathway Analysis (IPA®; Qiagen, Redwood City, CA, USA). All diseases related to the targets were retrieved from the Therapeutic

Table 3 Four categories of disease targets of the selected compounds from profiling

Target	No. of hit compound	Drugs[a]
Osteoporosis		
ABL1	2	Nilotinib, saracatinib, regorafenib
ER-α	4	17-α-ethinylestradiol, fulvestrant, β-estradiol
CSF1R	2	Nilotinib, sunitinib, pazopanib
MMP3	1	Marimastat
C-src	2	Dasatinib, AZM-475271, saracatinib,
MMP9	1	
MMP13	3	Marimastat
CDK9	1	BMS-387032, alvocidib
Prostate cancer		
Hsp90-α	15	Alvespimycin, retaspimycin, luminespib
MMP3	1	Marimastat
MET	1	Crizotinib, tivantinib, cabozantinib
AR	3	Testosterone enanthate, enzalutamide, 1-testosterone
MMP9	1	
RXR-α	4	Etretinate, tretinoin, bexarotene
MMP12	4	Marimastat
MMP13	3	Marimastat
MAP2K1	3	Selumetinib, trametinib, dabrafenib
Kidney diseases		
MMP9	1	
CA2	11	Ethoxyzolamide, dichlorphenamide, brinzolamide
P450scc	22	
MET	1	Crizotinib, tivantinib, cabozantinib
MIF	1	
sEH	2	
PPAR-γ	20	Icosapent, amlodipine/telmisartan, aleglitazar,
MMP12	4	Marimastat
KIF11	23	
MAPK14	19	Talmapimod, RO-3201195
CA9	1	Girentuximab, methazolamide, hydrochlorothiazide
Cardiovascular diseases		
JAK2	19	Tofacitinib, ruxolitinib
F2	8	Enoxaparin, desirudin, dabigatran etexilate
F10	15	Dalteparin, heparin, enoxaparin
REN	1	Aliskiren, aliskiren/valsartan, aliskiren/amlodipine
CA1	1	Ethoxyzolamide, dichlorphenamide, brinzolamide
ER-α	4	17-α-ethinylestradiol, fulvestrant, β-estradiol
MMP3	1	Marimastat
LTA4H	3	
THR-β	1	Amiodarone, levothyroxine, dextrothyroxine,
FGFR1	16	Pazopanib, nintedanib, regorafenib
PLA2G2A	7	Varespladib methyl, varespladib, indomethacin
FLT1	3	Sunitinib, pazopanib, axitinib

Table 3 continued

Target	No. of hit compound	Drugs[a]
FGFR2	2	Nintedanib, regorafenib, dexamethasone/thalidomide
CDK2	26	BMS-387032, alvocidib
EPHX2	2	
KDR	8	Sunitinib, cediranib, pazopanib
PPAR-γ	20	Icosapent, amlodipine/telmisartan, aleglitazar,
MMP12	4	Marimastat
MMP13	3	Marimastat
PIK3CG	12	Dactolisib, buparlisib,
GSK3-β	2	Enzastaurin
CDK9	1	BMS-387032, alvocidib
MAPK10	7	
NR1H2	4	
DHODH	7	Teriflunomide, leflunomide
PPAR-δ	8	Treprostinil, icosapent, bezafibrate
PPAR-α	2	Choline fenofibrate, aleglitazar, gemfibrozil
MAPK14	19	Talmapimod, RO-3201195
NR1H4	1	

[a] All drug information was obtained from IPA analysis and Drugbank

Target Database (TTD) [40] and DrugBank database [41]. The overall compound–target–pathway networks were generated using Cytoscape, version 3.2 (Cytoscape Consortium, USA). In the graphical networks, nodes represent the compounds, targets, and related diseases. The edges linking the compound-target and target-diseases represent their relationships and are marked with two types of lines. The related diseases are marked with different colors at the nodes. The targeted diseases pathway was mapped using the KEGGscape plugin of Cytoscape, version 3.2.

Results and discussion

Evaluation of constituents

In modern drug discovery, large compound libraries are compared, and the diversity of these libraries must be analyzed [42]. The constituents collected and synthesized from maca could be divided into eight compound classes (Fig. 1). The 40 compounds examined in this research were fished by targets (Fig. 2). The compounds with higher degree values were distributed across different categories, such as amide alkaloids (MA-24; 25), macaenes (MA-32; 33), and synthetic amides (MA-43; 44). Compounds that participate in more interactions than other components have a higher bioactivity value.

Network analysis

In total, 950 models were selected for in silico screening of the maca-DB. These models belong to 125 protein targets; 87 of those targets were validated by the TTD database, were involved in 60 pathways, and were targets of 41 maca constituents. As shown in Fig. 2, we chose three major disease areas (prostate cancer, osteoporosis, and kidney diseases) to validate the traditional medical action and the fished maca compounds.

Interpreting the mechanisms of action

An array of well-defined in-house structure and ligand-based pharmacophore models was selected from PharmaDB. For the profiling results, all biological functions of hit targets were annotated from TTD and DrugBank. The identified targets had variable pharmacologic usages, such as the treatment of osteoporosis (8 targets), prostate disease (9 targets), and kidney disease (11 targets). Some targets were related to cardiovascular diseases (CVD), such as hypertension, myocardial infarction, ischemic heart disease, and dyslipidemia (29 targets). Figure 3 and Table 3 provides an overview of the selected targets in the four categories of disease mentioned above. A total of 125 targets were mapped, and the IPA analysis indicated that 107 of them have been used to make drugs. The druggable list is presented in Additional file 1.

WEGA validation

The WEGA is suitable for large-scale parallel screening of a series of bioactive compounds; regardless of the conformations of the compounds, their targets can be experimentally determined. The results determined by shape showed that all binding models obtained with DS 4.5 had a high ligand-receptor structure binding value: all scores were above 0.5 (Additional file 2). Important molecular superimposition images are shown in Fig. 4.

Selected targets related to prostate cancer

All the gene interactions of these targets were analyzed using GeneMANIA (Fig. 5; Additional file 3). Epidemiological studies have found that consumption of maca could reduce the risk of prostate cancer, which might be associated with aromatic glucosinolate content [7, 8]. Animal experiments in mice [43] and rats [7, 44, 45] showed that maca reduced TE level in a dose-dependent manner and induced prostatic hyperplasia. Red maca aqueous extracts can also reduce ventral prostate size in normal and TE-treated rats [7].

In this study, nine targets annotated by the TTD database were related to prostate cancer. One of the most common targets used in the treatment of prostate diseases is the androgen receptor (AR). In some cell types, testosterone is converted by 5-alpha-reductase into dihydrotestosterone, which is an even more potent agonist for AR activation than testosterone [46]. AR is a sequence-specific DNA-binding protein involved in cellular

COMPOUND	COMPLEXITY	CYCLICITY	CID	AE	HD	HA	AB	ATMS	BNDS	SSSRS	AZ	RB	UE	NCC	XLOGP	MW
MA-1	42.579	37.903	1	2.61	1	1	6	25	25	1	6.12	15	4	0	0	345.31
MA-2	42.579	33.052	1	2.66	2	2	6	29	29	1	6.24	17	8	1	0	397.27
MA-3	42.579	33.043	1	2.66	1	3	6	29	29	1	6.24	17	9	0	0	395.25
MA-4	74.557	87.783	4	2.69	1	2	6	16	17	2	6.31	3	6	0	0	215.1
MA-5	42.579	34.283	1	2.63	1	2	6	28	28	1	6.18	17	7	0	0	383.29
MA-6	42.579	35.327	1	2.63	1	2	6	27	27	1	6.19	16	4	0	0	375.32
MA-7	42.579	35.601	1	2.6	1	1	6	27	27	1	6.11	17	5	0	0	371.32
MA-8	42.579	33.322	1	2.63	1	2	6	29	29	1	6.17	18	5	0	0	401.33
MA-9	42.579	35.596	1	2.6	1	1	6	27	27	1	6.11	17	6	0	0	369.31
MA-10	42.579	33.318	1	2.63	1	2	6	29	29	1	6.17	18	6	0	0	399.32
MA-11	42.579	35.588	1	2.6	1	1	6	27	27	1	6.11	17	7	0	0	367.29
MA-12	42.579	33.312	1	2.63	1	2	6	29	29	1	6.17	18	7	0	0	397.3
MA-13	42.579	34.556	1	2.6	1	1	6	28	28	1	6.11	18	4	0	0	387.36
MA-14	42.579	37.903	1	2.61	1	1	6	25	25	1	6.12	15	4	0	0	345.31
MA-15	42.579	35.605	1	2.6	1	1	6	27	27	1	6.11	17	4	0	0	373.34
MA-16	93.218	94.981	7	2.6	1	1	17	21	23	3	6.1	2	8	0	0	278.18
MA-17	93.218	92.647	7	2.59	1	1	17	22	24	3	6.09	2	8	0	0	292.2
MA-18	75.212	85.021	5	2.71	3	1	10	17	19	3	6.35	1	5	2	0	230.11
MA-19	42.579	34.289	1	2.63	1	2	6	28	28	1	6.18	17	6	0	0	385.3
MA-20	42.579	34.283	1	2.63	1	2	6	28	28	1	6.18	17	7	0	0	383.29
MA-21	42.579	34.283	1	2.63	1	2	6	28	28	1	6.18	17	7	0	0	383.29
MA-22	42.579	30.117	1	2.59	1	1	6	33	33	1	6.09	23	5	0	0	455.42
MA-23	42.579	35.605	1	2.6	1	1	6	27	27	1	6.11	17	4	0	0	373.34
MA-24	0	17.462	0	2.62	1	1	0	20	19	0	6.15	16	2	0	0	281.28
MA-25	0	14.092	0	2.64	2	1	0	25	24	0	6.2	19	5	0	0	347.29
MA-26	68.9	49.455	3	2.64	1	3	6	34	35	2	6.21	18	10	0	0	461.3
MA-27	42.579	32.632	1	2.6	1	1	6	30	30	1	6.1	20	5	0	0	413.37
MA-28	42.579	36.718	1	2.6	1	1	6	26	26	1	6.12	16	4	0	0	359.32
MA-29	78.345	85.075	6	2.92	4	4	0	17	18	2	6.82	1	3	4	0	244.07
MA-30	75.212	85.021	5	2.71	3	1	10	17	19	3	6.35	1	5	2	0	230.11
MA-31	74.557	87.783	4	2.69	1	2	6	16	17	2	6.31	3	6	0	0	215.1
MA-32	0	17.328	0	2.64	1	1	0	20	19	0	6.2	16	4	0	0	278.23
MA-33	0	17.335	0	2.64	1	1	0	20	19	0	6.2	16	3	0	0	280.24
MA-34	42.579	35.601	1	2.6	1	1	6	27	27	1	6.11	17	5	0	0	371.32
MA-35	42.579	34.283	1	2.63	1	2	6	28	28	1	6.18	17	7	0	0	383.29
MA-36	42.579	40.516	1	2.61	1	1	6	23	23	1	6.13	13	4	0	0	317.28
MA-37	42.579	37.584	1	2.64	1	2	6	25	25	1	6.2	14	4	0	0	347.29
MA-38	42.579	38.619	1	2.67	1	1	6	24	24	1	6.25	13	4	0	0	335.27
MA-39	42.579	37.063	1	2.63	1	1	6	24	24	1	6.58	13	4	0	0	351.24
MA-40	43.455	36.219	2	2.62	1	2	6	27	27	1	6.15	17	5	0	0	372.32
MA-41	43.455	33.515	2	2.64	1	2	6	28	28	1	6.54	17	5	0	0	406.28
MA-42	43.455	34.161	2	2.61	1	2	6	29	29	1	6.14	19	6	0	0	398.33
MA-43	99.634	90.467	9	2.64	1	2	12	26	27	2	6.19	10	8	0	0	351.22
MA-44	99.634	89.869	9	2.67	1	3	12	26	27	2	6.27	10	8	0	0	353.2
MA-45	95.265	88.964	8	2.68	1	3	12	24	25	2	6.29	8	8	0	0	325.17
MA-46	42.579	34.294	1	2.63	1	2	6	28	28	1	6.18	17	5	0	0	387.32
MA-47	42.579	31.785	1	2.65	1	2	6	29	29	1	6.55	17	5	0	0	421.28

Fig. 1 The diversity of compounds analyzed by the scaffold-based classification approach (SCA). CID means compound class ID, categories by complexity; the SCA also outputs the following structural descriptor values: (1) *Cyclicity* side chain value; (2) *AE* average electronegativity; (3) *HD* number of H-bond donors; (3) *HA* number of H-bond acceptors; (4) *AB* number of aromatic bonds; (5) *ATMS* number of non-H atoms; (6) *BNDS* number of non-H-involved bonds; (7) *SSSRS* number of the smallest set of smallest rings; (8) *AZ* average atomic numbers; (9) *RB* number of rotating bonds; (10) *MW* molecular weight

proliferation in prostate cancer and in the development of secondary sexual characteristics through activation by dihydrotestosterone [47]. AR is also involved in the regulation of the adhesion of prostate cancer cells to the extracellular matrix and to the invasion of prostate cancer cells through its influence on the expression of specific integrin subunits [48]. There is increasing evidence that the genus *Lepidium* could reduce the risk of prostate cancer development [49, 50]. Research also suggests that other cruciferous plants from the genus *Lepidium* could be used as important alternative treatments for prostate diseases [51]. Growth of the prostate is a hormone-mediated phenomenon regulated by both androgens and estrogens [52]. A recent report indicates that maca's effect on ventral prostate size may partly be a result of the action of glucosinolate metabolites on AR [28]. In this study, AR was fished by MA-4, MA-24, and MA-44 (Fig. 5a).

Stromelysin-1, also known as matrix metalloproteinase-3 (MMP-3), is an enzyme that activates other targeted matrix metalloproteinases (MMPs): MMP-9, MMP-12, and MMP-13 [53]. The expression of MMPs is primarily regulated at the level of transcription, where the promoter of the gene responds to various stimuli, including growth factors, cytokines, tumor promoters, and oncogene products [54]. MMPs are associated with various physiological and pathological processes, such as morphogenesis, angiogenesis, tissue repair, cirrhosis, arthritis, and metastasis [55]. MMPs also play a significant role in the development and metastasis of prostate cancer [56]. In particular, MMP-9 has been shown experimentally to be involved in prostate cancer [57]. These four targets share similar protein domains and were fished by MA-18, MA-25, MA-44, and MA-45 (Fig. 5b).

Proto-oncogene tyrosine-protein kinase Src (c-Src) is a non-receptor tyrosine kinase protein that may be

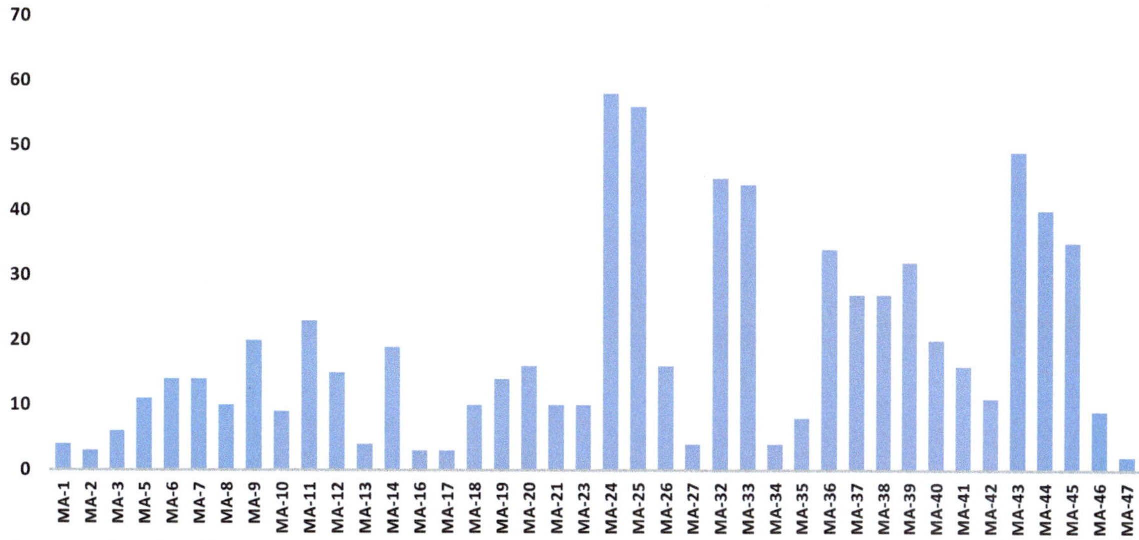

Fig. 2 Overview of number of hit compounds of the parallel pharmacophore screening against druggable targets in the field of diseases

involved in cancer progression by promoting other signals [58]. C-Src is highly expressed in malignant prostate cells [59]. When primary prostate cells were treated with a c-Src inhibitor in vitro, their proliferation, migration, and invasive potential were reduced [60].

As c-Src is a solid druggable target, several c-Src tyrosine kinase inhibitors have been utilized therapeutically [61]. Dasatinib has been approved for the treatment of chronic myeloid leukemia [62], which is an Src family inhibitor. Based on the binding results of those compounds that fished c-Src, we can predict that MA-24 and MA-25 may be pharmacologically similar to Dasatinib.

Selected targets related to kidney diseases

Renal tubular acidosis (RTA) is a metabolic acidosis caused by impaired excretion of acid by the kidney. Carbonic anhydrase II (CA2) is one of the 14 forms of human α carbonic anhydrases and the one with the highest catalytic activity. The physiological functions of CA2 include pH regulation, CO_2 and H_2CO_3 transport, and maintenance of H_2O and electrolyte balance. CA2 deficiency syndrome can lead to osteoporosis, RTA, and cerebral calcification.

In inherited CA2 deficiency, isolated proximal RTA presents with osteoporosis (owing to impaired osteoclast function), cerebral calcification, and variable levels of mental retardation. Although this form of inherited RTA is clinically more proximal, it can also present with a mixed proximal and distal phenotype, which reflects the presence of CA2 in cells all along the renal tubule. CA2 was fished by MA-18, MA-24, MA-38, MA-44, and MA-45 (Fig. 5c). Kidney status directly affects the reproductive function, especially sexual behavior. Oral administration of a purified lipidic extract from maca could enhance sexual behavior by increasing the number of complete intromissions in normal mice and decreasing the latent period of erection in erectile dysfunction male rats [63].

Selected targets related to osteoporosis

Osteoporosis is a skeletal fragility disorder and is common in elderly people. Its prevalence is increasing as more individuals are developing low bone mineral density [64]. The edible part of maca, the hypocotyl, has been widely used to treat osteoporosis [65]. Ethanol extract of maca has anti-osteoporotic activity and indicated maca alkaloids, steroids, glucosinolates, isothiocyanates, and macamides are probably responsible for its biological functions [19].

Estrogen receptor α (ER-α) binds to estrogens and regulates bone homeostasis and prevents postmenopausal bone loss [66, 67]. Estrogen deficiency is a major determinant of bone loss in postmenopausal women [68, 69]. In one ovariectomized rats experiment, ER-α was the predominant ER form expressed in mesenchymal stem cells [70]. Co-expression of ER-α with other genes indicates its activator function in the osteogenic differentiation of mesenchymal stem cells, which causes osteoporosis [71]. Estradiol, estrone, and raloxifene bind to the alpha receptor. However, because the ER's helix 12 domain plays a crucial role in determining its interactions with co-activators and co-repressors, different ER combinations may respond differently to various ligands, which may translate into tissue selective agonistic and antagonistic effects [72, 73]. For example, tamoxifen is an antagonist in the breast and is used as a breast cancer treatment, but it is

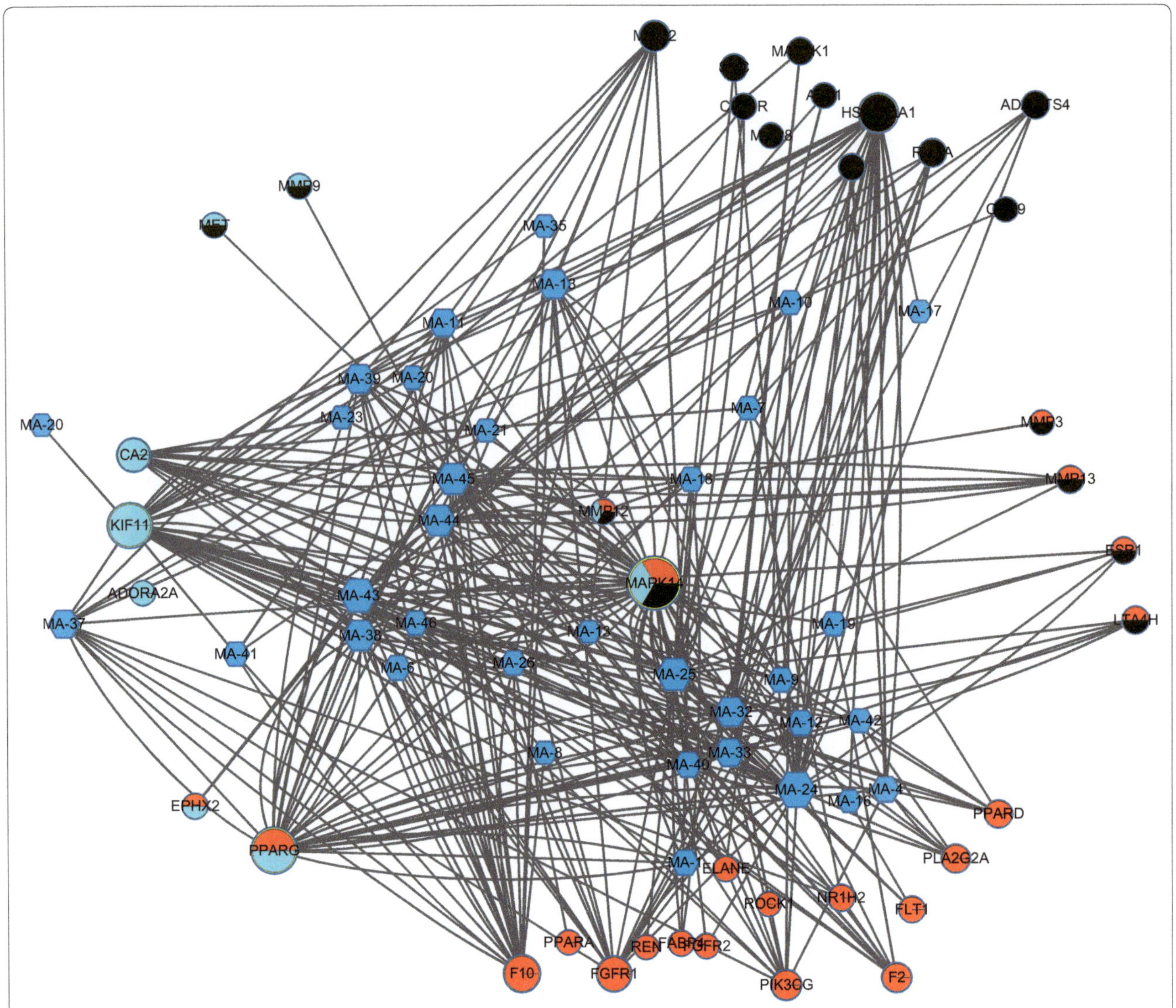

Fig. 3 The major pharmacologic network of maca. Hexagon, compounds; circle, targets (*red*: osteoporosis; *light blue*: kidney diseases; *deep blue*: prostate cancer)

an ER agonist in bone and therefore prevents osteoporosis [69]. Recent studies have suggested that maca contains phyto-estrogens, which may have estrogenic activity [74, 75]. We found that three compounds were connected to ER: MA-19, MA-24, and MA-25 (Fig. 5d).

Enzymatic cleavage by MMPs is involved in the destruction of articular cartilage, and the high expression of MMP-9 and MMP-13 could be detected in pathologic synovium and cartilage samples [76]. Several natural substances containing maca extract tested in vitro are effective agents, as evidenced by the strong regulation of MMP-9 and MMP-13 [77]. In osteoclast migration, MMPs control the cell–matrix interactions required in the model of osteoclast recruitment in primitive long bones [78]. As classical anti-osteoporotic agents, bisphosphonates are involved in the inhibition of the functions of several MMPs (MMP-3, -9, -12, and -13), which were mapped in this virtual screening.

Prediction of the function of maca compounds in the treatment of cardiovascular diseases

A total of 29 targets related to CVD were mapped. Maca could be used in the treatment of CVD characterized by atherogenic lipoprotein profile, and showed relevant angiotensin I-converting enzyme inhibitory activities, indicating potential anti-hypertension activity; however, the mechanisms of these activities are still to be clarified. This result indicated that maca might have significant potential for the treatment of CVD.

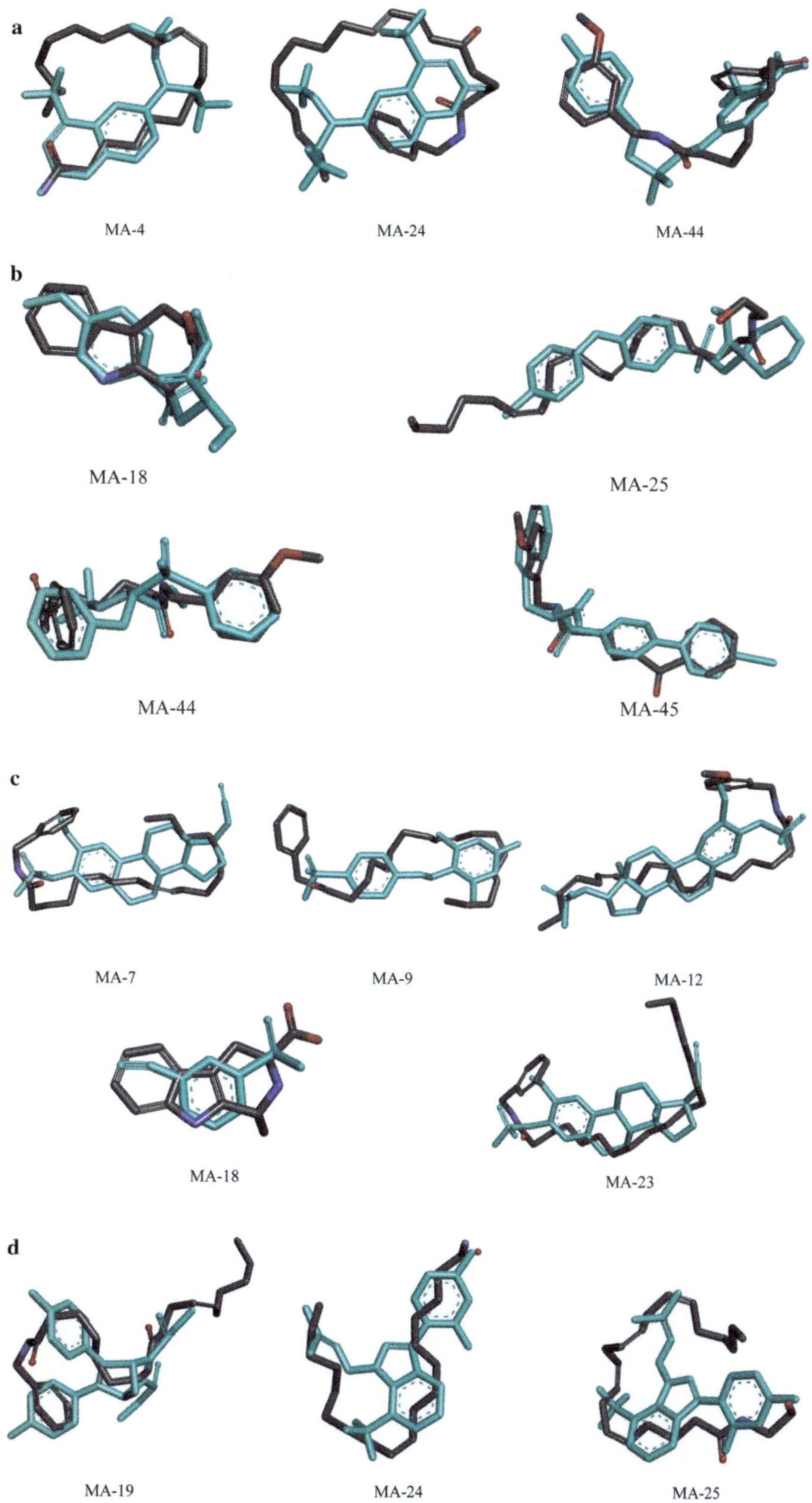

Fig. 4 Compounds from maca align with natural ligands from PDB structure (*light blue*) by WEGA (**a** matrix metalloproteinases; **b** androgen receptor; **c** carbonic anhydrase II; **d** estrogen receptor)

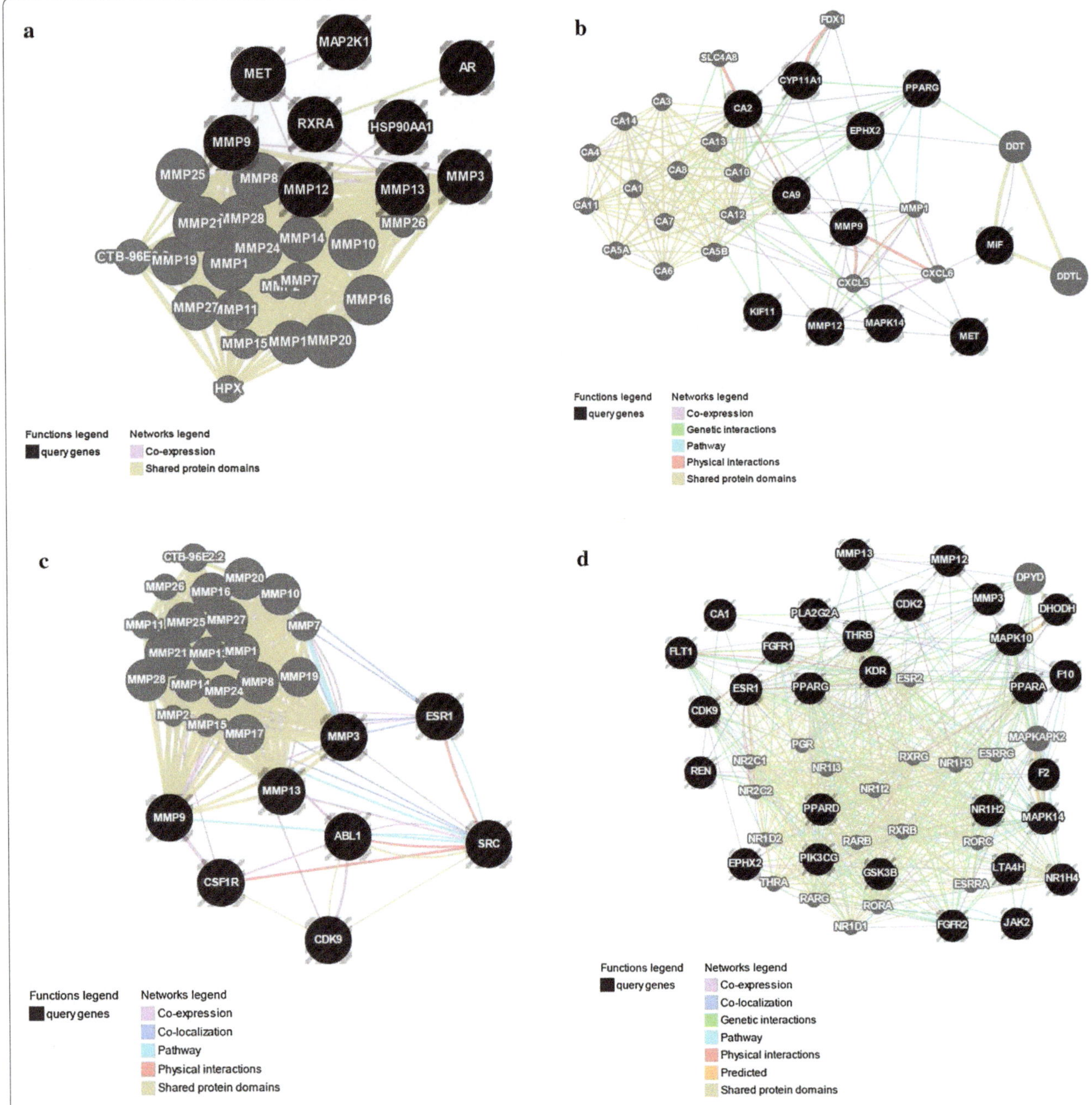

Fig. 5 Network images for the interaction of targets related to four disease categories fished by profiling (**a** prostate cancer; **b** kidney diseases; **c** osteoporosis; **d** cardiovascular diseases)

Kinase activity mediated by mitogen-activated protein kinase 14 (MAPK14), also called p38α, has been identified in many tissues [79]. p38α is mainly activated through MAPK kinase kinase cascades and exerts its biological function via downstream substrate phosphorylation [80]. Pharmacological and genetic inhibition of p38α has revealed its biological significance regarding physiological functions and its potential for targeting p38α in human diseases, especially CVD [81–83]. MAPK14 activity regulates myocyte cytokinesis and promotes cell-cycle exit during maturation in the newborn mouse heart [84]. MAPK14 has also been associated with cell-cycle arrest in mammalian cardiomyocytes [85], and its inhibition might be a strategy to promote cardiac regeneration in response to injury [86]. Furthermore, MAPK14 promoted myocyte apoptosis and cardiomyocyte hypertrophy, and targeted IRS-1-mediated Akt signaling and promoted myocyte death under chronic insulin stimulation in vitro [87, 88].

Peroxisome proliferator-activated receptors (PPARs) are a group of nuclear receptor proteins [89], including PPARα, PPARδ, and PPARγ, whose ligand and DNA-binding domains share 60–80 % homology [90, 91]. PPARs are widely expressed in the vasculature, myocardium, and the immune cells, such as monocytes and macrophages [92]. Additionally, PPAR-retinoid X receptor heterodimers repress CLOCK/BMAL1 gene expression [93]. Hence, PPARs could regulate the expression of a series of genes involved in metabolism that impact cardiovascular physiology [94]. Different PPAR isoforms are observed in various cardiovascular pathologies, such as atherosclerosis, hypertension, and cardiac hypertrophy [95]. Both PPARα and PPARγ are expressed in endothelial cells, vascular smooth muscle cells, and monocytes/macrophages [96, 97]. In atherosclerosis, activation of these two proteins reduces leukocyte recruitment and cell adhesion [98]. Both regulate cytokine-induced genes (such as VCAM-1 and tissue factor), and PPARα and PPARγ inhibit the expressions of tumor necrosis factor-α and MCP-1, respectively [99]. PPARδ activation decreases the expressions of MCP-1, ICAM-1, and inflammatory cytokines and attenuates atherosclerosis development [100].

The potential use of PPAR agonists and dual PPAR agonists, including PPARα/γ, PPARα/δ, and PPARδ/γ dual agonists, in the treatment of CVD has recently received attention [101]. Compounds that are capable of targeting more than one PPAR isotype and are effective at treating CVD have emerged as an interesting and efficient treatment approach. Both MAPK14 and PPARs are related to a series of maca compounds (Table 4).

Conclusion

In silico target fishing identified maca's traditional effects on treatment and prevention of osteoporosis, prostate cancer, and kidney diseases, and its potential function of treating cardiovascular diseases, as the most important of this herb's possible activities.

Table 4 Compounds fished by MAPK14 and PPARs

Targets related to CVD	Compounds
MAPK14	MA-1, 6, 9, 12, 21, 23, 24, 25, 36, 37, 38, 39, 40, 43
PPARα	MA-26
PPARγ	MA-1, 18, 24, 36
PPARδ	MA-4

Abbreviations

AR: androgen receptor; BMD: bone mineral density; CA2: carbonic anhydrase II; CHARMM: chemistry at Harvard macromolecular mechanics; c-Src: tyrosine-protein kinase Src; CST: cell signaling technology; CVD: cardiovascular disease; DS: discovery studio; ER-α: estrogen receptor α; IPA: ingenuity pathway analysis; KEGG: Kyoto encyclopedia of genes and genomes; LPE: latent period of erection; MAPK14: mitogen-activated protein kinase 14; MMFF94x: Merck molecular force field 94×; MMPs: matrix metalloproteinases; MOE: molecular operating environment; MSCs: mesenchymal stem cells; PDB: protein data bank; PPARs: peroxisome proliferator-activated receptors; RMSD: root mean square deviation; RTA: renal tubular acidosis; TE: testosterone enanthate; TTD: therapeutic target database; WEGA: weighted Gaussian algorithm.

Authors' contributions

HBL conceived and designed the study. FY, XLT and XY performed the experiments. FY analyzed the data and wrote the manuscript. All authors read and approved the final manuscript.

Author details

[1] Institute of Medicinal Plant Development, Chinese Academy of Medical Sciences, Peking Union Medical College, 151 Malianwa N, Haidian District, Beijing 100193, China. [2] Key Laboratory of Bioactive Substances and Resources Utilization of Chinese Herbal Medicine, Ministry of Education, Beijing 100193, China. [3] Research Center for Drug Discovery, School of Pharmaceutical Sciences, Sun Yat-sen University, 132 East Circle at University City, Guangzhou 510006, China.

Acknowledgements

We are very grateful to Dr. Jun Xu (Research Center for Drug Discovery, School of Pharmaceutical Sciences, Sun Yat-sen University, Guangzhou) for his valuable suggestions. We would like to thank Mr. Ke-hao Wu (College of Life Science, Hunan Normal University, Changsha) for assistance with data processing.

Competing interests

The authors declare that they have no competing interests.

References

1. Hermann M, Heller J. Andean roots and tubers: ahipa, arracacha, maca and yacon. Rome: Inernational Plant Genetic Resources Insititute; 1997. p. 1–199.
2. Esparza E, Hadzich A, Kofer W, Mithöfer A, Cosio EG. Bioactive maca (*Lepidium meyenii*) alkamides are a result of traditional Andean postharvest drying practices. Phytochemistry. 2015;116:138–48.
3. León J. The, "Maca" (Lepidium meyenii), A little known food plant of Peru. Econ Bot. 1964;18:122–7.
4. Gonzales GF, Singh VK, Govil JN, Ahmad K, Sharma RK. Biological effects of *Lepidium meyenii*, maca, a plant from the highlands of Peru. Nat Prod. 2007;1:209–34.
5. Sandoval M, Okuhama NN, Angeles FM, Melchor VV, Condezo LA, Lao J, Miller MJS. Antioxidant activity of the cruciferous vegetable Maca (*Lepidium meyenii*). Food Chem. 2002;79:207–13.
6. Piacente S, Carbone V, Plaza A, Zampelli A, Pizza C. Investigation of the tuber constituents of maca (*Lepidium meyenii* Walp.). J Agric Food Chem. 2002;50:5621–5.

7. Gonzales GF, Miranda S, Nieto J, Fernández G, Yucra S, Rubio J, Yi P, Gasco M. Red maca (*Lepidium meyenii*) reduced prostate size in rats. Reprod Biol Endocrinol. 2005;3:1–16.
8. Večeřa R, Orolin J, Škottová N, Kazdová L, Oliyarnik O, Ulrichová J, Šimánek V. The influence of maca (*Lepidium meyenii*) on antioxidant status, lipid and glucose metabolism in rat. Plant Food Hum Nutr. 2007;62:59–63.
9. Wu H, Kelley CJ, Pino-Figueroa A, Vu HD, Maher TJ. Macamides and their synthetic analogs: evaluation of in vitro FAAH inhibition. Bioorg Med Chem. 2013;21:5188–97.
10. Cicero AFG, Bandieri E, Arletti R. *Lepidium meyenii* Walp. improves sexual behaviour in male rats independently from its action on spontaneous locomotor activity. J Ethnopharmacol. 2001;75:225–9.
11. Ruiz-Luna AC, Salazar S, Aspajo NJ, Rubio J, Gasco M, Gonzales GF. *Lepidium meyenii* (Maca) increases litter size in normal adult female mice. Reprod Biol Endocrinol. 2005;3:1–16.
12. Lee KJ, Dabrowski K, Rinchard J, Gomez C, Guz L, Vilchez C. Supplementation of maca (*Lepidium meyenii*) tuber meal in diets improves growth rate and survival of rainbow trout *Oncorhynchus mykiss* (Walbaum) alevins and juveniles. Aquac Res. 2004;35:215–23.
13. Clément C, Kneubühler J, Urwyler A, Witschi U, Kreuzer M. Effect of maca supplementation on bovine sperm quantity and quality followed over two spermatogenic cycles. Theriogenology. 2010;74:173–83.
14. Gonzales C, Rubio J, Gasco M, Nieto J, Yucra S, Gonzales GF. Effect of short-term and long-term treatments with three ecotypes of *Lepidium meyenii* (MACA) on spermatogenesis in rats. J Ethnopharmacol. 2006;103:448–54.
15. Gasco M, Villegas L, Yucra S, Rubio J, Gonzales GF. Dose-response effect of Red Maca (*Lepidium meyenii*) on benign prostatic hyperplasia induced by testosterone enanthate. Phytomedicine. 2007;14:460–4.
16. Lembè DM, Gasco M, Gonzales GF. Fertility and estrogenic activity of Turraeanthus africanus in combination with *Lepidium meyenii* (Black maca) in female mice. Eur J Integr Med. 2012;4:e345–51.
17. Rubio J, Qiong W, Liu XM, Jiang Z, Dang HX, Chen SL, Gonzales GF. Aqueous extract of black maca (*Lepidium meyenii*) on memory impairment induced by ovariectomy in mice. Evid Based Complement Alternat Med. 2011;2011:253958.
18. Rubio J, Dang H, Gong M, Liu XM, Chen SL, Gonzales GF. Aqueous and hydroalcoholic extracts of Black Maca (*Lepidium meyenii*) improve scopolamine-induced memory impairment in mice. Food Chem Toxicol. 2007;45:1882–90.
19. Rosales-Hartshorn M. Maca: botanical medicine from the Andes. Adv Food Tech Nutr Sci Open J. 2015;1:e1–6.
20. Lentz A, Gravitt K, Carson CC, Marson L. Acute and chronic dosing of *Lepidium meyenii* (Maca) on male rat sexual behavior. J Sex Med. 2007;4:332–40.
21. Shin BC, Lee MS, Yang EJ, Lim HS, Ernst E. Maca (*L. meyenii*) for improving sexual function: a systematic review. BMC Complement Altern Med. 2010;10:44–50.
22. Dror O, Shulman-Peleg A, Nussinov R, Wolfson HJ. Predicting molecular interactions in silico: I. A guide to pharmacophore identification and its applications to drug design. Curr Med Chem. 2004;11:71–90.
23. Taha MO, Bustanji Y, Al-Bakri AG, Yousef AM, Zalloum WA, Al-Masri IM, Atallah N. Discovery of new potent human protein tyrosine phosphatase inhibitors via pharmacophore and QSAR analysis followed by in silico screening. J Mol Graph Model. 2007;25:870–84.
24. Muhammad I, Zhao JP, Dunbar DC, Khan IA. Constituents of *Lepidium meyenii* 'maca'. Phytochemistry. 2002;59:105–10.
25. Cui BL, Zheng BL, He K, Zheng QY. Imidazole alkaloids from *Lepidium meyenii*. J Nat Prod. 2003;66:1101–3.
26. Zhao JP, Muhammad I, Dunbar DC, Mustafa J, Khan IA. New alkamides from maca (*Lepidium meyenii*). J Agric Food Chem. 2005;53:690–3.
27. McCollom MM, Villinski JR, McPhail KL, Craker LE, Gafner S. Analysis of macamides in samples of Maca (*Lepidium meyenii*) by HPLC-UV-MS/MS. Phytochem Anal. 2005;16:463–9.
28. Tellez MR, Khan IA, Kobaisy M, Schrader KK, Dayan FE, Osbrink W. Composition of the essential oil of *Lepidium meyenii* (Walp.). Phytochemistry. 2002;61:149–55.
29. Gonzales GF, Gonzales-Castañeda C. The methyltetrahydro-β-carbolines in Maca (*Lepidium meyenii*). Evid Based Complement Alternat Med. 2009;6:315–6.
30. Ganzera M, Zhao J, Muhammad I, Khan IA. Chemical profiling and standardization of *Lepidium meyenii* (Maca) by reversed phase high performance liquid chromatography. Chem Pharm Bull. 2002;50:988–91.
31. Gonzales GF. Ethnobiology and ethnopharmacology of *Lepidium meyenii* (Maca), a plant from the Peruvian highlands. Evid Based Complement Alternat Med. 2012;2012:193496.
32. O'Boyle NM, Banck M, James CA, Morley C, Vandermeersch T, Hutchison GR. Open babel: an open chemical toolbox. J Cheminform. 2011;3:33–46.
33. Guner OF. Pharmacophore perception, development, and use in drug design, vol. 2. La Jolla: International Univeristy Line; 2000.
34. Giannakakou P, Gussio R, Nogales E, Downing KH, Zaharevitz D, Bollbuck B, Poy G, Sackett D, Nicolaou K, Fojo T. A common pharmacophore for epothilone and taxanes: molecular basis for drug resistance conferred by tubulin mutations in human cancer cells. Proc Natl Acad Sci USA. 2000;97:2904–9.
35. http://www.rcsb.org/pdb/home/home.do.
36. Yan X, Li J, Liu Z, Zheng M, Ge H, Xu J. Enhancing molecular shape comparison by weighted Gaussian functions. J Chem Inf Model. 2013;53:1967–78.
37. http://www.kegg.jp.
38. http://www.cellsignal.com/contents/science/cst-pathways/science-pathways.
39. Warde-Farley D, Donaldson SL, Comes O, Zuberi K, Badrawi R, Chao P, Franz M, Grouios C, Kazi F, Lopes CT, Maitland A, Mostafavi S, Montojo J, Shao Q, Wright G, Bader GD, Morris Q. The GeneMANIA prediction server: biological network integration for gene prioritization and predicting gene function. Nucleic Acids Res. 2010;38:W214–20.
40. Zhu F, Shi Z, Qin C, Tao L, Liu X, Xu F, Zhang L, Song Y, Liu XH, Zhang JX, Han BC, Zhang P, Chen YZ. Therapeutic target database update 2012: a resource for facilitating target-oriented drug discovery. Nucleic Acids Res. 2012;40:D1128–36.
41. Knox C, Law V, Jewison T, Liu P, Ly S, Frolkis A, Pon A, Banco K, Mak C, Neveu V, Djoumbou Y, Eisner R, Guo AC, Wishart DS. DrugBank 3.0: a comprehensive resource for 'omics' research on drugs. Nucleic Acids Res. 2011;39:D1035–41.
42. Xu J. A new approach to finding natural chemical structure classes. J Med Chem. 2002;45:5311–20.
43. Gonzales GF, Gasco M, Malheiros-Pereira A, Gonzales-Castañeda C. Antagonistic effect of *Lepidium meyenii* (red maca) on prostatic hyperplasia in adult mice. Andrologia. 2008;40:179–85.
44. Gonzales GF, Vasquez V, Rodriguez D, Maldonado C, Mormontoy J, Portella J, Pajuelo M, Villegas L, Gasco M, Mathur P. Effect of two different extracts of red maca in male rats with testosterone-induced prostatic hyperplasia. Asian J Androl. 2007;9:245–51.
45. Gasco M, Villegas L, Yucra S, Rubio J, Gonzales G. Dose-response effect of Red Maca (*Lepidium meyenii*) on benign prostatic hyperplasia induced by testosterone enanthate. Phytomedicine. 2007;14:460–4.
46. Davis SR, Worsley R. Androgen treatment of postmenopausal women. J Steroid Biochem. 2014;142:107–14.
47. Fu M, Wang CG, Reutens AT, Wang J, Angeletti RH, Siconolfi-Baez L, Ogryzko V, Avantaggiati ML, Pestell RG. p300 and p300/cAMP-response element-binding protein-associated factor acetylate the androgen receptor at sites governing hormone-dependent transactivation. J Biol Chem. 2000;275:20853–60.
48. Nagakawa O, Akashi T, Hayakawa Y, Junicho A, Koizumi K, Fujiuchi Y, Furuya Y, Matsuda T, Fuse H, Saiki I. Differential expression of integrin subunits in DU-145/AR prostate cancer cells. Oncol Rep. 2004;12:837–41.
49. Azimi H, Khakshur AA, Aghdasi I, Fallah-Tafti M, Abdollahi M. A review of animal and human studies for management of benign prostatic hyperplasia with natural products: perspective of new pharmacological agents. Inflamm Allergy Drug Targets. 2012;11:207–21.
50. Shrivastava A, Gupta VB. Various treatment options for benign prostatic hyperplasia: a current update. J Midlife Health. 2012;3:10–9.
51. Marti S, Fernandez CC, Perez-Fernandez R. Effect of an integral suspension of *Lepidium latifolium* on prostate hyperplasia in rats. Fitoterapia. 2004;75:187–91.
52. Lund TD, Munson DJ, Adlercreutz H, Handa RJ, Lephart ED. Androgen receptor expression in the rat prostate is down-regulated by dietary phytoestrogens. Reprod Biol Endocrinol. 2004;2:1–5.

53. Egeblad M, Werb Z. New functions for the matrix metalloproteinases in cancer progression. Nat Rev Cancer. 2002;2:161–74.
54. Matrisian LM. Metalloproteinases and their inhibitors in matrix remodeling. Trends Genet. 1990;6:121–5.
55. Eguchi T, Kubota S, Kawata K, Mukudai Y, Uehara J, Ohgawara T, Ibaragi S, Sasaki A, Kuboki T, Takigawa M. Novel transcription factor-like function of human matrix metalloproteinase 3 regulating the *CTGF/CCN2* gene. Mol Cell Biol. 2008;28:2391–413.
56. Lokeshwar BL. MMP inhibition in prostate cancer. Ann NY Acad Sci. 1999;878:271–89.
57. Kong DJ, Li YW, Wang ZW, Banerjee S, Sarkar FH. Inhibition of angiogenesis and invasion by 3,3′-diindolylmethane is mediated by the nuclear factor-κB downstream target genes *MMP-9* and *uPA* that regulated bioavailability of vascular endothelial growth factor in prostate cancer. Cancer Res. 2007;67:3310–9.
58. Devary Y, Gottlieb RA, Smeal T, Karin M. The mammalian ultraviolet response is triggered by activation of Src tyrosine kinases. Cell. 1992;71:1081–91.
59. Wheeler DL, Iida M, Dunn EF. The role of Src in solid tumors. Oncologist. 2009;14:667–78.
60. Park SI, Zhang J, Phillips KA, Araujo JC, Najjar AM, Volgin AY, Gelovani JG, Kim SJ, Wang Z, Gallick GE. Targeting Src family kinases inhibits growth and lymph node metastases of prostate cancer in an orthotopic nude mouse model. Cancer Res. 2008;68:3323–33.
61. Musumeci F, Schenone S, Brullo C, Botta M. An update on dual Src/Abl inhibitors. Future Med Chem. 2012;4:799–822.
62. Breccia M, Salaroli A, Molica M, Alimena G. Systematic review of dasatinib in chronic myeloid leukemia. Onco Targets Ther. 2013;6:257–65.
63. Zheng BL, He K, Kim CH, Rogers LL, Shao Y, Huang ZY, Lu Y, Yan SJ, Qien LC, Zheng QY. Effect of a lipidic extract from *lepidium meyenii* on sexual behavior in mice and rats. Urology. 2000;55:598–602.
64. Hodgson SF, Watts NB, Bilezikian JP, Clarke BL, Gray TK, Harris DW, Johnston CC, Kleerekoper M, Lindsay R, Luckey MM, McClung MR, Nankin HR, Petak SM, Recker RR. American association of clinical endocrinologists medical guidelines for clinical practice for the prevention and treatment of postmenopausal osteoporosis: 2001 edition, with selected updates for 2003. Endocr Pract. 2003;9:544–64.
65. Zhang YZ, Yu LJ, Ao MZ, Jin WW. Effect of ethanol extract of *Lepidium meyenii* Walp. on osteoporosis in ovariectomized rat. J Ethnopharmacol. 2006;105:274–9.
66. Dahlman-Wright K, Cavailles V, Fuqua SA, Jordan VC, Katzenellenbogen JA, Korach KS, Maggi A, Muramatsu M, Parker MG, Gustafsson JA. International union of pharmacology LXIV. Estrogen receptors. Pharmacol Rev. 2006;58:773–81.
67. Eriksen EF, Colvard DS, Berg NJ, Graham ML, Mann KG, Spelsberg TC, Riggs BL. Evidence of estrogen receptors in normal human osteoblast-like cells. Science. 1988;241:84–6.
68. Sims NA, Dupont S, Krust A, Clement-Lacroix P, Minet D, Resche-Rigon M, Gaillard-Kelly M, Baron R. Deletion of estrogen receptors reveals a regulatory role for estrogen receptors-β in bone remodeling in females but not in males. Bone. 2002;30:18–25.
69. Deroo BJ, Korach KS. Estrogen receptors and human disease. J Clin Invest. 2006;116:561–70.
70. Clark CR, MacLusky NJ, Parsons B, Naftolin F. Effects of estrogen deprivation on brain estrogen and progestin receptor levels and the activation of female sexual behavior. Horm Behav. 1981;15:289–98.
71. Zhou S, Zilberman Y, Wassermann K, Bain SD, Sadovsky Y, Gazit D. Estrogen modulates estrogen receptor α and β expression, osteogenic activity, and apoptosis in mesenchymal stem cells (MSCs) of osteoporotic mice. J Cell Biochem Suppl. 2001;81:144–55.
72. Bakas P, Liapis A, Vlahopoulos S, Giner M, Logotheti S, Creatsas G, Meligova AK, Alexis MN, Zoumpourlis V. Estrogen receptor α and β in uterine fibroids: a basis for altered estrogen responsiveness. Fertil Steril. 2008;90:1878–85.
73. Shang Y, Brown M. Molecular determinants for the tissue specificity of SERMs. Science. 2002;295:2465–8.
74. Rochira V, Balestrieri A, Madeo B, Baraldi E, Faustini-Fustini M, Granata AR, Carani C. Congenital estrogen deficiency: in search of the estrogen role in human male reproduction. Mol Cell Endocrinol. 2001;178:107–15.
75. Cutillo DM. Method for metabolic correction. US Patent 20,150,313,949. 2015.
76. Oh H, Yang S, Park M, Chun JS. Matrix metalloproteinase (MMP)-12 regulates MMP-9 expression in interleukin-1β-treated articular chondrocytes. J Cell Biochem. 2008;105:1443–50.
77. Akhtar N, Miller MJ, Haqqi TM. Effect of a Herbal-Leucine mix on the IL-1β-induced cartilage degradation and inflammatory gene expression in human chondrocytes. BMC Complement Altern Med. 2011;11:66–76.
78. Delaissé JM, Andersen TL, Engsig MT, Henriksen K, Troen T, Blavier L. Matrix metalloproteinases (MMP) and cathepsin K contribute differently to osteoclastic activities. Microsc Res Tech. 2003;61:504–13.
79. Lee JC, Laydon JT, McDonnell PC, Gallagher TF, Kumar S, Green D, McNulty D, Blumenthal MJ, Heys JR, Landvatter SW. A protein kinase involved in the regulation of inflammatory cytokine biosynthesis. Nature. 1994;372:739–46.
80. Han J, Lee JD, Bibbs L, Ulevitch RJ. A MAP kinase targeted by endotoxin and hyperosmolarity in mammalian cells. Science. 1994;265:808–11.
81. Alexa A. Characterisation of mapk14/mapk11 mediated cardioprotection using RNAi. Circulation. 2013;128:A12734.
82. Waterworth DM, Li L, Scott R, Warren L, Gillson C, Aponte J, Sarov-Blat L, Sprecher D, Dupuis J, Reiner A, Psaty BM, Tracy RP, Lin H, McPherson R, Chissoe S, Wareham N, Ehm MG. A low-frequency variant in MAPK14 provides mechanistic evidence of a link with myeloperoxidase: a prognostic cardiovascular risk marker. J Am Heart Assoc. 2014;3:e001074.
83. Muslin AJ. MAPK signalling in cardiovascular health and disease: molecular mechanisms and therapeutic targets. Clin Sci. 2008;115:203–18.
84. Liu Z, Fan HY, Wang Y, Richards JS. Targeted disruption of *Mapk14* (*p38 MAPK α*) in Granulosa cells and Cumulus cells causes cell-specific changes in gene expression profiles that rescue COC expansion and maintain fertility. Mol Endocrinol. 2010;24:1794–804.
85. Wagner EF, Nebreda ÁR. Signal integration by JNK and p38 MAPK pathways in cancer development. Nat Rev Cancer. 2009;9:537–49.
86. Jopling C, Boue S, Izpisua Belmonte JC. Dedifferentiation, transdifferentiation and reprogramming: three routes to regeneration. Nat Rev Mol Cell Biol. 2011;12:79–89.
87. Knowlton DL, Tang K, Henstock PV, Subramanian RR. miRNA alterations modify kinase activation in the IGF-1 pathway and correlate with colorectal cancer stage and progression in patients. J Cancer. 2011;2:490–502.
88. Földes G, Mioulane M, Wright JS, Liu AQ, Novak P, Merkely B, Gorelik J, Schneider MD, Ali NN, Harding SE. Modulation of human embryonic stem cell-derived cardiomyocyte growth: a testbed for studying human cardiac hypertrophy? J Mol Cell Cardiol. 2011;50:367–76.
89. Michalik L, Auwerx J, Berger JP, Chatterjee VK, Glass CK, Gonzalez FJ, Grimaldi PA, Kadowaki T, Lazar MA, O'Rahilly S, Palmer CN, Plutzky J, Reddy JK, Spiegelman BM, Staels B, Wahli W. International Union of Pharmacology LXI. Peroxisome proliferator-activated receptors. Pharmacol Rev. 2006;58:726–41.
90. Dreyer C, Krey G, Keller H, Givel F, Helftenbein G, Wahli W. Control of the peroxisomal β-oxidation pathway by a novel family of nuclear hormone receptors. Cell. 1992;68:879–87.
91. Ziouzenkova O, Perrey S, Marx N, Bacqueville D, Plutzky J. Peroxisome proliferator-activated receptors. Curr Atheroscler Rep. 2002;4:59–64.
92. Abdelrahman M, Sivarajah A, Thiemermann C. Beneficial effects of PPAR-γ ligands in ischemia-reperfusion injury, inflammation and shock. Cardiovasc Res. 2005;65:772–81.
93. Nakamura K, Inoue I, Takahashi S, Komoda T, Katayama S. Cryptochrome and period proteins are regulated by the CLOCK/BMAL1 Gene: crosstalk between the PPARs/RXRα-regulated and CLOCK/BMAL1-regulated system. PPAR Res. 2008;2008:348610.
94. Chandra V, Huang P, Hamuro Y, Raghuram S, Wang Y, Burris TP, Rastinejad F. Structure of the intact PPAR-γ-RXR-α nuclear receptor complex on DNA. Nature. 2008;456:350–6.
95. Asakawa M, Takano H, Nagai T, Uozumi H, Hasegawa H, Kubota N, Saito T, Masuda Y, Kadowaki T, Komuro I. Peroxisome proliferator-activated receptor γ plays a critical role in inhibition of cardiac hypertrophy in vitro and in vivo. Circulation. 2002;105:1240–6.
96. Marx N, Sukhova GK, Collins T, Libby P, Plutzky J. PPARα activators inhibit cytokine-induced vascular cell adhesion molecule-1 expression in human endothelial cells. Circulation. 1999;99:3125–31.

97. Marx N, Bourcier T, Sukhova GK, Libby P, Plutzky J. PPARγ activation in human endothelial cells increases plasminogen activator inhibitor type-1 expression PPARγ as a potential mediator in vascular disease. Arterioscler Thromb Vasc Biol. 1999;19:546–51.
98. Kersten S, Desvergne B, Wahli W. Roles of PPARs in health and disease. Nature. 2000;405:421–4.
99. Tham DM, Martin-McNulty B, Wang YX, Wilson DW, Vergona R, Sullivan ME, Dole W, Rutledge JC. Angiotensin II is associated with activation of NF-κB-mediated genes and downregulation of PPARs. Physiol Genomics. 2002;11:21–30.
100. Rival Y, Benéteau N, Taillandier T, Pezet M, Dupont-Passelaigue E, Patoiseau JF, Junquéro D, Colpaert FC, Delhon A. PPARα and PPARδ activators inhibit cytokine-induced nuclear translocation of NF-κB and expression of VCAM-1 in EAhy926 endothelial cells. Eur J Pharmacol. 2002;435:143–51.
101. Henke BR. Peroxisome proliferator-activated receptor α/γ dual agonists for the treatment of type 2 diabetes. J Med Chem. 2004;47:4118–27.

16

Acupuncture therapy for drug addiction

Farid Esmaeili Motlagh[1,2,3], Fatimah Ibrahim[1,2*], Rusdi Abd Rashid[3], Tahereh Seghatoleslam[3,4] and Hussain Habil[3]

Abstract

Acupuncture therapy has been used to treat substance abuse. This study aims to review experimental studies examining the effects of acupuncture on addiction. Research and review articles on acupuncture treatment of substance abuse published between January 2000 and September 2014 were searched using the databases ISI Web of Science Core Collection and EBSCO's MEDLINE Complete. Clinical trial studies on the efficacy of acupuncture therapy for substance abuse were classified according to substance (cocaine, opioid, nicotine, and alcohol), and their treatment protocols, assessments, and findings were examined. A total of 119 studies were identified, of which 85 research articles addressed the efficacy of acupuncture for treating addiction. There were substantial variations in study protocols, particularly regarding treatment duration, frequency of electroacupuncture, duration of stimulation, and choice of acupoints. Contradictory results, intergroup differences, variation in sample sizes, and acupuncture placebo effects made it difficult to evaluate acupuncture effectiveness in drug addiction treatment. This review also identified a lack of rigorous study design, such as control of confounding variables by incorporating sham controls, sufficient sample sizes, reliable assessments, and adequately replicated experiments.

Background

In 1997, the National Institutes of Health accepted acupuncture therapy as an acceptable procedure complementary to Western medicine [1]. Evidence for its therapeutic effects comes mainly from clinical practice and research into pain control, fibromyalgia, headaches, Parkinson's disease, schizophrenia, and depression [2]. Acupuncture therapy can be administered using either manual insertion of needles or electroacupuncture (EA), a mild electrical stimulation of acupoints. Extended acupuncture methods may involve finger pressure (acupressure) and laser therapy [3].

In 1985, Dr. M. Smith finalized the National Acupuncture Detoxification Association (NADA) protocol that is currently practiced in over 250 hospitals in the United Kingdom and United States [4]. In 1996, the World Health Organization accepted acupuncture as a treatment for drug abuse [5]. The latest modification to this treatment protocol was developed in 2005 by Dr. Ji Sheng from Peking University, Beijing, China [6]. Currently, more than 700 addiction treatment centers use acupuncture as an adjunctive procedure [7].

Prominent effects of acupuncture are increases in the levels of enkephalin, epinephrine, endorphin, serotonin, norepinephrine, and dopamine in the central nervous system and plasma [8] that might mediate substance abuse. Acupuncture has been used to treat addiction for three decades [2–89]. For example, auricular acupuncture (AA) is effective in treating alcohol and drug abuse in both Europe and the United States [4].

However, several clinical trials have indicated that acupuncture was not effective in treating addiction [2, 3, 31, 67, 69, 78–80]. Thus, the efficacy of the NADA protocol has been reassessed over the last decade [7]. Several factors have been studied to evaluate the efficacy of acupuncture therapy; for example, treatment protocol, choice of acupoints, duration of acupuncture, study design diversity, sample size, addiction history, and assessment techniques.

This study aims to review the published research on acupuncture therapy for substance abuse in relation to study type, authors, funding agencies, countries, agonist substances, and acupoints used for stimulation.

*Correspondence: fatimah@um.edu.my
[1] Department of Biomedical Engineering, Faculty of Engineering, University of Malaya, 50603 Kuala Lumpur, Malaysia
Full list of author information is available at the end of the article

Experimental studies published between January 2000 and September 2014 were systematically reviewed and analyzed to try to resolve the lack of agreement about acupuncture's efficacy for substance abuse.

Review

Literature search

A search of the ISI Web of Science Core Collection and EBSCOHost (MEDLINE Complete) databases for the period January 2000 to September 2014 was conducted to identify acupuncture clinical trials. Keywords, topics available in the databases, and titles were searched for the following terms: "acupuncture," "electroacupuncture," "acupoint stimulation," "transcutaneous," and "electrostimulation" as single words or combinations (total number of articles: 25 358). The results were refined to exclude non-English language materials. The preliminary findings of the first phase were refined by several parallel filters to identify documents relevant to acupuncture treatment of substance abuse. The operator between the filters was the "OR" command. Single, relevant words were selected for each filter and included any combination of the following: "alcohol," "addict," "opioid," "heroin," "cigarette," "nicotine," "tobacco," "cocaine," and "substance" as title, topic, keywords, or abstract text (total number of articles: 230) from both searched databases. The search results were collated and filtered to exclude proceedings papers and letters, yielding 161 studies. The abstracts of these documents were reviewed to exclude papers related to other addiction fields such as the Internet, food, or games; 119 documents comprised the refined, selected results. Three authors (FEM, RR, and TS) independently assessed studies for eligibility and crosschecked the material for study relevance. The publication selection process was shown in Fig. 1.

The articles were classified according to their specifications, including publication date, number of citations, source, authors, organization, and funding agencies. All original research papers were examined for their efficacy and method of treating different categories of addiction to agonist substances (e.g., cocaine, opioid and opiate, nicotine, alcohol, morphine). Original clinical trials that investigated the efficacy of acupuncture therapy were divided into six categories based on substance dependence (cocaine, opioid and opiate, nicotine, alcohol, morphine, and other substances) with a narrative review of their methods and results. Although morphine is an opioid, it has been assigned its own section because of the high number of publications on this topic. Heroin, methadone, and opiates are discussed in the opioid section.

The findings are discussed and compared according to type of addictive substance. There were 96 articles and 29 review papers; 83 articles were original investigations (76 of which were clinical trials of acupuncture efficacy), with 45 articles involving human beings and 38 involving animals. Figure 2 shows the percentage of all documents in each type of category. Original investigations of humans and animals were classified separately according to type of substance dependence. These articles placed more of an investigative emphasis on morphine and alcohol than on other substances.

The total number of citations for all documents was 1495 (mean = 15.83 and standard deviation = 15.27, citation range 2–87 by excluding 29 articles cited zero times or only once). The top ten most cited articles were shown in Table 1. The United States (43 articles) and China (40 articles) published almost 70 % of all articles. Among the Asian countries, China and South Korea published 59 articles, comprising 50 % of publications. Their funding agencies were also the top supporters in this field. Peking, Kyung Hee, and Daegu Haany Universities were the top three organizations, publishing 40 articles since 2000.

The published articles were associated with various research areas (Fig. 3). About 80 % of the articles focused on neuroscience and neurology, substance abuse, and integrative complementary medicine research areas. Published articles for each year were shown in Fig. 4.

Original experimental research articles were reviewed according to type of substance dependence (Fig. 2); the treatment method, subjects, objectives, and assessments of clinical trials for each group were shown in Tables 2, 3, 4, 5, 6, 7.

Cocaine

Avants and Margolin have evaluated the efficacy of AA for cocaine addiction treatment in four studies on human subjects. Although promising results were reported in their first study on 82 cocaine-dependent subjects [10], another study on 83 cocaine-dependent subjects found AA to be effective in reducing cocaine in only one of two trials [60]. When the original study was repeated with 620 subjects, no effect was found [61]. These researchers also conducted a study in 2005 on 40 cocaine abusers who had tested positive for the human immunodeficiency virus and were under methadone maintenance; no difference was found between the standard and reduced NADA protocols for cocaine use [59].

Three studies on rats were conducted to explore the effects of bilateral stimulation at the *Shenmen* (HT7) points. Modulation of the central dopaminergic system by acupuncture might be effective in preventing the behavioral effects of cocaine in rats [44]. By regulating neuronal activation in the nucleus accumbens (NAc) shell, acupuncture reduced stress-induced relapse [84]. The effect of acupuncture on the inhibition of cocaine-induced locomotor activity was mediated by A-fiber

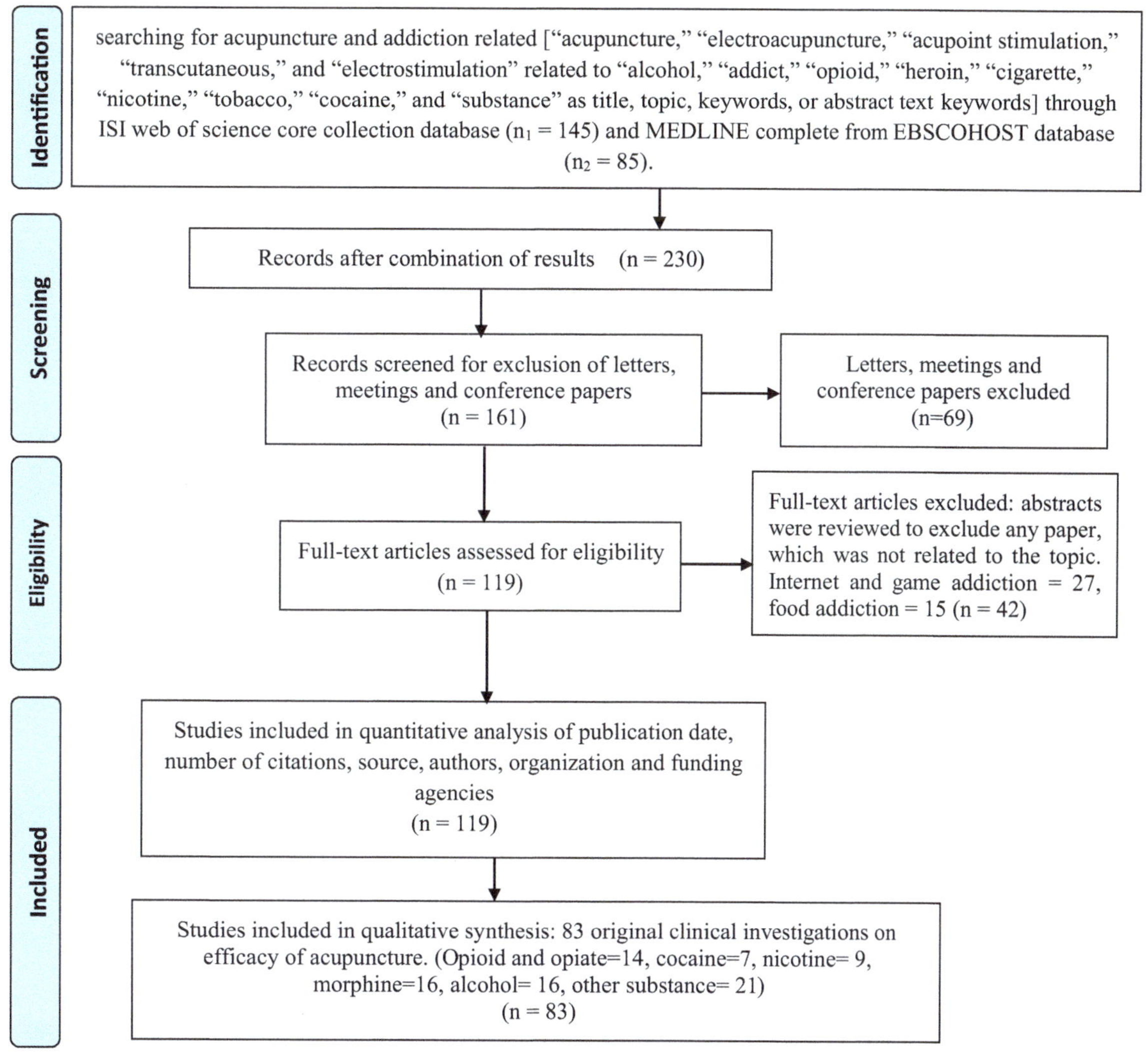

Fig. 1 Flow chart of selection process

activation of the ulnar nerve in rats [42]. See Table 2 for study details.

Opioids and opiates

In 2002, Montazeri investigated the efficacy of acupuncture at *Hegu* (LI4), *Neiguan* (PC6), *Shenmen* (HT7), *Taichong* (LR3), *Zusanli* (ST36), *Dazhui* (DU14), and *Baihui* (DU20) in 40 male adult heroin- or opium-addicted patients. The severity of withdrawal symptoms declined when acupuncture was used in rapid opiate detoxification [63]. Liu (2007) used functional magnetic resonance imaging to show that hypothalamus activation associated with manual acupuncture at *Zusanli* (ST36) was more robust in heroin addicts compared with healthy subjects [55]. EA (2 Hz) at *Zusanli* (ST36) and *Sanyinjiao* (SP6) was effective in reducing active responses elicited by discrete cues in rats [56]. The same EA treatment showed promise in treating heroin-seeking behaviors when combined with extinction therapy [33]. EA (2 Hz) at the same points—*Zusanli* (ST36) and *Sanyinjiao* (SP6)—activated the endogenous opioid cannabinoid and the dopamine systems in rats [81].

An evaluation of the event-related potentials of heroin addicts before and after acupuncture at *Neiguan* (PC6) and *Zusanli* (ST36) suggested that EA might potentially lower relapse rates by inhibiting attention bias to heroin [37]. The presentation of heroin cues could induce activation in craving-related brain regions, which are involved in reward, learning and memory, cognition, and emotion. Acupuncture at *Zusanli* (ST36) rapidly suppressed the activation of these specific brain regions related to craving [17]. Transcutaneous electric acupoint stimulation

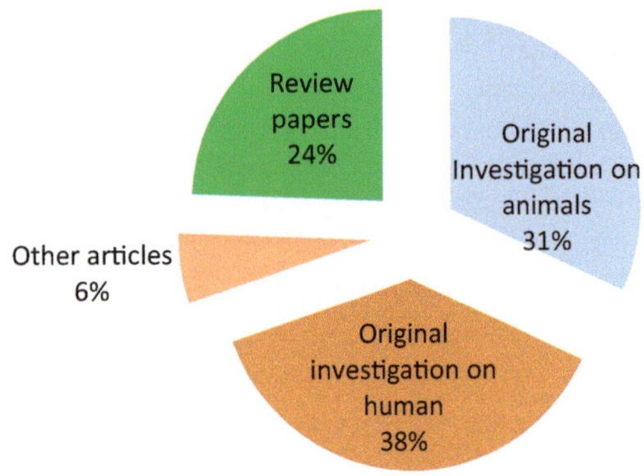

Article type	Number
Original investigation on rats	38
Original investigation on human	45
Other articles	7
Review papers	29
Total	119

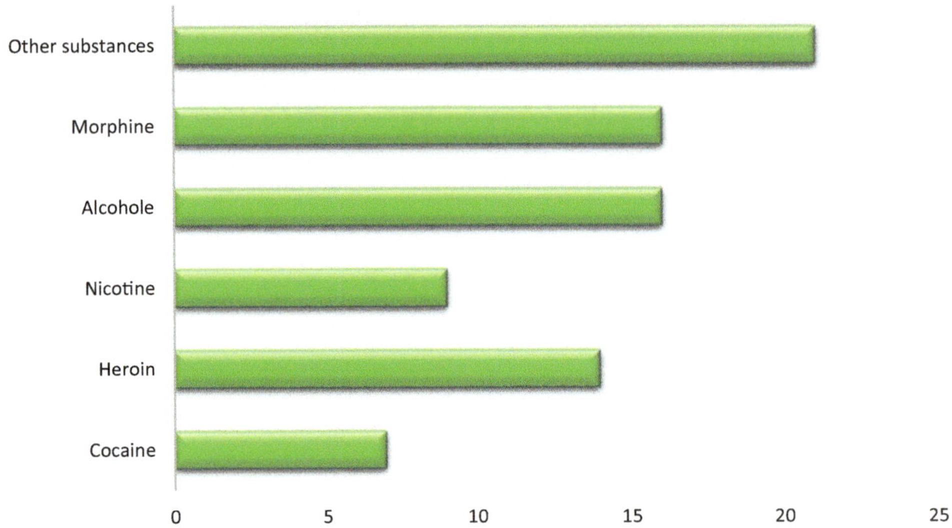

Fig. 2 Classification of selected articles into review papers and original investigations on humans and animals. The lower diagram shows the number of original clinical investigations according to substance. Morphine and alcohol have the most articles. Each of the columns is described separately in Tables 2, 3, 4, 5, 6, 7

was a possible adjunctive treatment to pharmacological treatments for heroin detoxification [62]. Acupuncture at *Dazhui* (GV14) and *Baihui* (DU20) prevented brain cell apoptosis in heroin-readdicted rats, normalized neuronal ultrastructure in the ventral tegmental area of heroin relapse rats, and protected nerve cells against injury in heroin relapse rats [32, 88].

Recent studies of acupuncture's effectiveness as an adjunct therapy in methadone maintenance programs have been controversial. In 2009, Bearn demonstrated a lack of effect for adjunctive methadone maintenance treatment with AA upon withdrawal severity or craving [11]. In 2013, Pei Lin showed a lack of AA effectiveness on the number of daily consumed cigarettes, relapse rate, and withdrawal symptoms, and examined patients' satisfaction and coping with AA as an adjunct treatment to methadone maintenance treatment among Malaysian subjects [57, 58]. However, Chan et al. [22] claimed that 2 weeks of acupuncture therapy reduced the daily dose of methadone and was also associated with greater improvement in sleep latency. See Table 3 for study details.

Nicotine

Acupuncture stimulation at *Zusanli* (ST36) exerted a therapeutic effect on nicotine detoxification [21] and acupuncture at *Zusanli* (ST36) or *Shenmen* (HT7) might attenuate anxiety-like behavior following nicotine withdrawal by modulating corticotrophin-releasing factor in the amygdala [20]. Smoking withdrawal symptoms could be ameliorated by acupuncture treatment [18]. In one study, acupuncture at *Shenmen* (HT7) attenuated

Table 1 Top 10 most cited articles from 2000 to 2014

Title	First author	Source title	Publication year	Total citations
Acupuncture: An evidence-based review of the clinical literature [90]	Mayer DJ	Annual Review of Medicine	2000	87
A randomized controlled trial of auricular acupuncture for cocaine dependence [10]	Avants SK	Archives of Internal Medicine	2000	67
Acupuncture for the treatment of cocaine addiction—a randomized controlled trial [61]	Margolin A	Journal of the American Medical Association	2002	66
Clinical research on acupuncture: Part I. What have reviews of the efficacy and safety of acupuncture told us so far? [91]	Birch S	Journal of Alternative and Complementary Medicine	2004	64
Peripheral neuropathy: Pathogenic mechanisms and alternative therapies [92]	Head, Kathleen A	Alternative Medicine Review	2006	50
Acupuncture and related interventions for smoking cessation [78]	White AR	Cochrane Database of Systematic Reviews	2006	43
A large randomized placebo controlled study of auricular acupuncture for alcohol dependence [16]	Bullock ML	Journal of Substance Abuse Treatment	2002	41
Peripheral electric stimulation inhibits morphine-induced place preference in rats [75]	Wang B; Luo, F	NeuroReport	2000	39
Acupuncture in clinical neurology [67]	Rabinstein AA	Neurologist	2003	37
Traditional Chinese medicine in treatment of opiate addiction [93]	Shi, Jie	Acta Pharmacologica Sinica	2006	34

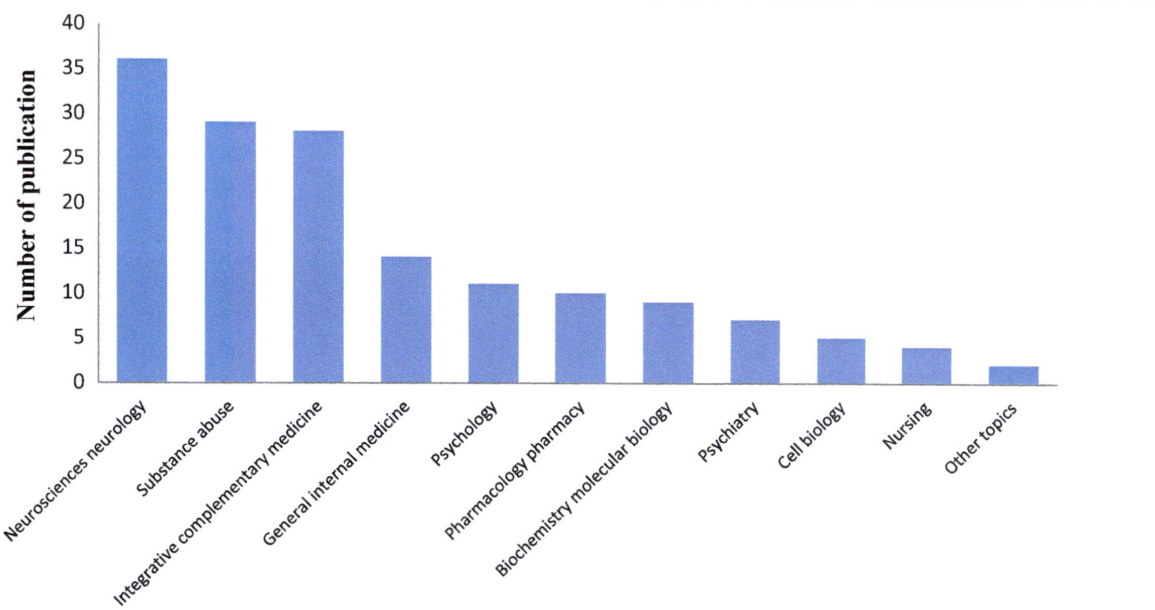

Fig. 3 Number of research articles in each area. Neuroscience, substance abuse, and complementary medicine are ranked highest

cigarette withdrawal symptoms more than acupuncture at *Shousanli* (LI10) [19]. Real acupuncture (as opposed to sham acupuncture) at *Shenmen* (HT7) alleviated cue-induced cravings through the regulation of activity in brain regions (medial prefrontal cortex, premotor cortex, amygdala, hippocampus, and thalamus) related to craving scores in the initial abstinence phase [38].

However, one study failed to find any effect of acupuncture on cotinine serum levels, carbon monoxide exhalation, and smoking quit rate in 59 smokers [83]. It has been suggested that DRD2 gene TaqI A polymorphism was related to AA response in smoking cessation treatment [65]. Auricular transcutaneous electrical neurostimulation relieved withdrawal symptoms and decreased

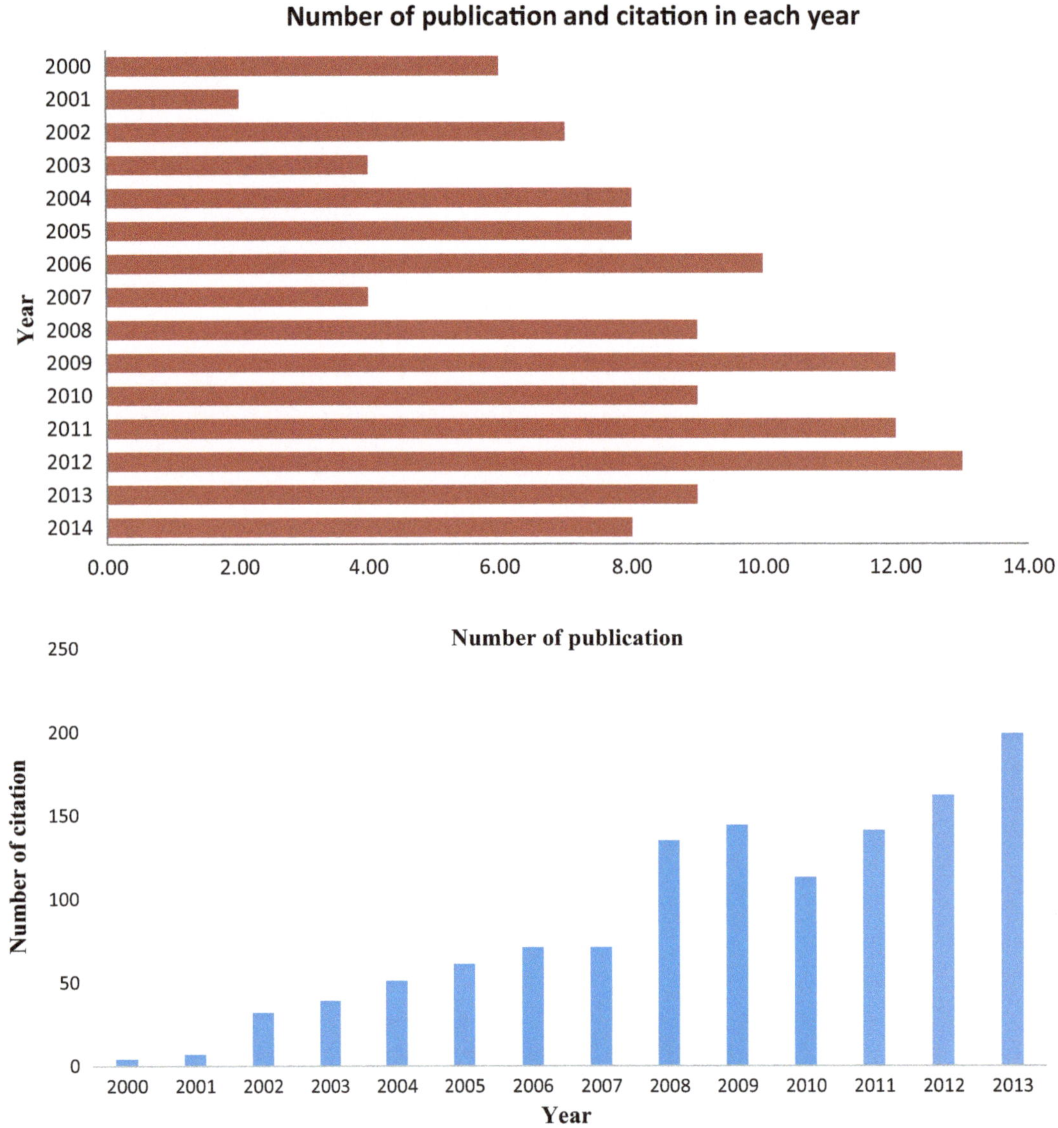

Fig. 4 Number of publications (*top*) and citations (*bottom*) per year. This figure shows that since 2008, the number of citations has increased to 200 per year. Before 2008, it was about 50 per year

anxiety and stress levels during the detoxification period in a study of six smokers [15]. Auricular transcutaneous electrostimulation therapy might be an acceptable alternative therapy for smoking cessation [72]. See Table 4 for study details.

Alcohol

Conflicting results from two large randomized single-blind, placebo-controlled trials suggested that acupuncture was not effective in reducing alcohol use [16, 39]. However, promising results have been found using acupuncture as an adjunctive treatment to carbamazepine medication to reduce the severity of alcohol withdrawal symptoms [39]. In one study, AA failed to reduce the duration and severity of alcohol withdrawal symptoms [43]; another study found no advantage for laser AA in treating alcohol withdrawal [74]. However, research indicated that laser therapy helps to promote the release of endorphins in the body and decreases discomfort accompanying alcohol withdrawal [87]. It might therefore be a safe and painless beneficial adjunct treatment for alcoholism [87].

Acupuncture at *Zusanli* (ST36) or *Sanyinjiao* (SP6) modulated postsynaptic neural activation in the striatum

Table 2 Original investigations of acupuncture therapy effects in cocaine-dependent subjects

Publication year; first author		Objectives	Subjects	Stimulated acupoints (acupuncture type, acupoints, frequency)	Assessments	Outcomes
2000	Avants [10]	To evaluate the AA efficacy in cocaine addiction treatment compared to needle-insertion and no-needle relaxation control conditions	82 Cocaine-dependent, methadone-maintained patients	Auricular acupuncture at 4 NADA points (sympathetic, lung, liver, and *Shenmen* (HT7)), 5 times a week for 8 weeks	Urine toxicology screens 3-times-weekly	Acupuncture showed positive results compared to control groups for treatment of cocaine dependence
2002	Margolin [60]	To Compare two cocaine addiction clinical trials of AA to explore consistency of treatment effects	165 Cocaine-dependent, methadone-maintained patients (Study 1, n = 82; Study 2, n = 83)	Auricular acupuncture at 4 NADA points (sympathetic, lung, liver, and *Shenmen* (HT7)), 5 times a week for 8 weeks	Urine toxicology screens 3-times-weekly, retention in treatment, treatment attendance, treatment credibility, therapeutic alliance, and acute effects	The results of two groups were controversial and no conclusion could be made regarding the effectiveness of AA
2002	Margolin [61]	To evaluate the AA efficacy in cocaine addiction treatment	620 Cocaine-dependent methadone-maintained patients. 412 Cocaine only and 208 opiates + cocaine	Auricular acupuncture at 4 NADA points (sympathetic, lung, liver, and *Shenmen* (HT7)), 5 times a week for 8 weeks	Urine toxicology during treatment and at the 3- and 6-month post randomization follow-up, and retention in treatment	acupuncture was not more effective than a needle insertion or relaxation control in reducing cocaine use
2005	Margolin [59]	To evaluate effects of acupuncture and spirituality, therapy in the treatment of HIV-positive drug users	40 HIV-seropositive, cocaine-dependent, methadone-maintained patients	Auricular acupuncture at 5 NADA points, 5 times weekly for 8 weeks	Urine toxicology twice weekly, depression and anxiety at pre- and post-treatment	acupuncture and a spirituality-focused psychotherapy was effective in reducing the cocaine use
2009	Lee and Bombi [44]	To investigate the effects of acupuncture on the repeated cocaine-induced neuronal and behavioral sensitization alternations	32 Male Sprague–Dawley rats, n = 15 acupuncture	Acupuncture bilaterally at *Shenmen* (HT7) for 1 min	Cocaine-induced locomotor activity and the expression of tyrosine hydroxylase (TH) in the brain	acupuncture was effective for inhibiting the behavioral effects of cocaine by possible modulation of the central dopaminergic system
2012	Yoon [84]	To investigate the effects of acupuncture on cocaine-seeking and the expression of c-Fos and the transcription factor cAMP response element-binding protein (CREB)	24 Male Sprague–Dawley rats, n = 6 EA	Acupuncture at *Shenmen* (HT7) as study and *Yangxi* (LI5) as control for 1 min	Cocaine-seeking behavior, surface expression, and phosphorylated CREB (pCREB) activation in the NAc shell	acupuncture attenuated stress-induced relapse by regulating neuronal activation in the NAc shell
2013	Kim and Seol Ah [42]	To explore the peripheral mechanisms underlying acupuncture treatment for drug addiction	12 Male Sprague–Dawley rats	Acupuncture at *Shenmen* (HT7) as study and *Yangxi* (LI5) as control for 1 min	Suppression of cocaine-induced locomotor activity	acupuncture inhibited the cocaine-induced locomotor activity

Acupoints in NADA protocol are located at (sympathetic: in the deltoid fossa at the junction of the infra-antihelix crus and the medial order of the helix, lung: in the center of the cavum concha, liver: located in the posterior to upper portion of the helix crus, kidney: in the cleft between the upper plateau, and the helix)

Table 3 Original investigations of acupuncture therapy effects in opioid- and opiate-dependent subjects

Publication year, first author		Objectives	Subjects	Stimulated acupoints. (acupuncture type, acupoints, frequency)	Assessments	Outcomes
2002	Montazeri, Kamran [63]	To identify the effects of body acupuncture on rapid opiate detoxification	40 Opioid addicts during ROD by naloxone, n = 20 acupuncture	Bilaterally acupuncture at *Hegu* (LI4), *Neiguan* (PC6), *Shenmen (HT7)*, *Taichong* (LR3), *Zusanli* (ST36), *Baihui* (DU20) and *Dazhui* (DU14) 30 min for 3 days	Severity of withdrawal reaction (Clinical Institute Narcotic Assessment (CINA) score)	acupuncture reduced the severity of withdrawal symptoms associated with rapid opiate detoxification
2007	Liu [55]	To investigate the activation in the hypothalamus associated with acupuncture stimulation	Six healthy men and six heroin addicts	Acupuncture at *Zusanli* (ST36) with rotation for 11 min	fMRI, Cortisol level and psychophysical responses, including the deqi sensation, anxiety, and sharp pain	Acupuncture caused activation of the hypothalamus among addicts
2009	Bearn [11]	To investigate AA effects as an adjunct to MMT upon withdrawal severity or craving	83 Opioid users under MMT	Acupuncture at 5 points of cartilage ridge area in the ear, 30–40 min for 14 days	Daily measures of withdrawal severity and craving using the short opiate withdrawal scale and an eight-item craving questionnaire	AA had no effect upon withdrawal severity or craving when provided as an adjunct to a standard methadone detoxification treatment
2010	Meade [62]	To evaluate the effectiveness of TEAS as an adjunctive treatment for inpatients receiving opioid detoxification	48 Men and women under detoxification with buprenorphine-naloxone	2 and 100 Hz TEAS at *Hegu* (LI4) and *Neiguan* (PC6), 30 min daily for 4 days	The addiction severity index, opioid withdrawal scale, brief pain inventory, the Pittsburgh sleep quality index, physical and mental health status by the medical outcomes survey	TEAS was effective in using drugs and improving the pain interference and physical health
2011	Xia [81]	To investigate the rewarding effect of EA	68 Male Sprague–Dawley rats	2 Hz EA at *Neiguan* (PC6) and *Zusanli* (ST36), 30 min for 5 days	Conditioned place preference (CPP)	EA was capable of inducing CPP in the rat via the activation of the endogenous opioid-, cannabinoid- and dopamine-systems
2011	Jiang [37]	To compare the changes of cognitive attention-related brain function before and after EA	Ten Heroin addicts and ten healthy subjects	2 Hz bilateral EA at *Neiguan* (PC6) and *Zusanli* (ST36)	ERP at 64 electrode spots before and after EA intervention task on the positive emotional clue (PEG), negative emotional clues (NEC), and heroin-related clue (HRC). The P200 amplitude components on (Fz, Cz, and Pz)	Electroacupuncture effectively inhibited the attention bias to heroin
2012	Cai [17]	To understand the influence of heroin cue exposure on brain activation	12 Heroin addicts and 12 healthy subjects	non-twirled acupuncture and twirled acupuncture at bilateral *Zusanli* (ST36) for 1 min	fMRI during heroin cue exposure	Acupuncture can rapidly suppress the activation of specific brain regions related to craving as an intervention for drug craving
2012	Liu [56]	To investigate the beneficial effects of EA on heroin-seeking behavior	40 Male Sprague–Dawley rats, n = 10 EA	2 Hz EA at *Zusanli* (ST36) and *Sanyinjiao* (SP6), once a day for 14 days during heroin abstinence	Contextual and discrete cue-induced reinstatement of active responses. Fos-positive nuclei detection in the nucleus accumbens (NACc) core and shell	acupuncture was effective in preventing relapse to drug addiction

Table 3 continued

Publication year, first author		Objectives	Subjects	Stimulated acupoints. (acupuncture type, acupoints, frequency)	Assessments	Outcomes
2013	Hu [33]	To investigate the effects of EA on the extinction of heroin-seeking behavior	18 Male Sprague–Dawley rats, n = 6 EA	2 Hz EA at *Zusanli* (ST36) and *Sanyinjiao* (SP6), once a day for 7 days	The extinction response of heroin associated cues and applied immunohistochemistry to detect FosB-positive nuclei in the nucleus accumbens core	Acupuncture enhanced extinction learning when combined with extinction therapy for the treatment of heroin addiction
2013	Lua, Pei Lin [57]	To find the effects of AA in number of consumed daily cigarettes, relapse rate, and withdrawal symptoms	40 MMT, 29 MMT + AA human subjects	Auricular acupuncture at 5 points NADA points, 3 times a week	Malay HOQOLBREF, withdrawal symptoms	Acupuncture adjunct to MMT was beneficial in managing addiction behaviors
2013	Lua, Pei Lin [58]	To examine the patients' satisfaction and coping with AA as an adjunct treatment to MMT	40 MMT, 29 MMT + AA human subjects	Auricular acupuncture at 5 points NADA points, 3 times a week	Patient satisfaction with pharmaceutical care questionnaire (PSPCQ) and Malay brief COPE-27	Acupuncture adjunct to MMT did not influence patient satisfaction and their coping ways
2014	Chan [22]	To examine the effectiveness of acupuncture for heroin addicts on methadone maintenance	60 Heroin addicts in MMP	EA at *Hegu* (LI4), *Zusanli* (ST36) and *Shenmen (HT7)*, twice a week for 4 weeks	Daily consumption of methadone, variations in the 36-item Short Form Health Survey-36 (SF-36) and the Pittsburgh Sleep Quality Index (PSQI) scores, and heroin craving	Acupuncture adjunct to MMT was useful in reducing the daily dose of methadone and great improvement in sleep latency at follow-up
2014	Hou [32]	To observe cell apoptosis in the hippocampus and frontal lobe of heroin readdicted rats by electron microscopy.	40 Wistar rats during the detoxificstion by methadone	Acupuncture at *Baihui* (GV20) and *Dazhui* (GV14), 30 min for 5 successive days	Morphology of nerve cells, Bax expression and Bcl-2 expression in the frontal cortex and hippocampus	Acupuncture was effective in preventing brain cell apoptosis in heroin readdicted rats
2014	Zhang [88]	To verify the relationship between acupuncture, neurotrophic factor expression and brain cell structural changes	32 Wistar rats, n = 16 acupuncture	Acupuncture at *Baihui* (DU20) and *Dazhui* (DU14) for 30 min, once a day for five consecutive days	The neuronal ultrastructure of the ventral tegmental area, brain-derived and glial cell line-derived neurotrophic factor expression in the ventral tegmental area	Acupuncture protected brain neurons against injury in rats with heroin relapse

Acupoints in NADA protocol are located at (sympathetic in the deltoid fossa at the junction of the infra-antihelix crus and the medial order of the helix, lung in the center of the cavum concha, liver located in the posterior to upper portion of the helix crus, kidney in the cleft between the upper plateau, and the helix)

Table 4 Original investigations of acupuncture therapy effects in nicotine-dependent subjects

Publication year; first author		Objectives	Subjects	Stimulated acupoints (acupuncture type, acupoints, frequency)	Assessments	Outcomes
2004	Chae [21]	To investigate the acupuncture effects on the functional alterations of the mesolimbic dopaminergic systems	35 Male Sprague–Dawley rats	Acupuncture at *Zusanli* (ST36), *Shenmen* (HT7), or *Taiyuan* (LU9) for 4 days	Nicotine-induced FLI in the striatum and the nucleus accumbens	acupuncture had a therapeutic effect on nicotine addiction
2005	Park [65]	To examine whether the DRD2 TaqI A polymorphism is associated with the response to acupuncture	231 Healthy Korean male smokers	AA at lung, throat, *Shenmen* (HT7), and endocrine points for 96 s, 3 times for a week	Cigarette consumption, the desire to smoke, and Genomic DNA extracted from blood samples	Acupuncture was effective to influence the DRD2 TaqI A polymorphism
2008	Chae [20]	To investigate the effect of acupuncture on anxiety-like behavior and corticotrophin-releasing factor (CRF) and neuropeptide Y (NPY) mRNA expression in the amygdala during nicotine withdrawal	38 Male Sprague–Dawley rats, n = 18 acupuncture	Acupuncture at *Zusanli* (ST36), *Shenmen* (HT7), 30 s for 3 days	The anxiogenic response by using an elevated plus maze. CRF and NPY mRNA levels by using reverse transcription polymerase chain reaction (RT-PCR) analysis	acupuncture attenuated anxiety-like behavior following nicotine withdrawal
2008	Bonnette [15]	To explore the effects of ATENS in combination with addiction education, behavioral training and coaching	6 Smokers	Acupuncture at 5 NADA protocol or 1-3 points, 5 times a week for 8 weeks	In-depth interviews for withdrawal symptoms, anxiety and stress levels	auriculotherapy relieved withdrawal symptoms and reduced anxiety and stress levels during the detoxification
2009	Yeh [83]	To evaluate the effects of a 6-week acupoint stimulation program for quitting	59 Smokers	Acuouncture at *Shenmen* (HT7), lung, stomach, mouth and endocrine and *Tim mee for* 20 min, once a week for 6 weeks	Demographic factors, serum cotinine, carbon monoxide exhalation, daily tobacco consumption, and quit smoking rate of participants before and after the 6-week intervention	Acupuncture showed no statistically significant effect on quitting smoking
2010	Thanavaro [72]	To explore the efficacy of ATET as an adjunctive treatment to intensive individual counseling on smoking cessation	29 Subjects	Auricular transcutaneous electrostimulation therapy at 10 areas on the pinna	The "Fagerstrom Test for Nicotine Dependence," the "What Are Your Triggers Test" and the "Why Do I Smoke Quiz."	individual counseling may produce smoking cessation rates comparable to counseling with pharmacotherapy
2010	Chae [18]	To investigate the effect of acupuncture on the selective attention to smoking-related visual cues	29 Smokers	Acupuncture, *Shenmen* (HT7), (NA)	The attentional bias and cigarette withdrawal scale	Acupuncture ameliorated the smoking withdrawal symptoms as well as the selective attention to smoking-related visual cues
2011	Chae [19]	To investigate effects of acupuncture on ameliorating cigarette withdrawal symptoms	29 Smokers, n = 15 acupuncture	Acupuncture at *Shenmen* (HT7) or *Shousanli* (LI10), 20 min for 3 days	The cigarette withdrawal scale (CWS), comparing the low-frequency/high-frequency (HF/LF) ratio in the HRV of the RA and SA groups	acupuncture attenuated withdrawal symptoms and smoking cues-induced autonomic responses
2013	Kang [38]	To investigate acupuncture effects on ameliorating cravings induced by smoking-related visual cues	25 Male smokers	Acupuncture at *Shenmen* (HT7) for 1 min	fMRI and craving scores to smoking-related visual cues were assessed before and after RA or sham treatment	acupuncture alleviated cue-induced cravings through the regulation of activity in brain regions involved in attention, motivation, and reward

Acupoints in NADA protocol are located at (sympathetic: in the deltoid fossa at the junction of the infra-antihelix crus and the medial order of the helix, lung: in the center of the cavum concha, liver: located in the posterior to upper portion of the helix crus, kidney: in the cleft between the upper plateau, and the helix)

Table 5 Original investigations of acupuncture therapy effects in alcohol-dependent subjects

Publication year; first author		Objectives	Subjects	Stimulated acupoints (acupuncture type, acupoints, frequency)	Assessments	Outcomes
2001	Yoshimoto [86]	To investigate the effect of EA on changes in alcohol-drinking behavior in rats challenged with restriction and immobilization stress	8–12 Male Sprague–Dawley rats	1 Hz and 100 Hz EA at *Zusanli* (ST 36) and *Shenshu* (BL 23) for 10 min, twice a week for 1–3 weeks	Time-access alcohol-drinking behavior, brain dopamine (DA) level	Acupuncture at *Zusanli* (ST 36) was more effective for reducing the increased alcohol-drinking behavior
2002	Bullock [16]	To report the clinical data on the efficacy of acupuncture for alcohol dependence	503 Alcoholics	AA at *Shenmen* (HT7), lung, sympathetic, and liver for 40 min, 6 days a week for 3 weeks	Alcohol use, depression, anxiety, functional status, and preference for therapy	acupuncture was not found to be effective in reduction of alcohol use alone
2002	Karst [39]	To investigate the acupuncture effects on alcohol withdrawal therapy with carbamazepine	34 Alcoholics	*AA at Sympathetic, Shenmen (HT7), kidney, liver, lung, Baihui* (GV20), extra1, and *He Gu* (Li4), daily for 10 days	Clinical Institute Withdrawal Assessment (CIWA-Ar-scale)	Acupuncture as an adjunctive treatment to carbamazepine medication shows promise for the treatment of alcohol withdrawal symptoms
2003	Trumpler [74]	To compare auricular laser and needle acupuncture with sham laser stimulation in reducing the duration of alcohol withdrawal	48 alcoholics undergoing alcohol withdrawal with clomethiazole n = 17 laser, n = 15 needle	AA (2-10 out of 24 points) for 30-45 min, laser AA at 24 pints (1 min for each point), 3-4 days	The duration of withdrawal symptoms (nurse-rated scale), duration of sedative prescription	Acupuncture showed no relevant benefit for alcohol withdrawal
2004	Zalewska-Kaszubska [87]	To intensify AA method by additional biostimulation of the whole organism	53 Alcoholics under daily helium–neon laser for neck biostimulation	Laser AA at concha points for 4 periods of ten times applied every 2nd day	The Beck Depression Inventory-Fast Screen (BDI-FS), beta-endorphin plasma concentration by using the radioimmunoassay (RIA)	laser therapy was useful as an adjunct treatment for alcoholism
2005	Kim [40]	To investigate the effects of acupuncture on alcohol withdrawal syndrome (AWS) and Fos-like immunoreactivity (FLI) in the striatum and the nucleus accumbens (NAC) of rats	24 Male Sprague–Dawley rats	Acupuncture at *Zusanli* (ST36) and *Sanyinjiao* (SP6) for 3 days	Alcohol withdrawal syndrome (AWS) and Fos-like immunoreactivity (FLI) in the striatum and the nucleus accumbens (NAC)	acupuncture was useful in the treatment of alcoholism by modulating post-synaptic neural activation in the striatum and NAC
2006	Yoshimoto [85]	To investigate the neuropharmacological mechanisms of oriental acupuncture	24 Male Sprague–Dawley rats, n = 16 acupuncture	unilateral or bilateral acupuncture at *Shenshu* (BU23) acupoint, 60 min	Dopamine (DA) and serotonin (5-HT) contents of the microdialysates in the ACC	Acupuncture was effective for treatment of emotional disorders and laconism by increasing and prolonging the activity of serotonergic neurons
2006	Zhao [89]	To investigate the effects of acupuncture on chronic ethanol-induced changes in extracellular dopamine levels in the nucleus accumbens shell	35 Male Sprague–Dawley rats, n = 21 sham or real acupuncture	Bilateral acupuncture at *Shenmen* (HT7) point or *Neiguan* (PC6) or tail) for 1 min	Extracellular dopamine levels in the nucleus accumbens shell (using in vivo microdialysis in unanesthetized rats)	Acupuncture at HT7 was effective to normalize the release of dopamine in the mesolimbic system following chronic ethanol treatment

Table 5 continued

Publication year; first author	Objectives	Subjects	Stimulated acupoints (acupuncture type, acupoints, frequency)	Assessments	Outcomes
2007 Kunz [43]	To compare auricular needle acupuncture with aromatherapy in reducing the duration and severity of symptoms of alcohol withdrawal with carbamazepine, oxcarbazepine, and benzodiazepines	74 alcoholics, n = 36 acupuncture, n = 38 aromatherapy	AA at 5 NADA points, 45 min for 5 days	Alcohol-withdrawal syndrome (AWS scale), subjective visual analog scale of craving and the Self-Assessment Manikin (SAM)	acupuncture was not more effective than the control therapy on alcohol withdrawal symptoms
2008 Overstreet [64]	To investigate the EA effects for reducing voluntary alcohol intake in alcohol-preferring rats	18 inbred alcohol-preferring P rats (IP), n = 9 EA	2 and 100 Hz EA at *Zusanli* (ST36) and *Sanyinjiao* (SP6) for 30 min	Alcohol intake	Acupuncture affected on alcohol intake in the alcohol-dependent IP rats
2009 Dos Santos [28]	To investigate the effects of EA over locomotor sensitization induced by ethanol in mice	12 Male Swiss mice	2 Hz EA at *Zusanli* (ST36) and/or *Neiguan* (PC6) for 10 min	The locomotor activity, the expression of homer1A mRNA assessed by PCR	EA modulated homer1A expression and glutamatergic plasticity
2010 Yang [82]	To evaluate the effects of HT7 acupuncture on VTA GABA neuron excitability, ethanol inhibition of VTA GABA neuron firing rate, and ethanol self-administration	32 Male Wistar rats	2 Hz EA at *Shenmen* (HT7) or *Neiguan* (PC6) for 1 min	Ethanol-Reinforced Responding, VTA GABA Neuron Activity, VTA GABA Neuron Firing Rate	acupuncture reduced ethanol suppression of VTA GABA neuron firing rate, and reduced ethanol self-administration without affecting sucrose consumption
2011 Li [50]	To demonstrate that SD rats escalated their ethanol intake and subsequently developed ethanol dependence under the IE procedure	26 Male Sprague–Dawley rats	2 and 100 HZ EA at *Zusanli* (ST36) for 20 min	Intake of and preference for ethanol	EA treatments decreased the intake of and preference for ethanol, without resulting in a rebound increase in ethanol intake when the EA treatments were terminated
2012 Li [49]	To test the hypothesis that EA suppression on alcohol consumption may be mediated by transcription factors, such as FosB/ΔFosB protein in reward-related brain regions	33 Male Sprague–Dawley rats	2 and 100 HZ EA at *Zusanli* (ST36), 30 min for 6 days	The expression of FosB/ΔFosB in several reward-related brain regions using immunohistochemistry	EA treatment effectively reduced ethanol consumption and preference in rats by down-regulation of FosB/ΔFosB in reward-related brain regions
2012 Escosteguy-Neto [29]	To investigate EA effects during ethanol withdrawal on CB1R immunoreactivity	12 Male Swiss mice	2 and 100 Hz EA at *Zusanli* (ST36)/*Neiguan* (PC6) or *Dazhui* (DU14)/*Baihui* (DU20), 10 min for 4 days	CB1R in the prefrontal cortex, striatum, hippocampus, amygdala and ventral tegmental area	EA inhibited CB1R upregulation which depended on acupoints association and frequency of stimulation
2012 Fallopa [30]	To investigate whether EA reverses locomotor sensitization induced by ethanol is parallel to ERK signaling	12 Male Swiss mice	2 and 100 Hz EA at *Zusanli* (ST36)/*Neiguan* (PC6) or *Dazhui* (DU14)/*Baihui* (DU20), 10 min for 4 days	pERK immune-histochemistry	EA increased CB1R in the prefrontal cortex, striatum, hippocampus, amygdala and ventral tegmental area

Acupoints in NADA protocol are located at (sympathetic: in the deltoid fossa at the junction of the infra-antihelix crus and the medial order of the helix, lung: in the center of the cavum concha, liver: located in the posterior to upper portion of the helix crus, kidney: in the cleft between the upper plateau, and the helix)

and NAc in rats [89]. Acupuncture at *Shenmen* (HT7) normalized dopamine release in the mesolimbic system [89], modulated mesolimbic dopamine release, and suppressed the reinforcing effects of ethanol [82]. Activation of the endogenous opiate system might be responsible for *Zusanli* (ST36) and *Sanyinjiao* (SP6) stimulation effects on alcohol intake in alcohol-dependent rats [64].

EA applied at *Zusanli* (ST36) was more effective than EA at *Shenshu* (BL23) at normalizing alcohol-drinking behavior in rats [86]; the activity of serotonergic neurons in the reward system pathway of the brain might be increased and prolonged by acupuncture [85]. EA at the combination *Zusanli* (ST36) and *Neiguan* (PC6) (but not at either point alone) prevented sensitization of the mesocorticolimbic pathway induced by ethanol in mice and modulated both the expression of the protein homer1A and glutamatergic plasticity [28]. EA (2 Hz) at *Zusanli* (ST36) could reduce voluntary intake of ethanol, but not sucrose, in rats [50] and 100 Hz EA treatment at *Zusanli* (ST36) effectively reduces preference for ethanol and its consumption in rats [49]. In one study, 2 Hz EA at *Zusanli* (ST36) and *Neiguan* (PC6) or 100 Hz EA at *Dazhui* (DU14) and *Baihui* (DU20) inhibited CB1R upregulation in ethanol-withdrawn mice [29]. The behavioral effects of 2 Hz EA at *Dazhui* (DU14) and *Baihui* (DU20), but not 100 Hz EA at *Zusanli* (ST36) and *Neiguan* (PC6), depended on extracellular signal-regulated kinase signaling [30]. See Table 5 for study details.

Morphine

Compared with 100 Hz, 2 Hz peripheral electric stimulation (PES) at *Zusanli* (ST36) and *Sanyinjiao* (SP6) inhibited the expression of morphine-induced conditioned place preference (CPP) (see [52] for information on CPP) via activation of opioid receptors [75]. One study found that the release and synthesis of enkephalin in the NAc was accelerated by 2 Hz stimulation of *Zusanli* (ST36) and *Sanyinjiao* (SP6) [53]. In addition, EA suppression of opiate addiction might involve the release of endogenous μ-, δ-, and κ-opioid agonists in the NAc shell [52] and might activate the cannabinoid, endogenous opioid, and dopamine systems to induce CPP in rats [81]. PES (100 Hz) at *Zusanli* (ST36) and *Sanyinjiao* (SP6) activated the suprasegmental δ- and κ-opioid receptors in the central nervous system, which cause the anticraving effects of PES in rats [70]. It was also found that the expression of preproenkephalin and preprodynorphin mRNAs in the NAc was mediated by 2 Hz or 100 Hz PES, with the release of endogenous μ-, δ-, and κ-opioid agonists to suppress morphine-induced CPP [71]. Stimulation at *Zusanli* (ST36) and *Sanyinjiao* (SP6) (100 Hz) for 30 min normalized the activity of ventral tegmental area dopamine neurons [34], downregulated p-cAMP response element binding, and accelerated dynorphin synthesis in the spinal cord [76].

Some research suggests that 2 Hz EA is a potential complementary therapy for improving immune dysfunction in opiate addicts [51] and that 2 Hz or 100 Hz EA facilitates the recovery of male sexual behavior in rats during morphine withdrawal [27]. Thirty minutes of EA of 2 Hz or 100 Hz at *Zusanli* (ST36) and *Sanyinjiao* (SP6) reversed the morphological alterations induced by chronic morphine administration [25]. In addition, by increasing NREM sleep, REM sleep, and total sleep time, EA could be a potential treatment for sleep disturbance during morphine withdrawal [48].

EA at *Shenshu* (BL23) attenuated the expression of the proto-oncogene c-Fos in the central nucleus of the amygdala [54]. Acupuncture at *Shenmen* (HT7) inhibited neurochemical and behavioral sensitization to morphine by decreasing dopamine release in the NAc [41]. Acupuncture at *Shenmen* (HT7) significantly suppressed morphine-induced increase in locomotor activity and Fos expression in the NAc and striatum [45]. Acupuncture at *Yanggu* (SI5) can reduce the reinstatement of morphine-seeking behaviors by mediating the gamma-aminobutyric acid receptor system [46, 47]. See Table 6 for study details.

Other substances

Studies of methamphetamine, cannabis, illicit/psychoactive drugs, and polydrug users are shown in Table 7. Twelve studies used the NADA 5-point protocol and AA as their treatment method. The findings indicated that people dependent on drugs preferred acupuncture treatment [9], which was associated with a decrease in psychological distress [12] and an increase in confidence [14], but showed no efficacy for drug consumption and withdrawal symptoms [9, 12–14]. However, the conflicting nature of the research findings remains a controversial issue. Although there was evidence against the effectiveness of acupuncture in drug addiction treatment [7, 35, 36], recent studies have shown an effect for AA [23, 24, 26, 68, 73] and transcutaneous electric acupoint stimulation [66] per se or as adjunct treatments. Issues of safety and placebo effects suggest the need for further research [26, 35, 36, 66]. See Table 7 for study details.

Conclusion

AA and NADA protocols failed to show a strong therapeutic effect for cocaine, nicotine, and alcohol addiction treatment. However, some studies discussed here

Table 6 Original investigations of acupuncture therapy effects in morphine-dependent subjects

Publication year; first author	Objectives	Subjects	Stimulated acupoints (acupuncture type, acupoints, frequency)	Assessments	Outcomes
2000 Wang [75]	To observe the effect of peripheral electric stimulation (PES) on morphine-induced Conditioned place preference CPP	57/82 Male Sprague–Dawley rats	2 and 100 Hz PES at *Zusanli* (ST36) and *Sanyinjiao* (SP6) for 30 min	Conditioned place preference	2 Hz PES could specifically inhibit the expression of morphine-induced CPP
2003 Shi [70]	To examine the effect of 100 Hz peripheral electric stimulation (PES) on the expression of morphine-induced CPP	48 Male Sprague–Dawley rats	100 Hz PES at *Zusanli* (ST36) and *Sanyinjiao* (SP6), 30 min a day for 3 days	Conditioned place preference	Repeated 100 Hz PES had anti-craving effects by activating supra-segmental δ- and κ-opioid receptors
2004 Shi [71]	To elucidate if preproenkephalin (PPE) and preprodynorphin (PPD) mRNAs in the nucleus accumbens (NAc) play a role in PES suppressing morphine-induced CPP	48 Male Sprague–Dawley rats	2 and 100 Hz PES at Zusanli (ST36) and Sanyinjiao (SP6), 30 min a day for 3 days	Conditioned place preference	PES suppressed both the expression of morphine-induced CPP and the reinstatement of extinguished CPP
2004 Cui [27]	To investigate the effect of EA on the sexual behavior of male rats undergoing morphine withdrawal	41 Male Sprague–Dawley rats	2 and 100 Hz EA at *Zusanli* (ST36) and *Sanyinjiao* (SP6), 30 min a day for 7 days	Total serum testosterone (TST) concentrations	EA facilitated the recovery of male sexual behavior and increased TST concentrations
2005 Kim [41]	To investigate the effect of acupuncture on repeated morphine-induced changes in extracellular dopamine levels	31 Male Sprague–Dawley rats	Acupuncture at *Shenmen* (HT7) for 1 min	Dopamine release in the nucleus accumbens and behavioral hyperactivity	Acupuncture decreased both dopamine release in the nucleus accumbens and behavioral hyperactivity
2005 Liu [54]	To evaluate the effect of EA on morphine withdrawal signs and c-Fos expression of the amygdala	21 Male Sprague–Dawley rats	100 Hz EA at *Shenshu* (BL23) for 30 min	Corticosterone levels and behavioral responses during EA stimulation	EA significantly reduced the signs of morphine withdrawal
2008 Chu [25]	To observe the effect of EA on chronic morphine-induced neuronal morphological changes in the ventral tegmental area (VTA)	12 Male Sprague–Dawley rats	2 and 100 Hz EA at *Zusanli* (ST36) and *Sanyinjiao* (SP6), 30 min for 3 days	The rough endoplasmic reticulum, membrane configuration of the nucleus and mitochondria, and structure of myelin sheath	EA reversed the morphological alterations induced by chronic morphine administration
2009 Hu [34]	To examine alterations in the firing rate of Dopamine neurons in 100 Hz EA treatment	40 Male Sprague–Dawley rats	100 Hz EA at *Zusanli* (ST36) and *Sanyinjiao* (SP6), 30 min for 10 days	Conditioned place preference	EA was effective for the treatment of opiate addiction by normalizing the activity of VTA DA neurons
2010 Liang [53]	To find the Role of enkephalin in the nucleus accumbens mediating the effects of EA	218 Male Sprague–Dawley rats	2 Hz EA at *Zusanli* (ST36) and *Sanyinjiao* (SP6), 30 min for 1-3 days	Conditioned place preference	EA up-regulated the mRNA level of preproenkephalin in the NAc
2010 Lee [45]	To investigate the effect of acupuncture on morphine-induced behavioral sensitization and the neuronal changes in NAc and striatum	14 Male Sprague–Dawley rats	Acupuncture at *Shenmen* (HT7), 1 min for 3 days	Morphine-induced changes of locomotor activity and Fos expression	acupuncture suppressed the morphine-induced increases in the locomotor activity and Fos expression in the NAc and striatum

Table 6 continued

Publication year; first author	Objectives	Subjects	Stimulated acupoints (acupuncture type, acupoints, frequency)	Assessments	Outcomes
2011 Li [48]	To observe whether EA could modulate the immune status of morphine dependence and withdrawal mice	40 Male BALB/c mice	2 Hz EA at *Zusanli* (ST36) and *Sanyinjiao* (SP6), 30 min for 5 days	Splenic T Lymphocyte Proliferation, IL-2 Production, $CD4^+/CD8^+$ Ratio	EA raised IL-2 and normalized chronic morphine exposure-induced immune dysfunctions
2011 Li [51]	To investigate the effect of 2 and 100 Hz EA of the sleep disturbance during morphine withdrawal	15 Male Sprague–Dawley rats	2 and 100 Hz EA at *Zusanli* (ST36) and *Sanyinjiao* (SP6), 30 min twice a day for 3 days	Electroencephalogram and electromyogram	EA decreased NREM/REM and total sleep time, while the sleep latency prolonged significantly during acute morphine withdrawal
2011 Wang [76]	To find the optimum protocol for EA effective for alleviating withdrawal syndrome	40 Male Sprague–Dawley rats	100 Hz EA at *Zusanli* (ST36) and *Sanyinjiao* (SP6) for 30 min	Conditioned place preference	EA down-regulated of p-CREB and accelerated of dynorphin synthesis in spinal cord
2011 Xia [81]	To investigate whether EA by itself will produce some rewarding effect	44 Male Sprague–Dawley rats	2 Hz EA at *Zusanli* (ST36) and *Sanyinjiao* (SP6) for 30 min	Conditioned place preference	EA was capable of inducing CPP in the rat via the activation of the endogenous opioid-, cannabinoid- and dopamine-systems
2012 Lee [47]	To investigate the role of acupuncture in the reinstatement of morphine seeking	15 Male Sprague–Dawley rats	Acupuncture, *Yanggu* (SI5) or *Yangxi* (LI5) for 1 min	Morphine reinstatement	acupuncture attenuated the reinstatement of morphine seeking behavior by blocking the GABA receptor antagonists
2013 Lee [46]	To investigate whether acupuncture could suppress the reinstatement of morphine-seeking behavior	28 Male Sprague–Dawley rats	Acupuncture, *Yanggu* (SI5) or *Yangxi* (LI5) or *Zusanli* (ST36) for 1 min	Morphine-seeking behavior	acupuncture suppressed morphine injection perfectly

Acupoints in NADA protocol are located at (sympathetic: in the deltoid fossa at the junction of the infra-antihelix crus and the medial order of the helix, lung: in the center of the cavum concha, liver: located in the posterior to upper portion of the helix crus, kidney: in the cleft between the upper plateau, and the helix)

Table 7 Original investigations of acupuncture therapy effects in poly-drug and other substance abusers (*NA* not available)

Publication year; first author		Objectives	Subjects	Stimulated acupoints (acupuncture type, acupoints, frequency)	Assessments	Outcomes
2000	Russell [68]	To compare the behavior of addicts in a treatment center with archived information from no-acupuncture (NA) patients	86 Patients (Methamphetamine was the primary drug of choice for 44)	AA at 5 NADA points, 45 min for 9 weeks	Program retention, new arrests incurred, drug-positive urinalysis results, and number of days needed to progress from entry level to secondary level treatment	Acupuncture improved program retention up to 30 days among methamphetamine-addicted patients
2000	Song Bernstein [14]	To explore the meaning of substance abusers' experience while receiving acupuncture as a part of the treatment for substance dependence	8 Human Subjects	AA, (NA), once a week	Interviews, researcher's field notes, and demographic data obtained from the participants' medical records	Acupuncture caused anticipation of pain, apprehension concerning a new experience, mood elevation, inability to describe the experience, physical sensation, relaxation, and improved sleep
2004	Berman [13]	To compare the experimental NADA-Acudetox protocol with a non-specific helix control protocol in a randomized trial	174 Inmates	Auricular acupuncture at 5 NADA points, 40 min for 4 weeks	A simple drug use questionnaire, the Acupuncture Treatment Assessment Scale (ATAS), a Swedish research version of the Symptom Check List 90	Acupuncture had no significant efficiency over the placebo
2005	Janssen [36]	To examine the utility of acupuncture treatment in reducing substance use in the marginalized, transient population	261 Humans	AA at 5 NADA points for 40 min	Questionnaire, Drug use symptomatology, severity of withdrawal symptoms	Acupuncture caused reduction in overall use of substances and decrease in intensity of withdrawal symptoms
2006	Tian [73]	To examine the efficacy of AA in addition to usual care in substance abuse treatment	17 Humans	AA at 5-points NADA, once a week for 6 consecutive weeks	The Hopkins Symptom Checklist (SCL-20) depression scale, brief substance craving scale	there was a positive response to the specific auricular acupressure treatment on psychological distress, craving, and drug/alcohol use measures
2007	Courbasson and Christine [26]	To evaluate the benefits of adding AA to a 21-day outpatient structured psychoeducational treatment program	185 Women with concurrent substance use problems, anxiety, and depression	AA at 5 points NADA for 45 min, 3 times a week	Physiological cravings for substances, depression, and anxiety	AA as an adjunct therapy to a comprehensive psychoeducational treatment was effective and more viable treatment alternative to anxiolytics

Table 7 continued

Publication year; first author		Objectives	Subjects	Stimulated acupoints (acupuncture type, acupoints, frequency)	Assessments	Outcomes
2009	Ashton [9]	To describe the characteristics of clients choosing AA or counseling to treat dependence at a UK self-referral center	162 Humans, n = 36 acupuncture, n = 126 counselling	AA at 5-points NADA, 45 min, once a week for 11 weeks	Psychometric variables (anxiety, depression, dependence severity, readiness to change), and alcohol and drug consumption	Acupuncture was preferred by clients and follow up assessments showed a significant decrease in psychological distress and reduction of alcohol consumption
2014, 2010	Chang and Bei-Hung [23, 24]	Examine the effects of acupuncture and related response (RR) on reducing craving	23 Acupuncture, 23 RR, 21 controls (homeless military veterans)	AA at 5-points NADA, 45 min twice a week	Degree of craving and anxiety levels	acupuncture and the relaxation reduced craving and anxiety levels
2011	Black, S. [7]	To test the hypothesis if AA reduces the anxiety associated with withdrawal from psychoactive drugs.	101 Patients recruited from an addiction treatment service	AA at 5-points NADA 45 min for 3 days	Anxiety state by using a pretest–posttest treatment design	The NADA protocol was not more effective than sham or treatment setting control in reducing anxiety
2012	Janssen [35]	To test the ability of maternal acupuncture treatment among mothers who use illicit drugs to reduce the frequency and severity of withdrawal symptoms among their newborns	50 Women using acupuncture, 39 women standard care	AA at 5-points NADA for 45 min	Days of neonatal morphine treatment for symptoms of neonatal withdrawal. Neonatal outcomes included admission to a neonatal ICU and transfer to foster care	length of treatment for neonatal abstinence syndrome showed no efficiency of acupuncture
2012	Penetar [66]	To investigate the effects of TEAS on drug addiction	9 Cocaine-dependent, 11 Cannabis-dependent	2 and 100 Hz at *Neiguan* (PC6)/*Waiguan* (TH5) and *Hegu* (LI4)/*Laogong* (PC8) stimulation, Twice-daily 30-minute sessions of for 3.5 days	Drug use and drug cravings, cue-induced craving EEG evaluation, and P300 ERP	TEAS did not reduce drug use or drug cravings, or alter the ERP peak voltage or latency but modulated several self reported measures of mood and anxiety
2014	Bergdah [12]	To describe patients' experiences of receiving AA during protracted withdrawal	15 Human subjects	AA at 5-points NADA 40 min, twice a week for 5 weeks	Interview	AA reinforced sense of relaxation and well-being, peacefulness and harmony, and new behaviors

Acupoints in NADA protocol are located at (sympathetic: in the deltoid fossa at the junction of the infra-antihelix crus and the medial order of the helix, lung: in the center of the cavum concha, liver: located in the posterior to upper portion of the helix crus, kidney: in the cleft between the upper plateau, and the helix)

indicate that acupuncture at *Shenmen* (HT7), *Zusanli* (ST36), and *Sanyinjiao* (SP6) acupoints can affect drug-induced physiological activities.

Authors' contributions

FEM, FI, RAR, and TS designed and conceived the study. FEM, RR, TS, FI, and RAR carried out the article searches. FEM performed the statistical analysis. FEM and TS wrote the manuscript. FI, RAR, and HH revised the manuscript. All authors read and approved the final manuscript.

Author details

[1] Department of Biomedical Engineering, Faculty of Engineering, University of Malaya, 50603 Kuala Lumpur, Malaysia. [2] Centre for Innovation in Medical Engineering, Faculty of Engineering, University of Malaya, 50603 Kuala Lumpur, Malaysia. [3] Centre of Addiction Sciences, University of Malaya, 21st Floor, Wisma Research and Development, Jalan Pantai Baru, 59200 Kuala Lumpur, Malaysia. [4] Shahid Beheshti University of Medical Sciences, Tehran, Iran.

Acknowledgements

We would like to acknowledge and thank the University of Malaya and Ministry of Higher Education for providing High Impact Research Grant, account codes E000007-20001 to fund this project.

Competing interests

The authors declare that they have no competing interests.

References

1. Pelletier KR, Marie A, Krasner M, Haskell WL. Current trends in the integration and reimbursement of complementary and alternative medicine by managed care, insurance carriers, and hospital providers. Am J Health Promot. 1997;12(2):112–22.
2. Jordan JB. Acupuncture treatment for opiate addiction: a systematic review. J Subst Abuse Treat. 2006;30(4):309–14. doi:10.1016/j.jsat.2006.02.005.
3. Lin JG, Chan YY, Chen YH. Acupuncture for the treatment of opiate addiction. Evid Based Complement Alternat Med. 2012;. doi:10.1155/2012/739045.
4. Cowan D. Methodological issues in evaluating auricular acupuncture therapy for problems arising from the use of drugs and alcohol. Acupunct Med. 2011;29(3):227–9. doi:10.1136/aim.2010.003772.
5. Organization WHO. WHO traditional medicine strategy 2002–2005. 2002.
6. Cui CL, Wu LZ, Luo F. Acupuncture for the treatment of drug addiction. Neurochem Res. 2008;33(10):2013–22. doi:10.1007/s11064-008-9784-8.
7. Black S, Carey E, Webber A, Neish N, Gilbert R. Determining the efficacy of auricular acupuncture for reducing anxiety in patients withdrawing from psychoactive drugs. J Subst Abuse Treat. 2011;41(3):279–87. doi:10.1016/j.jsat.2011.04.001.
8. Cabioglu MT, Ergene N, Tan U. Smoking cessation after acupuncture treatment. Int J Neurosci. 2007;117(5):571–8. doi:10.1080/00207450500535289.
9. Ashton H, Nodiyal A, Green D, Moore B, Heather N. Acupuncture or counselling: outcomes and predictors of treatment choice in a non-statutory addiction service. J Subst Use. 2009;14(3–4):151–60. doi:10.1080/14659890802659002.
10. Avants SK, Margolin A, Holford TR, Kosten TR. A randomized controlled trial of auricular acupuncture for cocaine dependence. Arch Intern Med. 2000;160(15):2305–12. doi:10.1001/archinte.160.15.2305.
11. Bearn J, Swami A, Stewart D, Atnas C, Giotto L, Gossop M. Auricular acupuncture as an adjunct to opiate detoxification treatment: effects on withdrawal symptoms. J Subst Abuse Treat. 2009;36(3):345–9. doi:10.1016/j.jsat.2008.08.002.
12. Bergdahl L, Berman AH, Haglund K. Patients' experience of auricular acupuncture during protracted withdrawal. J Psychiatr Ment Health Nurs. 2014;21(2):163–9. doi:10.1111/jpm.12028.
13. Berman AH, Lundberg U, Krook AL, Gyllenhammar C. Treating drug using prison inmates with auricular acupuncture: a randomized controlled trial. J Subst Abuse Treat. 2004;26(2):95–102. doi:10.1016/s0740-5472(03)00162-4.
14. Bernstein KS. The experience of acupuncture for treatment of substance dependence. In: J Nurs Scholarsh. Wiley, United States. 2000. http://search.ebscohost.com/login.aspx?direct=true&db=mdc&AN=12462821&site=ehost-live. Accessed 3 32.
15. Bonnette ML. Auricular transcutaneous electrical neuro-stimulation, addiction education, behavioral training, coaching support and the nicotine addiction treatment process. J Addict Nurs. 2008;19(3):130–40. doi:10.1080/10884600802305976.
16. Bullock ML, Kiresuk TJ, Sherman RE, Lenz SK, Culliton PD, Boucher TA, et al. A large randomized placebo controlled study of auricular acupuncture for alcohol dependence. J Subst Abuse Treat. 2002;22(2):71–7. doi:10.1016/s0740-5472(01)00217-3.
17. Cai X, Song X, Li C, Xu C, Li X, Lu Q. Acupuncture inhibits cue-induced heroin craving and brain activation. Neural Regen Res. 2012;7(33):2607–16. doi:10.3969/j.issn.1673-5374.2012.33.006.
18. Chae Y, Kang OS, Lee HJ, Kim SY, Lee H, Park HK, et al. Effect of acupuncture on selective attention for smoking-related visual cues in smokers. Neurol Res. 2010;32:S27–30. doi:10.1179/016164109x12537002793805.
19. Chae Y, Park H-J, Kang OS, Lee H-J, Kim S-Y, Yin C-S, et al. Acupuncture attenuates autonomic responses to smoking-related visual cues. Complement Ther Med. 2011;19:S1–7. doi:10.1016/j.ctim.2010.09.003.
20. Chae Y, Yeom M, Han J-H, Park H-J, Hahm D-H, Ac IS, et al. Effect of acupuncture on anxiety-like behavior during nicotine withdrawal and relevant mechanisms. Neurosci Lett. 2008;430(2):98–102. doi:10.1016/j.neulet.2007.10.026.
21. Chae YY, Yang CH, Kwon YK, Kim MR, Pyun KH, Hahm DH, et al. Acupuncture attenuates repeated nicotine-induced behavioral sensitization and c-Fos expression in the nucleus accumbens and striatum of the rat. Neurosci Lett. 2004;358(2):87–90. doi:10.1016/j.neulet.2003.12.121.
22. Chan YY, Lo WY, Li TC, Shen LJ, Yang SN, Chen YH, et al. Clinical efficacy of acupuncture as an adjunct to methadone treatment services for heroin addicts: a randomized controlled trial. Am J Chin Med. 2014;42(3):569–86. doi:10.1142/s0192415x14500372.
23. Chang BH, Sommers E, Herz L. Acupuncture and relaxation response for substance use disorder recovery. J Subst Use. 2010;15(6):390–401. doi:10.3109/14659890903580466.
24. Chang B-H, Sommers E. Acupuncture and relaxation response for craving and anxiety reduction among military veterans in recovery from substance use disorder. Am J Addict. 2014;23(2):129–36. doi:10.1111/j.1521-0391.2013.12079.x.
25. N-n Chu, Xia W, Yu P, Hu L, Zhang R, Cui C-L. Chronic morphine-induced neuronal morphological changes in the ventral tegmental area in rats are reversed by electroacupuncture treatment. Addict Biol. 2008;13(1):47–51. doi:10.1111/j.1369-1600.2007.00092.x.
26. Courbasson CMA, de Sorkin AA, Dullerud B, Van Wyk L. Acupuncture treatment for women with concurrent substance use and anxiety/depression—an effective alternative therapy? Fam Community Health. 2007;30(2):112–20.
27. Cui GH, Ren XW, Wu LZ, Han JS, Cui CL. Electroacupuncture facilitates recovery of male sexual behavior in morphine withdrawal rats. Neurochem Res. 2004;29(2):397–401. doi:10.1023/B:NERE.0000013743.53827.ad.
28. dos Santos JG, Filev R, Coelho CT, Yamamura Y, Mello LE, Tabosa A. Electroacupuncture inhibits ethanol-induced locomotor sensitization and alters homer1A mRNA Expression in mice. Alcohol Clin Exp Res. 2009;33(8):1469–75. doi:10.1111/j.1530-0277.2009.00977.x.
29. Escosteguy-Neto JC, Fallopa P, Varela P, Filev R, Tabosa A, Santos JG. Electroacupuncture inhibits CB1 upregulation induced by ethanol withdrawal in mice. Neurochem Int. 2012;61(2):277–85. doi:10.1016/j.neuint.2012.05.014.
30. Fallopa P, Escosteguy-Neto JC, Varela P, Carvalho TN, Tabosa AMF, Santos JG. Electroacupuncture reverses ethanol-induced locomotor sensitization and subsequent pERK expression in mice. Int J Neuropsychopharmacol. 2012;15(8):1121–33. doi:10.1017/s1461145711001325.
31. Gates S, Smith LA, Foxcroft DR. Auricular acupuncture for cocaine dependence. Cochrane Database Syst Rev. 2006(1). doi:10.1002/14651858.CD005192.pub2.

32. Hou XR, Zhang RJ, Lv H, Cai XH, Xie GC, Song XG. Acupuncture at Baihui and Dazhui reduces brain cell apoptosis in heroin readdicts. Neural Regen Res. 2014;9(2):164–70. doi:10.4103/1673-5374.125345.
33. Hu AR, Lai MJ, Wei JZ, Wang LN, Mao HJ, Zhou WH, et al. The effect of electroacupuncture on extinction responding of heroin-seeking behavior and FosB expression in the nucleus accumbens core. Neurosci Lett. 2013;534:252–7. doi:10.1016/j.neulet.2012.12.021.
34. Hu L, Chu NN, Sun LL, Zhang R, Han JS, Cui CL. Electroacupuncture treatment reverses morphine-induced physiological changes in dopaminergic neurons within the ventral tegmental area. Addict Biol. 2009;14(4):431–7. doi:10.1111/j.1369-1600.2009.00163.x.
35. Janssen PA, Demorest LC, Kelly A, Thiessen P, Abrahams R. Auricular acupuncture for chemically dependent pregnant women: a randomized controlled trial of the NADA protocol. Subst Abuse Treat Prev Policy. 2012;. doi:10.1186/1747-597x-7-48.
36. Janssen PA, Demorest LC, Whynot EM. Acupuncture for substance abuse treatment in the downtown eastside of Vancouver. J Urban Health. 2005;82(2):285–95. doi:10.1093/jurban/jti054.
37. Jiang YP, Liu H, Xu P, Wang Y, Lu GH. Effect of electro-acupuncture intervention on cognition attention bias in heroin addiction abstinence-a dot-probe-based event-related potential study. Chin J Integr Med. 2011;17(4):267–71. doi:10.1007/s11655-011-0698-y.
38. Kang OS, Kim SY, Jahng GH, Kim H, Kim JW, Chung SY, et al. Neural substrates of acupuncture in the modulation of cravings induced by smoking-related visual cues: an FMRI study. Psychopharmacology. 2013;228(1):119–27. doi:10.1007/s00213-013-3015-y.
39. Karst M, Passie T, Friedrich S, Wiese B, Schneider U. Acupuncture in the treatment of alcohol withdrawal symptoms: a randomized, placebo-controlled inpatient study. Addict Biol. 2002;7(4):415–9. doi:10.1080/1355621021000006017.
40. Kim JH, Chung JY, Kwon YK, Kim KJ, Yang CH, Hahm DH, et al. Acupuncture reduces alcohol withdrawal syndrome and c-Fos expression in rat brain. Am J Chin Med. 2005;33(6):887–96. doi:10.1142/s0192415x0500348x.
41. Kim MR, Kim SJ, Lyu YS, Kim SH, Lee YK, Kim TH, et al. Effect of acupuncture on behavioral hyperactivity and dopamine release in the nucleus accumbens in rats sensitized to morphine. Neurosci Lett. 2005;387(1):17–21. doi:10.1016/j.neulet.2005.07.007.
42. Kim SA, Lee BH, Bae JH, Kim KJ, Steffensen SC, Ryu Y-H, et al. Peripheral afferent mechanisms underlying acupuncture inhibition of cocaine behavioral effects in rats. PLoS One. 2013;. doi:10.1371/journal.pone.0081018.
43. Kunz S, Schulz M, Lewitzky M, Driessen M, Rau H. Ear acupuncture for alcohol withdrawal in comparison with aromatherapy: a randomized-controlled trial. Alcohol Clin Exp Res. 2007;31(3):436–42. doi:10.1111/j.1530-0277.2006.00333.x.
44. Lee B, Han S-M, Shim I. Acupuncture attenuates cocaine-induced expression of behavioral sensitization in rats: possible involvement of the dopaminergic system in the ventral tegmental area. Neurosci Lett. 2009;449(2):128–32. doi:10.1016/j.neulet.2008.10.089.
45. Lee B, Shim I, Lee H, Yin CS, Park HK, Yang JS, et al. Morphine-induced locomotor response and Fos expression in rats are inhibited by acupuncture. Neurol Res. 2010;32:S107–10. doi:10.1179/016164109x12537002794444.
46. Lee BH, Lim SC, Jeon HJ, Kim JS, Lee YK, Lee HJ, et al. Acupuncture suppresses reinstatement of morphine-seeking behavior induced by a complex cue in rats. Neurosci Lett. 2013;548:126–31. doi:10.1016/j.neulet.2013.05.026.
47. Lee BH, Ma JH, In S, Kim HY, Yoon SS, Jang EY, et al. Acupuncture at SI5 attenuates morphine seeking behavior after extinction. Neurosci Lett. 2012;529(1):23–7. doi:10.1016/j.neulet.2012.09.020.
48. Li HY, Zhang R, Cui CL, Han JS, Wu LZ. Damage of splenic T lymphocyte proliferation and differentiation and its normalization by electroacupuncture in morphine-dependent mice mode. Evid Based Complement Alternat Med. 2011;. doi:10.1155/2011/424092.
49. Li J, Sun YA, Ye JH. Electroacupuncture decreases excessive alcohol consumption involving reduction of FosB/Delta FosB levels in reward-related brain regions. PLoS One. 2012;7(7):12. doi:10.1371/journal.pone.0040347.
50. Li J, Zou YH, Ye JH. Low frequency electroacupuncture selectively decreases voluntarily ethanol intake in rats. Brain Res Bull. 2011;86(5–6):428–34. doi:10.1016/j.brainresbull.2011.08.013.
51. Li YJ, Zhong F, Yu P, Han JS, Cui CL, Wu LZ. Electroacupuncture treatment normalized sleep disturbance in morphine withdrawal rats. Evid Based Complement Alternat Med. 2011;. doi:10.1093/ecam/nep133.
52. Liang J, Li YJ, Ping XJ, Yu P, Zuo YF, Wu LZ, et al. The possible involvement of endogenous ligands for mu-, delta- and kappa-opioid receptors in modulating morphine-induced CPP expression in rats. Peptides. 2006;27(12):3307–14. doi:10.1016/j.peptides.2006.08.011.
53. Liang J, Ping XJ, Li YJ, Ma YY, Wu LZ, Han JS, et al. Morphine-induced conditioned place preference in rats is inhibited by electroacupuncture at 2 Hz: role of enkephalin in the nucleus accumbens. Neuropharmacology. 2010;58(1):233–40. doi:10.1016/j.neuropharm.2009.07.007.
54. Liu S, Zhou WH, Liu HF, Yang GD, Zhao WK. Electroacupuncture attenuates morphine withdrawal signs and c-Fos expression in the central nucleus of the amygdala in freely moving rats. Brain Res. 2005;1044(2):155–63. doi:10.1016/j.brainres.2005.02.075.
55. Liu S, Zhou WH, Ruan XZ, Li RH, Lee TT, Weng XC, et al. Activation of the hypothalamus characterizes the response to acupuncture stimulation in heroin addicts. Neurosci Lett. 2007;421(3):203–8. doi:10.1016/j.neulet.2007.04.078.
56. Liu S, Zhu FL, Lai MJ, Sun LM, Liu YJ, Zhou WH. Electroacupuncture suppresses discrete cue-evoked heroin-seeking and Fos protein expression in the nucleus accumbens core in rats. Evid Based Complement Alternat Med. 2012;. doi:10.1155/2012/286404.
57. Lua PL, Talib NS. Auricular acupuncture for drug dependence: an open-label randomized investigation on clinical outcomes, health-related quality of life, and patient acceptability. Altern Ther Health Med. 2013;19(4):28–42.
58. Lua PL, Talib NS, Ismail Z. Methadone maintenance treatment versus methadone maintenance treatment plus auricular acupuncture: impacts on patient satisfaction and coping mechanism. J Pharm Pract. 2013;26(6):541–50. doi:10.1177/0897190013489574.
59. Margolin A, Avants SK, Arnold R. Acupuncture and spirituality-focused group therapy for the treatment of HIV-positive drug users: a preliminary study. J Psychoactive Drugs. 2005;37(4):385–90.
60. Margolin A, Avants SK, Holford TR. Interpreting conflicting findings from clinical trials of auricular acupuncture for cocaine addiction: does treatment context influence outcome? J Altern Complement Med. 2002;8(2):111–21. doi:10.1089/107555302317371398.
61. Margolin A, Kleber HD, Avants SK, Konefal J, Gawin F, Stark E, et al. Acupuncture for the treatment of cocaine addiction—a randomized controlled trial. JAMA. 2002;287(1):55–63. doi:10.1001/jama.287.1.55.
62. Meade CS, Lukas SE, McDonald LJ, Fitzmaurice GM, Eldridge JA, Merrill N, et al. A randomized trial of transcutaneous electric acupoint stimulation as adjunctive treatment for opioid detoxification. J Subst Abuse Treat. 2010;38(1):12–21. doi:10.1016/j.jsat.2009.05.010.
63. Montazeri K, Farahnakian M, Saghaei M. The effect of acupuncture on the acute withdrawal symptoms from rapid opiate detoxification. Acta Anaesthesiol Sin. 2002;40(4):173–7.
64. Overstreet DH, Cui CL, Ma YY, Guo CY, Han JS, Lukas SE, et al. Electroacupuncture reduces voluntary alcohol intake in alcohol-preferring rats via an opiate-sensitive mechanism. Neurochem Res. 2008;33(10):2166–70. doi:10.1007/s11064-008-9791-9.
65. Park HJ, Kim ST, Yoon DH, Jin SH, Lee SJ, Lee HJ, et al. The association between the DRD2 TaqI A polymorphism and smoking cessation in response to acupuncture in Koreans. J Altern Complement Med. 2005;11(3):401–5. doi:10.1089/acm.2005.11.401.
66. Penetar DM, Burgos-Robles A, Trksak GH, MacLean RR, Dunlap S, Lee DYW, et al. Effects of transcutaneous electric acupoint stimulation on drug use and responses to cue-induced craving: a pilot study. Chin Med. 2012;. doi:10.1186/1749-8546-7-14.
67. Rabinstein AA, Shulman LM. Acupuncture in clinical neurology. Neurologist. 2003;9(3):137–48. doi:10.1097/00127893-200305000-00002.
68. Russell LC, Sharp B, Gilbertson B. Acupuncture for addicted patients with chronic histories of arrest—a pilot study of the consortium treatment center. J Subst Abuse Treat. 2000;19(2):199–205. doi:10.1016/s0740-5472(00)00118-5.
69. Samuels N, Gropp C, Singer SR, Oberbaum M. Acupuncture for psychiatric illness: a literature review. Behav Med. 2008;34(2):55–62. doi:10.3200/bmed.34.2.55-64.
70. Shi XD, Ren W, Wang GB, Luo F, Han JS, Cui CL. Brain opioid-receptors are involved in mediating peripheral electric stimulation-induced inhibition

of morphine conditioned place preference in rats. Brain Res. 2003;981(1–2):23–9. doi:10.1016/s0006-8993(03)02798-7.

71. Shi XD, Wang GB, Ma YY, Ren W, Luo F, Cui CL, et al. Repeated peripheral electrical stimulations suppress both morphine-induced CPP and reinstatement of extinguished CPP in rats: accelerated expression of PPE and PPD mRNA in NAc implicated. Brain Res Mol Brain Res. 2004;130(1–2):124–33. doi:10.1016/j.molbrainres.2004.07.016.
72. Thanavaro JL, Delicath TA. Auricular Transcutaneous Electrostimulation Therapy and Intensive Counseling for the Treatment of Smoking Cessation in a Primary Care Practice. J Addict Nurs. 2010;21(4):215–24. doi:10.3109/10884602.2010.515694.
73. Tian XW, Krishnan S. Efficacy of auricular acupressure as an adjuvant therapy in substance abuse treatment: a pilot study. Altern Ther Health Med. 2006;12(1):66–9.
74. Trumpler F, Oez S, Stahli P, Brenner HD, Juni P. Acupuncture for alcohol withdrawal: a randomized controlled trial. Alcohol. 2003;38(4):369–75. doi:10.1093/alcalc/agg091.
75. Wang B, Luo F, Xia YQ, Han JS. Peripheral electric stimulation inhibits morphine-induced place preference in rats. NeuroReport. 2000;11(5):1017–20. doi:10.1097/00001756-200004070-00024.
76. Wang GB, Wu LZ, Yu P, Li YJ, Ping XJ, Cui CL. Multiple 100 Hz electroacupuncture treatments produced cumulative effect on the suppression of morphine withdrawal syndrome: central preprodynorphin mRNA and p-CREB implicated. Peptides. 2011;32(4):713–21. doi:10.1016/j.peptides.2010.12.006.
77. Wen H, Cheung S. Treatment of drug addiction by acupuncture and electrical stimulation. Asian J Med. 1973;9:138–41.
78. White AR, Rampes H, Campbell JL. Acupuncture and related interventions for smoking cessation. Cochrane Database Syst Rev. 2006;. doi:10.1002/14651858.CD0000009.pub2.
79. White AR, Rampes H, Liu JP, Stead LF, Campbell J. Acupuncture and related interventions for smoking cessation. Cochrane Database Syst Rev. 2011;. doi:10.1002/14651858.CD000009.pub3.
80. White AR, Rampes H, Liu JP, Stead LF, Campbell J. Acupuncture and related interventions for smoking cessation. Cochrane Database Syst Rev. 2014;. doi:10.1002/14651858.CD000009.pub4.
81. Xia W, Chu NN, Liang J, Li YJ, Zhang R, Han JS, et al. Electroacupuncture of 2 Hz Has a rewarding effect: evidence from a conditioned place preference study in rats. Evid Based Complement Alternat Med. 2011;. doi:10.1093/ecam/nen043.
82. Yang CH, Yoon SS, Hansen DM, Wilcox JD, Blumell BR, Park JJ, et al. Acupuncture Inhibits GABA neuron activity in the ventral tegmental area and reduces ethanol self-administration. Alcohol Clin Exp Res. 2010;34(12):2137–46. doi:10.1111/j.1530-0277.2010.01310.x.
83. Yeh M-L, Chang C-Y, Chu N-F, Chen H-H. A 6-week acupoint stimulation intervention for quitting smoking. Am J Chin Med. 2009;37(5):829–36.
84. Yoon SS, Yang EJ, Lee BH, Jang EY, Kim HY, Choi SM, et al. Effects of acupuncture on stress-induced relapse to cocaine-seeking in rats. Psychopharmacology. 2012;222(2):303–11. doi:10.1007/s00213-012-2683-3.
85. Yoshimoto K, Fukuda F, Hori M, Kato B, Kato H, Hattori H, et al. Acupuncture stimulates the release of serotonin, but not dopamine, in the rat nucleus accumbens. Tohoku J Exp Med. 2006;208(4):321–6. doi:10.1620/tjem.208.321.
86. Yoshimoto K, Kato B, Sakai K, Shibata M, Yano T, Yasuhara M. Electroacupuncture stimulation suppresses the increase in alcohol-drinking behavior in restricted rats. Alcohol Clin Exp Res. 2001;25(6):63S–8S.
87. Zalewska-Kaszubska J, Obzejta D. Use of low-energy laser as adjunct treatment of alcohol addiction. Lasers Med Sci. 2004;19(2):100–4. doi:10.1007/s10103-004-0307-9.
88. Zhang RJ, Cai XH, Song XG, Dong CY, Hou XR, Lv L. Normalization of ventral tegmental area structure following acupuncture in a rat model of heroin relapse. Neural Regen Res. 2014;9(3):301–7. doi:10.4103/1673-5374.128228.
89. Zhao RJ, Yoon SS, Lee BH, Kwon YK, Kim KJ, Shim I, et al. Acupuncture normalizes the release of accumbal dopamine during the withdrawal period and after the ethanol challenge in chronic ethanol-treated rats. Neurosci Lett. 2006;395(1):28–32. doi:10.1016/j.neulet.2005.10.043.
90. Mayer DJ. Acupuncture: an evidence-based review of the clinical literature. Annu Rev Med. 2000;51(1):49–63.
91. Birch S, Hesselink JK, Jonkman FA, Hekker TA, Bos A. Clinical research on acupuncture: part 1. What have reviews of the efficacy and safety of acupuncture told us so far? The. J Altern Complement Med. 2004;10(3):468–80.
92. Head KA. Peripheral neuropathy: pathogenic mechanisms and alternative therapies. Alternative medicine review. 2006;11(4):294.
93. Shi J. LU L. Traditional Chinese medicine in treatment of opiate addiction1. Acta Pharmacol Sin. 2006;27(10):1303–8.

17

Comparison of chemical profiles and effectiveness between Erxian decoction and mixtures of decoctions of its individual herbs: a novel approach for identification of the standard chemicals

H. P. Cheung[1], S. W. Wang[1], T. B. Ng[2], Y. B. Zhang[1], L. X. Lao[1], Z. J. Zhang[1], Y. Tong[1], F. W. S. Chung[1] and S. C. W. Sze[1*]

Abstract

Background: Identification of bioactive standard chemicals is a major challenge in the study of the Chinese medicinal formula. In particular, the chemical components may interact differently depending on the preparative methods, therefore affecting the amounts of bioactive components and their pharmacological properties in the medicinal formula. With the use of Erxian decoction (EXD) as a study model—a well-known Chinese medicinal formula for treating menopausal symptoms, a novel and rapid approach in seeking standard chemicals has been established by differentially comparing the HPLC profiles and the menopause-related biochemical parameters of combined decoction of EXD (EXD-C) and mixtures of the decoctions of its individual herbs (EXD-S).

Methods: The levels of six chemicals, which exerted actions on the HPO axis, have been measured in EXD-C and EXD-S by HPLC. Twelve-month-old female Sprague-Dawley rats were employed and treated with EXD-C and EXD-S. Their endocrine functions after treatment were evaluated by determining the ovarian mRNA levels of aromatase, a key enzyme for estradiol biosynthesis. The effect of the antioxidant regimen was determined by the hepatic superoxide dismutase-1 (SOD), catalase (CAT) and glutathione peroxidase (GPx-1) mRNA levels.

Results: The amounts of mangiferine, ferulic acid, jatrorrhizine and palmatine in EXD-S were twofold higher than those in EXD-C. EXD-S was more effective in stimulating ovarian aromatase and the expression of the antioxidant enzymes compared with EXD-C.

Conclusion: Mangiferine, ferulic acid, jatrorrhizine and palmatine are suitable for use as standard chemicals for quality evaluation of EXD according to our approach. EXD-S could be more effective than EXD-C.

Keywords: Standard chemicals, Chinese medicine formula, Erxian decoction, Menopause, Novel approach

Background

The clinical use of Chinese medicine (CM) formulas for treating chronic diseases and aging-related disorders has been gaining momentum in recent years. The multiple pharmacological properties of CM formula are proved to be contributed by the multiple bioactive chemicals in a CM formula through multiple mechanisms [1]. Thus, seeking bioactive and standard chemical is crucial for quality control evaluation of CM formulas. While the contemporary analytic techniques allow us to isolate and detect multiples chemical components from CM

*Correspondence: stephens@hku.hk
[1] School of Chinese Medicine, Li Ka Shing Faculty of Medicine, The University of Hong Kong, 10 Sassoon Road, Pokfulam, Hong Kong, SAR, China
Full list of author information is available at the end of the article

formulas simultaneously, identification of bioactive and standard chemicals remains a tedious task.

Due to the complexity of the chemicals in a CM formula, the potential interaction and the subsequent changes in the pharmacological properties have drawn the attention of many researchers in the field [1]. Interactions leading to changes in the chemical components of TCM may arise during the processing of herbal materials or during the decoction procedures [2]. Conventionally, different herbal materials in a Chinese medicinal formula are decocted together to yield the medicinal extract, which can be regarded as a "combined decoction". To the contrary, individual herbs can be decocted separately and mixed together to compose a medicinal formula. This is particularly common in the recent development of herbal formulations, extracts of individual herbal material can be concentrated in the form of granules, and the medicinal formula can be reconstituted by mixing the corresponding amounts of granules [3]. The resulting decoction is thus regarded as a mixture of decoctions of separated individual herbs (separated decoction)". However, due to the difference in their decoction processes, there will be variations in the chemical components of the "combined decoction" and "separated decoction". It is known that during the decoction process, the chemicals from different herbs may interact to affect the solubility, conversion of chemical structures, or may lead to generation of new chemicals or precipitation [3]. For example, results obtained from a previous study revealed that the component of 1,5-dicaffeoylquinic acid in the Tibetan herb (*Saussurea laniceps*) was transesterificated into 1,3-dicaffeoylquinic acid during boiling in water [4]. These interactions may affect the amounts of bioactive components in the medicinal formula, and thus the pharmacological properties. On the one hand, the discrepancy between the chemical components and the pharmacological properties between "combined decoction" and "separated decoction" has raised concerns about the variation in quality and therapeutic efficacy of decoctions prepared using different methods. On the other hand, such discrepancy may hint the bioactive components contributing to the pharmacological properties, thus opening up the possibility of a novel and rapid approach for identification of the chemical standards of CM formulas for quality control purpose.

In this study, Erxian decoction (EXD), an anti-menopausal Chinese medicine formula, was selected as a study model to demonstrate the feasibility of our approach for identification of the chemical standards of CM formulas. Erxian decoction (EXD) is a popular TCM formula that has been clinically used for relieving menopausal syndrome for more than 60 years [5]. Our previous EXD studies have used a LC-DAD-ESI-MS/MS method in characterising the key chemical constitutents of EXD absorbed or metabolised in vivo during the treatment of menopausal syndromes [6]. Knowing that the causes of menopausal syndromes involves the hypothalamus-pituitary-ovary (HPO) axis, target compounds of this study were identified and differentiated by their presence in the major organs of the HPO axis (i.e. brain and ovary) and serum. Six chemicals from EXD that may contribute to relief of menopausal syndrome were selected: mangiferine, ferulic acid, icariin, jatrorrhizine, palmatine and berberine [6]. Therefore, the levels of mangiferine, ferulic acid, icariin, jatrorrhizine, palmatine and berberine in both EXD-C and EXD-S were determined and compared by HPLC profiles. Besides chemical analysis, it has been found in human that during menopause, the expression of aromatase, a key enzyme for ovarian estradiol production, and the activities of some antioxidant enzymes, including superoxide dismutase-1 (SOD1), and glutathione peroxidase (GPx-1), underwent a decrease leading to a decline of ovarian estrogen production and serum estrogen level [7]. In addition, our previous study also demonstrated that EXD relieved menopausal syndrome via up-regulation of the mRNA levels of ovarian aromatase and hepatic antioxidant enzymes catalase (CAT) in twelve-month-old naturally aging SD-rats with lower serum estradiol levels compared with those of 3-month-old young SD-rat [5]. Therefore, we evaluated and compared the pharmacological properties of EXD-C and EXD-S for alleviating menopause by measurement of their mRNA levels of ovarian aromatase and hepatic antioxidant enzymes SOD-1, CAT, and GPx-1 after drug treatment. Results and approach obtained from this study could be applied in quality control studies of other existing CM formulas, which ensure the use of high-quality CM formulas clinically. The following shows our approach for selecting the standard markers for quality control of CM formulas: (i) the standard markers should be present at target sites/organs in vivo; (ii) the standard markers should be associated with pharmacological and clinical effects of CM formulas; (iii) the amounts of standard markers should have twofold differences for different decoction processing (EXD-S: separate decoction of EXD vs EXD-C: combined decoction of EXD).

Methods

Herbal materials and preparation of different decoctions of EXD

One kilogram of the six component herbs of EXD namely *Herba Epimedii, Rhizoma Curculiginis, Radix Morindae officinalis, Cortex Phellodendri, Radix Anemarrhenae,* and *Radix Angelicae sinensis* (composition ratio = 12:12:10:10:9:9) were decocted together with distilled water in 10:1 (v/w) ratio at 100 °C for 1 h to prepare "combined decoction of EXD" (EXD-C), the extraction was repeated twice. The procedures were the same as those described in our previous publication [5]. For preparation of "mixtures of EXD individual herbs decoction" (EXD-S), the component herbs in the amounts according to above composition ratio of EXD-C were decocted separately instead and reconstituted afterward. The extraction was also repeated twice. Both of the herbal extracts, EXD-C and EXD-S, were filtered and lyophilized in a freeze drier (Labconco, Freezone). The dried powdered extracts were stored at −80 °C before use. The herbal materials were collected from various sources and their identity was confirmed by Dr YanBo Zhang (one of the authors), School of Chinese medicine, the University of Hong Kong.

Quality control and high performance liquid chromatography (HPLC)

To evaluate the consistency of the quality of EXD-S and EXD-C extracts, three batches of 0.5 g powder of extracts were extracted with 10 ml 75% methanol in a water bath at 60 °C for 15 min, followed by ultrasonication for 30 min. The extracts were centrifuged at 15,700×*g* and filtered with 0.45 μm Millex® syringe filter (Millipore). Six standard chemicals namely mangiferine, ferulic acid, icariin, jatrorrhizine, palmatine and berberine which are well-known compounds in EXD [5] were employed for quantitation. The HPLC profiles of the EXD-S and EXD-C were generated using Water 600S HPLC system (Waters) with a reverse-phase column (XBridge® C18, 5 μl, 250 mm × 4.6 mm i.d., Waters, USA). The mobile phase consisted of acetonitrile (solvent A) and 0.05% SDS in 0.1% acetic acid (solvent B). A programmed gradient was used for elution with 5–30% A in 0–30 min, 30% A in 30–35 min, 30–50% A in 35–40 min, 50–55% A in 40–65 min. The injection volume was 10 μl and flow rate was 1 ml/min. The ultraviolet (UV) absorbance from 200 to 400 nm was measured with a diode array detector (DAD). Chromatograms were generated at 345 nm to observed most number of peaks. The peak integration and quantitation were analyzed with the Waters Empower 2 software (Waters), the procedures were the same as those described in our previous publication [5].

Animals

Twelve-month old female Sprague-Dawley (SD)-rats with low serum estradiol levels were employed as the animal model [5]. Animals were purchased at the age of 8 months from the Laboratory Animal Units, the University of Hong Kong and housed at an ambient temperature of 24 °C with a relative humidity of 50–65% and 12-h light–dark cycles till the required age. The rats were acclimated for four months and their serum estradiol levels were monitored before the experiment. The experiments had been approved by the Committee on the Use of Live Animals in Teaching and Research (CULATR) of the Li Ka Shing Faculty of Medicine, the University of Hong Kong.

Drug administration and organ harvesting

Rats were arbitrarily divided into six groups with ten animals each. EXD-S and EXD-C extracts dissolved in 2 ml of water (0.76 and 1.52 g/kg) were administered via gavage tubing daily for 6 weeks. The control group received an equal volume of water instead of drug. At the end of the experiment, the rats were euthanized by an intraperitoneal injection of pentobarbital (200 mg/kg). The ovaries and livers were collected and stored at −80 °C until further experiment.

RNA extraction and quantitative real-time PCR

The RNA extraction and quantitative real-time PCR were performed according to the previous methods published by our group [5]. In brief, total RNA was isolated from the ovary and liver using the TRIZOL® reagent according to instructions of the manufacturer (Invitrogen Life Technologies). The purity and concentration of RNA were determined by the absorbance at 260/280 nm and at 260 nm, respectively. The cDNA was transcribed from 1 μg of total RNA using random hexamers (Promega) and reverse transcriptase II (Invitrogen Life Technologies) following the manufacturer's instructions. Quantitative real-time PCR was performed for the expression of aromatase (Cyp19), CAT, SOD-1, glutathione peroxidase 1 (GPx-1) genes and beta-actin (β-actin) as housekeeping control using the Platinum® quantitative PCR SuperMIX-UDG (Invitrogen Life Technologies) in a final reaction volume of 25 μl in 0.25 X SYBR green (Molecular Probes®, Invitrogen Life Technologies) according to the manufacturer's protocol. The sequences of the PCR primers are described in our previous study [5]. The target genes were amplified with the following programme: pre-incubation at 94 °C for 15 min, followed by 40 cycles of incubation at 94 °C for 20 s, 57 °C for 20 s and 72 °C for 20 s. Following the amplification process, a melting curve analysis was performed by raising the temperature from 72 to 95 °C at a rate of 1 °C/5 s to ensure the specificity of PCR products. Quantitation of PCR product was performed by comparing with the standard curve (plot of number of threshold cycle (Ct) value against log of standard amount with a series of 20-fold dilution), and the results were expressed as Ct value. Quantity of the target genes was normalized with the housekeeping gene β-actin for relative quantitation. The experiments were repeated in triplicate for analysis.

Statistical analysis

For the peaks in HPLC profiles of EXD-S and EXD-C, relative standard deviation (RSD) was calculated. For PCR experiments, data were expressed as mean ± SEM. Statistically analysis was performed using One-way ANOVA followed by Tukey's Multiple Comparison Test. A p value <0.05 in a comparison was considered statistically significant. Statistical analysis was performed with GraphPad Prism 4® software (GraphPad Software).

Results

HPLC profiles of EXD-S and EXD-C

The peaks from chromatograms generated at 345 nm show most detectable peaks were integrated. The chromatograms of EXD-S and EXD-C annotated with the six standard chemicals are shown in Fig. 1. Three batches of EXD-S and EXD-C were injected. The amounts of the six standard chemicals were determined from the standard curve and are listed in Table 1. The contents of all the six marker chemicals were found to decrease to different extents in EXD-C (Fig. 2). The content of mangiferin in EXD-S and EXD-C demonstrated a 2.09-fold difference. The decrease in content of three berberine-type alkaloids (jatrorrhizine, palmatine and berberine) in EXD-C varied from 3.44-old for jatrorrhizine, 30.17-fold for palmatine and 1.62-fold for berberine. The content of ferulic acid in EXD-C decreased by 2.46-fold and the amount of icariin showed a 1.17-fold decrease in EXD-C (Fig. 3). For all the six standard chemicals, the RSD values calculated were within 5%, indicating consistency in the quality of the sample injected and reproducibility of the HPLC profile, as well as excluding the influence of any unknown variability or instability found in the composition of the active constituents in the molecular investigation of the EXD extract.

Effects of EXD-S and EXD-C on expression of Cyp19, CAT, SOD and GPx-1 at transcriptional level

After treatment with EXD-S and EXD-C for 6 weeks, the expression of ovarian Cyp19, SOD, CAT and hepatic GPx-1 was regulated differently. From the results, both treatments with EXD-S and EXD-C at high doses significantly stimulated the expression of ovarian Cyp19 gene, which encodes the key enzyme aromatase for estrogen secretion. ($p < 0.01$ compared with control group in Tukey's Multiple Comparison Test following One-way ANOVA). The stimulatory effect on up-regulation of Cyp19 was most prominent in EXD-S at high dose, which is in line with our previous finding [5], in which the expression level of Cyp19 gene was significantly higher than that of EXD-C at high dose ($p < 0.001$ compared with control group in Tukey's Multiple Comparison Test following One-way ANOVA) (Fig. 4).

The effects of EXD-S and EXD-C were less prominent on the gene expression of hepatic antioxidant enzymes. The relative mRNA levels of CAT after treatment of EXD were slightly higher than that of control by around 1.5-fold, without statistical significance. EXD-S treatment at both dosages displayed a trend of increase in CAT expression compared with EXD-C, but again no significant differences were detected (Fig. 5).

The mRNA levels of SOD-1 and GPx-1 in all treatment groups were comparable to that of control. However, in EXD-S (low dose) treated group, the hepatic mRNA expression of SOD-1 was significantly higher than that of EXD-C (low dose) group (Fig. 6). EXD-S at high dose also displayed a tendency of increase in the mRNA level of hepatic GPx-1 compared with that of EXD-C groups, but such tendency was devoid of statistically significant difference (Fig. 7).

Discussion

The effects of different decoction methods on chemical profiles of anti-menopausal EXD formula have been demonstrated by HPLC, with the six selected chemicals that have been present at HPO-axis in vivo revealed from our previous publication [6]. Results obtained from HPLC profile revealed that all the six chemicals including mangiferin, ferulic acid, icariin, jatrorrhizine, palmatine and berberine were higher in content in EXD-S than that in EXD-C (Figs. 2, 3), the HPLC profile of EXD-S is the same as that in our previous publication [5]. Such changes in chemical profiles may be due to the interaction of different components during the decoction process. For instance, the chemical components may enhanced the solubility of each other when decocted together thus increasing the final content of chemicals in the extract [8]. On the contrary, they may precipitate with each other forming insoluble complex leading to loss of bioactive components [8]. It is known that alkaloids like berberine, palmatine and jatrorrhizine would form precipitate with the flavone baicalin [9]. Alkaloids may also precipitate with organic acids forming insoluble salts [8]. It is possible that the alkaloids species in combined decoction of EXD (EXD-C) may precipitate with organic acid from its different ingredient herbs like ferulic acid, flavonoid compounds such as icariin or other undetected flavone species and are lost from EXD-C. Also, bioactive components can be converted by chemical reactions like hydrolysis of glycosides. In the combined decoction of EXD (EXD-C), hydrolysis may be facilitated to remove the sugar units from the flavonoids glycoside icariin, leading to decrease in its content [2].

Mangiferine, ferulic acid, jatrorrhizine and palmatine were confirmed as the key chemical markers for quality control of anti-menopausal EXD according to our proposed approach. Because (i) they have been present at HPO axis, revealed by our previous study; (ii) their pharmacological effects are related to menopause. As it has

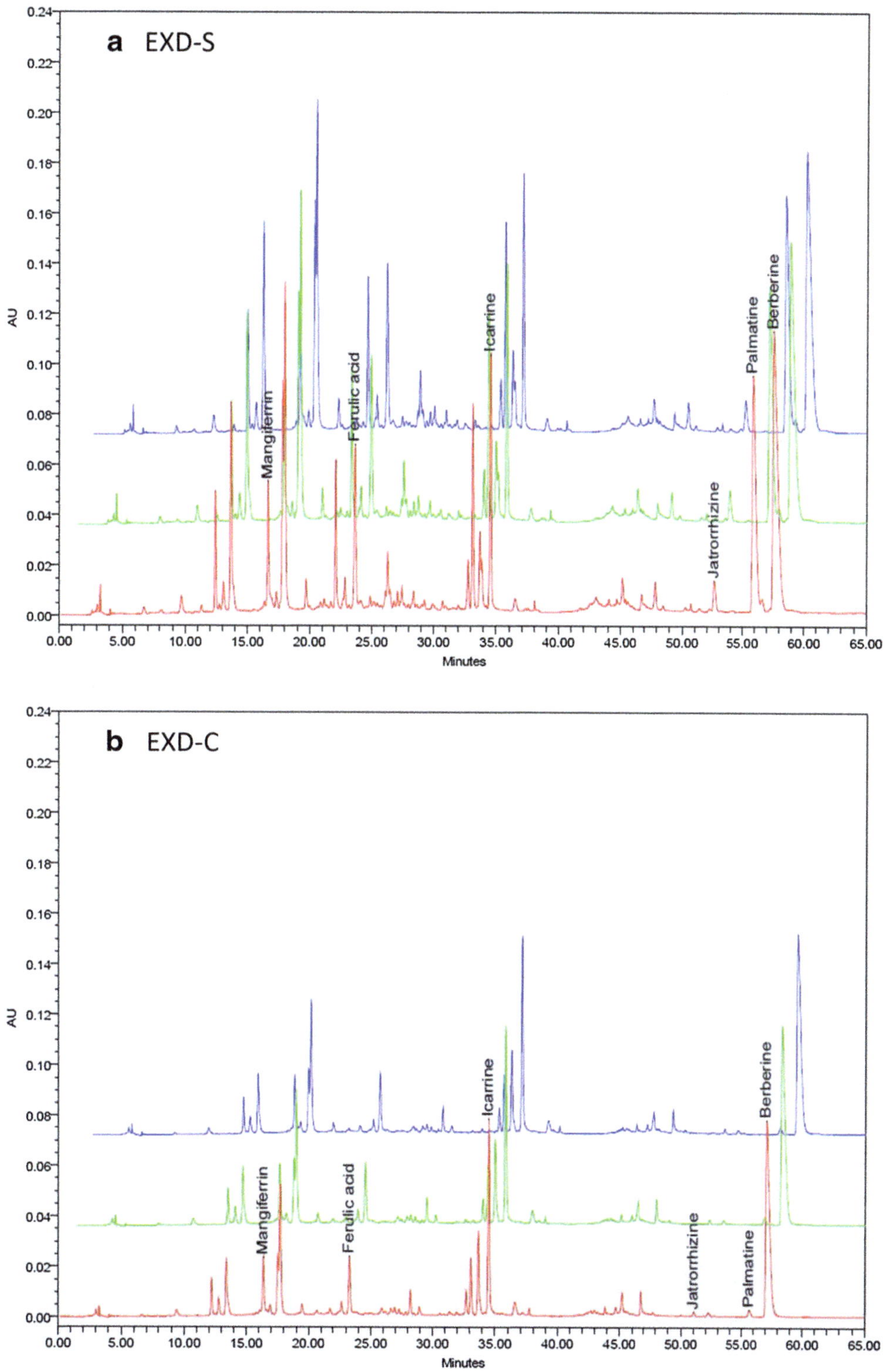

Fig. 1 Overlaid HPLC chromatograms of **a** EXD-S [4] and **b** EXD-C from three repeated injections extracted at 345 nm. The peaks of six standard chemicals were annotated as mangiferine, ferulic acid, icariin, jatrorrhizine, palmatine and berberine, in a chorological order of retention time

been reported that along with aging and menopause, the antioxidant enzymes is down-regulated, and the estrogen secretion through aromatase is hampered [6]. These four chemical markers possess antioxidant activities [10–13]. Besides, ferulic acid were also reported to have estrogenic properties, its treatment increases the bone mineral

Table 1 The contents of six standard chemicals of EXD in three injections of EXD-S and EXD-C

Injection	Mangiferin (mg/g)	Ferulic acid (mg/g)	Icariin (mg/g)	Jatrorrhizine (mg/g)	Palmatine (mg/g)	Berberine (mg/g)
EXD-S1	1.368	0.4871	1.731	0.1004	1.083	1.615
EXD-S2	1.371	0.4896	1.744	0.1010	1.090	1.617
EXD-S3	1.382	0.4996	1.745	0.1014	1.092	1.628
Mean	1.374	0.4921	1.740	0.1010	1.089	1.620
RSD (%)	0.57	1.34	0.46	0.48	0.46	0.43
EXD-C1	0.6581	0.1983	1.498	0.02865	0.03577	1.000
EXD-C2	0.6610	0.1980	1.493	0.03009	0.03661	1.001
EXD-C3	0.6583	0.2034	1.479	0.02947	0.03592	1.003
Mean	0.6591	0.1999	1.490	0.02940	0.03610	1.001
RSD (%)	0.24	1.53	0.65	2.45	1.23	0.17
Mean ratio	2.085	2.462	1.168	3.435	30.17	1.618

The results are expressed as mg or chemicals per g of EXD extract. RSD values were calculated for each chemical from three injections and the mean ratio represents the ratio of amount of chemicals in EXD-S to that of EXD-C

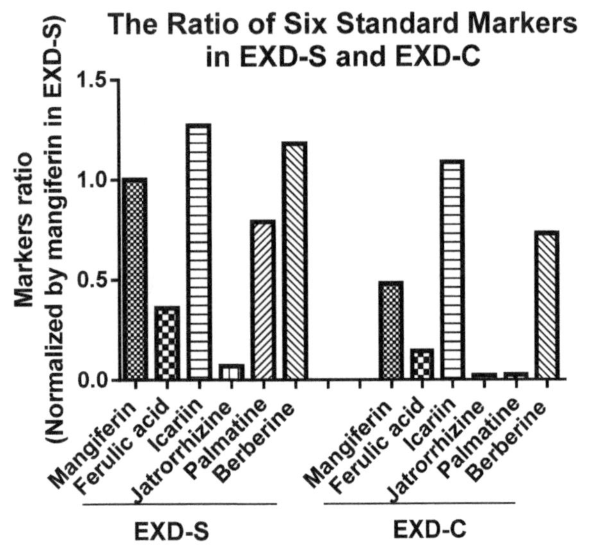

Fig. 2 The ratio of six standard markers in EXD-S and EXD-C

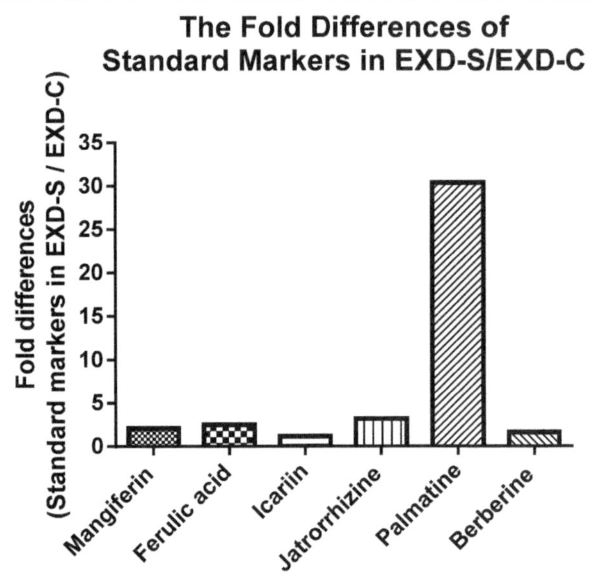

Fig. 3 The fold differences of standard markers in EXD-S/EXD-C

density in ovariectomized female rats of the Sprague-Dawley strain with slightly increasing the serum levels of estrogen [14]. In addition, it has been shown to be effective in treating hot flashes in menopausal women [15]; (iii) the amounts of these four chemical markers in EXD-S are twofold higher than those in EXD-C, thus different decoction methods could be easily revealed by different amounts of these four markers in HPLC profile (Fig. 3). In particular, palmatine is almost 30.38-fold higher in EXD-S compared with EXD-C (Fig. 3), which will be further biologically characterized in our further experiment.

Besides chemical analysis, the effects of EXD-S and EXD-C on ovarian aromatase mRNA expression and hepatic antioxidant enzymes were evaluated, which has also been proven as the targets of EXD by our group previously [5]. As anticipated, EXD stimulated ovarian aromatase (Cyp19) expression the transcriptional level at high dose (1.76 g/kg). The up-regulation of Cyp19 mRNA level in EXD-S-treated rats was significantly almost twofold higher than that of EXD-C, which may have been due to the overall increase in bioactive components in EXD-S as revealed from the HPLC profiles. It is known that the bioactive components in EXD such as mangiferin, berberine, palmatine and jatrorrhizine possess antioxidant activities [10–13]. Besides, icariin and ferulic acid were also reported to have estrogenic properties [14, 16]. The lower amounts of these bioactive compounds in EXD-C may explain the decreased bioactivity of EXD-C

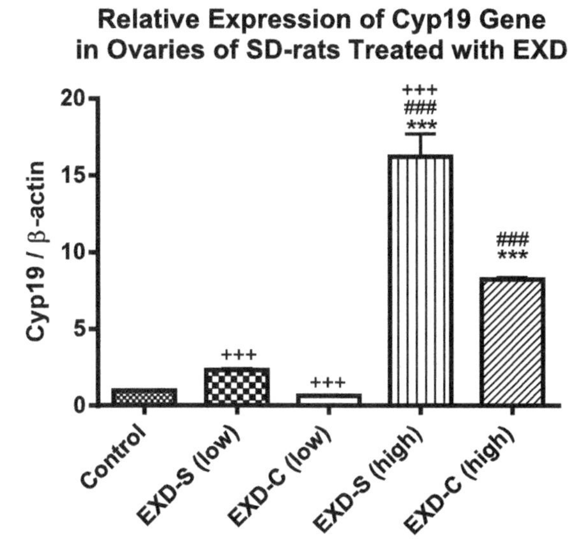

Fig. 4 The relative expression of Cyp19 gene at transcriptional level in ovaries of SD-rats treated with different EXD decoctions. Data were normalized by control group and expressed as mean ± SEM. Control: control group (fed with water); EXD-S: SD-rats treated with separate decoction of EXD at 0.76 g/kg (low) and 1.52 g/kg (high); EXD-C: SD-rats treated with combined decoction of EXD at 0.76 g/kg (low) and 1.52 g/kg (high). ***$p < 0.001$ compared with Control;$^{###}p < 0.001$ compared with EXD-C (low);$^{+++}p < 0.001$ compared with EXD-C (high) (Tukey's Multiple Comparison Test following One-way ANOVA) (n = 3)

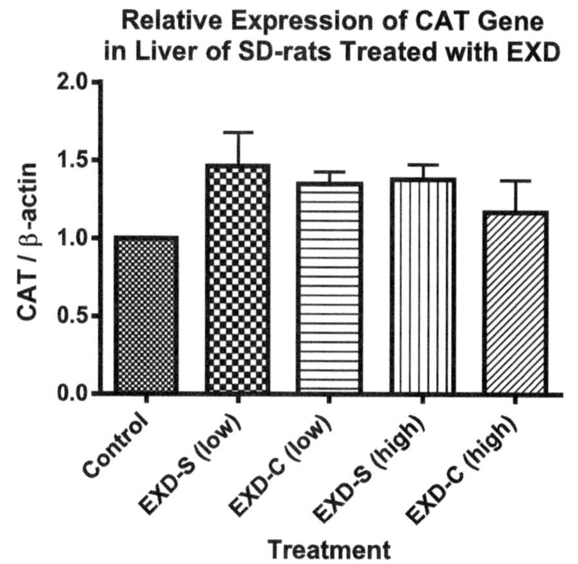

Fig. 5 The relative expression of CAT gene at transcriptional level in livers of SD-rats treated with different EXD decoctions. Data were normalized by control group and expressed as mean ± SEM. Control: control group (fed with water); EXD-S: SD-rats treated with separate decoction of EXD at 0.76 g/kg (low) and 1.52 g/kg (high); EXD-C: SD-rats treated with combined decoction of EXD at 0.76 g/kg (low) and 1.52 g/kg (high). No statistical significances were detected among groups (Tukey's Multiple Comparison Test following One-way ANOVA) (n = 3)

in vivo. The effects of EXD-S on mRNA level of hepatic antioxidants are in line with our previous findings [5]. In our previous study, EXD could significantly up-regulate CAT expression at the transcriptional level [5]. In this study, both EXD-S and EXD-C elicited around 1.5-fold of increase in the mRNA level of CAT, although no statistical significance was detected. Consistent with the results of Cyp19 expression, EXD-S showed a stronger tendency of stimulation of CAT and GPx-1 than EXD-C. The mRNA level of SOD-1 in EXD-S-treated group was significantly higher than that of the group treated with low dosages of EXD-C. These again support the better pharmacological properties of EXD-S than EXD-C.

In a TCM formula, the complexity of chemical components imposes difficulties in the identification of standard chemicals for quality control. The observation of differences in the chemical profiles of EXD-S and EXD-C in relation to their bioactivity has opened up the possibility of a novel and rapid approach to identify the standard chemicals in CM formulas. Since the pharmacological properties of a medicinal formula are conferred by the chemical components, which may change as a result of different decoction conditions. By comparing the HPLC profiles of the decoctions, the differentially extracted components would be those responsible for the observed discrepancy in bioactivity. This would facilitate the identification and selection of bioactive components as standard chemicals out of the complex herbal mixture. In a study on Radix *Scutellariae* (Huangqin) decoction, an increase in the amount of the bioactive compound baicalin was observed in the combined decoction [17]. In another study on Tangkuei Liu Huang Decoction, the amount of baicalin was higher in separate decoctions than that of combined decoction [18]. These findings suggest that the bioactive components in a herbal extract can be affected by the decoction method as well as the herbal interaction between different herbs. The decoction methods would also affect the pharmacological properties. In some studies, the combined decoction may have better therapeutic efficacy and vice versa [19, 20]. Whether the component herbs of a Chinese medicinal formula should be decocted separately or in combination together depends on different individual formulas, but the decoction of herbal materials is often an inevitable process for the preparation of most of the CM prescriptions. The evaluation of chemical profiles as well as the pharmacological properties of different processing methods may indicate a novel approach for identifying the standard chemicals of the CM formula. In this study, the feasibility of such approach is evaluated by differential comparison

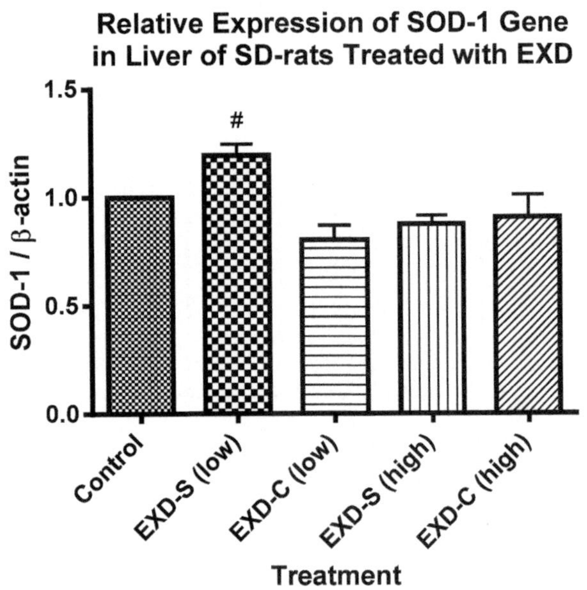

Fig. 6 The relative expression of SOD-1 gene at transcriptional level in livers of SD-rats treated with different EXD decoctions. Data were normalized by control group and expressed as mean ± SEM. Control: control group (fed with water); EXD-S: SD-rats treated with separate decoction of EXD at 0.76 g/kg (low) and 1.52 g/kg (high); EXD-C: SD-rats treated with combined decoction of EXD at 0.76 g/kg (low) and 1.52 g/kg (high). $^{\#}p < 0.05$ compared with EXD-C (low) (Tukey's Multiple Comparison Test following One-way ANOVA) (n = 3)

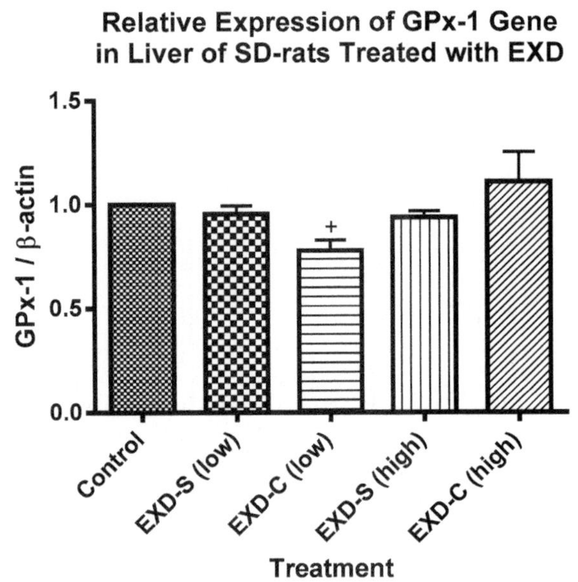

Fig. 7 The relative expression of GPx-1 gene at transcriptional level in livers of SD-rats treated with different EXD decoctions. Data were normalized by control group and expressed as mean ± SEM. Control: control group (fed with water); EXD-S: SD-rats treated with separate decoction of EXD at 0.76 g/kg (low) and 1.52 g/kg (high); EXD-C: SD-rats treated with combined decoction of EXD at 0.76 g/kg (low) and 1.52 g/kg (high). $^{+}p < 0.05$ compared with EXD-C (high) (Tukey's Multiple Comparison Test following One-way ANOVA) (n = 3)

of the HPLC profile of EXD-S and EXD-C in relation to the pharmacological properties. Eventually, this approach can be coupled with analytic techniques to identify the differentially extracted components obtained by different decoction methods.

In future developments, such approach may be polished by further validations with a more comprehensive pharmacological screening platform, and further evaluation of the feasibility of this approach can be conducted with other Chinese medicinal formulas. The four key chemicals, including mangiferine, ferulic acid, jatrorrhizine and palmatine, found in EXD could be further investigated in vitro and in vitro to identify their combined effects as a mixture of four in treating menopausal syndromes.

Conclusions

In this study, the HPLC profiles of EXD-S and EXD-C have been evaluated with six known marker chemicals, which exerted actions on the HPO axis. All six chemicals were present at a higher level in EXD-S than in EXD-C. Four of them, including mangiferine, ferulic acid, jatrorrhizine and palmatine, were demonstrated to be suitable standard chemicals for quality control of EXD according to our novel and rapid approach. Both EXD-S and EXD-C displayed stimulatory effects on the expression of ovarian aromatase and hepatic SOD-1, with the effect of EXD-S being more potent. The changes of pharmacological activity in relation to the changes in chemical profiles of EXD decoction demonstrated the feasibility of a novel and rapid approach for identification of bioactive standard compounds from TCM formulas.

Abbreviations

TCM: traditional Chinese medicine; EXD: Erxian decoction; EXD-S: mixtures of EXD individual herbs decoction; EXD-C: combined decoction of EXD; SD-rat: Sprague Dawley-rat; CAT: catalase; SOD-1: superoxide dismutase 1; GPx-1: glutathione peroxidase; Ct: threshold cycle; RSD: relative standard deviation; HPLC: high performance liquid chromatography; HPO: hypothalamus-pituitary-ovary.

Authors' contributions

SCWS, YBZ, ZJZ and YT conceived and designed the study. HPC and SWW conducted the experiment and analyses. HPC, FWSC and SCWS wrote the manuscript. LXL and ZJZ provided invaluable comments. SCWS and TBN revised the manuscript. All authors read and approved the final manuscript.

Author details

[1] School of Chinese Medicine, Li Ka Shing Faculty of Medicine, The University of Hong Kong, 10 Sassoon Road, Pokfulam, Hong Kong, SAR, China. [2] School of Biomedical Science, Faculty of Medicine, The Chinese University of Hong Kong, Shatin, N.T., Hong Kong, SAR, China.

Acknowledgements

This study was partially supported by grants from the Seed Funding Programme for Basic Research (Project Number 201211159146 and 201411159213), the University of Hong Kong. We thank Mr Keith Wong and Ms Cindy Lee for their technical assistances.

Competing interests

The authors declare that they have no competing interests.

References

1. Zhang LH. Studies of active ingredients of Chinese traditional compound medicine (CTCM) (我對中藥複方有效成分研究的一些看法). Prog Chem (化學進展). 1999;2(11):186–8.
2. Cai BC, Qin KM, Wu H, Cai H, Lu TL, Zhang XD. Chemical mechanism during Chinese medicine processing (中藥炮制過程化學機理研究). Prog Chem (化學進展). 2012;24(4):637–49.
3. Deng YY, Gao WY, Chen HX, Wu SS. 中藥複方合煎與分煎的差異性研究進展. Chin Tradit Herb Drugs (中草藥). 2005;36(12):1909–11.
4. Yi T, Lo H, Zhao Z, Yu Z, Yang Z, Chen H. Comparison of the chemical composition and pharmacological effects of the aqueous and ethanolic extracts from a Tibetan "Snow Lotus" (*Saussurea laniceps*) herb. Molecules. 2012;17(6):7183–94.
5. Sze SCW, Tong Y, Zhang YB, Zhang ZJ, Lau AS, Wong HK, Tsang KW, Ng TB. A novel mechanism: Erxian decoction, a Chinese medicine formula, for relieving menopausal syndrome. J Ethnopharmacol. 2009;123(1):27–33.
6. Hu YM, Wang YT, Sze SCW, Tsang KW, Wong HK, Liu Q, Zhong LD, Tong Y. Identification of the major chemical constituents and their metabolites in rat plasma and various organs after oral administration of effective Erxian decoction (EXD) fraction by liquid chromatography-mass spectrometry. Biomed Chromatogr. 2010;24(5):479–89.
7. Okatani Y, Morioka N, Wakatsuki A, Nakano Y, Sagara Y. Role of the free radical-scavenger system in aromatase activity of the human ovary. Horm Res. 1993;39(Suppl 1):22–7.
8. Yuan ST, Du HY, Xia C. Effect of separated and combined decoction of Chinese medicinal formula on solubility of components (中藥複方湯劑分煎合煎對溶出效果的影響). Chin J Inf Tradit Chin Med (中國中醫藥訊息雜誌). 1999;6(7):29–32.
9. Yi L, Xu X. Study on the precipitation reaction between baicalin and berberine by HPLC. J Chromatogr B. 2004;810(1):165–8.
10. Sato T, Kawamoto A, Tamura A, Tatsumi Y, Fujii T. Mechanism of antioxidant action of pueraria glycoside (PG)-1 (an isoflavonoid) and mangiferin (a xanthonoid). Chem Pharm Bull (Tokyo). 1992;40(3):721–4.
11. Kaewpradub N, Dej-adisai S, Yuenyongsadwad S. Antioxidant and cytotoxic activities of Thai medicinal plants named Khaminkhruea: *Arcangelisia flava*, *Coscinium blumeanum* and *Fibraurea tinctoria*. Songklanakarin J Sci Technol. 2005;27(Suppl. 2):455–67.
12. Yokozawa T, Ishida A, Kashiwada Y, Cho EJ, Kim HY, Ikeshiro Y. Coptidis Rhizoma: protective effects against peroxynitrite-induced oxidative damage and elucidation of its active components. J Pharm Pharmacol. 2004;56(4):547–56.
13. Rackova L, Majekova M, Kost'alova D, Stefek M. Antiradical and antioxidant activities of alkaloids isolated from *Mahonia aquifolium*. Structural aspects. Bioorg Med Chem. 2004;12(17):4709–15.
14. Sassa S, Kikuchi T, Shinoda H, Suzuki S, Kudo H, Sakamoto S. Preventive effect of ferulic acid on bone loss in ovariectomized rats. In Vivo. 2003;17(3):277–80.
15. Philp HA. Hot flashes–a review of the literature on alternative and complementary treatment approaches. Altern Med Rev. 2003;8(3):284–302.
16. Ye HY, Lou YJ. Estrogenic effects of two derivatives of icariin on human breast cancer MCF-7 cells. Phytomedicine. 2005;12(10):735–41.
17. Chen JZ, Lu GY, Luo XM, Ye L, Chen JM. Comparison of baicalin, paeoniflorin and glycyrrhetic acid in different decoctions of Huangqin decoction (黃芩湯分煎液與合煎液中黃芩苷，芍藥苷和甘草酸含量的比較). Chin Tradit Patent Drugs (中成藥). 2008;30(9):1330–3.
18. Jin FY, Zhong ZL, Zhang LY, Liang GY, Cao PX, Yang YQ. Comparison of the content of baicalin in the different decoctions of TangKuei six yellow decoction (當歸六黃湯分煎樣品與合煎樣品中黃芩苷含量的比較). Lishizhen Med Materia Medica Res (時珍國醫國藥). 2009;20(3):681–2.
19. Gao L, Xie M, Sun MY. Experimental research on the anti-febrile effect of mingled decoction and separated decoction of *Bupleurium* roots and *Scutellaria* root on the fever induced by LPS in rats (柴芩合煎液與分煎液對LPS 誘導的大鼠發熱模型的影響). Chin J Exp Tradit Med Formulae (中國實驗方劑學雜誌). 2003;9(6):22–5.
20. Wang XT, Lu Y, Hu YL, Hou SK. Effect of separated and combined decoction of Chinese medicinal extract on mastitis in dairy cattle (分煎和合煎對中藥乳康灌注液治療奶牛乳腺炎效果的影響). Anim Husb Vet Med (畜牧與獸醫). 2008;40(3):69–71.

18

Chemical compositions, chromatographic fingerprints and antioxidant activities of Citri Exocarpium Rubrum (*Juhong*)

Yang Zhao[1,2], Chun-Pin Kao[3], Chi-Ren Liao[1], Kun-Chang Wu[1], Xin Zhou[2], Yu-Ling Ho[4*] and Yuan-Shiun Chang[1,5*]

Abstract

Background: Citri Exocarpium Rubrum (CER), which is known as *Juhong* in Chinese, is the dried exocarp of *Citrus reticulata* Blanco and its cultivars (Fam. Rutaceae) and is currently used in Chinese medicine to protect the stomach and eliminate *dampness* and phlegm. The main aim of this study was to develop a high-performance liquid chromatography ultraviolet mass spectrometry (HPLC-UV-MS) method for determining the chemical compositions and fingerprint of CER. We also evaluated the antioxidant properties of CER based on its 2,2-diphenyl-1-picrylhydrazyl (DPPH) free radical scavenging activity, ferric ion reducing antioxidant power (FRAP) and trolox equivalent antioxidant capacity (TEAC) assays.

Methods: Ten CER samples were collected from Hong Kong and mainland China. Each CER sample was extracted using an ultrasonic extraction method. Chromatographic separation was achieved using a conventional Dikma Inspire C18 column with photo diode array detection (190–400 nm). Hesperidin, nobiletin and tangeretin were quantified based on the UV signal observed at 330 nm. The column was eluted with a mobile phase consisting of water and acetonitrile (15–55%) over 55 min. Fingerprints combined with similarity and principal component analyses were used to classify the herbs. The DPPH free radical scavenging activity, FRAP and ABTS properties of the different CER samples were assayed. Bivariate correlation analysis was performed to investigate the correlation between the characteristic peaks and their antioxidant capacities.

Results: Limit of detection (LOD), limit of quantification (LOQ), linearity, inter-day precision, intra-day precision, repeatability, stability and recovery of the developed method were validated, and the method was subsequently used to determine the contents of hesperidin, nobiletin and tangeretin, and to acquire the fingerprints of the CER samples. Seventeen characteristic peaks were found in the fingerprints, and eleven of them were identified. Bivariate correlation analysis revealed correlations between the characteristic peaks and the antioxidant activities of the samples.

Conclusion: An HPLC-UV-MS method was developed and validated after a detailed investigation on extraction of chemical compounds from CER using different solvents and extraction times. None of the peaks was correlated with the DPPH free radical scavenging activity or ferric reducing capacity. Most of the peaks were correlated well with the ABTS radical scavenging capacity.

*Correspondence: elaine@sunrise.hk.edu.tw; yschang@mail.cmu.edu.tw
[1] Department of Chinese Pharmaceutical Sciences and Chinese Medicine Resources, College of Biopharmaceutical and Food Sciences, China Medical University, Taichung 40402, Taiwan
[4] Department of Nursing, Hungkuang University, Taichung 43302, Taiwan
Full list of author information is available at the end of the article

Background

Citri Exocarpium Rubrum (CER), which is known as *Juhong* in Chinese, is the dried exocarp of *Citrus reticulata* Blanco and its cultivars (Fam. Rutaceae), and this material is used in Chinese medicine to protect the stomach and eliminate *dampness* and phlegm [1]. CER has been reported to exhibit antioxidant activity [2] and induce apoptosis in human lung cancer cells [3]. Hesperidin, nobiletin and tangeretin are the main bioactive components of CER, and these compounds have been reported to have several properties, e.g. including antioxidant [4], anti-inflammatory [5] and anticancer activities [5, 6]. However, hesperidin is the only one of these compounds currently described as a chemical marker for quality assessment of CER in the 2015 edition of the Chinese Pharmacopoeia [1], which stipulates that the content of the marker should not be less than 1.7%. Several quantitative quality control methods have been reported for CER and CER-related commercial products [7–9]. However, the quality of herbal materials cannot be thoroughly or accurately evaluated based on the quantification of one or two chemical components. Fingerprinting analysis, which represents a much more accurate form of quality control analysis has therefore been introduced and accepted by the World Health Organization (WHO) as an effective strategy for assessing the quality of herbal medicines [10–13].

The aim of this study was to develop a high-performance liquid chromatography ultraviolet mass spectrometry (HPLC-UV-MS) method to determine the hesperidin, nobiletin and tangeretin contents in different CER samples, as well as developing a deeper understanding of the chemical profiles of these materials. Similarity and principal component analyses (PCA) were also performed based on the contents of hesperidin, nobiletin and tangeretin, as well as the PA/W (peak area divided by sample weight) values of the 17 characteristic peaks. The antioxidant activities of the CER samples were evaluated and subjected to a fingerprint-efficacy correlation process.

Methods

Chemicals, solvents and herbal materials

Hesperidin, nobiletin and tangeretin were purchased from Shanghai R & D Center for Standardization of Traditional Chinese Medicines (China). LC-grade methanol and acetonitrile were purchased from the branch company of Merck in Taipei, Taiwan. Purified water was prepared with Milli-Q system (Millipore, Milford, MA, USA). All other reagents used in the present study were of analytical grade. Ten batches of CER herbal materials were collected from Hong Kong and mainland China, which were marked as L-CER-01–L-CER-04 (from local in Hong Kong) and CER-01–CER-06 (from mainland China). All the samples were authenticated by professor Yuan-Shiun Chang and the specimens have been deposited in Department of Chinese Pharmaceutical Sciences and Chinese Medicine Resources, School of Pharmacy, China Medical University.

Preparation of herbal materials and reference compounds

CER samples were dried in a shade place and were ground into fine powder (20 mesh) using a grinder with a knife blade. Two hundred milligrams of each CER powder was carefully weighed into a tube. Methanol (20 mL) was then added into the tube. Each sample was then extracted using an ultrasonic cleaner (Delta DC400H) at a frequency of 40 kHz at 25 °C for 30 min. The extract was centrifuged (UX-17414-21 Cole-Parmer™ MS-3400 Variable Speed Clinical Centrifuge, USA) for 10 min at 2000×*g* and the supernatant was then transferred into a volumetric flask. The procedure was repeated for one more time and the supernatants were combined. The final volume was made up to 50 mL with methanol which was then filtered through a 0.45 μm PVDF syringe filter (VWR Scientific, Seattle, WA) for analysis.

The reference compounds of hesperidin, nobiletin and tangeretin were weighed and dissolved in methanol at 499.2, 11.94 and 5.0288 mg/L (stock solutions), respectively. The stock solutions were then diluted to 31.20–499.20 mg/L for hesperidin, 0.75–11.94 mg/L for nobiletin and 0.31–5.03 mg/L for tangeretin, respectively for establishment of calibration curves. An aliquot of 10 μL of each solution was used for HPLC and HPLC-ESI-MS analyses.

HPLC analysis

HPLC analyses were performed on a Waters 2695 HPLC system (Waters Corporation, USA) equipped with Waters 2998 photodiode array detector (PDA), Waters e2695 separations module and column heater module. A Dikma Inspire, C18 column (250 mm × 4.6 mm i.d., 5 μm) was used. The mobile phase consisted of water (A) and acetonitrile (B). The optimized elution conditions were as follow: 0–10 min, 15–20% B; 10–25 min, 20% B; 25–35 min, 20–40%; 35–55 min, 40–55%. The flow rate was 1 mL/min and the injection volume was 10 μL. UV spectra were acquired from 190 to 400 nm. The autosampler and column compartment were maintained at 25 and 35 °C, respectively.

HPLC-ESI-MS analysis

HPLC-ESI-MS analyses were performed on a TSQ Quantum Access Max Triple Stage Quadrupole Mass Spectrometer (Thermo Fisher Scientific Inc., Waltham, MA, USA) with an Accela 1250 UHPLC system equipped with an Accela 1250 PDA detector, an Accela HTC PAL autosampler, and an Accela 1250 binary pump. The column and elution conditions used were the same as that described in the section, "HPLC analysis", except that the flow rate was set at 0.20 mL/min with a split ratio. Ultra-high pure helium (He) and high purity nitrogen (N_2) were used as collision gas and nebulizer, respectively. The optimized parameters in negative/positive ion modes were as follows: ion spray voltage, −2.5 kV/3.5 kV; auxiliary gas, 40 arbitrary units; sheath gas, 15 arbitrary units; capillary temperature, 350 °C; vaporizer temperature, 300 °C; capillary offset, −30 V/30 V. Spectra were recorded in the range of *m/z* 100–1500 for full scan data, meanwhile, the normalized collision energy was tested from 25 to 45% for MS^2 data with dependent scan.

Antioxidant activities

DPPH assay

The DPPH free radical-scavenging activity of each sample was assayed according to published articles [14–16] with minor modifications. In brief, a 0.3 mM solution of methanolic DPPH was freshly prepared. An aliquot (50 μL) of each sample (with appropriate enrichment or dilution if necessary) was added to 150 μL of methanolic DPPH solution to initiate the reaction. Discolorations were measured at 517 nm after reaction for 30 min at room temperature in the dark. Measurements were performed in triplicate. The %DPPH quenched was calculated according to the following equation:

$$\%\,\text{DPPH quenched} = (A_{control} - A_{sample}) \times 100 / A_{control} - A_{blank}$$

where $A_{control}$, A_{sample}, and A_{blank} represent the absorbance of the control, the selected antioxidant sample at certain concentration, and the blank, respectively, measured at 517 nm. EC_{50} values calculated denote the concentration of a sample required to decrease the absorbance by 50%. The antioxidant capacity was expressed as μmol butylated hydroxytoluene (BHT) equivalents/gram of dried CER sample.

FRAP assay

The ability to reduce ferric ions was measured based on the methods reported in previous papers [16, 17] with minor revisions. Briefly, 30 μL of each sample (with appropriate enrichment or dilution if necessary) was added to 200 μL of FRAP reagent (10 parts of 300 mM sodium acetate buffer at pH 3.6, 1 part of 10.0 mM 2,4,6-tripyridyl-s-triazine (TPTZ) solution, and 1 part of 20.0 mM $FeCl_3 \cdot 6H_2O$ solution), and the reaction mixture was placed at room temperature for 5 min. Fresh working solutions of $FeSO_4 \cdot 7H_2O$ were used for calibration. The antioxidant capacity of reducing ferric ions of each sample was expressed as μ mol Fe^{2+} equivalents per gram of dried CER sample.

TEAC assay

The ABTS free radical-scavenging activity of each sample was assayed according to the method described in published papers [16, 18] with minor modifications. A mixture (1:1, v/v) of ABTS (7.0 mM) and potassium persulfate (6 mM) was allowed to react overnight at room temperature in the dark to form radical cation $ABTS^{+}$. The mixture was then diluted with water to reach absorbance values between 1.0 and 1.5 at 731 nm (constant initial absorbance values must be used for standard and samples) as working solution. An aliquot (50 μL) of each sample (with appropriate enrichment or dilution if necessary) was mixed with the working solution (150 μL), and the decrease of absorbance was measured at 731 nm after 10 min. EC_{50} values calculated denote the concentration of a sample required to decrease the absorbance by 50%. The antioxidant capacity was expressed as μmol BHT equivalents/gram of dried CER sample.

Data analysis

Similarity analysis

Similarity values of the chromatographic fingerprints obtained from CER samples were calculated using the following two formulas:

$$\text{Correlation coefficient} = \frac{\sum_{i=1}^{n}(X_i - \bar{X}_i)(Y_i - \bar{Y}_i)}{\sqrt{\sum_{i=1}^{n}(X_i - \bar{X}_i)^2 (Y_i - \bar{Y}_i)^2}}$$

$$\text{Angle cosin} = \frac{\sum_{i=1}^{n} X_i Y_i}{\sqrt{\sum_{i=1}^{n} X_i^2}\sqrt{\sum_{i=1}^{n} Y_i^2}}$$

where, X_i and Y_i represented the peak area of the characteristic peak in each sample and the peak area of the characteristic peak in reference fingerprint generated, respectively.

Principal component analysis (PCA)

The data obtained from chromatographic fingerprints were analyzed with Solo (Eigenvector Research, Inc.,Wenatchee, WA). Normalize (2-Norm, length = 1) and mean center were used for data reprocessing before PCA was performed.

One-way ANOVA and correlation analyses

Differences in mean values of antioxidant assays for different CER samples were obtained by one-way ANOVA. Pearson r correlation coefficients between the peak areas of the seventeen characteristic peaks and their antioxidant capacities were calculated by SPSS software (version 17.0, IBM Corporation, USA). *P* values less than 0.05 were considered statistically significant.

Results and discussion

Optimization of extraction method

The extraction solvents were optimized taking the extraction efficiency of hesperidin, nobiletin and tangeretin as indexes. Methanol, 50% methanol, ethanol and 50% ethanol were investigated with ultrasonic extraction at room temperature. The powder of CER (0.2 g) was extracted with 20 mL of different solvents for twice (30 min for once). As a result, the contents of the three analytes obtained by methanol were the highest compared with the values obtained from other solvents. Furthermore, the three analytes were almost extracted completely (>99%) for the second time (Additional files 1 and 2).

Optimization of chromatographic conditions

Different mobile phase systems, methanol–water and acetonitrile–water elution systems were tested to obtain sharp and symmetrical peaks. Good resolution, baseline, sharp and symmetrical peaks were obtained by acetonitrile–water system. Two other columns (Grace Alltima C18 and Waters XBridge Shield RP18) were screened before Dikma Inspire, C18 column (250 mm × 4.6 mm i.d., 5 μm) was finally selected as the column of choice (Additional file 3). PDA full scan (190–400 nm) was used to acquire all the main peaks and finally 330 nm was selected as detection wavelength. Representative chromatographic fingerprints obtained from CER-01 and L-CER-04 were shown in Fig. 1, in which characteristic peaks were marked as 1–17. Different column temperatures at 20, 25, 30 and 35 °C were also investigated. Although chromatograms detected at different temperatures didn't show obvious differences, 35 °C was selected as the preferable one to minimize the influences from fluctuating room temperature on the chromatograms. In the process of gradient optimization, gradient time, gradient procedure and initial composition of the mobile phase were taken into consideration. Eventually, the gradient procedure was finalized, as described in "HPLC analysis" section.

Validation of quantitative analytical method

The HPLC method was validated by defining its limit of detection (LOD), limit of quantification (LOQ), linearity, inter-day precision, intra-day precision, repeatability, stability and recovery characteristics.

Calibration curves were plotted based on a linear regression analysis of the integrated peak areas (*y*) versus the concentrations (*x*, mg/L) of hesperidin, nobiletin

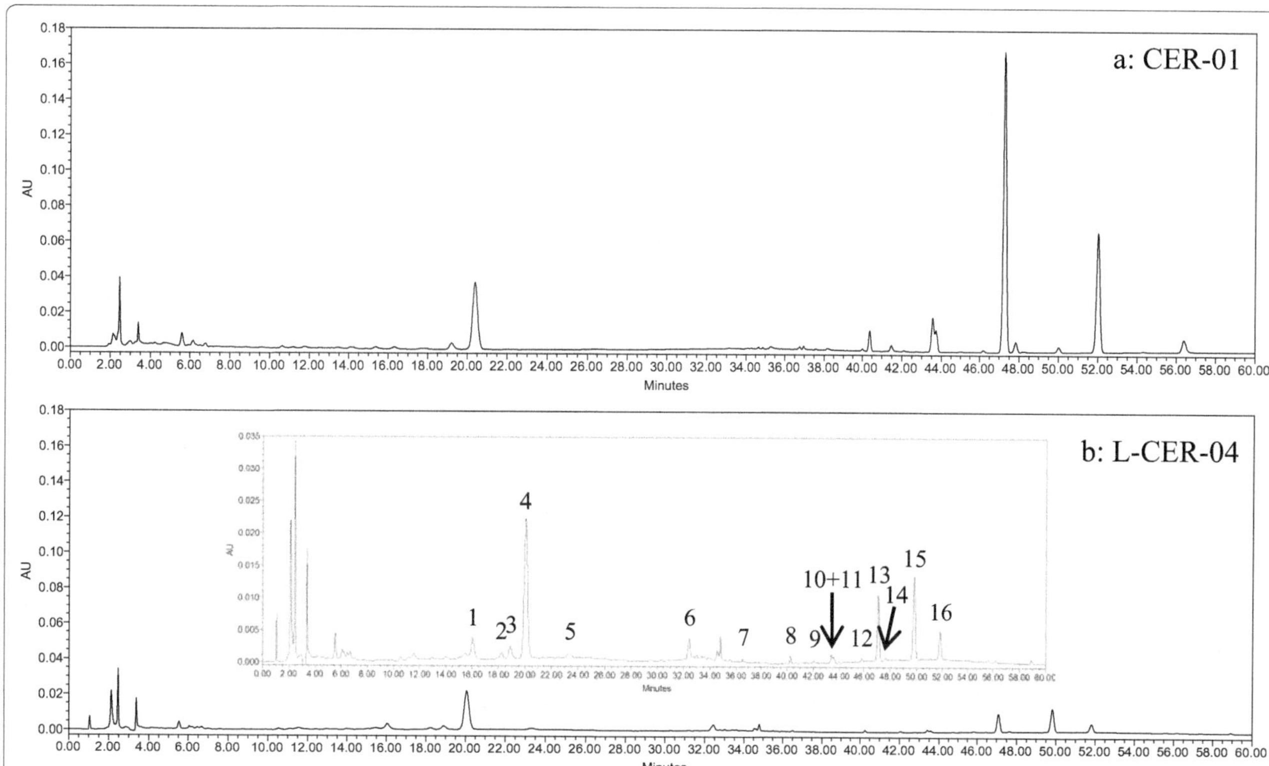

Fig. 1 Representative chromatograms of CER-01 (**a**) and CER-04 (**b**) detected at 330 nm. Seventeen characteristic peaks are marked as 1–17

and tangeretin at five different levels. The LOD and LOQ values were determined amongst the baseline noise for all three of the analytes under the optimized chromatographic conditions according to the International Union of Pure and Applied Chemistry (IUPAC) definition. The LOD values were determined as the concentration of each analyte required to generate a signal with a single-to-noise (S/N) ratio of 3:1, whereas the LOQ was defined as the concentration of each analyte required to generate a signal with an S/N ratio of 10:1. The regression equations, correlation coefficients, linear ranges, LODs and LOQs for hesperidin, nobiletin and tangeretin are shown in Table 1. The correlation coefficients (R^2) of hesperidin, nobiletin and tangeretin were greater than 0.99, indicating good linearity.

Intra- and inter-day variations were chosen to determine the precision of our newly developed method. For the intra-day variability test, one of the mixed standard solutions (hesperidin, 124.80 mg/mL; nobiletin, 2.99 mg/mL; tangeretin, 1.26 mg/mL) was analyzed five times within 1 day, whereas one of the mixed standard solutions was examined in triplicate on a daily basis for three consecutive days for the inter-day variability test. Repeatability was evaluated by analyzing five different working solutions prepared from the same sample (L-CER-01). The stability of the method was determined by the repeated analysis of the same sample solution at different times during a 24 h period of storage at room temperature. The RSD values for the retention times and peak areas of hesperidin, nobiletin and tangeretin were taken as the measurements of precision and stability. The RSDs of the retention times and contents (mg/g) were taken as the measurements of repeatability. All of the RSD values for the retention times and peak areas (or contents) were found to be less than 2.00 and 3.00%, respectively (Table 2).

The recovery of our newly developed method was determined using spiked CER samples. A small portion (0.2 g) of L-CER-04 was individually spiked with 7.0056 mg of hesperidin, 0.1393 mg of nobiletin and 0.0467 mg of tangeretin. Five replicate samples were extracted and analyzed according to the procedures described above. As shown in Table 3, the mean recoveries (n = 5) of hesperidin, nobiletin and tangeretin were 104.92% ± 0.67, 95.87 ± 0.72 and 96.58 ± 2.08, respectively.

Validation of the chromatographic fingerprinting method

The chromatographic fingerprinting method was validated for its inter- and intra-day precisions, repeatability and stability. The inter-day precision was evaluated by running five consecutive injections of the same test sample within 1 day. The intra-day precision was evaluated by analyzing the same test sample in triplicate each day for 3 consecutive days. The repeatability of the method was examined by determining five different solutions prepared from the same botanical sample (L-CER-04). The stability was examined by analyzing the same sample

Table 1 Regression data, LODs and LOQs for the three analytes assayed in HPLC-UV chromatograms

Analyte	Calibration curve[a]	R^2	Linear range (mg/L)	LOD[b] (ng/mL)	LOQ[c] (ng/mL)
1	$y = 3.0149x - 21.812$	0.9994	31.20–499.20	418.8	128.6
2	$y = 41.396x - 4.1898$	0.9995	0.75–11.94	6.8	24.7
3	$y = 50.822x + 3.2433$	0.9996	0.31–5.03	12.0	40.8

1 Hesperidin, *2* Nobiletin, *3* Tangeretin

[a] *y* is the peak area in UV chromatograms detected in 330 nm, *x* is the concentration (mg/L) of the analyte

[b] LOD refers to the limit of detection, s/n = 3

[c] LOQ refers to the limit of quantification, s/n = 10

Table 2 Results of precision, repeatability and stability of the three analytes, expressed as RSD (%)

Analyte	Precision				Repeatability (n = 5)		Stability (n = 6)	
	Intra-day RSD (%) (n = 5)		Inter-day RSD (%) (n = 9)		RSD (%)		RSD (%)	
	t_R^a	PA[b]	t_R	PA	t_R	Contents (mg/g)	t_R	PA
1	0.32	0.39	1.39	2.98	0.52	0.94	1.08	1.65
2	0.42	0.44	1.76	1.31	0.07	1.08	0.72	2.71
3	0.47	0.49	1.65	1.69	0.07	0.88	1.53	1.34

1 Hesperidin, *2* Nobiletin, *3* Tangeretin

[a] Refers to retention time

[b] Refers to peak area

Table 3 Recoveries of the three analytes using L-CER-04 as tested sample

Analytes	Sample weight (g)	Original (mg)	Added (mg)	Found (mg)	Recovery (%)	Mean recovery ± SD
1	0.2029	6.9687	7.0056	14.3330	105.12	104.92 ± 0.67
	0.2014	6.9172	7.0056	14.3097	105.52	
	0.2023	6.9481	7.0056	14.2179	103.77	
	0.2013	6.9137	7.0056	14.2663	104.95	
	0.2065	7.0923	7.0056	14.4638	105.22	
2	0.2029	0.1416	0.1393	0.2745	95.41	95.87 ± 0.72
	0.2014	0.1405	0.1393	0.2738	95.71	
	0.2023	0.1411	0.1393	0.2748	95.97	
	0.2013	0.1404	0.1393	0.2756	97.06	
	0.2065	0.1441	0.1393	0.2767	95.22	
3	0.2029	0.0557	0.0467	0.1009	96.91	
	0.2014	0.0556	0.0467	0.1008	96.65	
	0.2023	0.0547	0.0467	0.1006	98.14	96.58 ± 2.08
	0.2013	0.0546	0.0467	0.1005	98.13	
	0.2065	0.0568	0.0467	0.1003	93.06	

1 Hesperidin, *2* Nobiletin, *3* Tangeretin

solution at different time points (0, 2, 4, 8, 16 and 24 h). The results of these experiments expressed in two forms, including (1) the RSDs of the relative retention times (RRT) and relative peak areas (RPA) of each characteristic peak relative to the reference peak (nobiletin); and (2) the similarity values for the chromatographic fingerprints of the different samples relative to the reference values, which were calculated using the formulas discussed in the "Data analysis" section. The RSD values were all less than 5%, whereas the similarity values were all greater than 0.99, indicating that our newly developed chromatographic fingerprinting method is satisfactory for the analysis of the samples.

Quantitative determination of hesperidin, nobiletin and tangeretin contents of the CER samples

Our newly developed HPLC-UV method was used to quantify the different amounts of hesperidin, nobiletin and tangeretin in several different batches of CER. Calibration curves were generated for these compounds using reference compound and used to calculate the hesperidin, nobiletin and tangeretin contents in different samples (Table 4).

The contents of hesperidin, nobiletin and tangeretin in different samples varied from 23.8 to 79.6 mg/g, 0.587 to 15.7 mg/g and 0.222 to 6.03 mg/g, respectively. The differences in contents of hesperidin in different CER samples were small, whereas the differences in contents of nobiletin and tangeretin changed considerably.

All of the CER samples collected from mainland China were found to have higher hesperidin, nobiletin and tangeretin contents than those collected locally from Hong Kong. CER-01 had the highest content of hesperidin between all the samples tested in the current study at 79.6 mg/g, whereas CER-04 had the highest contents of nobiletin and tangeretin at 15.7 and 6.03 mg/g, respectively. The lowest content of hesperidin was found in L-CER-01 at 23.8 mg/g, whereas the lowest contents of nobiletin and tangeretin were both found in L-CER-03 at 0.588 and 0.222 mg/g, respectively.

Assignment of the characteristic peaks

Figure 1 shows the 17 characteristic peaks detected at 330 nm in the CER-01 and L-CER-04 samples. The structures responsible for these peaks were identified based on their MS and MS^2 behaviors and a comparison of these data with those in the literature (Table 5). The MS conditions were optimized and the data were collected in the negative and positive ESI modes.

Peak 2 had a retention time of 18.3 min and a UV absorption maximum of 282 nm. Although this compound did not give intense mass ions in the negative or positive ionization mode, it was unequivocally identified as naringin based on a comparison of its absorption wavelength and retention time data with those of the reference compound. The identity of this peak was further confirmed by the addition of a standard solution of naringin to the CER extract.

Peak 4 had a retention time of 20.1 min and a UV absorption maximum at 283 nm. MS analysis in the negative ionization mode revealed $[M-H]^-$ and $[2M-H]^-$ ions with an *m/z* values of 609 and 1219. The fragmentation pattern of the former of these two ions was studied by MS^2 analysis, which revealed a series of product ions

Table 4 Contents (mg/g dry weight, mean ± SD) of hesperidin, nobiletin and tangeretin in different CER samples

Sample no.	Content (mg/g dry weight) (Mean ± SD)			Moisture content (%)
	Hesperidin	Nobiletin	Tangeretin	
L-CER-01	23.7940 ± 0.4782	0.9882 ± 0.0047	0.5086 ± 0.0034	11.86
L-CER-02	48.9356 ± 0.1245	0.8221 ± 0.0121	0.3308 ± 0.0024	11.99
L-CER-03	39.3195 ± 0.2017	0.5771 ± 0.0109	0.2155 ± 0.0055	13.39
L-CER-04	42.6070 ± 0.5382	0.7187 ± 0.0109	0.3069 ± 0.0049	8.14
CER-01	79.5846 ± 0.5380	14.6451 ± 0.0889	5.6522 ± 0.0329	9.33
CER-02	73.2414 ± 0.5380	14.6177 ± 0.6494	5.5453 ± 0.2511	9.60
CER-03	71.6286 ± 0.0907	14.9612 ± 0.0022	5.7574 ± 0.0011	9.20
CER-04	73.7426 ± 0.2926	15.6881 ± 0.0637	6.0309 ± 0.0244	8.39
CER-05	41.2002 ± 0.2510	2.3286 ± 0.0193	1.2122 ± 0.0103	7.96
CER-06	39.7620 ± 0.0302	6.2006 ± 0.0090	4.0030 ± 0.0051	11.58

with *m/z* values of 301 $[M\text{-Rutinosyl}-H]^-$, 286 $[M\text{-Rutinosyl}-CH_3-H]^-$, 257 $[M\text{-Rutinosyl}-CO_2-H]^-$, 242 $[M\text{-Rutinosyl}-CO_2-CH_3-H]^-$ and 134 $[M\text{-Rutinosyl}-CO_2-CH_3-C_6H_4O_2-H]^-$. MS analysis of peak 4 in the positive ionization mode revealed a series of protonated molecular ion peaks with *m/z* values of 611 $[M+H]^+$, 1243 $[2M+Na]^+$, 465 $[M\text{-Rhamnosyl}+H]^+$ and 303 $[M\text{-Rutinosyl}+H]^+$. The MS^2 fragmentation of the first of these four peaks gave six fragment ions with *m/z* values of 303 $[M\text{-Rutinosyl}+H]^+$, 285 $[M\text{-Rutinosyl}-H_2O+H]^+$, 270 $[M\text{-Rutinosyl}-H_2O-CH_3+H]^+$, 195 $[M\text{-Rutinosyl}-C_6H_4O_2+H]^+$ and 177 $[M\text{-Rutinosyl}-C_6H_4O_2-H_2O+H]^+$. This peak was unequivocally identified as hesperidin based on a comparison of its MS data with the data from the reference compound and the literature [7, 19].

Peak 5 had a retention time of 23.3 min and a UV absorption maximum of 283 nm. MS analysis in the negative ionization mode gave a peak with an *m/z* value of 609 $[M-H]^-$. In contrast, analysis in the positive ionization mode gave four peaks with *m/z* values of 611 $[M+H]^+$, 633 $[M+Na]^+$, 465 $[M\text{-Rhamnosyl}+H]^+$ and 303 $[M\text{-Rutinosyl}+H]^+$. The peak was identified as neohesperidin.

Peak 10 gave a retention time of 43.6 min with UV absorption maxima at 214, 241 and 330 nm. MS analysis in the negative ion mode did not give a major mass ion signal. In contrast, MS analysis in the positive ion mode revealed several mass ions with *m/z* values of 373 $[M+H]^+$, 395 $[M+Na]^+$, 767 $[2M+Na]^+$, 358 $[M-CH_3+H]^+$, 343 $[M-CH_2O+H]^+$ and 312 $[M-H_2O-CO-CH_3+H]^+$. The first of these peaks was subjected to MS^2 fragmentation analysis, which resulted in three fragment ions with *m/z* values of 343 $[M-CH_2O+H]^+$, 312 $[M-H_2O-CO-CH_3+H]^+$ and 297 $[M-H_2O-CO-CH_2O+H]^+$. This peak was identified as sinensetin based on a comparison of its MS data with the data from the literature [20, 21]. Peak 11 co-eluted with peak 10 with a retention time of 43.73 min and UV absorption maxima at 270, 295 and 341 nm. In a similar manner to peak 10, MS analysis of peak 11 in the negative ion mode revealed no major peak. However, MS analysis in the positive ion mode revealed a molecular ion peak with an *m/z* value of 343 $[M+H]^+$ along with several other ions with *m/z* values of 707 $[2M+Na]^+$, 328 $[M-CH_3+H]^+$, 313 $[M-CH_2O+H]^+$ and 285 $[M-CH_2O-CO+H]^+$. The molecular ion peak with an *m/z* value of 343 was subjected to MS^2 analysis, which resulted in two major daughter ions with *m/z* values of 313 $[M-CH_2O+H]^+$ and 285 $[M-CH_2O-CO+H]^+$. This peak was identified as tetramethyl-*O*-isoscutellarein by comparing its MS data with those from the literature [20].

Peak 12 eluted with a retention time of 46.3 min and gave two UV absorption maxima at 208 and 336 nm. MS analysis in the negative ion mode did not reveal any major peaks, whereas analysis in positive ion mode revealed two protonated molecular ion peaks with *m/z* values of 403 $[M+H]^+$ and 373 $[M-CH_2O+H]^+$. The former of these two peaks was subjected to MS^2 fragmentation analysis, which revealed several fragment ions with *m/z* values of 373 $[M-CH_2O+H]^+$, 388 $[M-CH_3+H]^+$, 355 $[M-CH_2O-H_2O+H]^+$ and 327 $[M-CH_2O-H_2O-CO+H]^+$. A comparing of these data with the data from a reference compound and the literature [21] revealed that this peak was hexamethoxyflavone.

Peak 13 eluted with a retention time of 47.1 min and gave a UV absorption maximum of 333 nm. MS analysis in the negative ion mode revealed no obvious peak, whereas analysis in the positive ion mode revealed a protonated molecular ion with an *m/z* value of 403 $[M+H]^+$, as well as two other peaks with *m/z* values of 388 $[M-CH_3+H]^+$ and 373 $[M-CH_2O+H]^+$. MS^2 fragmentation analysis of the protonated molecular ion peak with an *m/z* value of 403 revealed several daughter peaks with

Table 5 Assignment of the characteristic peaks

No.	RT (min)	UV (nm)	MS in neg. mode	MS in pos. mode	MS^2 in neg. mode	MS^2 in pos. mode	Assignment	References
1	15.2	283	/	/	/	/	Unknown	/
2	18.3	282	/	/	/	/	Naringin	/
3	19.2	253, 347	607 $[\text{M–H}]^-$	609 $[\text{M+H}]^+$ 631 $[\text{M+Na}]^+$ 463 $[\text{M-Rhamnosyl+H}]^+$ 301 $[\text{M-Rutinosyl+H}]^+$	299 $[\text{M-Rutinosyl-H}]^-$	301 $[\text{M-Rutinosyl+H}]^+$	Unknown	/
4	20.1	283	609 $[\text{M–H}]^-$ 1219 $[\text{2M–H}]^-$	611 $[\text{M+H}]^+$ 1243 $[\text{2M+Na}]^+$ 465 $[\text{M-Rhamnosyl+H}]^+$ 303 $[\text{M-Rutinosyl+H}]^+$	301 $[\text{M-Rutinosyl-H}]^-$ 286 $[\text{M-Rutinosyl-CH}_3\text{–H}]^-$ 257 $[\text{M-Rutinosyl-CO}_2\text{–H}]^-$ 242 $[\text{M-Rutinosyl-CO}_2\text{-CH}_3\text{-H}]^-$ 134 $[\text{M-Rutinosyl-CO}_2\text{–CH}_3\text{–C}_6\text{H}_4\text{O}_2\text{–H}]^-$	303 $[\text{M-Rutinosyl+H}]^+$ 285 $[\text{M-Rutinosyl-H}_2\text{O+H}]^+$ 270 $[\text{M-Rutinosyl–H}_2\text{O–CH}_3\text{+H}]^+$ 195 $[\text{M-Rutinosyl–C}_6\text{H}_4\text{O}_2\text{+H}]^+$ 177 $[\text{M-Rutinosyl–C}_6\text{H}_4\text{O}_2\text{–H}_2\text{O+H}]^+$	Hesperidin	[7, 19]
5	23.3	283	609 $[\text{M–H}]^-$	611 $[\text{M+H}]^+$ 633 $[\text{M+Na}]^+$ 465 $[\text{M-Rhamnosyl+H}]^+$ 303 $[\text{M-Rutinosyl+H}]^+$	/	/	Neohesperidin	/
6	32.4	254, 347	723 $[\text{M–H}]^-$ 695 $[\text{M–CO–H}]^-$	725 $[\text{M+H}]^+$ 747 $[\text{M+Na}]^+$	417 $[\text{M-306–H}]^-$	419 $[\text{M-306+H}]^+$	Unknown	/
7	36.5	210, 257, 342	/	/	/	/	Unknown	/
8	40.3	203, 269, 345	/	373 $[\text{M+H}]^+$ 395 $[\text{M+Na}]^+$ 358 $[\text{M–CH}_3\text{+H}]^+$ 343 $[\text{M–CH}_2\text{O+H}]^+$	/	343 $[\text{M–CH}_2\text{O+H}]^+$	Unknown	/
9	42.2	206, 253, 270, 355	/	403 $[\text{M+H}]^+$ 425 $[\text{M+Na}]^+$ 388 $[\text{M–CH}_3\text{+H}]^+$ 373 $[\text{M–CH}_2\text{O+H}]^+$	/	373 $[\text{M–CH}_2\text{O+H}]^+$	Unknown	/
10	43.6	214, 241, 330	/	373 $[\text{M+H}]^+$ 395 $[\text{M+Na}]^+$ 767 $[\text{2M+Na}]^+$ 358 $[\text{M–CH}_3\text{+H}]^+$ 343 $[\text{M–CH}_2\text{O+H}]^+$ 312 $[\text{M–H}_2\text{O–CO–CH}_3\text{+H}]^+$	/	343 $[\text{M–CH}_2\text{O+H}]^+$ 312 $[\text{M–H}_2\text{O–CO–CH}_3\text{+H}]^+$ 297 $[\text{M–H}_2\text{O–CO–CH}_2\text{O+H}]^+$	Sinensetin	[20, 21]
11	43.7	270, 295, 341	/	343 $[\text{M+H}]^+$ 707 $[\text{2M+Na}]^+$	/	313 $[\text{M–CH}_2\text{O+H}]^+$ 285 $[\text{M–CH}_2\text{O–CO+H}]^+$	Tetramethyl-O-isoscutellarein	[20]

Table 5 continued

No.	RT (min)	UV (nm)	MS in neg. mode	MS in pos. mode	MS² in neg. mode	MS² in pos. mode	Assignment	References
				328 $[M-CH_3+H]^+$ 313 $[M-CH_2O+H]^+$ 285 $[M-CH_2O-CO+H]^+$				
12	46.3	208, 336	/	403 $[M+H]^+$ 373 $[M-CH_2O+H]^+$	/	388 $[M-CH_3+H]^+$ 373 $[M-CH_2O+H]^+$ 355 $[M-CH_2O-H_2O+H]^+$ 327 $[M-CH_2O-H_2O-CO+H]^+$	Hexamethoxyflavone	[21]
13	47.1	333	/	403 $[M+H]^+$ 388 $[M-CH_3+H]^+$ 373 $[M-CH_2O+H]^+$	/	388 $[M-CH_3+H]^+$ 373 $[M-CH_2O+H]^+$ 343 $[M-2CH_2O+H]^+$ 313 $[M-3CH_2O+H]^+$ 283 $[M-4CH_2O+H]^+$ 239 $[M-C_{10}H_{12}O_2+H]^+$ 211 $[M-C_{10}H_{12}O_2-CO+H]^+$	Nobiletin	[7, 20, 22]
14	47.7	266, 322	/	343 $[M+H]^+$ 365 $[M+Na]^+$ 328 $[M-CH_3+H]^+$ 313 $[M-CH_2O+H]^+$	/	313 $[M-CH_2O+H]^+$ 299 $[M-CO_2+H]^+$	Tetramethyl-O-scutellarein	[20]
15	50.1	253, 343	/	433 $[M+H]^+$ 455 $[M+Na]^+$ 496 $[M+Na+CH_3CN]^+$ 418 $[M-CH_3+H]^+$ 403 $[M-CH_2O+H]^+$	/	403 $[M-CH_2O+H]^+$ 373 $[M-2CH_2O+H]^+$ 345 $[M-2CH_2O-CO+H]^+$	3,5,6,7,8,3′,4′-Heptamethoxyflavone	[7, 20]
16	51.8	270, 323	/	373 $[M+H]^+$ 395 $[M+Na]^+$ 358 $[M-CH_3+H]^+$	/	343 $[M-CH_2O+H]^+$ 283 $[M-3CH_2O+H]^+$ 312 $[M-CH_3-H_2O-CO+H]^+$	Tangeretin	[7, 20, 22]
17	56.5	203, 254, 282, 341	/	389 $[M+H]^+$ 411 $[M+Na]^+$ 374 $[M-CH_3+H]^+$ 359 $[M-CH_2O+H]^+$	/	374 $[M-CH_3+H]^+$ 359 $[M-CH_2O+H]^+$	5-Hydroxy-6,7,8,3′,4′-pentamethoxyflavone	[7]

m/z values of 373 $[M-CH_2O+H]^+$, 388 $[M-CH_3+H]^+$, 343 $[M-2CH_2O+H]^+$, 313 $[M-3CH_2O+H]^+$, 283 $[M-4CH_2O+H]^+$, 239 $[M-C_{10}H_{12}O_2+H]^+$ and 211 $[M-C_{10}H_{12}O_2-CO+H]^+$. A comparison of these data with those obtained from a reference compound and the literature [7, 20, 22] revealed that this peak was nobiletin.

Peak 14 eluted with a retention time of 47.7 min and gave two UV absorption maxima at 266 and 322 nm. MS analysis in the negative ion mode did not reveal any major peak, whereas analysis in the positive ion mode gave several peaks with *m/z* values of 343 $[M+H]^+$, 365 $[M+Na]^+$, 328 $[M-CH_3+H]^+$ and 313 $[M-CH_2O+H]^+$. The peak with an *m/z* value of 343 $[M+H]^+$ was subjected to MS^2 fragmentation analysis and gave two daughter ions with *m/z* values of 313 $[M-CH_2O+H]^+$ and 299 $[M-CO_2+H]^+$. This peak was identified as tetramethyl-*O*-scutellarein based on a comparison of its data with those described in the literature [20].

Table 6 Similarity values of each sample compared to the reference fingerprint generated

Sample no.	Similarity			
	Correlation coefficient		Angle cosin	
	Mean[a]	Median[b]	Mean	Median
L-CER-01	0.2414	0.1666	0.4666	0.4017
L-CER-02	0.4443	0.5450	0.5903	0.6573
L-CER-03	0.4422	0.5300	0.6050	0.6599
L-CER-04	0.4327	0.5146	0.6124	0.6602
CER-01	0.8866	0.7544	0.9126	0.8247
CER-02	0.8873	0.7536	0.9140	0.8251
CER-03	0.8856	0.7535	0.9116	0.8238
CER-04	0.8853	0.7562	0.9116	0.8257
CER-05	0.7290	0.8199	0.8180	0.8767
CER-06	0.7193	0.7427	0.7929	0.8098

[a] The reference fingerprint was generated with mean values of the samples

[b] The reference fingerprint was generated with median vales of the samples

Peak 15 gave a retention time of 50.1 min and two UV absorption maxima at 253 and 343 nm. MS analysis in the negative ion mode revealed no major ions. However, MS analysis in the positive ion mode revealed five peaks with *m/z* values of 433 $[M+H]^+$, 455 $[M+Na]^+$, 496 $[M+Na+CH_3CN]^+$, 418 $[M-CH_3+H]^+$ and 403 $[M-CH_2O+H]^+$. The peak with an *m/z* value of 433 $[M+H]^+$ was subjected to MS^2 analysis, resulting in three major daughter ions with *m/z* values of 403 $[M-CH_2O+H]^+$, 373 $[M-2CH_2O+H]^+$ and 345 $[M-2CH_2O-CO+H]^+$. This peak was tentatively identified as 3,5,6,7,8,3′,4′-heptamethoxyflavone based on a comparison with data from the literature [7, 20].

Peak 16 eluted with a retention time of 51.8 min and two UV absorption maxima at 270 and 323 nm. MS analysis in the negative ion mode revealed no major peaks, whereas analysis in the positive ion mode revealed three major peaks with *m/z* values of 373 $[M+H]^+$, 395 $[M+Na]^+$ and 358 $[M-CH_3+H]^+$. The protonated molecular ion with an *m/z* value of 373 $[M+H]^+$ was subjected to MS^2 fragmentation analysis, which resulted in three daughter peaks with *m/z* values of 343 $[M-CH_2O+H]^+$, 283 $[M-3CH_2O+H]^+$ and 312 $[M-CH_3-H_2O-CO+H]^+$. This peak was identified as tangeretin based on a comparison of these data with those reported in the literature [7, 20, 22], as well as the data obtained from the reference compounds.

Peak 17 gave a retention time of 56.5 min with four UV absorption maxima at 203, 254, 282 and 343 nm. No major peaks were observed by MS analysis in the negative ion mode, whereas analysis in the positive ion mode revealed four peaks with *m/z* values of 389 $[M+H]^+$, 411 $[M+Na]^+$, 374 $[M-CH_3+H]^+$ and 359 $[M-CH_2O+H]^+$. The peak with an *m/z* value of 389 $[M+H]^+$ was subjected to MS^2 fragmentation analysis, resulting in two daughter ions with *m/z* values of 359 $[M-CH_2O+H]^+$ and 374 $[M-CH_3+H]^+$. This peak was tentatively identified as 5-hydroxy-6,7,8,3′,4′-pentamethoxyflavone based on a comparison of these data with the data from the literature [7].

Peak 1 eluted with a retention time of 15.2 min and a UV absorption maximum of 283 nm. Peak 7 had a retention time of 36.5 min and three UV absorption maxima at 210, 257 and 342 nm. However, neither of these two peaks gave any major ions when they were analyzed by MS in the negative and positive ionization modes.

Peak 3 had a retention time of 19.2 min with two UV absorption maxima at 253 and 347 nm. MS analysis in the negative ion mode revealed a deprotonated molecular ion peak with an *m/z* value of 607 $[M-H]^-$. The subsequent fragmentation of this peak by MS^2 analysis resulted in a daughter peak with an *m/z* value of 299 $[M\text{-Rutinosyl}-H]^-$. MS analysis in the positive ion mode resulted in four major peaks with *m/z* values of 609 $[M+H]^+$, 631 $[M+Na]^+$, 463 $[M\text{-Rhamnosyl}+H]^+$ and 301 $[M\text{-Rutinosyl}+H]^+$. MS^2 fragmentation analysis of the first of these four peaks resulted in a daughter ion with an *m/z* value of 301 $[M\text{-Rutinosyl}+H]^+$.

Peak 6 eluted with a retention time of 32.4 min and two UV absorption maxima at 254 and 347 nm. Analysis in negative ion mode revealed two peaks with *m/z* values of 732 $[M-H]^-$ and 695 $[M-CO-H]^-$. The subsequent fragmentation of the former of these two peaks by MS^2 analysis gave a daughter ion with an *m/z* value of 417 $[M\text{-}306-H]^-$. MS analysis in the positive ion mode resulted in two peaks with *m/z* values of 725 $[M+H]^+$ and 747 $[M+Na]^+$. The MS^2 fragmentation of the former of these two peaks resulted in a daughter peak with an *m/z* value of 419 $[M\text{-}306+H]^+$.

Peak 8 had a retention time of 40.3 min and gave three UV absorption maxima at 203, 269 and 345 nm. MS analysis in the negative ion mode did not reveal any major peaks, whereas analysis in the positive ion mode gave four peaks with *m/z* values of 373 $[M+H]^+$, 395 $[M+Na]^+$, 358 $[M-CH_3+H]^+$ and 343 $[M-CH_2O+H]^+$. The first of these four peaks was subjected to MS^2 analysis, which resulted in a major daughter peak with an *m/z* value of 343 $[M-CH_2O+H]^+$.

Peak 9 had a retention time of 42.2 min with four UV absorption maxima at 206, 253, 270 and 355 nm. MS analysis in the negative ionization mode revealed major peaks whereas analysis in the positive ion mode revealed four peaks with *m/z* values of 403 $[M+H]^+$, 425 $[M+Na]^+$, 388 $[M-CH_3+H]^+$ and 373 $[M-CH_2O+H]^+$. The peak observed with an *m/z* value of 403 $[M+H]^+$ was subjected to MS^2 fragmentation analysis, resulting in a daughter peak with an *m/z* value of 373 $[M-CH_2O+H]^+$.

Despite of best efforts, we were unable to identify peaks 1, 3, 6–9.

Fingerprinting and chemometrics

In this study, all the CER samples were compared with the corresponding reference samples (generated from all the CER samples) based on their calculated similarity values (Table 6). We also performed PCA based on the contents of three specific analytes, as well as the PA/W values of the remaining 14 characteristic peaks. This operation can be thought of as revealing the internal structure of the data in a way that explains the variance of the samples.

Fingerprinting analysis was conducted using the 17 characteristic peaks shown in the overlapped chromatograms (Fig. 2). These peaks were used as variables to calculate the similarity values. The results of this process showed that the similarity values of the L-CER samples (0.24–0.66) were lower than those of the CER samples (0.72–0.91), indicating that the chemical profiles of the CER samples were similar to that of the reference fingerprint. Based on the contents and PA/W values of the different samples, we determined that the hesperidin, nobiletin and tangeretin contents of the L-CER samples were lower than those of the CER samples. Furthermore, the CER samples contained 10–30 times as much nobiletin and tangeretin as the L-CER samples. Peaks 1, 6 and 7 were not detected in most of the CER samples, however, they were found to be particularly prominent in the L-CER samples. None of the L-CER samples contained a signal corresponding to peak 17 (5-hydroxy-6,7,8,3′,4′-pentamethoxyflavone), which was found in all the CER samples. Although all of the L-CER samples purchased in pharmacies in Hong Kong were actually imported from mainland China, they all showed considerable differences in the chemical profiles. For example, the hesperidin contents of the CER samples were around two times higher than those of the L-CER samples. Further work should therefore be conducted to determine whether these differences in the chemical compositions of the samples could lead to differences in their efficacies in clinical practice.

In this study, the variables for each sample in the PCA consisted of their hesperidin, nobiletin and tangeretin contents, as well as the PA/W values of the remaining 14 characteristic peaks. The resulting data were exported to Excel (Microsoft, Inc., Belleview, WA, USA) to form a two-dimensional matrix (10 samples versus 17 variables), which cumulatively accounted for 94.31 of the total variance, based on which PCA scores plot (Fig. 3) was generated. CER-01, CER-02, CER-03, CER-04 and CER-06 were tightly clustered to the left of the plot, with PC1 scores around −0.6. L-CER-02, L-CER-03 and L-CER-04 were tightly clustered in the lower right of the plot with high PC2 scores. CER-05 was the only CER sample to be found at some distance from the other CER samples, although it was close to the L-CER samples. L-CER-01 was positioned in the upper right of the plot and far away from all of the other samples giving it the highest PC2 score. The loading plot of a variable on a PC generally reflects the extent to which that variable contributes to the PC, and how well the PC accounts for variations in the variable over the data points. The loading results also described the relationships between different variables.

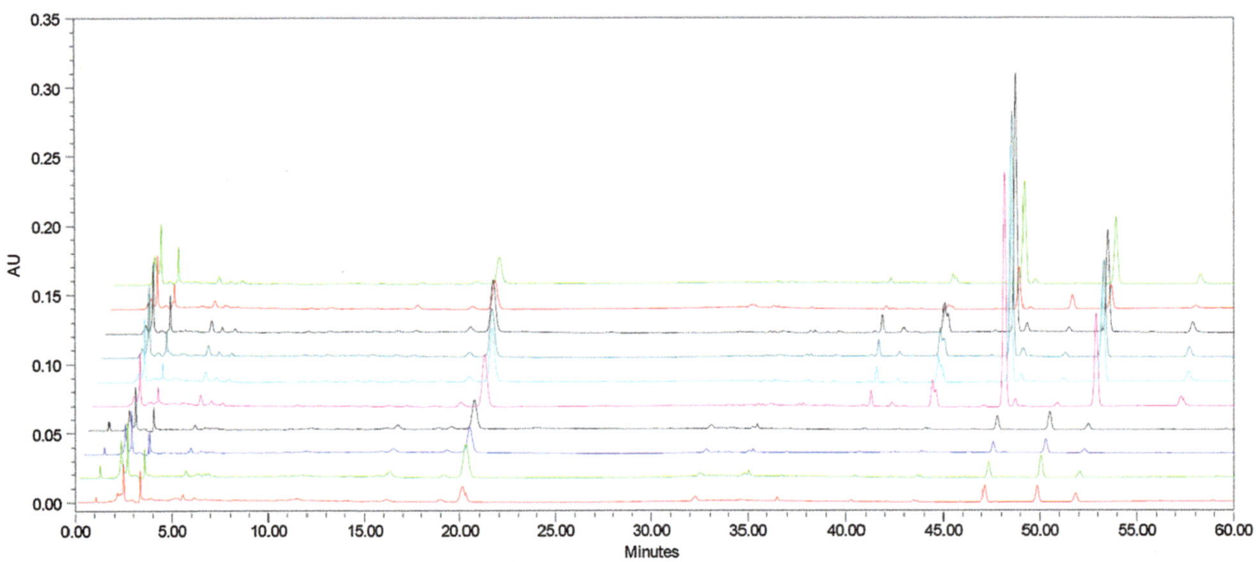

Fig. 2 Overlapped chromatographic fingerprints of the testes CER samples

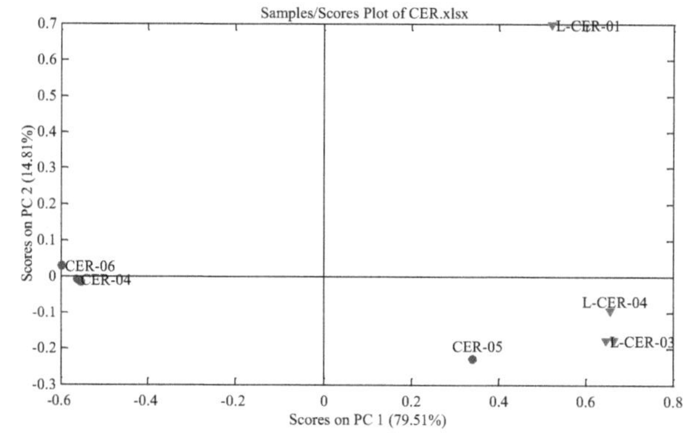

Fig. 3 PCA scores plot of CER samples based on the first two components

PC1 loadings plot indicated that peak 8, peaks 10 and 11 (sinensetin and tetramethyl-*O*-isoscutellarein), peak 14 (tetramethyl-*O*-scutellarein) and peak 17 (5-hydroxy-6,7,8,3′,4′-pentamethoxyflavone) had made a negative contribution to the positions of the samples tested in PC1. In contrast, peak 1, peak 5 (neohesperidin), peak 6 and peak 15 (3,5,6,7,8,3′,4′-heptamethoxyflavone) had made a positive contribution to PC1. In other words, samples with higher contents or PA/W values of peak 8, peaks 10 and 11 (sinensetin and tetramethyl-*O*-isoscutellarein), peak 14 (tetramethyl-*O*-scutellarein) and peak 17 (5-hydroxy-6,7,8,3′,4′-pentamethoxyflavone) would be positioned to the left of the scores plot. Meanwhile, samples with higher contents or PA/W values of peak 1, peak 5 (neohesperidin), peaks 6 and 15 (3,5,6,7,8,3′,4′-heptamethoxyflavone) would be positioned to the right of the scores plot. In this study, CER-01, CER-02, CER-03, CER-04 and CER-06 had high PA/W values for peak 8, peak 10 + 11 (sinensetin and tetramethyl-*O*-isoscutellarein), peak 14 (tetramethyl-*O*-scutellarein) and peak 17 (5-hydroxy-6,7,8,3′,4′-pentamethoxyflavone), and were consequently positioned to the left of the scores plot. In contrast, all of the L-CER samples had high PA/W values for peak 5 (neohesperidin), peak 6 and peak 15 (3,5,6,7,8,3′,4′-heptamethoxyflavone). The hesperidin, nobiletin and tangeretin contents of CER-05 and the PA/W values of the other characteristic peaks resembled those of the L-CER samples more closely than those of the CER samples.

The loading plot for PC2 showed that peak 1, peak 3, peak 5 (neohesperidin), peak 10 + 11 and peak 15 were having the greatest influence on the samples on the PC2 positions. Peak 5 (neohesperidin) made a positive contribution to the positions, whereas peak 1, peak 3, peak 10 + 11 and peak 15 made a negative contribution to these positions. L-CER-01 had the highest value for peak 5 (neohesperidin) of all of the samples tested in the current study.

Antioxidant activity of CER samples

2,2-Diphenyl-1-picrylhydrazyl (DPPH) assay

The DPPH free radical scavenging activities of the CER samples are shown in Fig. 4a. Each sample was tested at three different concentrations. CER-06 had the highest value at 173.005 μmol butylated hydroxytoluene equivalent (BHTE)/g of dried sample, followed by L-CER-01 at 164.741 μmol BHTE/g of dried sample. L-CER-03 had the lowest value at 68.818 μmol BHTE/g of dried sample, followed by L-CER-02 at 94.372 μmol BHTE/g of dried sample. The EC_{50} values of the samples were calculated and the results are shown in Fig. 4b. Materials with the lowest EC_{50} value exhibited the greatest free radical-scavenging activity. Although the DPPH radical-scavenging activities of all the CER samples tested in the current study were lower than that of BHT, the results showed that the different samples exhibited different radical-scavenging abilities.

Ferric ion reducing antioxidant power (FRAP) assay

The FRAP values (expressed as Fe^{2+} equivalents) were used to determine the ferric reducing activities of the different CER samples (Fig. 5). The values were between 19.887 (L-CER-03) and 43.890 (CER-06) μmol Fe^{2+} equivalents/g of dried CER sample. The value obtained for BHT was the highest of all of the samples tested at 275.01 μmol Fe^{2+} equivalents/g of BHT. The ferric reducing activities of all of the CER samples were less than that of BHT.

Trolox equivalent antioxidant capacity (TEAC) assay

The antioxidant activities of the CER samples were determined using the TEAC method, which gave values in the range of 27.120 to 58.391 μmol BHTE/g of dried sample (Fig. 6a). L-CER-03 showed the highest value of all of the samples tested at 58.391 μmol BHTE/g of dried sample, whereas CER-06 gave the lowest value at 27.120 μmol BHTE/g of dried sample. The EC_{50} values were calculated and the results are displayed in Fig. 6b. The differences in the antioxidant activities of the different CER samples were attributed to differences in their chemical compositions.

Correlation analysis

Pearson r correlation values were calculated using bivariate correlation analysis because we only evaluated 10 CER samples in the present study, and we were therefore unable to determine whether these samples did or did not obey a Gaussian distribution. The results of this analysis are shown in Table 7, where "−" and "+" have been used to represent negative and positive correlations, respectively. Peaks 03, 04, 08, 10, 11, 13, 14, 16 and 17 positively correlated with the ABTS radical scavenging activity,

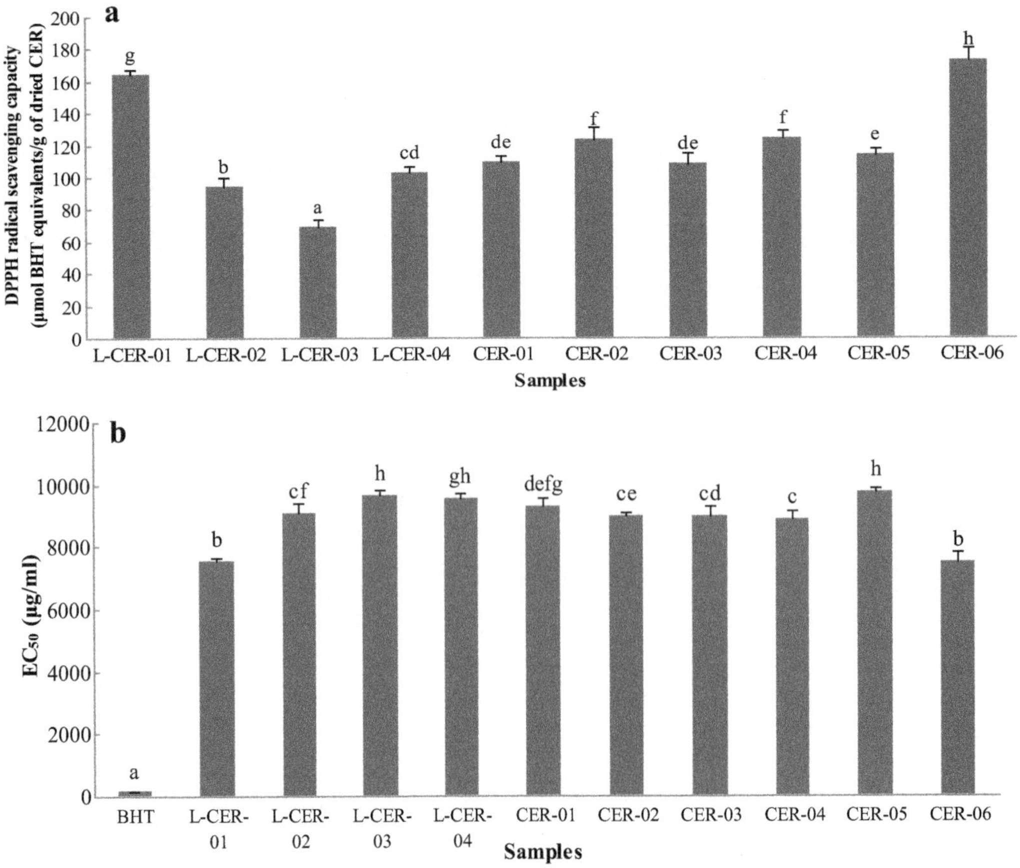

Fig. 4 DPPH radical scavenging capacity of CER samples (**a**) and EC_{50} values of BHT and CER samples (**b**). *Different letters* represent significant differences ($P < 0.05$)

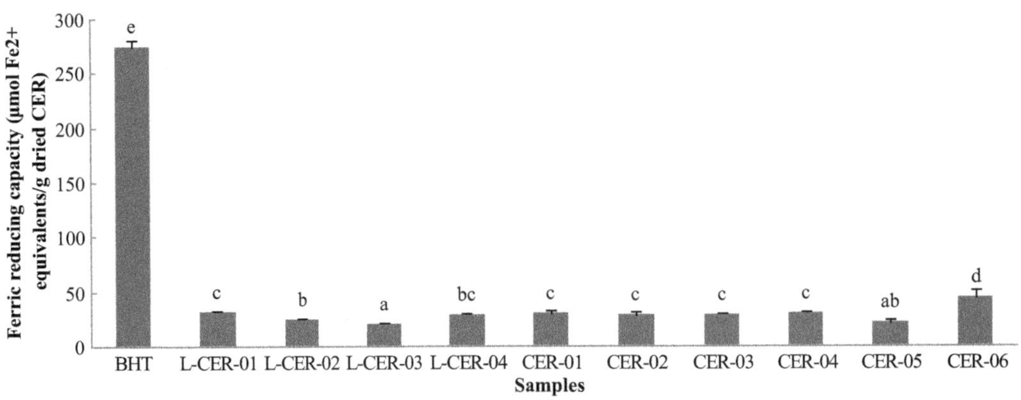

Fig. 5 Ferric reducing capacity of CER samples. The values are expressed as mol Fe^{2+} equivalents per gram of dried CER sample (mean ± SD). *Different letters* represent significant differences ($P < 0.05$)

whereas peaks 01, 06 and 15 negatively correlated with the ABTS radical scavenging activity. None of the peaks correlated with the DPPH free radical scavenging or ferric reducing activity.

Conclusion

An HPLC-UV-MS method has been developed and validated after a detailed investigation on extraction of chemical compounds from CER using different solvents

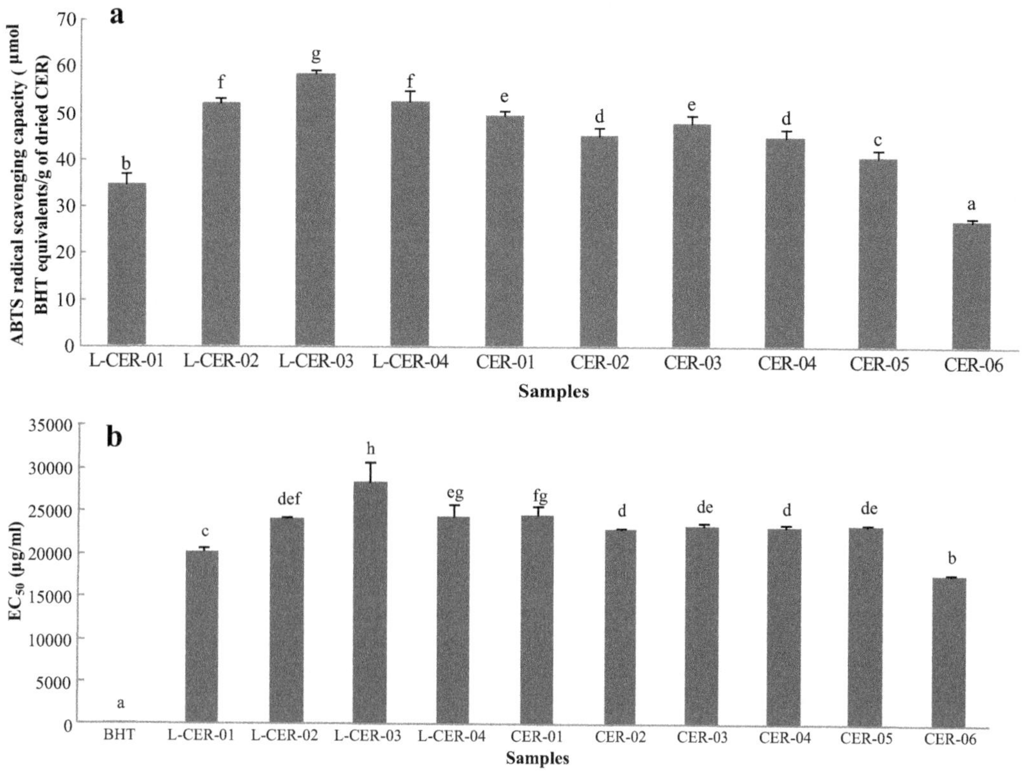

Fig. 6 ABTS radical scavenging capacity of CER samples (**a**) and EC_{50} values of BHT and CER samples (**b**). *Different letters* represent significant differences ($P < 0.05$)

Table 7 Spearman's correlation between the characteristic peaks of each CER sample and its antioxidant capacities

Peak no.	Correlation coefficient		
	DPPH free radical scavenging capacity	Ferric reducing capacity	ABTS radical scavenging capacity
Peak 01	−0.575	0.446	−0.760**
Peak 02	−0.290	0.174	−0.406
Peak 03	0.152	−0.224	0.697**
Peak 04	−0.055	0.079	0.709**
Peak 05	0.138	0.450	−0.510
Peak 06	−0.307	0.533	−0.792**
Peak 07	−0.252	0.511	−0.743
Peak 08	0.527	−0.042	0.952**
Peak 09	−0.115	0.394	0.612
Peak 10 + 11	0.503	−0.030	0.976**
Peak 12	−0.018	0.395	0.638*
Peak 13	0.503	−0.030	0.976**
Peak 14	–	–	0.915**
Peak 15	−0.418	0.697	−0.709*
Peak 16	0.503	−0.030	0.976**
Peak 17	0.550	−0.306	0.932**

* $P < 0.05$

** $P < 0.01$

and extraction times. None of the peaks correlated with the DPPH free radical scavenging activity or ferric reducing capacity. In contrast, most of the peaks correlated well with the ABTS radical scavenging capacity.

Authors' contributions

YLH, YSC and XZ designed the study. YZ, CPK, CRL and KCW performed the experiments. YZ wrote the manuscript. YSC revised the manuscript. All authors read and approved the manuscript.

Author details

[1] Department of Chinese Pharmaceutical Sciences and Chinese Medicine Resources, College of Biopharmaceutical and Food Sciences, China Medical University, Taichung 40402, Taiwan. [2] Key Laboratory for Information System of Mountainous Areas and Protection of Ecological Environment, Guizhou Normal University, Guiyang 550001, China. [3] Department of Nursing, Hsin Sheng College of Medical Care and Management, Taoyuan 32544, Taiwan. [4] Department of Nursing, Hungkuang University, Taichung 43302, Taiwan. [5] Chinese Crude Drug Pharmacy, China Medical University Hospital, Taichung 40402, Taiwan.

Acknowledgements

The authors would like to acknowledge the grant support from Hong Kong Chinese Materia Medica Standard Office, Department of Health, Hong Kong, for this study. (HKCMMS-CMU-Phase VII to YS Chang).

Competing interests

The authors declare that they have no competing interests.

References

1. The State Pharmacopoeia Commission of The People's Republic of China. Pharmacopoeia of the People's Republic of China. Beijing: Chemical Industry Press; 2015. p. 602–3.
2. Yu MW, Lou SN, Chiu EM, Ho CT. Antioxidant activity and effective compounds of immature calamondin peel. Food Chem. 2013;136:1130–5.
3. Xiao H, Yang CS, Li S, Jin H, Ho CT, Patel T. Monodemethylated polymethoxyflavones from sweet orange (*Citrus sinensis*) peel inhibit growth of human lung cancer cells by apoptosis. Mol Nutr Food Res. 2009;53:398–406.
4. Yi ZB, Yu Y, Liang YZ, Zeng B. In vitro antioxidant and antimicrobial activities of the extract of *Pericarpium Citri Reticulatae* of new Citrus cultivar and its main flavonoids. LWT-Food Sci Technol. 2008;41:597–603.
5. Manthey JA, Grohmann K, Guthrie N. Biological properties of citrus flavonoids pertaining to cancer and inflammation. Curr Med Chem. 2001;8:135–53.
6. Attaway JA. Citrus juice flavonoids with anticarcinogenic and antitumor properties. Food Phytochem Cancer Prev. 1994;19:240–8.
7. Liu EH, Zhao P, Duan L, Zheng GD, Guo L, Yang H, Li P. Simultaneous determination of six bioactive flavonoids in Citri Reticulatae Pericarpium by rapid resolution liquid chromatography coupled with triple quadrupole electrospray tandem mass spectrometry. Food Chem. 2013;141:3977–83.
8. Zhang J, Gao W, Liu Z, Zhang Z. Identification and simultaneous determination of twelve active components in the methanol extract of traditional medicine Weichang'an Pill by HPLC-DAD-ESI-MS/MS. Iran J Pharm Res. 2013;12:15–24.
9. Yu JW, Deng KY, Peng T, Zhu BY, Liu HY. Simultaneous determination of six ingredients in Huoxiang Zhengqi oral liquid by UPLC. Zhongguo Zhong Yao Za Zhi. 2013;38:2314–7.
10. Zhao Y, Sun JH, Yu LL, Chen P. Chromatographic and mass spectrometric fingerprinting analyses of *Angelica sinensis* (Oliv.) Diels-derived dietary supplements. Anal Bioanal Chem. 2013;405:4477–85.
11. Zhao Y, Kao CP, Chang YS, Ho YL. Quality assessment on Polygoni Multiflori Caulis using HPLC/UV/MS combined with principle component analysis. Chem Cent J. 2013;7:106.
12. Sun JH, Chen P. Chromatographic fingerprint analysis of yohimbe bark and related dietary supplements using UHPLC/UV/MS. J Pharm Biomed Anal. 2012;61:142–9.
13. Zhao Y, Chen P, Lin LZ, Harnly JM, Yu LL, Li ZW. Tentative identification, quantitation, and principal component analysis of green pu-erh, green, and white teas using UPLC/DAD/MS. Food Chem. 2011;126:1269–77.
14. Cheng ZH, Moore J, Yu LL. High-throughput relative DPPH radical scavenging capacity assay. J Agric Food Chem. 2006;54:7429–36.
15. Yi T, Lo HW, Zhao ZZ, Yu ZL, Yang ZJ, Chen HB. Comparison of the chemical composition and pharmacological effects of the aqueous and ethanolic extracts from a Tibetan "Snow Lotus" (*Saussurea laniceps*) herb. Molecules. 2012;17:7183–94.
16. Yi T, Chen QL, He XC, So SW, Lo YL, Fan LL, et al. Chemical quantification and antioxidant assay of four active components in Ficus hirta root using UPLC-PAD-MS fingerprinting combined with cluster analysis. Chem Cent J. 2013;7:115.
17. Benzie Iris FF, Strain JJ. The ferric reducing ability of plasma (FRAP) as a measure of "antioxidant powder": the FRAP assay. Anal Biochem. 1996;239:70–6.
18. Stratil P, Klejdus B, Kuban V. Determination of total content of phenolic compounds and their antioxidant activity in vegetables—evaluation of spectrophotometric methods. J Agric Food Chem. 2006;54:607–16.
19. Roowi S, Crozier A. Flavonoids in tropical citrus species. J Agric Food Chem. 2011;59:12217–25.
20. Wang DD, Wang J, Huang XH, Tu Y, Ni KY. Identification of polymethoxylated flavones from green tangerine peel (*Pericarpium Citri Reticulatae Viride*) by chromatographic and spectroscopic techniques. J Pharm Biomed Anal. 2007;44:63–9.
21. Dugo P, Mondello L, Dugo L, Stancanelli R, Dugo G. LC-MS for the identification of oxygen heterocyclic compounds in citrus essential oils. J Pharm Biomed Anal. 2000;24:147–54.
22. Zhang JY, Zhang Q, Zhang HX, Ma Q, Lu JQ, Qiao YJ. Characterization of polymethoxylated flavonoids (PMFs) in the peels of 'Shatangju' Mandarin (*Citrus reticulate* Blanco) by online high-performance liquid chromatography coupled to photodiode array detection and electrospray tandem mass spectrometry. J Agric Food Chem. 2012;60:9023–34.

19

The influence of duodenally-delivered Shakuyakukanzoto (*Shao Yao Gan Cao Tang*) on duodenal peristalsis during endoscopic retrograde cholangiopancreatography: a randomised controlled trial

Haruka Fujinami[1], Shinya Kajiura[2], Jun Nishikawa[2], Takayuki Ando[2] and Toshiro Sugiyama[2*]

Abstract

Background: Anti-cholinergic agents may be used to inhibit duodenal peristalsis, but they may have adverse effects. Shakuyakukanzoto (*Shao Yao Gan Cao Tang*) has an anti-spasmodic effect and has been used before for oesophagogastroduodenoscopy and colonoscopy. This randomised clinical trial aimed to evaluate the inhibitory effect of Shakuyakukanzoto on duodenal peristalsis, and its usefulness when administered into the duodenum just before endoscopic retrograde cholangiopancreatography (ERCP).

Methods: Participants were recruited between June 2008 and December 2010. All were aged ≥18 years and provided written informed consent. Exclusion criteria were: acute pancreatitis, a history of ischemic heart disease, prostatic hypertrophy or glaucoma, and altered/postsurgical upper gastrointestinal anatomy. The recruited participants were randomly assigned to the Shakuyakukanzoto group and control group. Shakuyakukanzoto 100 mg/mL solution or placebo (warm water) was administered directly as a spray into the duodenum during endoscopy. Efficacy was evaluated by observing the extent of duodenal peristalsis and assessing the difficulty of cannulating the common bile duct, the required time (RT) from administration to inhibition of duodenal peristalsis and the stop duration time (DT, the duration for which peristalsis was inhibited). Side effects were evaluated by measuring serum potassium concentration after ERCP.

Results: Of 28 participants, 15 were assigned to the Shakuyakukanzoto group and 13 to the control group. Duodenal peristalsis was inhibited in eight of the 10 eligible participants (80.0%) in the Shakuyakukanzoto group and none (0%) of the nine eligible participants in the control group ($P = 0.026$). In the Shakuyakukanzoto group, mean RT (±standard deviation) was 76.0 ± 23.9 s and DT was 11.3 ± 4.2 min. No adverse effects were observed in the Shakuyakukanzoto group during or after ERCP.

Conclusion: Duodenal peristalsis can be inhibited by spraying Shakuyakukanzoto solution directly into the duodenum.

Trial registration UMIN Clinical Trials Registry (UMIN-CTR) UMIN000011469

*Correspondence: tsugi@med.u-toyama.ac.jp
[2] Department of Gastroenterology, Graduate School of Medicine and Pharmaceutical Science, University of Toyama, Sugitani 2630, Toyama City, Toyama 930-0194, Japan
Full list of author information is available at the end of the article

Background

Endoscopic retrograde cholangiopancreatography (ERCP) has become increasingly important in the diagnosis and treatment of pancreatic and biliary diseases [1]. It is important to obtain a clear view, without duodenal peristalsis, to perform ERCP safely and effectively. Antispasmodics such as hyoscine-*N*-butylbromide or glucagon are often used to inhibit duodenal spasm [2], but their systemic use may cause adverse events, including dry mouth, urinary retention, orthostatic hypotension, palpitations, hyperglycaemia and anaphylaxis. Furthermore, these drugs are contraindicated in participants with ischaemic heart disease, prostatic hypertrophy, glaucoma and diabetes mellitus [3, 4].

Shakuyakukanzoto (*Shao Yao Gan Cao Tang*), an aqueous mixture of extracts of *Paeoniae radix* (*Shakuyaku, Shao Yao*) and *Glycyrrhizae radix* (*Kanzo, Gan Cao*), is reported to rapidly reduce abdominal pain and muscular cramps [5, 6], and suppress contraction of the ileum [7]. We have previously reported the inhibitory effect of Shakuyakukanzoto on duodenal peristalsis during ERCP [8], a finding that was later corroborated by Sakai et al. [9]. This randomised clinical trial aimed to evaluate the inhibitory effect of Shakuyakukanzoto on duodenal peristalsis and its utility when administered directly into the duodenum just before ERCP.

Methods

Study design

This was a prospective, randomised, placebo-controlled trial to investigate the effectiveness of Shakuyakukanzoto solution on intestinal peristalsis. A CONSORT flow diagram of the study protocol is presented in Fig. 1 [10]. The study was approved by the Ethics Committee of the University of Toyama, Toyama, Japan (Additional file 1), and informed consent was obtained from all participants (Additional file 2). Participants scheduled for ERCP at Toyama University Hospital were invited at this study between June 2008 and December 2010. Inclusion criteria were: (1) participants ≥18 years old, with (2) the capacity to provide written informed consent. Exclusion criteria were: (1) acute active pancreatitis; (2) a history of ischemic heart disease, prostatic hypertrophy or glaucoma, and (3) altered or postsurgical upper gastrointestinal anatomy. Randomization was achieved by a computer-generated list of numbers to assign group allocation.

ERCP

Endoscopic retrograde cholangiopancreatography was performed by one of four trained endoscopists, each with at least 5 years of experience (HF, SK, JN and TA). Images of all procedures were recorded digitally. All participants were administered midazolam 5 mg (Astellas Pharma Inc., Tokyo, Japan) intravenously before the procedure, and heart rate and peripheral oxygen saturation were monitored by pulse oximetry during the procedure. We prepared a 100 mg/mL Shakuyakukanzoto solution by dissolving 5.0 g Shakuyakukanzoto extract (TJ-68; Tsumura Co., Tokyo, Japan) in 50 mL of warm water, while 50 mL of warm water was used as the placebo control. Both solutions were administered at 36 °C by spraying directly towards the major papilla of the duodenum through the endoscope. Those cases with no duodenal peristalsis at the major papilla were excluded from the study, and the study drug was not administered.

Evaluation of duodenal peristalsis

We measured duodenal peristalsis during ERCP using a four-grade scoring system of the degree of peristalsis and the difficulty of cannulation previously described by Niwa et al. [11]. The four scores used were as follows: (+0) no peristalsis of the duodenum during ERCP, cannulation was easy to perform; (+1) slight peristalsis of the duodenum, cannulation was easy to perform; (+2) moderate peristalsis of the duodenum, cannulation was difficult to perform; and (+3) severe peristalsis of the duodenum, cannulation could not be performed.

Efficacy and side effects of Shakuyakukanzoto solution

The primary efficacy was inhibition of duodenal peristalsis, calculated as the proportion of participants scoring either +0 or +1 after treatment. To further assess the effects of Shakuyakukanzoto solution, we reviewed the digital recordings of ERCP to measure the required time (RT) from administration of the study drug until peristalsis was diminished, and the duration time (DT) of inhibition of peristalsis (Fig. 2). As hypokalaemia has been reported as a side effect of Shakuyakukanzoto [12], we measured serum potassium concentration before and 24 h after ERCP.

Statistical analysis

The primary outcome criterion was the efficacy rate of Shakuyakukanzoto compared with placebo. The sample size calculation for this study was based on the effective rate achieved in a previous trial, with the response rates in the Shakuyakukanzoto and control groups expected to be 70 and 10%, respectively. The no-peristalsis rate was expected to be 40% [9, 13]. The target sample size required to detect a difference in the response rate between the groups with a significance level of 5% and a power 90% was 13 per group, including a 40% dropout rate. Data are expressed as mean ± standard deviation (SD). Either Fisher's exact test or Student's *t* test were used to compare paired data. A *P* value less than 0.05 was considered statistically significant. All statistical analyses

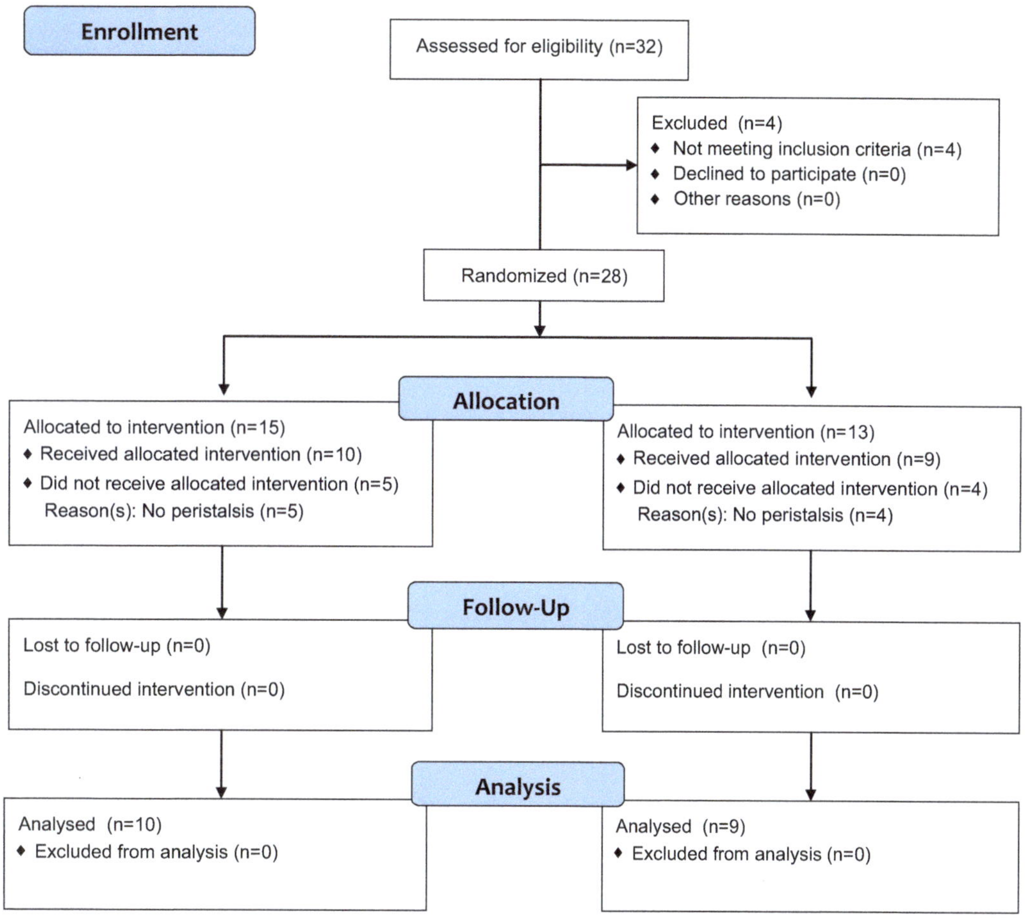

Fig. 1 CONSORT flow diagram of enrolled and randomised participants. Recruitment, group allocation and retention of study participants

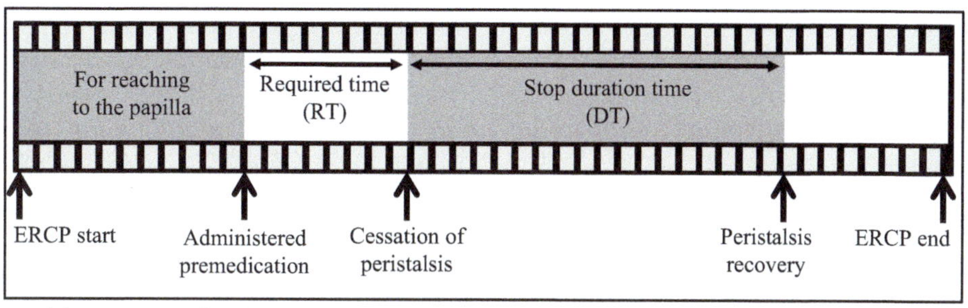

Fig. 2 Required time and duration time of study drug during ERCP. Required time (RT): from study drug administration to cessation of peristalsis. Stop duration time (DT): from cessation to recovery of peristalsis. Both were obtained from the digital recording made of each ERCP

were performed using the Statview 5.0 (Abacus Concepts Inc., Berkeley, CA, USA).

Results

In total, 149 ERCP procedures were performed during the study period, and 32 participants were enrolled into the study. Four were excluded due to exacerbation of acute pancreatitis and/or cholangitis. The remaining 28 participants fulfilled the inclusion criteria and were randomly allocated to one of the two groups: 15 participants to the Shakuyakukanzoto group and 13 to the placebo control group. Five participants in the Shakuyakukanzoto group and four in the control group were excluded as no duodenal peristalsis was evident at duodenoscopy.

Consequently, we subjected the data of 10 and nine participants from the Shakuyakukanzoto and control groups to analysis, respectively. Participants' demographic and clinical characteristics are summarised in Table 1. There was no significant difference in sex, mean age or indication for ERCP between the groups. Duodenal peristalsis was inhibited in eight of the 10 participants (80.0%) in the Shakuyakukanzoto group and none (0%) of the control group ($P = 0.026$; Table 2). Mean RT and DT for Shakuyakukanzoto were 76.0 ± 23.9 s and 12.4 ± 5.0 min, respectively. There was no significant difference in the serum potassium concentration in the Shakuyakukanzoto group before or after the procedure (4.1 ± 0.3 mEq/L versus 4.3 ± 0.3 mEq/L, respectively, $P = 0.192$; Table 2).

Discussion

To the best of our knowledge, this is the first placebo-controlled study that has shown that Shakuyakukanzoto is an effective and safe anti-spasmodic premedication for ERCP. In a previous observational study [9], Shakuyakukanzoto acted as an anti-spasmodic agent and abolished duodenal peristalsis in the majority of participants to whom it was administered, but this was not a randomised, controlled study and the extent of suppression of peristalsis was not measured. In this study, we excluded participants in whom duodenal peristalsis was not evident at duodenoscopy, and assessed peristalsis and its influence on the technical difficulty of cannulating the common bile duct using the scoring system previously described by Niwa et al. [11].

Gastrointestinal peristalsis may be an impediment to accurate endoscopic examination. Intramuscular or intravenous administration of an anti-cholinergic agent such as hyoscine-*N*-butyl bromide is generally required to abolish peristalsis [14]. Administration of an anti-cholinergic drug may, however, cause potentially serious complications, including cardiovascular events, urinary retention and ocular hypertension [4]. Glucagon may also be used to reduce peristalsis, but while it has fewer adverse effects on the cardiovascular system, it may induce hyperglycaemia [15]. Therefore, these drugs are not recommended for participants with cardiac disease, glaucoma, prostatic hyperplasia or diabetes mellitus [4, 15].

Shakuyakukanzoto has two active components. Paeoniflorin is a bioactive component of *Paeoniae radix*, and reportedly exhibits anti-coagulant [16], neuromuscular blocking [17–23], immunoregulating [24] and anti-hyperglycaemic effects [25]. Glycyrrhizic acid is a bioactive component of *Glycyrrhizae radix* and is reported to have anti-inflammatory [26] and hepatoprotective activity [27], and inhibit anti-platelet aggregation [28] and formation of peptic ulcers [29, 30]. These two components may exert synergistic effects. Although paeoniflorin is poorly absorbed in the gastrointestinal tract and has low bioavailability [31, 32], its absorption is significantly improved when administered orally in Shakuyakukanzoto solution [33].

Rather than administering standard anti-spasmodic drugs, or administering Shakuyakukanzoto orally, we sprayed Shakuyakukanzoto directly into the duodenum during duodenoscopy, and found that duodenal peristalsis was inhibited in 80% of cases. These effects were likely observed because the *Glycyrrhizae radix* reportedly inhibits acetylcholine-induced contraction and the contractile machinery of smooth muscle, while *Paeoniae radix* inhibits neurogenic contraction in the small bowel (the latter reportedly inhibits peristalsis in guinea pig ileum and in mouse jejunum and ileum) [7, 34]. Although paeoniflorin and glycyrrhizin may be ineffective when applied individually, they are recognised to block neuromuscular synapses when applied in combination in animal models [21].

Peppermint oil, a major constituent of which is menthol, also inhibits the contraction of smooth muscle of the gastrointestinal tract [35–37]. Instillation

Table 1 Participants' demographic and clinical characteristics

	Shakuyakukanzoto group	Control group	*P* value
Participants	10 (52.6)	9 (47.4)	
Male	7 (70.0)	6 (66.7)	1.000[a]
Age (years old)	69.1	71.2	0.708[b]
Diagnostic ERCP	7 (36.8)	3 (15.8)	0.179[a]
Therapeutic ERCP	3 (15.8)	6 (31.6)	

Data are presented as number (proportion, %) or mean ± standard deviation

[a] Fisher's exact test was used to assess statistical significance

[b] Student's *t* test was used to assess statistical significance

Table 2 Efficacy and safety of *Shakuyakukanzoto*

	Shakuyakukanzoto group	Control group
Ceased peristalsis	8 (80.0)	0 (0)
Required time (s)	76.0 ± 23.9	ND
Stop duration time (min)	11.3 ± 23.9	ND
Potassium concentration (mEq/L)		
Before procedure	4.1 ± 0.3	4.0 ± 0.3
24 h after procedure	4.3 ± 0.3	4.2 ± 0.2

**ND* no data. The required time and stop duration time in the control group were not measured because inhibition of duodenal peristalsis was not achieved with the placebo

Data are presented as number (proportion, %) or mean ± standard deviation of peppermint oil into the colon during colonoscopy reduces spasm and reduces the need for intramuscular or intravenous anti-spasmodic agents during endoscopic examination [13, 38, 39]. The mechanism of smooth muscle relaxation brought about by peppermint oil has been investigated in models using the smooth muscle of guinea pigs and mice.

The brown colour of Shakuyakukanzoto solution might affect endoscopic examination by obscuring the entrance to the common bile duct; however, ductal cannulation was possible in all cases in which Shakuyakukanzoto was administered. Nevertheless, its distinctive colour made blinding of the study to the endoscopist impractical.

The intraluminal administration of a rapidly acting agent that directly affects smooth muscle has obvious advantages over the systemic administration of an anticholinergic drug. In this study, we evaluated the efficacy of Shakuyakukanzoto administered directly into the duodenum immediately before ERCP. We have also found that Shakuyakukanzoto sprayed directly onto the duodenal papilla significantly reduced serum amylase concentration 1 h and 1 day after ERCP [40]. Although we assessed only ERCP, our findings might also apply to other endoscopic examinations, such as upper endoscopy, balloon endoscopy and colonoscopy.

Conclusion

Duodenal peristalsis can be inhibited by spraying Shakuyakukanzoto solution directly into the duodenum.

Abbreviations

DT: stop duration time; ERCP: endoscopic retrograde cholangiopancreatography; RT: required time.

Authors' contributions

HF, SK, JN, TA and TS conceived and designed the study protocol. HF, SK, JN and TA collected data and endoscopic examination. HF, SK and JN conducted the clinical trial. HF wrote and revised the manuscript. All authors read and approved the final manuscript.

Author details

[1] Department of Endoscopy, Toyama University Hospital, Toyama, Japan.
[2] Department of Gastroenterology, Graduate School of Medicine and Pharmaceutical Science, University of Toyama, Sugitani 2630, Toyama City, Toyama 930-0194, Japan.

Competing interests

The authors declare that they have no competing interests.

References

1. Schofl R, Haefner M. Diagnostic cholangiopancreatography. Endoscopy. 2003;35:145–55.
2. Chang FY, Guo WS, Liao TM, Lee SD. A randomized study comparing glucagon and hyoscine N-butyl bromide before endoscopic retrograde cholangiopancreatography. Scand J Gastroenterol. 1995;30:283–6.
3. Mintzer J, Burns A. Anticholinergic side-effects of drugs in elderly people. J R Soc Med. 2000;93:457–62.
4. Ai M, Yamaguchi T, Odaka T, Mitsuhashi K, Shishido T, Yan J, et al. Objective assessment of the antispasmodic effect of shakuyaku-kanzo-to (TJ-68), a Chinese herbal medicine, on the colonic wall by direct spraying during colonoscopy. World J Gastroenterol. 2006;12:760–4.
5. Hinoshita F, Ogura Y, Suzuki Y, Hara S, Yamada A, Tanaka N, et al. Effect of orally administered shao-yao-gan-cao-tang (Shakuyaku-kanzo-to) on muscle cramps in maintenance hemodialysis patients: a preliminary study. Am J Chin Med. 2003;31:445–53.
6. Hyodo T, Taira T, Kumakura M, Yamamoto S, Yoshida K, Uchida T, et al. The immediate effect of Shakuyaku-kanzo-to, traditional Japanese herbal medicine, for muscular cramps during maintenance hemodialysis. Nephron. 2002;90:240.
7. Maeda T, Shinozuka K, Baba K, Hayashi M, Hayashi E. Effect of shakuyaku-kanzoh-toh, a prescription composed of shakuyaku (Paeoniae Radix) and kanzoh (Glycyrrhizae Radix) on guinea pig ileum. J Pharmacobiodyn. 1983;6:153–60.
8. Fujinami H, Hirano K, Sugiyama T. Assessment of diminished peristalsis using shakuyakukanzoto (TJ-68) as premedication for endoscopic retrograde cholangiopancreatography (ERCP). DDW-Japan. Sapporo; 2006.
9. Sakai Y, Tsuyuguchi T, Ishihara T, Kato K, Tsuboi M, Ooka Y, et al. Confirmation of the antispasmodic effect of shakuyaku-kanzo-to (TJ-68), a Chinese herbal medicine, on the duodenal wall by direct spraying during endoscopic retrograde cholangiopancreatography. J Nat Med. 2009;63:200–3.
10. Schulz KF, Altman DG, Moher D. CONSORT Group: CONSORT 2010 statement: updated guidelines for reporting parallel group randomised trials. Int J Surg. 2011;9:672–7.
11. Niwa H, Nakamura T, Fujino M. Endoscopic observation on gastric peristalsis and pyloric movement (in Japanese with English abstract). Gastroenterol Endosc. 1975;17:236–42.
12. Kinoshita H, Okabayashi M, Kaneko M, Yasuda M, Abe K, Machida A, et al. Shakuyaku-kanzo-to induces pseudoaldosteronism characterized by hypokalemia, rhabdomyolysis, metabolic alkalosis with respiratory compensation, and increased urinary cortisol levels. J Altern Complement Med. 2009;15:439–43.
13. Hiki N, Kaminishi M, Yasuda K, Uedo N, Honjo H, Matsuhashi N, et al. Antiperistaltic effect and safety of L-menthol sprayed on the gastricmucosa for upper GI endoscopy: a phase III, multicenter, randomized, double-blind, placebo-controlled study. Gastrointest Endosc. 2011;73:932–41.
14. Sissons GR, McQueenie A, Mantle M. The ocular effects of hyoscine-n-butylbromide ("Buscopan") in radiological practice. Br J Radiol. 1991;64:584–6.
15. Mochiki E, Suzuki H, Takenoshita S, Nagamachi Y, Kuwano H, Mizumoto A, et al. Mechanism of inhibitory effect of glucagon on gastrointestinal motility and cause of side effects of glucagon. J Gastroenterol. 1998;33:835–41.
16. Ishida H, Takamatsu M, Tsuji K, Kosuge T. Studies on active substances in herbs used for Oketsu ('stagnant blood') in Chinese medicine. VI. On the anticoagulative principle in Paeoniae Radix. Chem Pharm Bull. 1987;35:849–52.
17. Dezaki K, Kimura I, Miyahara K, Kimura M. Complementary effects of paeoniflorin and glycyrrhizin on intracellular Ca2 + mobilization in the nerve-stimulated skeletal muscle of mice. Jpn J Pharmacol. 1995;69:281–4.
18. Kimura M, Kimura I, Muroi M, Nakamura T, Shibata S. Depolarizing effects of glycyrrhizin-derivatives relating to the blend effects with paeoniflorin in mouse diaphragm muscle. Jpn J Pharmacol. 1986;41:263–5.
19. Kimura M, Kimura I, Kimura M. Decreasing effects by glycyrrhizin and paeoniflorin on intracellular Ca2 + -aequorin luminescence transients with or without caffeine in directly stimulated-diaphragm muscle of mouse. Jpn J Pharmacol. 1985;39:387–90.
20. Kimura M, Kimura I, Nojima H. Depolarizing neuromuscular blocking action induced by electropharmacological coupling in the combined effect of paeoniflorin and glycyrrhizin. Jpn J Pharmacol. 1985;37:395–9.

21. Kimura M, Kimura I, Takahashi K, Muroi M, Yoshizaki M, Kanaoka M, et al. Blocking effects of blended paeoniflorin or its related compounds with glycyrrhizin on neuromuscular junctions in frog and mouse. Jpn J Pharmacol. 1984;36:275–82.
22. Kimura M, Kimura I, Takahashi K. The neuromuscular blocking actions of coclaurine derivatives and of paeoniflorin derivatives. Planta Med. 1982;45:136.
23. Kimura M, Kimura I, Nojima H. The electropharmacological mechanisms of depolarizing neuromuscular blocking effects induced by the combination of paeoniflorin and glycyrrhizin. Jpn J Pharmacol. 1981;31(Suppl):72.
24. Liang J, Zhou A, Chen M, Xu S. Negatively regulatory effects of paeoniflorin on immune cells. Eur J Pharmacol. 1990;183:901–2.
25. Hsu FL, Lai CW, Cheng JT. Antihyperglycemic effects of paeoniflorin and 8-debenzoylpaeoniflorin, glucosides from the root of Paeonia lactiflora. Planta Med. 1997;63:323–5.
26. Inoue H, Mori T, Shibata S, Koshihara Y. Modulation by glycyrrhetinic acid derivatives of TPA-induced mouse ear oedema. Br J Pharmacol. 1989;96:204–10.
27. van Rossum TG, Vulto AG, de Man RA, Brouwer JT, Schalm SW. Review article: glycyrrhizin as a potential treatment for chronic hepatitis C. Aliment Pharmacol Ther. 1998;12:199–205.
28. Tawata M, Aida K, Noguchi T, Ozaki Y, Kume S, Sasaki H, et al. Anti-platelet action of isoliquiritigenin, an aldose reductase inhibitor in licorice. Eur J Pharmacol. 1992;212:87–92.
29. van Marle J, Aarsen PN, Lind A, van Weeren-Kramer J. Deglycyrrhizinised liquorice (DGL) and the renewal of rat stomach epithelium. Eur J Pharmacol. 1891;72:219–25.
30. Baker ME. Licorice and enzymes other than 11 betahydroxysteroid dehydrogenase: an evolutionary perspective. Steroids. 1994;59:136–41.
31. Xu S, Chen C, Chen G. The pharmacokinetics of paeoniflorin. Eur J Pharmacol. 1990;183:2390.
32. Takeda S, Isono T, Wakui Y, Matsuzaki Y, Sasaki H, Amagaya S, et al. Absorption and excretion of paeoniflorin in rats. J Pharm Pharmacol. 1995;47:1036–40.
33. Chen LC, Chou MH, Lin MF, Yang LL. Pharmacokinetics of paeoniflorin after oral administration of Shao-yao Gan-chao Tang in mice. Jpn J Pharmacol. 2002;88:250–5.
34. Sato Y, Akao T, He JX, Nojima H, Kuraishi Y, Morota T, et al. Glycycoumarin from Glycyrrhizae Radix acts as a potent antispasmodic through inhibition of phosphodiesterase 3. J Ethnopharmacol. 2006;105:409–14.
35. Nair B. Final report on the safety assessment of Mentha piperita (peppermint) oil, Mentha piperita (peppermint) leaf extract, Mentha piperita (peppermint) leaf, and Mentha piperita (peppermint) leaf water. Int J Toxicol. 2001;20:61–73.
36. Hills JM, Aaronson PI. The mechanism of action of peppermint oil on gastrointestinal smooth muscle. An analysis using patch clamp electrophysiology and isolated tissue pharmacology in rabbit and guinea pig. Gastroenterology. 1991;101:55–65.
37. Micklefield G, Jung O, Greving I, May B. Effects of intraduodenal application of peppermint oil (WS (R) 1340) and caraway oil (WS (R) 1520) on gastroduodenal motility in healthy volunteers. Phytother Res. 2003;17:135–40.
38. Asao T, Mochiki E, Suzuki H, Nakamura J, Hirayama I, Morinaga N, et al. An easy method for the intraluminal administration of peppermint oil before colonoscopy and its effectiveness in reducing colonic spasm. Gastrointest Endosc. 2001;53:172–7.
39. Imagawa A, Hata H, Nakatsu M, Yoshida Y, Takeuchi K, Inokuchi T, et al. Peppermint oil solution is useful as an antispasmodic drug for esophagogastroduodenoscopy, especially for elderly patients. Dig Dis Sci. 2012;57:2379–84.
40. Fujinami H, Kajiura S, Ando T, Mihara H, Hosokawa A, Sugiyama T. Direct spraying of shakuyakukanzoto onto the duodenal papilla: a novel method for preventing pancreatitis following endoscopic retrograde cholangiopancreatography. Digestion. 2015;91:42–5.

Permissions

All chapters in this book were first published in CM, by BioMed Central; hereby published with permission under the Creative Commons Attribution License or equivalent. Every chapter published in this book has been scrutinized by our experts. Their significance has been extensively debated. The topics covered herein carry significant findings which will fuel the growth of the discipline. They may even be implemented as practical applications or may be referred to as a beginning point for another development.

The contributors of this book come from diverse backgrounds, making this book a truly international effort. This book will bring forth new frontiers with its revolutionizing research information and detailed analysis of the nascent developments around the world.

We would like to thank all the contributing authors for lending their expertise to make the book truly unique. They have played a crucial role in the development of this book. Without their invaluable contributions this book wouldn't have been possible. They have made vital efforts to compile up to date information on the varied aspects of this subject to make this book a valuable addition to the collection of many professionals and students.

This book was conceptualized with the vision of imparting up-to-date information and advanced data in this field. To ensure the same, a matchless editorial board was set up. Every individual on the board went through rigorous rounds of assessment to prove their worth. After which they invested a large part of their time researching and compiling the most relevant data for our readers.

The editorial board has been involved in producing this book since its inception. They have spent rigorous hours researching and exploring the diverse topics which have resulted in the successful publishing of this book. They have passed on their knowledge of decades through this book. To expedite this challenging task, the publisher supported the team at every step. A small team of assistant editors was also appointed to further simplify the editing procedure and attain best results for the readers.

Apart from the editorial board, the designing team has also invested a significant amount of their time in understanding the subject and creating the most relevant covers. They scrutinized every image to scout for the most suitable representation of the subject and create an appropriate cover for the book.

The publishing team has been an ardent support to the editorial, designing and production team. Their endless efforts to recruit the best for this project, has resulted in the accomplishment of this book. They are a veteran in the field of academics and their pool of knowledge is as vast as their experience in printing. Their expertise and guidance has proved useful at every step. Their uncompromising quality standards have made this book an exceptional effort. Their encouragement from time to time has been an inspiration for everyone.

The publisher and the editorial board hope that this book will prove to be a valuable piece of knowledge for researchers, students, practitioners and scholars across the globe.

List of Contributors

Beikang Ge, Zhen Zhang and Zhong Zuo
School of Pharmacy, Faculty of Medicine, The Chinese University of Hong Kong, Shatin, New Territories, Hong Kong, China

Kelly Yin-Ching Lam, Gallant Kar-Lun Chan and Ping Yao
Division of Life Science, and Center for Chinese Medicine, The Hong Kong University of Science and Technology, Clear Water Bay Road, Hong Kong, China

Chuen-Fai Ku and Hong-Jie Zhang
School of Chinese Medicine, Hong Kong Baptist University, Hong Kong, China

Huai-You Wang, Huang-Quan Lin, Tina Ting-Xia Dong and Karl Wah-Keung Tsim
HKUST Shenzhen Research Institute, Hi-Tech Park, Nanshan, Shenzhen, Guangdong Province, China

Jihye Kim, Boncho Ku and Keun Ho Kim
KM Fundamental Research Division, Korea Institute of Oriental Medicine, 1672 Yuseongdae-ro, Yuseong-gu, Daejeon 34054, Republic of Korea

Hui-Fang Chiu
Department of Chinese Medicine, Taichung Hospital Ministry of Health and Well-being, Taichung, Taiwan.

Ying-Hua Wu, Kamesh Venkatakrishnan and Chin-Kun Wang
School of Nutrition, Chung Shan Medical University, Taichung, Taiwan

You-Cheng Shen
School of Health Diet and Industry Management, Chung Shan Medical University, Taichung, Taiwan

Shing-Jung Wang
Division of Research and Development, Standard Foods Corporation, Taipei, Taiwan

Kwan-Yat Zee, Pui Sze Chan, Johnson Chun Sing Ho, Stanley Man Lung Lai, Esmonde Francis Corbet and Wai Keung Leung
Kwan-Yat Zee, Pui Sze Chan and Johnson Chun Sing Ho contributed equally to this work Faculty of Dentistry, The University of Hong Kong, Hong Kong, SAR, China

Natthanan Taechakulwanijya
Graduate School, Faculty of Pharmaceutical Sciences, Khon Kaen University, Khon Kaen 40002, Thailand

Natthida Weerapreeyakul
Faculty of Pharmaceutical Sciences, Khon Kaen University, Khon Kaen 40002, Thailand

Sahapat Barusrux
Faculty of Associate Medical Sciences, Khon Kaen University, Khon Kaen 40002, Thailand

Sirithorn Siriamornpun
Department of Food Technology and Nutrition, Mahasarakham University, Mahasarakham 44000, Thailand

Yantao Li, Wanjun Lin, Jiajun Huang, Ying Xie and Wenzhe Ma
State Key Laboratory of Quality Research in Chinese Medicine, Macau University of Science and Technology, Taipa, Macao, China

Ji-Min Cheng and Lei Hu
Department of Ophthalmology, Affiliated Hospital of Taishan Medical University, Shandong, China

Xiao-Qian Liu and Xiu-Mei Zhang
Department of Pharmacology, School of Medicine, Shandong University, Jinan, Shandong, China

Jorn-Hon Liu
Department of Ophthalmology, Cheng Hsin General Hospital, Taipei, Taiwan

Wynn Hwai-Tzong Pan
Institute of Pharmacology, School of Medicine, National Yang-Ming University, Taipei, Taiwan.

Hsiao-Ming Chao
Department of Ophthalmology, Cheng Hsin General Hospital, Taipei, Taiwan
Institute of Pharmacology, School of Medicine, National Yang-Ming University, Taipei, Taiwan
Department of Chinese Medicine, School of Chinese Medicine, China Medical University, Taichung, Taiwan

Rui-Qi Yue, Jun Xu and Alan Ho
School of Chinese Medicine, Hong Kong Baptist University, Hong Kong, China

Ying-Yu Huang, Min Li, Quan-Bin Han and Liang-Feng Liu
Mr. & Mrs. Ko Chi Ming Centre for Parkinson's Disease Research (CPDR), Hong Kong Baptist University, Kowloon Tong, Hong Kong SAR

Ying Wei, Mihui Li, Qingli Luo, Jing Sun Yubao Lv and Jingcheng Dong
Department of Integrative Medicine, Huashan Hospital, Fudan University, 12 Middle Urumqi Road, Shanghai 200040, China
Institute of Integrated Traditional Chinese and Western Medicine, Fudan University, 12 Middle Urumqi Road, Shanghai 200040, China

Muhammadjan Abduwaki and Mammat Nurahmat
Department of Integrative Medicine, Huashan Hospital, Fudan University, 12 Middle Urumqi Road, Shanghai 200040, China
Xinjiang Uygur Medical College, 370 West Beijing Road, Hotan, Xinjiang 848000, China

Junling Deng, Kaweng Sitou, Ru Yan and Yuanjia Hu
State Key Laboratory of Quality Research in Chinese Medicine, Institute of Chinese Medical Sciences, University of Macau, Macao, China

Yongping Zhang
Guiyang College of Traditional Chinese Medicine, Guiyang, Guizhou, China

Shi Wei Wang1, Yan Bo Zhang, Liang Zhang, Jing Su, Hei Kei Wong, Ho Pan Cheung, Yao Tong and Stephen Cho Wing Sze
School of Chinese Medicine, LKS Faculty of Medicine, The University of Hong Kong, 10 Sassoon Road, Pokfulam, Hong Kong SAR

Fei Hua Wu
Department of Pharmacology, China Pharmaceutical University, Nanjing, China

Ai Hua Liu
School of Chinese Medicine, LKS Faculty of Medicine, The University of Hong Kong, 10 Sassoon Road, Pokfulam, Hong Kong SAR
Department of Physiology, School of Basic Medicine, Shanghai University of Traditional Chinese Medicine, Shanghai, China

Tzi Bun Ng
School of Biomedical Sciences, Faculty of Medicine, The Chinese University of Hong Kong, Shatin, N.T., Hong Kong SAR

Huifeng Zhu, Yuan Wang, Jinghuan Wang, Shan Feng, Xian Yang and Tao Wang
College of Pharmaceutical Sciences and Traditional Chinese Medicine, Southwest University, Chongqing 400715, China
Chongqing Engineering Research Center for Pharmacological Evaluation, POB 400715, Chongqing, China

Zhiqiang Liu
Department of Pharmacy, The First People's Hospital of Neijiang, Neijiang 641000, China

Dong Wan
Department of Emergency, The First Affiliated Hospital of Chongqing Medical University, POB 400016, Chongqing, China

You Hua Chen, Chun Hua Liu, Lu Wang and Xi Chen
Jiangsu Key Laboratory of TCM Evaluation and Translational Research, China Pharmaceutical University, 639 Longmian Road, Nanjing 210009, China

Hai Fang Chen
Jiangsu Key Laboratory of TCM Evaluation and Translational Research, China Pharmaceutical University, 639 Longmian Road, Nanjing 210009, China
Key Laboratory of Modern Preparation of TCM of Ministry of Education, Jiangxi University of Traditional Chinese Medicine, Nanchang 330004, China

Bo Yang Yu and Jin Qi
Department of Complex Prescription of Traditional Chinese Medicine, State Key Laboratory of Natural Medicines, China Pharmaceutical University, 639 Longmian Road, Nanjing 211198, China

Fan Yi, Xiao-lei Tan and Hai-bo Liu
Institute of Medicinal Plant Development, Chinese Academy of Medical Sciences, Peking Union Medical College, 151 Malianwa N, Haidian District, Beijing 100193, China
Key Laboratory of Bioactive Substances and Resources Utilization of Chinese Herbal Medicine, Ministry of Education, Beijing 100193, China

Xin Yan
Research Center for Drug Discovery, School of Pharmaceutical Sciences, Sun Yat-sen University, 132 East Circle at University City, Guangzhou 510006, China

Fatimah Ibrahim
Department of Biomedical Engineering, Faculty of Engineering, University of Malaya, 50603 Kuala Lumpur, Malaysia
Centre for Innovation in Medical Engineering, Faculty of Engineering, University of Malaya, 50603 Kuala Lumpur, Malaysia

Farid Esmaeili Motlagh
Department of Biomedical Engineering, Faculty of Engineering, University of Malaya, 50603 Kuala Lumpur, Malaysia
Centre for Innovation in Medical Engineering, Faculty of Engineering, University of Malaya, 50603 Kuala Lumpur, Malaysia
Centre of Addiction Sciences, University of Malaya, 21st Floor, Wisma Research and Development, Jalan Pantai Baru, 59200 Kuala Lumpur, Malaysia

Rusdi Abd Rashid and Hussain Habil
Centre of Addiction Sciences, University of Malaya, 21st Floor, Wisma Research and Development, Jalan Pantai Baru, 59200 Kuala Lumpur, Malaysia

Tahereh Seghatoleslam
Centre of Addiction Sciences, University of Malaya, 21st Floor, Wisma Research and Development, Jalan Pantai Baru, 59200 Kuala Lumpur, Malaysia
Shahid Beheshti University of Medical Sciences, Tehran, Iran

H. P. Cheung, S. W. Wang, Y. B. Zhang, L. X. Lao, Z. J. Zhang, Y. Tong, F. W. S. Chung and S. C. W. Sze
School of Chinese Medicine, Li Ka Shing Faculty of Medicine, The University of Hong Kong, 10 Sassoon Road, Pokfulam, Hong Kong, SAR, China

T. B. Ng
School of Biomedical Science, Faculty of Medicine, The Chinese University of Hong Kong, Shatin, N.T., Hong Kong, SAR, China

Chi-Ren Liao and Kun-Chang Wu
Department of Chinese Pharmaceutical Sciences and Chinese Medicine Resources, College of Biopharmaceutical and Food Sciences, China Medical University, Taichung 40402, Taiwan

Xin Zhou
Key Laboratory for Information System of Mountainous Areas and Protection of Ecological Environment, Guizhou Normal University, Guiyang 550001, China

Yang Zhao
Department of Chinese Pharmaceutical Sciences and Chinese Medicine Resources, College of Biopharmaceutical and Food Sciences, China Medical University, Taichung 40402, Taiwan
Key Laboratory for Information System of Mountainous Areas and Protection of Ecological Environment, Guizhou Normal University, Guiyang 550001, China

Chun-Pin Kao
Department of Nursing, Hsin Sheng College of Medical Care and Management, Taoyuan 32544, Taiwan

Yu-Ling Ho
Department of Nursing, Hungkuang University, Taichung 43302, Taiwan

Yuan-Shiun Chang
Department of Chinese Pharmaceutical Sciences and Chinese Medicine Resources, College of Biopharmaceutical and Food Sciences, China Medical University, Taichung 40402, Taiwan. Chinese Crude Drug Pharmacy, China Medical University Hospital, Taichung 40402, Taiwan

Haruka Fujinami
Department of Endoscopy, Toyama University Hospital, Toyama, Japan

Shinya Kajiura, Jun Nishikawa, Takayuki Ando and Toshiro Sugiyama
Department of Gastroenterology, Graduate School of Medicine and Pharmaceutical Science, University of Toyama, Sugitani 2630, Toyama City, Toyama 930-0194, Japan

Index